evolve

:• To access your Student Resources, visit the web address below:

http://evolve.elsevier.com/Ruppel

- **WebLinks**
  Links to places of interest on the web specific to respiratory care.

- **Content Updates**
  Find out the latest information about pulmonary function testing.

- **Case Studies**
  Apply your knowledge with additional real life scenarios.

- **Frequently Asked Questions**
  Additional material to enhance the textbook content.

- **Links to Related Products**
  See what else Elsevier has to offer in a specified field of interest.

Manual of

Pulmonary

Function Testing

Manual of

Pulmonary Function Testing

Eighth Edition

Gregg L. Ruppel MEd, RRT, RPFT, FAARC
Director,
Pulmonary Function Laboratory,
St. Louis University Hospital,
St. Louis, Missouri

Mosby
An Affiliate of Elsevier

With 91 illustrations

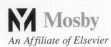
An Affiliate of Elsevier

11830 Westline Industrial Drive
St. Louis, Missouri 63146

Manual of Pulmonary Function Testing, Eighth Edition 0-323-02006-2

NOTICE

Pharmacology is an ever-changing field. Standard safety precautions must be followed, but as
new research and clinical experience broaden our knowledge, changes in treatment and drug
therapy may become necessary or appropriate. Readers are advised to check the most current
product information provided by the manufacturer of each drug to be administered to verify
the recommended dose, the method and duration of administration, and contraindications.
It is the responsibility of the licensed prescriber, relying on experience and knowledge of the
patient, to determine dosages and the best treatment for each individual patient. Neither the
publisher nor the author assumes any liability for any injury and/or damage to persons
or property arising from this publication.

Previous editions copyrighted 1998, 1994, 1991, 1986, 1982, 1979, 1975.

Acquisitions Editor: Mindy Copeland
Developmental Editor: Shelly Dixon
Publishing Services Manager: Pat Joiner
Project Manager: Gena Magouirk
Designer: Kathi Gosche

Printed in China.

Last digit in print number is: 9   8   7   6   5   4   3   2

For Carol, Paul, Katie, and Karen

Contributors

Carl Mottram, RRT, RPFT, FAARC
Coordinator,
Pulmonary Function Laboratories and Pulmonary Rehabilitation,
Assistant Professor of Medicine,
Mayo Clinic,
Rochester, Minnesota

Deborah White, RRT, RPFT
Washington University School of Medicine,
Department of Pediatrics/Pulmonary & Allergy,
Chief Technologist,
Pulmonary Function Laboratory,
St. Louis Children's Hospital,
St. Louis, Missouri

Preface

The primary functions of the lungs are oxygenation of mixed venous blood and removal of carbon dioxide. Gas exchange depends on the integrity of the entire cardiopulmonary system, including airways, pulmonary blood vessels, alveoli, respiratory muscles, and respiratory control mechanisms. A few pulmonary function tests assess individual parts of the cardiopulmonary system. However, most pulmonary function tests measure the status of the lungs' components in an overlapping way.

This eighth edition describes many common pulmonary function tests, their techniques, and the pathophysiology that may be evaluated by each test. Spirometry, lung volume measurements, diffusing capacity, and blood gas analysis are discussed as the basic tests of lung function. Also included are chapters on ventilation and ventilatory control and cardiopulmonary exercise tests. A new chapter (Chapter 8) has been added to discuss pediatric and infant pulmonary function testing. Bronchial challenge, metabolic measurements, disability determination, and preoperative evaluation are covered in a chapter on specialized test regimens (Chapter 9). Pulmonary function testing equipment and quality assurance are addressed in separate chapters.

This eighth edition elaborates on material presented in the first seven editions. Changes to this edition reflect suggestions from the users of previous editions. New to this edition is the aforementioned chapter on pediatric pulmonary function tests and an expanded discussion of cardiopulmonary exercise testing. Learning objectives for entry-level and advanced practitioners have been added at the start of each chapter. Each test section includes criteria for acceptability and interpretive strategies. The criteria are organized to help those performing pulmonary function tests adhere to recognized standards. These criteria are based largely on the most recent recommendations of the American Thoracic Society and the clinical practice guidelines of the American Association for Respiratory Care. The interpretive strategies are presented as a series of questions that can be used as a starting point for test interpretation. Chapter 10 includes information on some newer portable spirometers designed for use in primary care practices. Chapter 11 addresses calibration, quality control, quality assurance, and safety issues. It includes the current equipment recommendations of the American Thoracic Society, as well as safety guidelines from the Centers for Disease Control and Prevention. Case studies are included in most chapters as examples of the performance and interpretation of specific tests.

As in previous editions, each chapter includes self-assessment questions. The questions in this edition are new and are divided into entry-level and advanced categories. The answers may be found in Appendix A. A Selected Bibliography at the end of each chapter is arranged according to topics within the chapter, including standards and guidelines. As in previous editions, reference equations, nomograms, and sources for reference values are found in the appendixes, along with information on the use of reference values. Sample calculations for lung volumes, plethysmography, diffusion, and exercise tests are included in the appendixes.

This manual is intended to serve as a text for students of pulmonary function testing and as a reference for technologists and physicians. Because of the variety of methods and equipment used in pulmonary function evaluation, some tests are discussed in general terms. For this reason, readers are encouraged to use the Selected Bibliographies provided.

The presentation of indications, pathophysiology, and clinical significance of various tests presumes a basic understanding of cardiopulmonary anatomy and physiology. Again, readers are urged to refer to the General References included in the Selected Bibliography sections to refresh their background knowledge of lung function. The terminology used is that of the American College of Chest Physicians–American Thoracic Society (ACCP-ATS) Joint Committee on Pulmonary Nomenclature. In some instances, test names reflect common usage that does not follow the ACCP-ATS recommendations.

Gregg L. Ruppel, MEd, RRT, RPFT, FAARC

Acknowledgments

My thanks to Drs. William Kistner, John Winter, and James Wiant for their encouragement in the development of the original text. My special thanks to Drs. Roger Secker-Walker, Susan Marshall, and Gerald Dolan for comments and constructive criticism in the preparation of the revised editions. Special thanks also go to Ronald Gilmore and Jack Tandy for their contributions to the illustrations in previous editions. A note of thanks also to Thomas Anderson, MEd, RRT; David Shelledy, MA, RRT; Patricia Dent, BS, MS, RPT; and Barbara Disborough, MA, RRT, for their reviews of and suggestions for the fourth edition. Louis Metzger, RPFT; Donald Barker, BS, PA, RPFT; David Hoover, RRT, RPFT; Randall Krohn; James Kemp, MD; Alan Hibbett, RPFT; and Michael Snow, RPFT—all provided guidance and suggestions for the fifth edition. Cesar Keller, MD, and Deborah Stanger, RD, provided insight for case studies for the sixth edition. Robert Brown, RRT, RPFT, and Deborah White, RRT, RPFT, suggested significant changes for the seventh edition. Carl Mottram, RRT, RPFT, FAARC, and Deborah White, RRT, RPFT, both contributed to the eighth edition.

My appreciation for illustrations provided for this and previous editions goes to the following companies:

Abbott Critical Care Systems
Biochem International, Inc.
Collins Medical (Ferraris Cardiorespiratory)
HealthScan Products, Inc.
I-STAT Corporation
Jones Medical Instrument Company
Marquette Medical Systems
Medical Graphics, Inc.
Nellcor Puritan Bennett (Melville), Ltd.
Nonin Medical, Inc.
Novametrix Medical Systems, Inc.
Pulmonary Data Services, Inc. (Ferraris Medical, Inc.)
QRS Diagnostic, LLC
Radiometer America, Inc.
Hans Rudolph, Inc.
SDI Diagnostics
SensorMedics Corporation (VIASYS Healthcare)
Spirometrics Medical Equipment Company
Vitalograph Medical Instrumentation

Contents

Manual of

Pulmonary Function Testing

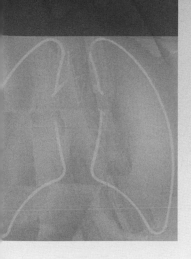

CHAPTER 1

INDICATIONS FOR PULMONARY FUNCTION TESTING

OBJECTIVES

After studying this chapter and reviewing the figures and tables, you should be able to do the following:

Entry-level

1. Categorize pulmonary function tests according to specific purposes
2. Identify at least one indication for spirometry, lung volumes, and diffusing capacity
3. List one obstructive and one restrictive pulmonary disorder
4. Relate pulmonary history to indications for performing pulmonary function tests

Advanced

1. Identify three indications for exercise testing
2. Name at least two diseases in which air trapping may occur
3. Describe the use of a technologist-adapted protocol for pulmonary function studies

This chapter provides an overview of pulmonary function testing. Common pulmonary function tests are introduced, and the indications for each test are discussed. Diseases that commonly require pulmonary function tests are described, and guidelines regarding patient preparation and assessment are presented. Adequate patient preparation, physical assessment, and pulmonary history help the tests provide answers to clinical questions. The importance of patient instruction in obtaining valid data is discussed. These topics are developed more fully in subsequent chapters.

Pulmonary Function Tests

Many different tests are used to evaluate lung function. These tests can be divided into categories based on the aspect of lung function they measure (Table 1-1). Although the tests can be performed alone, they are often performed in combination. Figure 1-1 shows a sample pulmonary function test report that includes spirometry, lung volumes, and diffusing capacity in

TABLE 1-1   Categories of Pulmonary Function Tests

A. Airway function
   1. Simple spirometry
      a. VC, expiratory reserve volume (ERV), inspiratory capacity (IC)
   2. Forced vital capacity maneuver
      a. FVC, FEV_1, FEF, PEF
         (1) Prebronchodilator and postbronchodilator
         (2) Prebronchochallenge and postbronchochallenge
      b. MEFV curves, $\dot{V}_{max_x}$
         (1) Prebronchodilator and postbronchodilator
         (2) Prebronchochallenge and postbronchochallenge
   3. Maximal voluntary ventilation (MVV)
   4. Maximal inspiratory/expiratory pressures (MIP/MEP)
   5. Airway resistance (Raw) and compliance (C_1)
B. Lung volumes and ventilation
   1. Functional residual capacity (FRC)
      a. Open-circuit (N_2 washout)
      b. Closed-circuit/rebreathing (He dilution)
      c. Thoracic gas volume (V_{TG})
   2. Total lung capacity (TLC), residual volume (RV), RV/TLC ratio
   3. Minute ventilation, alveolar ventilation, and dead space
   4. Distribution of ventilation
      a. Multiple-breath N_2
      b. He equilibration
      c. Single-breath techniques
C. Diffusing capacity tests
   1. Single-breath (breath holding)
   2. Steady state
   3. Other techniques
D. Blood gases and gas exchange tests
   1. Blood gas analysis and blood oximetry
      a. Shunt studies
   2. Pulse oximetry
   3. Capnography
E. Cardiopulmonary exercise tests
   1. Simple noninvasive tests
   2. Tests with exhaled gas analyses
   3. Tests with blood gas analyses
F. Metabolic measurements
   1. Resting energy expenditure (REE)
   2. Substrate utilization

Name:	Public, John Q.	Age:	65	Sex:	Male
ID:	123456789	Height:	71.5	Race:	Caucasian
Doctor:	Smith	Weight:	237	Date:	1/2/2003

		Predrug			Postdrug		
SPIROMETRY	Pred	Actual	%Pred	Actual	%Pred	%Chg
FVC (L)	4.72	4.00	85			
FEV_1 (L)	3.24	2.90	90			
FEV_1/FVC (%)	69	73				
$FEF_{25\%-75\%}$ (L/sec)	4.46	2.16	48			
FEF_{max} (L/sec)	8.95	6.21	69			
$FEF_{50\%}/FIF_{50\%}$ (%)	111	131				
MVV	126	108	86			
MIP	−104	−59	57			
MEP	202	111	55			
LUNG VOLUMES						
SVC (L)	4.72	4.42	94			
TLC Pleth (L)	7.31	7.89	108			
RV Pleth (L)	2.59	3.47	134			
RV/TLC Pleth (%)	35	44	126			
V_{TG} (L)	4.14	4.01	97			
ERV (L)	1.55	0.54	35			
IC (L)	3.17	3.87	122			
DIFFUSION						
DL_{CO} (ml/min/mm Hg)	26.30	28.92	110			
$DL_{CO_{corr}}$ (ml/min/mm Hg)	26.30	29.35	112			
DL/V_A (ml/min/mmHgL)	3.60	4.78				
V_A (L)	7.31	6.16	84			
AIRWAY RESISTANCE						
Raw (cm H_2O/L/sec)	1.25	1.13	90			
SGaw (L/sec/cm H_2O/L)	0.22	0.20	91			

Technologist's Comments
  Spirometry meets ATS criteria, and MVV, MIP, MEP were all acceptable.
  Lung volumes by plethysmography were acceptable and reproducible.
  DL_{CO}: Breath hold time longer than 11 seconds; corrected for 14.4 Hb.

Impression:
  All maneuvers were performed acceptably except for the diffusing capacity test.
  Spirometry is within normal limits with no evidence of obstruction. The patient's maximal
    inspiratory and expiratory pressures were moderately reduced.
  Lung volumes by plethysmography show a small increase in the residual volume and RV/TLC
    ratio consistent with air trapping.
  Diffusing capacity is normal despite a prolonged breath hold.
  Airway resistance and conductance are normal.
Interpretation: Essentially normal spirometry, but with decreased maximal pressures. Some
  evidence of air trapping. Normal diffusing capacity. Recommend clinical correlation of
  decreased respiratory muscle function.

Figure 1-1 *Sample pulmonary function test report.* Patient information is usually listed at the top. Lung function tests are grouped by category in the left column. The first data column contains patient's predicted (expected) values. The second column contains measured values obtained during testing. The third column contains the percent of predicted value for each test (actual/predicted × 100). The next three columns are blank because the patient was not retested after using the bronchodilator. Following the tabular data are sections containing the technologist's comments and the physician's impression and interpretation. Physician's signature is usually at the bottom.

TABLE 1-2 Indications for Spirometry

Spirometry may be indicated to:
A. Detect the presence or absence of lung disease
   1. History of pulmonary symptoms
      a. Dyspnea, wheezing
      b. Cough, phlegm production
      c. Chest pain, orthopnea
   2. Physical indicators
      a. Decreased breath sounds
      b. Chest wall abnormalities
   3. Abnormal laboratory findings
      a. Chest x-ray study
      b. Blood gases
B. Quantify the extent of known disease on lung function
   1. Pulmonary disease
      a. Chronic obstructive pulmonary disease
      b. Asthma
      c. Cystic fibrosis
      d. Interstitial diseases
   2. Cardiac disease (congestive heart failure)
   3. Neuromuscular disease (Guillain-Barré syndrome)
C. Measure effects of occupational or environmental exposure
   1. Smoking
   2. Working in hazardous or dusty environments
D. Determine beneficial or negative effects of therapy
   1. Bronchodilators or steroids
   2. Cardiac drugs (antiarrhythmics, diuretics)
   3. Lung resection, reduction, or transplant
   4. Pulmonary rehabilitation
E. Assess risk for surgical procedures
   1. Lung resection (lobectomy, pneumonectomy)
   2. Thoracic procedures (sternotomy)
   3. Abdominal procedures
F. Evaluate disability or impairment
   1. Social security or other compensation programs
   2. Legal or insurance evaluations

a format that is commonly used. Determining which tests to do depends on the *clinical question* to be answered. This question may be explicit, such as "Does the patient have *asthma*?" or less obvious, such as "Does this patient, who needs abdominal surgery, have any pulmonary disease that might complicate the procedure?" In either case, indications for specific tests are useful (Table 1-2).

AIRWAY FUNCTION TESTS

The most basic test of pulmonary function is the measurement of vital capacity (VC). This test simply measures the largest volume of air that can be moved into or out of the lungs. In the mid-1800s, Hutchinson developed a simple water-sealed *spirometer* that allowed measurement of VC. Hutchinson popularized the concept of using VC to assess lung function. He observed that VC was related to the standing height of the patient. He also developed tables to estimate

Pulmonary function data are usually grouped into categories as seen in Figure 1-1. The patient's demographic data (age, height, sex, race, etc.) are usually at the top of the report. The PFT data are presented in three columns. These columns show the predicted (expected) values, measured values obtained during testing, and the percent of predicted values for each test (actual/ predicted × 100). Be sure to identify which column is actual and which is predicted. The first data column contains patient's predicted (expected) values.

the expected VC for a healthy patient. The VC was usually graphed on chart paper, which allowed subdivisions of the VC to be identified (see Chapter 2).

Forced vital capacity (FVC) is a refinement of the simple VC test. During the 1930s, Barach observed that patients with asthma or *emphysema* exhaled more slowly than healthy patients. He noted that airflow out of the lungs was important in detecting *obstruction* of the airways. Barach used a rotating chart drum *(kymograph)* to display VC changes as a *spirogram*. He even evaluated the effects of *bronchodilator* medications using the forced expiratory spirogram.

Around 1950, Gaensler began using a microswitch in conjunction with a water-sealed spirometer to time FVC. He observed that healthy patients consistently exhaled approximately 80% of their FVC in 1 second, and almost all of the FVC in 3 seconds. He used the forced expired volume in the first second (FEV_1) to assess *airway obstruction*. In 1955, Leuallen and Fowler demonstrated a graphic method used to assess airflow. They measured airflow between the 25% and 75% points on a forced expiratory spirogram. This measure was described as the maximal midexpiratory flow rate (MMFR). This and similar measurements have been used to describe airflow from both healthy and airflow-obstructed patients. To standardize terminology, the MMFR is now referred to as the forced expiratory flow 25%-75% ($FEF_{25\%-75\%}$).

In addition to displaying FVC as a volume-time spirogram, it can also be represented by plotting airflow against volume. In the late 1950s, Hyatt and others began using the flow-volume display to assess airway function. The tracing was termed the maximal expiratory flow volume (MEFV) curve. By combining it with an inspiratory maneuver, a closed loop was displayed. This figure was called the *flow-volume loop* (see Chapter 2).

Peak expiratory flow (PEF) is measured using either a flow-sensing spirometer or a *peak flow meter*. In the 1960s, Wright popularized the use of peak flow to monitor asthmatic patients. Peak flow can be readily assessed from the flow-volume loop as well. Recently, portable peak flow meters that allow monitoring at home, as well as in the hospital or clinic, have been developed.

The FVC and its components, along with flow-volume loops and peak flow, are all used to measure response to bronchodilator medications (see Chapter 2). Tests are repeated before and after inhalation of a bronchodilator, and the percentage of change calculated. The same tests may be used to assess airway response after a challenge to the airways. These tests are referred to as *bronchial challenge* or *bronchial provocation* tests. The challenge may be in the form of an inhaled agent (e.g., *methacholine*) or a physical agent (e.g., exercise). In either case, airflow is assessed before and after the challenge. The percent change (normally a decrease) after challenge is calculated (see Chapter 9).

Maximal voluntary ventilation (MVV) was described as early as 1941. Cournand and Richards originally called it the maximal breathing capacity. In the MVV test, the patient breathes rapidly and deeply for 12 to 15 seconds. The volume of air exchanged is expressed in liters per minute. The MVV gives an estimate of the peak ventilation available to meet physiologic demands.

Measurement of respiratory muscle strength is accomplished by assessing maximal inspiratory pressure (MIP) and maximal expiratory pressure (MEP). This is done using either a pressure *transducer* or a simple aneroid *manometer*. MIP and MEP are important adjuncts to spirometry for monitoring respiratory muscle function in a variety of pulmonary and nonpulmonary diseases.

Airway resistance (Raw) measurements date back to the development of the body *plethysmograph* in the early 1950s. Comroe, Dubois, and others perfected a technique that provided estimates of *alveolar* pressure. The patient sits in an airtight box called a plethysmograph (see Chapter 10). The plethysmograph calculates pressure drop across the airways related to flow at the mouth (see Chapter 2). This technique originally required complicated monitoring and recording devices. The microprocessor has simplified the measurement of the required signals so that plethysmography is now widely used. The same equipment can also be used to measure thoracic gas volume (V_{TG}).

Lung *compliance* is measured by passing a small balloon into the esophagus to measure pleural pressure. Intrapleural pressure can then be related to volume changes to estimate the distensibility of the lung (see Chapter 2). Other less invasive techniques are available but not widely used.

LUNG VOLUME AND VENTILATION TESTS

Measurement of lung volume dates back to the early 1800s, well before Hutchinson's development of spirometry. Various techniques have been used to estimate the volume of gas remaining in the lung after a complete exhalation. Davy used a hydrogen dilution technique to estimate residual air. This technique was later improved by Meneely and Kaltreider using helium (He) instead of hydrogen. Around the same time, Darling, Cournand, and Richards began using oxygen breathing to wash nitrogen (N_2) out of the lungs. The collection and analysis of the volume of exhaled N_2 allowed the functional residual capacity (FRC) to be estimated. Using simple spirometry and FRC determinations allows total lung capacity (TLC) and residual volume (RV) to be calculated. The other commonly used method for measuring lung volumes uses the body plethysmograph to measure V_{TG} or FRC. Estimation of lung volumes from chest radiographs is possible but is not widely used.

Closed-circuit (He dilution) and open-circuit (N_2 washout) techniques are both widely used to measure FRC. Besides determining lung volumes, each technique provides useful information about distribution of ventilation within the lungs. The pattern of N_2 washout can be displayed graphically. The time required for He to equilibrate during *rebreathing* provides a similar index of the evenness of ventilation. In the early 1950s and 1960s, Fowler developed a single-breath N_2-washout technique. This method plotted N_2 concentration in expired air after a single breath of 100% oxygen. The single-breath N_2 washout provided information about gas distribution in the lungs. It also allowed estimates of the lung volume at which airway closure occurred when the patient exhaled completely (see Chapter 3).

Measurement of resting ventilation requires only a simple gas-metering device and a means of collecting expired air. Portable computerized spirometers allow *minute ventilation, tidal volume* (V_T) and breathing rate to be readily measured in almost any setting. Determination of *alveolar ventilation* or *dead space* (wasted ventilation) requires measurement of arterial partial pressure of carbon dioxide ($PaCO_2$) in addition to total ventilation. Alternately, the partial pressure of carbon dioxide (PCO_2) can be estimated from expired CO_2. The availability of blood gas analyzers and exhaled CO_2 analyzers makes these measurements routine.

DIFFUSING CAPACITY TESTS

The basis for the modern single-breath *diffusing capacity (DL$_{CO}$)* test was described by August and Marie Krogh in 1911. They showed that small but measurable differences existed between inspired and expired gas containing *carbon monoxide (CO)*. This change could be related to the uptake of gas across the lung. Although they used the method to test a series of patients, they did not employ the single-breath technique for clinical purposes. Around 1950, Forrester and colleagues revisited the method. They developed it as a tool to measure the gas exchange capacity of the lung. About the same time, Filley and others were promoting other techniques using CO to measure diffusing capacity. Most of these techniques allowed patients to breathe normally, rather than hold their breath. These methods are called steady-state techniques. Each method has certain limitations. However, the single-breath technique is the most widely used and standardized in the United States (see Chapter 5).

BLOOD GASES AND GAS EXCHANGE TESTS

Measurement of gases (O$_2$ and CO$_2$) in the blood began with volumetric methods used since the early 1900s. In 1957, Sanz introduced the glass *electrode* to measure *pH* of fluids potentiometrically. In 1958, Severinghaus added an outer jacket containing a *bicarbonate buffer* to the glass electrode. The electrode-buffer was separated from the blood being analyzed by a membrane that was permeable to CO$_2$. This allowed the pressure of CO$_2$ in the blood to be measured as a pH change in the electrode. In 1956 Leland Clark covered a platinum electrode with a polypropylene membrane. When a voltage was applied to the electrode, O$_2$ was reduced at the platinum *cathode* in proportion to its partial pressure. These three electrodes (pH, Pco$_2$, and partial pressure of oxygen [Po$_2$]) are the basis of modern blood gas analyzers. Today, blood gas analysis is available using portable instruments with miniature electrodes. Electrodes to measure *electrolytes* (K^{++}, Na^{++}, Cl$^-$) are also included in some blood gas analyzer systems.

Blood *oximetry* was developed during World War II to monitor the effects of exposure to high-altitude flight. During the 1960s, spectrophotometric analyzers that could measure the total *hemoglobin (Hb)*, along with oxyhemoglobin and *carboxyhemoglobin (COHb)* levels, were perfected. Blood oximetry testing has been combined with blood gas analysis so that both can be accomplished with a single instrument. *Pulse oximetry* was developed in the 1970s as a result of efforts to monitor cardiac rate by using a light beam to sense pulsatile blood flow. It was quickly discovered that the pulse could be sensed, and changes in light *absorption* could also be used to estimate arterial oxygen saturation.

Capnography, or monitoring of exhaled carbon dioxide, was developed in conjunction with the *infrared* gas analyzer (see Chapter 10). This sensitive and rapidly responding analyzer allows exhaled CO$_2$ to be monitored continuously. Most critical care units, operating rooms, and emergency departments use some combination of blood gas analysis, pulse oximetry, and capnography for patient monitoring. Blood gas analysis is an integral part of routine pulmonary function testing because it is the definitive test of the basic functions of the lung.

CARDIOPULMONARY EXERCISE TESTS

The simplest types of exercise tests are those in which the patient performs work and only noninvasive measurements are made. Such measurements include heart rate and rhythm monitoring using an electrocardiogram. Other simple, noninvasive measurements are blood pressure and respiratory rate monitoring. Analysis of exhaled gas is noninvasive, but the patient does have to breathe through a *mouthpiece* or mask. Ventilation and V$_T$ can be estimated by collecting the exhaled air. Analysis of expired gases permits *oxygen consumption* and

CO_2 production to be measured. When invasive measures (blood gas analysis, arterial catheters, pulmonary artery catheters) are used, the entire range of physiologic variables that affect exercise can be monitored. Computers allow sophisticated measurements to be made rapidly while the patient continues to exercise (*breath-by-breath* gas analysis).

◼ METABOLIC MEASUREMENTS

Measurement of energy expenditure and caloric requirements dates to the early 1900s. *Basal metabolic rate (BMR)* was measured by allowing a patient to rebreathe from a volume spirometer containing added oxygen. Plotting the rate at which oxygen was consumed could derive an estimate of energy expenditure. A similar approach is taken today, except that oxygen consumption and carbon dioxide production are monitored using gas analyzers. *Resting energy expenditure (REE)* has replaced BMR as the primary variable related to metabolic needs. Although BMR was used to detect disorders that affected *metabolism,* REE is used to manage critically ill patients whose caloric requirements may be difficult to estimate.

Indications for Pulmonary Function Testing

Each category of pulmonary function testing includes specific reasons why each test may be necessary. These reasons for testing are called *indications.* Some pulmonary function tests have well-defined indications. The same indications that apply to one type of test (e.g., spirometry) may apply to other categories as well.

◼ SPIROMETRY

Spirometry is the pulmonary function test performed most often because it is indicated in many situations (Table 1-2). Spirometry is often performed as a screening procedure. It may be the first test to indicate the presence of pulmonary disease. Spirometry is recommended as the "gold standard" for diagnosis of obstructive lung disease by the National Lung Health Education Program (NLHEP), the National Heart, Lung and Blood Institute (NHLBI), and the World Health Organization (WHO). However, spirometry alone may not be sufficient to completely define the extent of disease, response to therapy, preoperative risk, or level of impairment. Spirometry must be performed correctly because of the serious impact its results can have on the patient's life.

◼ LUNG VOLUMES

Lung volume determination usually includes the VC and its subdivisions, along with the FRC. From these two basic measurements, the remaining lung volumes and capacities can be calculated (see Chapters 2 and 3). Lung volumes are almost always measured in conjunction with spirometry, although the indications for them are distinct (Table 1-3). The most common reason for measuring lung volumes is to identify restrictive lung disease. A reduced VC suggests *restriction,* particularly if airflow is normal. Measurement of FRC and determination of TLC are necessary to confirm restriction. If TLC is abnormally reduced, restriction is present. The severity of the restrictive process is determined by the extent of reduction of the TLC. TLC and its components can be determined by several methods. For patients with obstructive lung diseases (*chronic obstructive pulmonary disease [COPD],* asthma), lung volumes measured by body plethysmography may be indicated (see Chapter 3).

TABLE 1-3   **Indications for Lung Volume Determination**

Lung volume determinations may be indicated to:
A. Diagnose or assess the severity of restrictive lung disease (reduced TLC)
B. Differentiate between obstructive and restrictive disease patterns
C. Assess response to therapy
   1. Bronchodilators, steroids
   2. Lung transplantation, resection, reduction
   3. Radiation or chemotherapy
D. Make preoperative assessments of patients with compromised lung function
E. Determine or evaluate disability
F. Assess gas trapping by comparison of plethysmographic lung volumes with gas dilution lung volumes
G. Standardize other lung function measures (i.e., specific conductance)

DIFFUSING CAPACITY

Diffusing capacity is measured by having the patient inhale a low concentration of CO and a *tracer* gas to determine gas exchange within the lungs (DL_{CO}). Several methods of evaluating the uptake of CO from the lungs are available, but the single-breath technique ($DL_{CO}sb$) is most commonly used. This method is also called the breath-hold technique because CO transfer is measured during 10 seconds of breath holding. DL_{CO} is usually measured in conjunction with spirometry and lung volumes. Although most pulmonary and cardiovascular diseases reduce DL_{CO} (Table 1-4), it may be increased in some cases (see Chapter 5). DL_{CO} testing is commonly used to monitor diseases caused by dust. These are conditions in which lung tissue is infiltrated by substances such as asbestos that disrupt the normal structure of the gas exchange units. DL_{CO} testing is also used to evaluate pulmonary involvement in systemic diseases such as rheumatoid arthritis. DL_{CO} measurements are often included in the evaluation of patients with obstructive lung disease.

BLOOD GASES

Blood gas analysis is often done in conjunction with pulmonary function studies. Blood is drawn from a peripheral artery without being exposed to air (i.e., anaerobically). The radial artery is often used for a single arterial puncture or indwelling catheter. Blood gas analysis includes measurement of hydrogen ion activity (pH), along with PCO_2 and PO_2. The same specimen CO may be used for blood oximetry to measure total Hb, oxyhemoglobin saturation (O_2Hb), carboxyhemoglobin (COHb), and *methemoglobin (MetHb)*.

   Blood gas analysis is the ideal measure of pulmonary function because it assesses the two primary functions of the lung (oxygenation and CO_2 removal). Evaluation of any pulmonary disorder may be considered a reason for performing blood gas analysis. Very specific indications for blood gas analysis are widely used (Table 1-5). Blood gas analysis is most commonly used to determine the need for supplemental oxygen and to manage patients who require ventilatory support. Some pulmonary function measurements require blood gas analysis as an integral part of the test (i.e., *shunt* or dead space studies). Blood gas analysis is invasive; noninvasive measurements of oxygenation or gas exchange are often preferred if they are safer or less costly. Many noninvasive techniques (e.g., pulse oximetry) rely on blood gas analysis to verify their validity (see Chapter 6).

TABLE 1-4   Indications for DL_{CO}

Diffusing capacity (DL_{CO}) measurements may be indicated to:
A. Evaluate or follow the progress of parenchymal lung diseases
    1. Dusts (asbestos, silica, metals)
    2. Organic agents (allergic alveolitis)
    3. Drugs (amiodarone, bleomycin)
B. Evaluate pulmonary involvement in systemic diseases
    1. Rheumatoid arthritis
    2. Sarcoidosis
    3. Systemic lupus erythematosus (SLE)
    4. Systemic sclerosis
    5. Mixed connective tissue disease
C. Evaluate obstructive lung disease
    1. Follow the progression of disease
       a. Emphysema
       b. Cystic fibrosis
    2. Differentiate types of obstruction
       a. Emphysema
       b. Chronic bronchitis
       c. Asthma
    3. Predict arterial desaturation during exercise in COPD
D. Evaluate cardiovascular diseases
    1. Primary pulmonary hypertension
    2. Acute or recurrent pulmonary thromboembolism
    3. Pulmonary edema and congestive heart failure
E. Quantify disability associated with interstitial lung disease
F. Evaluate pulmonary hemorrhage, polycythemia, or left-to-right shunts (increased DL_{CO})

■ EXERCISE TESTS

Physical exercise stresses the heart, lungs, and the pulmonary and peripheral circulatory systems. Exercise testing allows simultaneous evaluation of the cellular, cardiovascular, and ventilatory systems. Cardiopulmonary exercise tests can be used to determine the level of fitness or extent of *dysfunction*. Appropriately designed tests can determine the role of cardiac or pulmonary involvement. Understanding the physiologic basis for the patient's inability to exercise is key to offering effective therapy. Table 1-6 lists some indications for exercise tests.

Equipment used to measure oxygen consumption and CO_2 production during exercise can also measure resting metabolic rates. This allows estimates of caloric needs in patients who are critically ill. Indications for performing studies of REE are detailed in Chapter 9.

Patterns of Impaired Pulmonary Function

Patients are usually referred to the pulmonary function laboratory to evaluate signs or symptoms of lung disease. In some instances, the clinician may wish to exclude a specific diagnosis such as asthma. Indications for different categories of pulmonary function tests

TABLE 1-5 **Indications for Blood Gas Analysis**

Blood gas analysis and/or blood oximetry may be indicated to:

A. Evaluate adequacy of lung function
    1. Ventilation
        a. Pa_{CO_2}
    2. Acid-base status
        a. pH
        b. Pa_{CO_2}
    3. Oxygenation and oxygen-carrying capacity
        a. Pa_{O_2}
        b. Total Hb, O_2Hb, COHb, MetHb
    4. Intrapulmonary shunt
    5. V_D/V_T ratio
B. Determine need for supplemental oxygen (for clinical or reimbursement purposes)
    1. Presence or severity of resting hypoxemia
    2. Exercise desaturation
    3. Nocturnal desaturation
    4. Adequacy of oxygen prescription
C. Monitor ventilatory support
    1. Assess or follow respiratory failure
    2. Adjust therapy to improve oxygenation (PEEP, CPAP, pressure support)
D. Document the severity or progression of known pulmonary disease
E. Provide data to correct or corroborate other pulmonary function measurements
    1. Correct $D_{L_{CO}}$ measurements (Hb and COHb)
    2. Determine accuracy of pulse oximetry, transcutaneous monitors, or indwelling blood gas devices

PEEP, Positive end-expiratory pressure; *CPAP,* continuous positive airway pressure.

have been described previously. Sometimes, patients display patterns during testing that are consistent with a specific diagnosis. This section presents an overview of some commonly encountered forms of impaired pulmonary function.

OBSTRUCTIVE AIRWAY DISEASES

An obstructive airway disease is one in which airflow into or out of the lungs is reduced. This simple definition includes a variety of pathologic conditions. Some of these conditions are closely related regarding how they cause airway obstruction. For example, mucus hypersecretion is a component of *chronic bronchitis,* asthma, and *cystic fibrosis (CF),* although their causes are distinct.

Chronic Obstructive Pulmonary Disease

The term *COPD* is often used to describe long-standing airway obstruction caused by emphysema, chronic bronchitis, or asthma. These three conditions may be present alone or in combination (Figure 1-2). *Bronchiectasis* is sometimes considered a component of COPD. COPD is characterized by *dyspnea* at rest or with exertion, often accompanied by a productive cough. Delineation of the type of obstruction depends on the history, physical examination, and pulmonary function studies. Unfortunately, the term *COPD* is used to describe the clinical findings of dyspnea or cough without attention to the actual cause. This may lead to

TABLE 1-6 Indications for Exercise Testing

Exercise testing may be indicated to:
A. Determine the level of cardiorespiratory fitness
B. Document or diagnose exercise limitation as a result of fatigue, dyspnea, or pain
   1. Cardiovascular diseases
      a. Myocardial ischemia or dyskinesis
      b. Cardiomyopathy
      c. Congestive heart failure
      d. Peripheral vascular disease
   2. Pulmonary diseases
      a. Airway obstruction or hyperreactivity
      b. Interstitial lung disease
      c. Pulmonary vascular disease
   3. Mixed cardiovascular, pulmonary, or unknown etiologies
C. Evaluate adequacy of arterial oxyhemoglobin saturation
   1. Exercise desaturation/hypoxemia
   2. Oxygen prescription
   3. Right-to-left shunt
D. Assess preoperative risk, particularly lung resection or reduction
E. Assess disability, particularly related to occupational lung disease
F. Evaluate therapeutic interventions such as heart or lung transplantation

inappropriate therapy. Other similar terms *include chronic obstructive lung disease (COLD)* and *chronic airway obstruction (CAO).*

Emphysema

Emphysema means "air trapping" and is defined morphologically. The air spaces distal to the terminal bronchioles are abnormally increased in size. The walls of the alveoli undergo destructive changes. This destruction results in overinflation of lung units. If the process mainly involves the respiratory bronchioles, the emphysema is termed *centrilobular.* If the alveoli are also involved, the term *panlobular emphysema* is used to describe the pattern. These distinctions require examination of lung tissue either by biopsy or at postmortem. Because this is often impractical, emphysema is suspected when there is airway obstruction with air trapping. Physical assessment, chest x-ray studies, and pulmonary function studies are the primary diagnostic tools. Spirometry (FVC, FEV_1, and $FEV_{1\%}$) is used to determine the presence and extent of obstruction. Lung volumes (TLC, RV, and RV/TLC%) define the pattern of air trapping or hyperinflation caused by emphysema. DL_{CO} and blood gas analyses are useful in tracking the degree of gas exchange abnormality in emphysema. Exercise testing may be necessary if the emphysema patient is suspected of oxygen desaturation with exertion, or to plan pulmonary rehabilitation.

    Emphysema is caused primarily by cigarette smoking. Repeated inflammation of the respiratory bronchioles results in tissue destruction. As the disease advances, more and more alveolar walls are destroyed. Loss of elastic tissue results in airway collapse, air trapping, and *hyperinflation.* Some emphysema is caused by the absence of a protective enzyme, α_1-antitrypsin. The lack of this enzyme is caused by a genetic defect. α_1-Antitrypsin inhibits proteases in the blood from attacking healthy tissue. Deficiency of α_1-antitrypsin causes gradual destruction of alveolar walls resulting in panlobular emphysema. Chronic exposure to environmental pollutants can also contribute to the development of emphysema. The natural aging of the

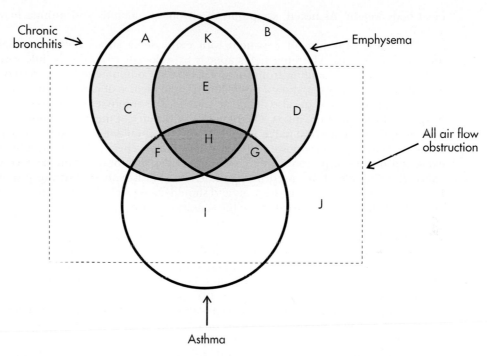

Figure 1-2 *Nonproportional diagram depicting the relationship between various components of COPD.*
Emphysema, chronic bronchitis, and asthma overlap to varying degrees (*shaded areas*). Chronic obstruction in small airways and all airway obstructive diseases (*large dashed square*) also overlap. **A,** Patients with chronic bronchitis but no airflow obstruction. **B,** Patients with anatomic changes related to emphysema, but no obstruction. **C,** Patients with chronic cough and airflow obstruction. **D,** Patients with emphysema and obstruction as demonstrated by spirometry. **E,** Combined chronic bronchitis and emphysema, commonly occurring in the same patient as a result of cigarette smoking. **F,** Combined chronic bronchitis and asthma. **G,** Combined emphysema and asthma. **H,** Combined asthma, chronic bronchitis, and emphysema. **I,** Patients with asthma manifested by reversible obstruction (spirometry or peak flow). **J,** Other forms of airway obstruction, including cystic fibrosis, bronchiolitis obliterans, or upper airway abnormalities (e.g., vocal cord dysfunction) are not considered part of COPD. **K,** Patients with cough and morphologic evidence of emphysema, but no obstruction. (Modified from American Thoracic Society: Standards for the diagnosis and care of patients with chronic obstructive pulmonary disease, *Am J Respir Crit Care Med* 152:S77-S120, 1995.)

lung also causes some changes that resemble the disease entity. The natural decline of elastic recoil in the lung reduces maximal airflow and increases lung volume as people age. Surgical removal of lung tissue sometimes causes the remaining lung to over-inflate.

The main symptom of emphysema is breathlessness, either at rest or with exertion. *Hypoxemia* may contribute to this dyspnea, particularly in advanced emphysema. However, the destruction of alveolar walls also causes loss of the capillary bed. Ventilation-perfusion matching may be relatively well preserved in patients with emphysema. As a result, oxygen levels may be only slightly decreased. This type of patient is sometimes called the pink puffer. As the disease advances, the loss of alveolar surface causes a decreased ability to oxygenate mixed venous blood. DL_{CO} is reduced. The patient becomes increasingly breathless, particularly with exertion. Muscle wasting seems to be common in emphysema, and patients are often below their ideal body weight. As noted, symptoms of chronic bronchitis and asthma may be present as well.

The chest x-ray film of a patient with emphysema shows flattened diaphragms and increased air spaces. The lung fields appear hyperlucent (dark) with little vascularity. The heart appears to be hanging from the great vessels. Computerized tomography (CT) scans, especially spiral CT scans, show a three-dimensional picture of enlarged air spaces and loss of supporting tissue. CT scans also delineate whether the emphysematous changes are localized or spread throughout the lungs. The physical appearance of the chest confirms what is shown radiographically. The chest wall is immobile with the shoulders elevated. The diameter of the chest is increased anteroposteriorly (so-called barrel chest). There is little *diaphragmatic* excursion during inspiration. Intercostal retractions may be prominent. Accessory muscles (neck and shoulders) are used to lift the chest wall. Breath sounds are distant or absent. Patients may need to support the arms and shoulders to catch their breath. Breathing is often done through pursed lips to alleviate the sensation of dyspnea.

Chronic Bronchitis

Chronic bronchitis is diagnosed by clinical findings. It is present when there is excessive mucus production, with a productive cough on most days, for at least 3 months for 2 years or more. The diagnosis is made by excluding other diseases that also result in excess mucus production. These include cystic fibrosis, *tuberculosis,* abscess, tumors, or bronchiectasis.

Chronic bronchitis, like emphysema, is caused primarily by cigarette smoking. It may also result from chronic exposure to environmental pollutants. Chronic bronchitis causes the mucus glands lining the airways to hypertrophy and increase in number. There is also chronic inflammation of the bronchial wall with infiltration of leukocytes and lymphocytes. The number of ciliated epithelial cells decreases. This causes impairment of mucus flow in the airways. Similar changes occur in respiratory bronchioles. Excessive mucus and poor clearance make the patient susceptible to repeated infections. Some patients who have chronic bronchitis caused by cigarette smoking experience a decrease in cough and mucus production after smoking cessation. Some airway changes, however, usually persist. Spirometry is useful in evaluating the extent of airway obstruction due to bronchitic changes. DL_{CO} may be helpful in distinguishing emphysema and chronic bronchitis; bronchitis patients may have preserved DL_{CO}, while emphysema patients tend to have reduced DL_{CO}.

Chronic cough is the defining symptom of chronic bronchitis. Some patients do not consider cough abnormal and refer to it as "smoker's cough" or "morning cough." In addition to cough, chronic bronchitis may produce dyspnea, particularly with exertion. Blood gas abnormalities usually accompany chronic bronchitis. Ventilation-perfusion mismatching causes hypoxemia. If hypoxemia persists, the patient may develop secondary polycythemia. *Cyanosis* may be present due to the combination of arterial *desaturation* and increased Hb levels. Chronic hypoxemia may also lead to right-sided heart failure *(cor pulmonale).* Advanced chronic bronchitis is also often accompanied by CO_2 retention *(hypercapnia).*

Unlike the emphysema patient, the patient with chronic bronchitis may show few clinical signs of underlying disease. Body weight may be normal or increased with minimal changes to the chest wall. Patients with bronchitis may appear normal except for cough and dyspnea. The chest x-ray film in chronic bronchitis differs markedly from that in emphysema. The congested airways are easily visible. The heart may appear enlarged with the pulmonary vessels prominent. The diaphragms may appear normal or flattened, depending on the degree of air trapping present. If there is right-sided heart failure, swelling *(edema)* of the lower extremities is often present.

Pulmonary infections can seriously aggravate chronic bronchitis. The appearance of the sputum produced can help predict worsening function. If it is normally white, a change to discolored sputum indicates the beginning of an infection. This may be accompanied by worsened hypoxemia and shortness of breath. Early treatment can potentially reverse an otherwise serious complication. Failure to manage the chest infection can result in severe hypoxemia and hypercapnia, with exacerbation of right-sided heart failure. Acute respiratory failure superimposed on chronic failure is the most common cause of death in patients with COPD.

Bronchiectasis

Bronchiectasis is pathologic dilatation of the bronchi. It results from destruction of the bronchial walls by severe, repeated infections. The terms *saccular, cystic,* and *tubular* are used to describe the appearance of the bronchi. Most bronchiectasis involves prolonged episodes of infection. Bronchiectasis is common in CF, as well as following bronchial obstruction by a tumor or foreign body. When the entire bronchial tree is involved, it is assumed that the disease is inherited or caused by developmental abnormalities.

The main clinical feature of bronchiectasis is a very productive cough. The sputum is usually purulent and foul smelling. *Hemoptysis* is also common. Frequent bronchopulmonary infections lead to gas exchange abnormalities similar to those of chronic bronchitis. Right-sided heart failure follows advancement of the disease. Chest x-ray studies, bronchograms, and CT scans are used to identify the type and extent of the disease. As in chronic bronchitis, spirometry may be useful for assessing the degree of obstruction and response to therapy.

Treatment of bronchiectasis includes vigorous bronchial hygiene. Regular antibiotic therapy is used to manage the repeated infections. *Bronchoscopy* and surgical *resection* are sometimes required to manage localized areas of infection. Patients with recurrent hemoptysis may require resection of the offending lobe.

Management of Chronic Obstructive Pulmonary Disease

COPD is a leading cause of morbidity and mortality throughout the world. COPD often includes components of emphysema and chronic bronchitis (Figure 1-2). This association most likely is due to the common risk factor of cigarette smoking. *Hyperreactive* airways disease (asthma) may also be present. Reversibility of obstruction, however, is usually less than in uncomplicated asthma. Bronchiectasis and bronchiolitis are also commonly found in patients with COPD.

An essential ingredient in COPD management is *early diagnosis.* The NLHEP and the WHO both recommend spirometry as a primary tool in early detection of chronic airflow limitation. Spirometry is recommended for all smokers over the age of 45 and for anyone with chronic cough, dyspnea on exertion, mucus hypersecretion, or wheezing.

Treatment of COPD begins with smoking cessation and avoiding irritants that inflame the airways. The rate of decline in lung function (FEV$_1$) in smokers is approximately twice that of nonsmokers. Smoking cessation decreases the accelerated decline. Other measures aimed at keeping the airways open are also important. Inhaled bronchodilators, especially β-agonists, are commonly used. Combinations of β-adrenergic and *anticholinergic* bronchodilators, together with inhaled *corticosteroids,* provide relief to many patients with COPD. This is often the case, even when there is little improvement in airflow assessed by spirometry. Some patients require oral steroids (e.g., prednisone) to manage chronic inflammation. Antibiotics are commonly used at the first sign of respiratory infections. Digitalis and *diuretics* are most often prescribed for the management of cor pulmonale.

Breathing retraining, bronchial hygiene measures, and physical reconditioning are important therapeutic modalities in addition to pharmacologic management. Breathing retraining is especially important for the patient with advanced COPD. Grossly altered pulmonary mechanics favor hyperinflation and use of accessory muscles. Training in the use of the diaphragm for slow, relaxed breathing can significantly improve gas exchange. Pulmonary rehabilitation, particularly physical reconditioning, permits many patients with otherwise debilitating disease to maintain their quality of life.

Supplemental (O_2) therapy is indicated in COPD when the patient's oxygen tension at rest or during exercise is less than 55 mm Hg. Oxygen may also be prescribed when signs of cor pulmonale are present. Many patients desaturate only with exertion. Exercise testing is the only reliable method of detecting exertional desaturation. Low-flow O_2 therapy can be implemented by a number of methods, including portable systems. Chronic O_2 supplementation has been shown to improve survival in patients with COPD.

Single-lung transplantation has recently been used for patients with end-stage COPD who are younger than 60 years old. Although *lung transplantation* causes immediate improvement in pulmonary function, it is expensive. The cost of hospitalization and follow-up care may be prohibitive. In addition, lack of donor organs means that many patients with COPD die while awaiting transplantation. The prognosis for those receiving lung transplants is generally good. In some transplant recipients, a severe form of airway obstruction *(bronchiolitis obliterans)* has been found to occur in the transplanted lung. The reason for this obstructive process is unclear, but the progression is rapid. Spirometry is used to monitor transplant recipients to detect early changes associated with bronchiolitis obliterans.

Lung volume reduction surgery (LVRS) has also been used to treat end-stage COPD. In this procedure, lung tissue that is poorly perfused is surgically removed. This allows the remaining lung units to expand with improved ventilation-perfusion matching. This technique works particularly well when there are large areas of trapped gas with little perfusion (bullae). The procedure can be performed by *sternotomy,* or using a flexible thoracoscope. With both methods, lung volumes (TLC and RV) are reduced and spirometry and gas exchange improve. Spirometry, lung volume measurement, and blood gas analysis are used to monitor changes in these patients.

Hyperreactive Airways Disease: Asthma

Asthma is characterized by reversible airway obstruction. Obstruction is characterized by inflammation of the mucosal lining of the airways, *bronchospasm,* and increased airway secretions. Bronchospasm is usually reversed by inhalation of bronchodilators but may be persistent and severe in some patients. Inflammation may be the essential element in the asthmatic response. Increased airway responsiveness is related to inhalation of antigens, viral infections, air pollution, or occupational exposure. Spirometry is the most useful tool for detecting reversible airway obstruction. Improvement in the FEV_1 or FVC (see Chapter 2) is the hallmark of reversibility. Airway resistance (Raw) and specific airway conductance (SGaw) are also useful in evaluation of reversible obstruction. Peak expiratory flow (PEF), measured using portable peak flow meters, can provide immediate information for a clinician or patient to modify therapy.

Asthma can occur at any age but often begins during childhood. Even infants can have hyperreactive airways (see Chapter 8). Some asthmatic children outgrow the disease, but in others the disease continues into adulthood. In some individuals, asthma begins after age 40. There appears to be a hereditary component to asthma; many cases occur in patients who have a family history of asthma or allergic disorders.

Agents or events that cause an asthmatic episode are called *triggers* (Table 1-7). Antigens such as animal dander, pollens, and dusts are the most common triggers. Other common triggers include exposure to air pollutants, exercise in cold or dry air, occupational exposure to dusts or fumes, and viral upper respiratory infections. Aspirin or other drugs can also trigger

TABLE 1-7   Asthma Triggers

A. Allergic agents
   1. Pollens
   2. Animal dander (proteins)
   3. House dust mites
   4. Molds
B. Nonallergic agents
   1. Viral infections
   2. Exercise
   3. Cold air
   4. Air pollutants (sulfur, nitrogen dioxides)
   5. Cigarette smoke
   6. Drugs (aspirin, beta-blockers)
   7. Food additives
   8. Emotional upset
C. Occupational exposure
   1. Toluene 2,4-diisocyanate (TDI)
   2. Cotton, wood dusts
   3. Grain
   4. Metal salts
   5. Insecticides

asthma, as can food additives (e.g., metabisulfites), or emotional upset (e.g., crying, laughing). All of these triggers act on the hyperresponsive airway to produce the symptoms of asthma.

The most common presentation of asthma includes *wheezing*, cough, and shortness of breath. The severity of asthmatic episodes varies, even in the same individual at different times. In many patients, airway function is relatively normal between intermittent episodes or attacks. Some patients have only cough or chest tightness that subsides spontaneously. However, severe episodes may be life threatening. In its worst presentation, asthma causes continuous chest tightness and wheezing that may not respond to the usual therapy. Dyspnea and cough can both be extreme, and if unresolved they can progress to respiratory failure.

During an attack there is usually wheezing, noisy breathing, and prolonged expiratory times. If the attack is severe, there may be significant air trapping, similar to the pattern seen in patients with emphysema. Accessory muscles of ventilation are used, and breathing may be labored. Spirometry or peak flows provide a simple means of tracking response to bronchodilators. Arterial blood gas testing may be necessary during severe asthmatic episodes. Hypoxemia is commonly present because of ventilation-perfusion mismatching. This usually results in a *respiratory alkalosis,* but evidence of *respiratory acidosis* suggests impending ventilatory failure.

Bronchial provocation tests using methacholine, *histamine,* exercise, or hyperventilation are often used to make the diagnosis of hyperreactive airways in patients who appear normal but have episodic symptoms. Skin testing is also used to demonstrate *sensitivity* to inhaled antigens.

Management of Asthma

The first step in asthma management is avoiding known triggers. In some instances this is easily accomplished. However, in the case of air pollution or occupational exposure, avoiding the offending substance may be expensive or impossible. Asthma education usually focuses on helping the affected individual identify and avoid triggers.

Pharmacologic management of asthma is usually based on a combination of bronchodilator, steroid, and antiinflammatory therapy. For many patients with mild asthma, an adrenergic bronchodilator from a metered-dose inhaler *(MDI)* may be the only treatment required. A variety of β-agonists are available in oral and inhaled forms. In severe asthma, long-acting β-adrenergic bronchodilators (such as salmeterol) are usually inhaled on a dosing schedule. Anticholinergic bronchodilators (such as ipratropium bromide) have become widely prescribed for use in conjunction with β-agonists. Ipratropium may be preferred in patients who experience tachycardia or tremor caused by adrenergic drugs. Although most β-agonists have a rapid onset of action (5 to 15 minutes), ipratropium typically takes 30 to 60 minutes for peak effect to occur. *Theophylline* preparations are still widely used in combination with inhaled bronchodilators. Long-acting theophylline drugs (12 to 24 hours) are often prescribed.

Corticosteroids are useful for acute or chronic asthma that responds poorly to conventional bronchodilators. Steroids act primarily as antiinflammatory agents in the airways and may allow adrenergic drugs to bronchodilate more effectively. Systemic corticosteroids have a number of adverse side effects, including reduction in bone density and adrenal suppression. Inhaled steroid preparations may eliminate the need for oral forms during chronic therapy. Several different preparations are now available in MDIs. Combinations of inhaled steroids and β-adrenergic bronchodilators seem to be very effective at preventing asthma symptoms. Children and adolescents may not respond to inhaled steroids. Inhaled steroids have relatively few side effects; fungal infection of the oral cavity is a common problem. Inhaled steroids decrease bone density, and their effect on growth in children is not completely understood.

Cromolyn sodium or *nedocromil* are used to prophylactically prevent *bronchoconstriction.* They cannot be used for acute episodes but may decrease the amount of corticosteroids or bronchodilators necessary. Cromolyn derivatives are available as a nebulized solution, inhaled powder, or MDI.

Leukotriene receptor antagonists also work to reduce airway inflammation. They block the release of leukotrienes, which potentiate inflammatory mediators. These drugs may be effective in cases in which inhaled steroids are not, and have been successfully used in conjunction with steroids. Some patients may better accept oral preparations of leukotriene antagonists.

Perhaps the most significant new tool in the management of asthma is the portable peak flow meter (see Chapter 2). This device allows simple monitoring of airway function by the patient at home, as well as by caregivers in a variety of settings. Measurement of peak flow provides objective data to guide both the patient and physician in modifying bronchodilator therapy or seeking early treatment.

Cystic Fibrosis

Cystic fibrosis (CF) is a disease that primarily affects the mucus-producing apparatus of the lungs and pancreas. CF is an inherited disorder, transmitted as an autosomal recessive trait. In whites, it occurs in approximately 1 in 2000 live births. CF was once considered a pediatric disease because affected individuals rarely lived to adulthood. Improved detection and aggressive treatment have increased the median survival age well into adulthood.

CF is characterized by malabsorption of food because of pancreatic insufficiency and progressive *suppurative* pulmonary disease. In infancy and early childhood, gastrointestinal manifestations seem to predominate. As the child gets older, respiratory complications related to the tenacious mucus production take over. Other organ systems may be involved as well. Children with CF tend to remain chronically infected with respiratory *pathogens,* such as *Staphylococcus aureus* or *Pseudomonas aeruginosa.*

Clinical manifestations of CF include chronic cough and sinusitis, bronchiectasis, and *atelectasis.* Hemoptysis and *pneumothorax* are common. Pulmonary function studies may be used to follow the progression of the disease. Spirometry (FEV_1) is frequently measured as an index of the need for lung transplantation. Chest x-ray studies show changes consistent with bronchiectasis and *honeycombing*. Atelectasis commonly affects entire lobes as a result of mucus impaction. Other complications center on gastrointestinal manifestations (e.g., bowel obstruction and vitamin deficiencies). Most individuals with CF are diagnosed in infancy or early childhood based on elevated sweat chloride levels. Occasionally, some young adults are not diagnosed until after age 15. In many instances, adolescents or even adults are misdiagnosed as having asthma or related pulmonary diseases. Misdiagnosis usually occurs in individuals who have mild CF with few complications.

Management of Cystic Fibrosis

Removal of the excess mucus produced in CF is the primary focus of management. This usually requires bronchial hygiene measures and pharmacologic intervention. Bronchodilators are used to reverse bronchospasm that commonly accompanies chronic inflammation. A genetically engineered enzyme is now used to reduce mucus viscosity in CF patients. This enzyme (rhDNase) is administered via an aerosol. This reduces the viscosity of secretions and improves airflow. Corticosteroids are used to combat both pulmonary inflammation and bronchial hyperreactivity. Continuous or intermittent antibiotics are also a mainstay of care in the patient with CF. Proper nutrition is similarly very important in managing CF. Pancreatic insufficiency increases the patient's metabolic rate, even though nutrients are poorly absorbed in the intestine. Pancreatic enzyme supplements and vitamins are required, particularly in children with CF. For individuals with severe CF, lung transplantation has become a lifesaving treatment. Pulmonary function studies are routinely used to assess lung function following transplantation.

Upper or Large Airway Obstruction

Many obstructive diseases involve the medium or *small airways*. Sometimes airway obstruction occurs in the upper airways (nose, mouth, pharynx) or in the large thoracic airways (trachea, mainstem bronchi). Obstruction can also occur where the upper and lower airways meet at the vocal cords. When obstruction occurs below the vocal cords, the degree of obstruction may vary with changes in thoracic pressure. This occurs because the airways themselves change size as thoracic pressure rises or falls. Obstructive processes above the vocal cords are not influenced by thoracic pressures but may still vary with airflow depending on the type of lesion involved. Regardless of the location of the problem, *large airway obstruction* results in increased work of breathing. Upper airway obstruction is frequently diagnosed using the flow-volume loop or measurements of airway resistance (see Chapter 2).

Vocal cord dysfunction or damage can result in significant airway obstruction. The vocal cords are normally held open or abducted during inspiration. When damaged, the vocal cords move toward the midline, narrowing the airway opening. This type of obstruction limits flow primarily during inspiration. In some cases, expiratory flow may be reduced as well, but inspiratory flow is typically lower. Common causes of vocal cord dysfunction include laryngeal muscle weakness or mechanical damage as sometimes occurs during intubation of the trachea. Severe infections involving the larynx can leave scar tissue on the vocal cords or supporting structures. Vocal cord dysfunction often mimics asthma. It may become notably worse when ventilation is increased, as happens during exercise. *Neuromuscular* disorders can cause paralysis of the vocal cords, also resulting in variable extrathoracic airway obstruction (see Chapter 2).

Tumors are a common cause of large airway obstruction. Lesions that invade the trachea or mainstem bronchi can significantly diminish airflow. The decrease in flow is directly related to the decrease in cross-sectional area of the airway. If the airway lumen (i.e., the part not obstructed) varies in cross-sectional area with inspiration and expiration, the obstruction is described as variable. During inspiration, thoracic pressure decreases and large airways increase their cross-sectional area. During expiration, the opposite occurs. If the airway is partially obstructed by a tumor, airflow will be decreased during inspiration and expiration, but more so during expiration. If the tumor reduces the cross-sectional area of the airway but does not vary with the phase of breathing, the obstruction is fixed. In this instance both inspiratory and expiratory flows are reduced approximately equally (see Chapter 2). Tumors in the upper airway may cause variable or fixed obstruction. If an extrathoracic tumor causes the airway cross section to vary with breathing, inspiratory flow is usually reduced.

Neuromuscular disorders that affect the muscles of the upper airway can also affect airway patency. When the muscles of the pharynx or larynx are relaxed (reduced muscle tone), airway collapse may occur during the inspiratory phase of breathing. Any disorder that affects innervation of pharyngeal muscles can cause similar obstructive patterns. Abnormal airflow patterns are sometimes seen in patients who have *obstructive sleep apnea,* although flow measurements cannot predict sleep apnea. *Myasthenia gravis* affects the muscles of respiration, including the muscles of the upper airway. Generalized weakness of these muscles can result in variable extrathoracic obstruction.

Both upper and large airway obstruction commonly result from trauma to the airways. These can occur as the result of motor vehicle accidents or falls. Scarring or stenosis of the trachea may also occur after prolonged endotracheal intubation or tracheostomy. The typical pattern is one of fixed obstruction, although some lesions do vary with the phase of breathing. Granulomatous disease, such as *sarcoidosis* or tuberculosis, can occasionally cause upper airway obstruction. Extrinsic airway compression can also reduce airflow. *Goiters* or *mediastinal* infections are the most common culprits that compress the airways in this way.

Management of Upper or Large Airway Obstruction

Treatment of lesions that produce upper or large airway obstruction is aimed at reversing the offending process. For vocal cord dysfunction, stopping inappropriate therapy (e.g., steroids) is the first step. Speech therapy and breathing retraining have been demonstrated to reduce inspiratory obstruction. In severe cases, a mixture of helium and oxygen (80% He–20% O_2) may be needed to alleviate dyspnea and interrupt the episode. Treatment of neuromuscular disease such as myasthenia gravis often reverses the associated airway obstruction.

Tumors usually require resection. Some *neoplasms* can be managed only by radiation or *chemotherapy.* In either case, spirometry with flow-volume curves (see Chapter 2) is used to assess airway obstruction. Surgical repair of trauma to the upper or large airways directly relieves airway obstruction and reduces the work of breathing.

■ RESTRICTIVE LUNG DISEASE

Restrictive lung disease is characterized by reduction of lung volumes. The VC and TLC are both reduced below the lower limit of normal. Any process that interferes with the bellows action of the lungs or chest wall can cause restriction. Restriction is often associated with (1) *interstitial lung diseases,* including *idiopathic fibrosis,* pneumoconioses, and sarcoidosis; (2) disease of the chest wall and *pleura;* (3) neuromuscular disorders; and (4) *congestive heart failure (CHF).*

Idiopathic Pulmonary Fibrosis

Idiopathic pulmonary fibrosis (IPF) is characterized by alveolar wall inflammation resulting in fibrosis. Vascular changes are usually associated with *pulmonary hypertension.* The patient has increasing exertional dyspnea. On the chest x-ray film, *infiltrates* are visible and advanced IPF shows a honeycombing pattern.

IPF often follows the use of medications such as *bleomycin,* cyclophosphamide, methotrexate, or *amiodarone.* IPF is also associated with a number of autoimmune diseases. Rheumatoid arthritis, systemic *lupus* erythematosus (SLE), and *scleroderma* all produce alveolar wall inflammation and *fibrotic* changes. As each disease progresses, lung volumes are reduced. These reductions in VC and TLC occur as fibrosis causes the lungs to become stiff. Measurement of pulmonary compliance (see Chapter 2) is sometimes helpful in quantifying the effects of the fibrosis. DL_{CO} (see Chapter 5) is often reduced due to ventilation-perfusion mismatching. The same process also causes hypoxemia at rest that worsens with exertion.

Management of IPF relies primarily on corticosteroids (prednisone). Long-term therapy is usually indicated with large initial doses, followed by tapering and then maintenance. Immunosuppressive agents are sometimes used in conjunction with steroids in difficult cases. In the most severe presentations, lung transplantation may be required. Spirometry, lung volume measurements, and DL_{CO} are routinely used to monitor the patient's progress and response to therapeutic interventions.

Pneumoconioses

Pneumoconiosis is lung impairment caused by inhalation of dusts. Certain types of dust exposure have been shown to result in pneumoconioses (Table 1-8). Dust particles in the size range between 0.5 and 5.0 microns are considered most dangerous because they are deposited throughout the lung. A carefully taken history, including work history, is essential. (See Pulmonary History in the Preliminaries to Patient Testing section). Most pneumoconioses are characterized by pulmonary fibrosis and chest x-ray abnormalities. Pulmonary function studies typically reveal a restrictive pattern with reduction in DL_{CO}.

Silicosis, caused by inhalation of silica dust, is common. Silica is deposited in the lung and ingested by macrophages. This results in the formation of nodules around bronchioles and blood vessels. As the silicosis advances, fibrosis occurs. The patient usually has cough and dyspnea. In addition to restriction shown by pulmonary function studies, some airways may also be obstructed. As nodules increase in size to more than 1 cm, the condition is labeled progressive massive fibrosis (PMF). PMF is usually accompanied by hypoxemia and pulmonary hypertension. Treatment of silicosis is directed at relieving hypoxemia and managing right-sided heart failure.

TABLE 1-8   Common Pneumoconioses

Dust	Pneumoconiosis	Occupation
Iron	Siderosis	Welder, miner
Tin	Stannosis	Metal worker
Barium	Baritosis	Miner, metallurgist, ceramics worker
Silica	Silicosis	Sandblaster, brick maker, coal miner
Asbestos	Asbestosis	Brake/clutch manufacturer, shipbuilder, steam fitter, insulator
Talc	Talcosis	Ceramics worker, cosmetics maker
Beryllium	Berylliosis	Alloy maker, electronic tube maker, metal worker
Coal	Coal worker's pneumoconiosis	Coal miner

Asbestosis results from inhalation of asbestos fibers. Asbestos has been commonly used in the manufacture of insulating materials, brake linings, roofing materials, and fire-resistant textiles. As with most pneumoconioses, the risk of developing asbestosis is related to the intensity and duration of exposure. The onset of symptoms is usually delayed for 20 years. Cigarette smoking has been shown to shorten the period between exposure and onset of symptoms. Inhaled asbestos fibers are engulfed by alveolar macrophages. Fibrosis in alveolar walls and around bronchioles develops. The visceral pleura may also show fibrous deposits. Plaques, made up of collagenous connective tissue, are often found on the parietal pleura. The patient experiences dyspnea on exertion. Pulmonary function tests show restriction and impaired *diffusion* (DL_{CO}). The chest x-ray film may show irregular densities in the lower lung fields, fibrotic changes (honeycombing), and diaphragmatic calcifications. COPD and lung cancer are also common in patients with asbestosis and are related to cigarette smoking. Treatment consists of assessment with pulmonary function tests (especially diffusing capacity) and relief of symptoms.

Coal worker's pneumoconiosis (CWP) is caused by an accumulation of coal dust in the lungs. It should not be confused with *black lung*, which is a legal term used to describe any chronic respiratory disease in a coal miner. Some coal contains silica, but CWP begins with a reaction to an accumulation of dust, called a *coal macule*. These macules are usually found in the upper lobes. The black coal pigment is deposited around the respiratory bronchioles. Diagnosis of CWP is made by history and chest x-ray film interpretation. Onset of symptoms caused by CWP usually occurs in advanced cases. Coal workers often have respiratory symptoms and physiologic findings consistent with COPD. These symptoms may be related more to cigarette smoking than to coal dust exposure. CWP causes fibrosis, restriction on pulmonary function tests, hypoxemia, and pulmonary hypertension. As in the case of other pneumoconioses, treatment is aimed at relief of the symptoms.

Sarcoidosis

Sarcoidosis is a granulomatous disease that affects multiple organ systems. The disease appears most often in the second through fourth decades. It occurs more commonly in African Americans, especially in women. The granuloma found in sarcoidosis is composed of macrophages, epithelioid cells, and other inflammatory cells. This granulomatous lesion may resolve with little or no structural change, or it may develop fibrosis in the target organ.

Symptoms of sarcoidosis include fatigue, muscle weakness, fever, and weight loss. Other symptoms involve the specific organ system in which the granulomatous changes occur. The lungs and lymph nodes of the mediastinum are frequently involved in patients who have sarcoidosis. Dyspnea and cough are the most common presenting symptoms. Chest x-ray films usually show enlargement of the *hilar* and mediastinal lymph nodes. Interstitial infiltrates may also be present. Other systems commonly involved in sarcoidosis include the skin, eyes, musculoskeletal system, heart, and central nervous system.

Pulmonary function tests show a pattern of restriction, with relatively normal flows. Diffusing capacity is usually not reduced except when there is advanced fibrosis of lung tissue. Arterial blood gas measurements may be normal, or there may be hypoxemia. Stress testing may show worsened gas exchange. It is not unusual for sarcoidosis in the early stages to show completely normal lung function. Diagnosis of sarcoidosis is sometimes made via clinical findings and chest x-ray examination, but biopsy of affected tissue is often necessary. This may involve mediastinoscopy or fiberoptic bronchoscopy.

Management of sarcoidosis includes medications to treat symptoms such as fever, skin lesions, or arthralgia. Serious complications involving worsening pulmonary function are usually treated with corticosteroids.

DISEASES OF THE CHEST WALL AND PLEURA

Several disorders involving the chest wall or pleura of the lungs result in restrictive patterns on pulmonary function studies. Conditions affecting the thorax include *kyphoscoliosis* and obesity. Pleural diseases include *pleurisy,* pleural *effusions,* and pneumothorax.

Kyphoscoliosis is a condition that involves abnormal curvature of the spine both anteriorly *(kyphosis)* and laterally *(scoliosis).* Patients who have kyphoscoliosis show rib cage distortion that can lead to recurrent infections as well as blood gas abnormalities. Depending of the degree of spinal curvature, the patient may have normal lung function or restriction. Ventilation may be normal. Lung compression usually causes ventilation-perfusion mismatching and hypoxemia. In severe cases, there may be hypercapnia and respiratory acidosis. Treatment of the disorder involves prevention of infections and relief of hypoxemia, if present. Surgical correction is necessary in many cases, and pulmonary function studies are used to evaluate patients both preoperatively and postoperatively.

Obesity restricts ventilation, especially when the obesity is severe. Increased mass of the thorax and abdomen interferes with the bellows action of the chest wall, as well as excursion of the diaphragm. Obesity is also related to a more general syndrome that consists of hypercapnia and hypoxemia, sleep apnea, and decreased respiratory drive. These findings are sometimes called the *obesity-hypoventilation* syndrome. Chronic hypoxemia in this syndrome results in polycythemia, pulmonary hypertension, and cor pulmonale. Not all patients who are obese show the signs of obesity-hypoventilation syndrome. However, pulmonary function studies often show restriction in proportion to the excess weight. Weight reduction relieves many of the associated symptoms. Respiratory stimulants, tracheostomy, and continuous positive airway pressure (CPAP) are used to manage the obstructive sleep apnea component.

Pleurisy and pleural effusions can each result in restrictive ventilatory patterns. Pleurisy is characterized by deposition of a fibrous *exudate* on the pleural surface. It is associated with other pulmonary diseases such as pneumonia or lung cancer. Pleurisy is often accompanied by chest discomfort or pain and may precede the development of pleural effusions. Pleural effusion is an abnormal accumulation of fluid in the pleural space. This fluid may be either a *transudate* or an exudate. Transudate occurs when there is an imbalance in the hydrostatic or oncotic pressures, as occurs in congestive heart failure (CHF). Exudates are associated with infections or with inflammation as in lung carcinoma. Patients with pleural effusions usually have symptoms that relate to the extent of the effusion. Small effusions often go unnoticed. If the effusion is large, there may be atelectasis from compression of lung tissue, and associated blood gas changes. Pulmonary function tests show restriction as a result of volume loss. In some cases, there is restriction caused by splinting as a result of pain. Treatment of pleurisy and pleural effusions is directed toward the underlying cause. Large or unresolved pleural effusions often require thoracentesis or chest tube drainage. Patients with painful pleural involvement may have difficulty performing spirometry or breath holding as required for DL_{CO}.

Pneumothorax is a condition in which air enters the pleural space. This air leak may be due to a perforation of the lung itself or of the chest wall (e.g., chest trauma). Small pneumothoraces may not cause any symptoms. Large pneumothoraces result in severe dyspnea and chest pain. Physical examination of the patient reveals decreased chest movement on the affected side. Breath sounds are usually absent. A chest x-ray study shows a shift of the mediastinum away from the pneumothorax. Small pneumothoraces usually resolve without treatment as gas is reabsorbed from the pleural space. Large air leaks usually require a chest tube with appropriate drainage to allow lung re-expansion.

Pulmonary function tests are usually contraindicated in the presence of pneumothorax. However, undiagnosed pneumothorax may present a risk if pulmonary function studies are performed. Maneuvers that generate high intrathoracic pressures (i.e., FVC, MVV, MIP/MEP) can aggravate an untreated pneumothorax. The potential for development of a *tension pneumothorax* exists when these maneuvers are performed. In a tension pneumothorax, air enters the pleural space but cannot escape. Increasing pressure compresses the opposite lung, as well as the heart and great vessels. Compression of the mediastinum interferes with venous return to the heart and can cause a rapid drop in blood pressure. A tension pneumothorax can be fatal if not treated immediately. Patients referred for pulmonary function studies that have known or suspected pneumothoraces should be tested very carefully. In many instances, the information obtained may not justify the risk to the patient.

■ NEUROMUSCULAR DISORDERS

Diseases that affect the spinal cord, peripheral nerves, neuromuscular junctions, and the respiratory muscles can all cause a restrictive pattern of pulmonary function. Most of these disorders result in an inability to generate normal respiratory pressures. The VC and TLC are usually reduced. Some chronic neuromuscular disorders are associated with decreased lung compliance. Blood gas abnormalities, particularly hypoxemia, may result if the degree of involvement is severe. Stiff lungs and rapid respiratory rates often result in respiratory alkalosis *(hyperventilation)*. Progressive muscle weakness results in *hypoventilation* and respiratory failure.

Diaphragmatic paralysis may be bilateral or unilateral. Bilateral paralysis may be the end stage of various disorders. The most prominent finding is *orthopnea,* or shortness of breath in the supine position. In the upright position, the patient has a marked increase in VC and improvement in gas exchange. Simple spirometry in the supine and sitting positions can demonstrate the functional impairment. Unilateral paralysis usually results from damage to one of the phrenic nerves (e.g., trauma, surgery, or tumor). As with bilateral paralysis, there is a marked change in VC from supine to sitting position. Diagnosis of the affected side may require chest x-ray, or examination under fluoroscopy. Reduced inspiratory pressures (see Chapter 2) may suggest diaphragmatic involvement.

Amyotrophic lateral sclerosis (ALS, or Lou Gehrig's disease) affects the anterior horn cells of the spinal cord. Progressive muscle weakness results in a gradual decrease in VC and TLC. Pulmonary function studies may be done serially to assess the progression of the disease.

Guillain-Barré syndrome is a progressive disease involving the peripheral nerves. Lower extremity weakness ascends to the upper extremities and face. There may be marked respiratory muscle weakness along with weakness of the pharyngeal and laryngeal muscles. Serial measurements of the VC, MIP, and MEP are used to follow the disease progression.

Myasthenia gravis is an abnormality of neuromuscular transmission. It particularly affects muscles innervated by the bulbar nuclei (i.e., face, lips, throat, neck). The patient with myasthenia gravis has pronounced fatigability of the muscles. Speech and swallowing difficulties can occur with prolonged exercise of the associated muscles. Progression of a myasthenic crisis can be assessed using VC and respiratory pressures. Analysis of the flow-volume curve (see Chapter 2) may be helpful in detecting upper airway obstruction brought on by muscular weakness.

■ CONGESTIVE HEART FAILURE

Congestive heart failure is often used synonymously with left *ventricular* failure. Failure of the left ventricle may be caused by systemic hypertension, coronary artery disease, or aortic insufficiency. CHF may also be associated with *cardiomyopathy,* congenital heart defects, and left-to-right shunts. In each case, fluid backs up in the lungs. The pulmonary venous system becomes engorged. Fluid may spill into the alveolar spaces (pulmonary edema) or the pleural space (effusion).

The patient who has CHF usually has shortness of breath on exertion, cough, and fatigue. If coronary artery disease is the cause of CHF, there may be chest pain *(angina)* as well. Exertional dyspnea is related to pulmonary venous congestion. The fluid overload in the lungs reduces lung volume and makes the lungs stiff (decreased compliance). Dyspnea is usually worse when the patient is supine (i.e., orthopnea). This orthopnea results from increased pulmonary vascular congestion with increased venous return. Dyspnea brought on by CHF may be difficult to distinguish from other causes (e.g., chronic pulmonary disease). The chest x-ray film usually shows increased pulmonary congestion. The heart (left ventricle) may appear enlarged, particularly if systemic hypertension in the cause.

Treatment of CHF is directed at the underlying cause. Relief of systemic hypertension can reduce the myocardial workload. This is usually accomplished by vasodilator therapy. Reducing fluid retention is also important in managing CHF. Diuretics such as furosemide (Lasix) are commonly used to reduce the *afterload* on the ventricle. Oxygen therapy may also help reduce myocardial workload, especially if there is hypoxemia. If the cause of CHF is an arrhythmia, *antiarrhythmic* agents are typically used. Inotropic agents such as dobutamine may be used to increase myocardial contractility, especially after an acute infarction. Pulmonary function tests, particularly lung volumes and DL_{CO}, may be used to monitor the effects of treatment.

LUNG TRANSPLANTATION

Lung transplantation has evolved as an effective treatment for end-stage lung disease. Lung transplantation has been used for patients with CF, primary pulmonary hypertension, and COPD (Table 1-9). Double lung transplants are usually performed in patients who have CF, generalized bronchiectasis, or in some types of COPD. Heart-lung transplants have been used for *Eisenmenger's syndrome,* pulmonary hypertension with cor pulmonale, and end-stage lung disease coexisting with severe heart disease. Single-lung transplantation has been used effectively in patients with COPD who are younger than approximately 60 years old. Single-lung transplantation offers the benefit that two recipients can share a single donor's organs. Survival rates for lung transplant recipients have steadily improved. Longer survival is mainly due to more potent antirejection drugs (e.g., *cyclosporine*) and better adjunctive therapy.

TABLE 1-9 Indications for Lung Transplantation

Transplant type	Disease state
Heart-lung	Eisenmenger's syndrome, severe cardiac defect
	Pulmonary hypertension, cor pulmonale
	End-stage lung disease, coexisting severe cardiac disease
Double-lung	Cystic fibrosis
	Generalized bronchiectasis
	COPD with severe chronic bronchitis or extensive bullae
Single-lung	Restrictive fibrotic lung disease
	Eisenmenger's syndrome (less severe cardiac anomalies)
	COPD
	Primary pulmonary hypertension

Modified from American Thoracic Society: Lung transplantation, *Am Rev Respir Dis* 147:772-776, 1993.

Pulmonary function tests are used to both assess potential transplant candidates and follow them postoperatively.

Preoperative evaluation consists of documentation of the severity of the specific disease process. Spirometry, lung volumes, DL_{CO}, and blood gas analysis are all used to rank the level of dysfunction. The same tests are also used to detect sudden worsening of lung function that might necessitate rapid intervention. Cardiopulmonary exercise testing may be indicated to determine the extent of the physiologic abnormality. For example, a patient with border-line pulmonary hypertension at rest may develop severe hypertension during even mild exertion.

Most transplantation programs list patients as prospective candidates when their pulmonary disease has advanced beyond predefined limits. An extended wait for lung transplantation is a direct result of the shortage of donor organs. Patients are often referred for transplant evaluation when a major decline in their condition is observed. The term *transplant window* has been used to describe the time period during which the patient is sick enough to require transplantation, but healthy enough to have a reasonable chance of success.

Posttransplant follow-up relies heavily on pulmonary function tests. Spirometry has been used extensively to monitor improvements resulting from transplantation. Recipients of double-lung transplants often show lung function values approaching those of normal patients within a few months. Blood gas changes usually occur immediately after surgery. Single-lung transplant (SLT) recipients show similar gains. However, because SLT patients retain a native lung, improvement in pulmonary function is usually less than when both lungs are replaced. Interpretation of spirometry, lung volumes, and blood gases in SLT patients is often complicated by the presence of the native lung along with the transplanted lung.

Besides monitoring improved lung function, pulmonary function tests are used to detect rejection and the development of bronchiolitis obliterans. Rejection may be difficult to distinguish from other pulmonary complications (e.g., pneumonia) in patients who are immunosuppressed. There is some evidence that spirometric changes (FVC, FEV_1, $FEF_{25\%-75\%}$) may signal episodes of acute rejection. Chronic rejection is thought to be associated with the development of bronchiolitis obliterans. This pattern is characterized by the development of severe airflow limitation in the transplanted lung. Spirometry, particularly indices of small airway function, may provide the earliest signs of bronchiolitis obliterans.

Preliminaries to Patient Testing

Several preliminary steps precede any pulmonary function study. These include patient preparation, physical measurements and assessment, brief pulmonary history, and instructions to the patient in the performance of specific test maneuvers. In addition, pulmonary function tests are usually done in an ordered sequence. The testing sequence may be determined by laboratory policy, or it may be adapted for specific needs using a predefined protocol.

PATIENT PREPARATION

Patient preparation for pulmonary function studies consists mainly of instructions given to the patient in advance of the actual test session. These instructions focus on taking or withholding specific medications, refraining from smoking, and other guidelines related to specific tests (e.g., exercise tests, blood gases).

WITHHOLDING MEDICATIONS

Patients referred for evaluation of airflow limitation are often already taking bronchodilators or related drugs. If response to bronchodilator is to be assessed, bronchodilators should be withheld at least 4 to 6 hours before testing. The exact length of time to withhold a bronchodilator is dictated by the onset of action and duration of the drug. Guidelines for withholding specific bronchodilators are presented in detail in Chapter 2. It may be impossible for some patients to withhold their bronchodilators. The patient should be instructed to take the bronchodilator when breathing problems require it.

Care should be taken when instructing outpatients about withholding medications. Some patients may be unable to correctly identify all of their medications. Hence, it may be difficult for them to correctly withhold only bronchodilators. Some patients incorrectly withhold all medications. This may cause serious problems for patients who rely on insulin (diabetic patients), antiarrhythmics, or antihypertensives used for high blood pressure. If the patient is uncertain, it may be preferable to not withhold any medications.

SMOKING CESSATION

Patients referred for pulmonary function tests should be asked to refrain from smoking for 24 hours before the test. Smoking cessation is especially important if DL_{CO} tests or arterial blood gas tests are ordered. Smoking has been shown to reduce diffusing capacity. Smoking raises the level of CO in the blood, which also interferes with the measurement of diffusing capacity. Increased CO in the blood (COHb) makes it difficult to interpret O_2 saturation measured by pulse oximetry (see Chapter 6).

OTHER PATIENT PREPARATION ISSUES

Patients referred for pulmonary function tests should probably be advised not to eat a large meal immediately before their appointment. The same is true if the patient will be exercising as part of the evaluation. If the patient is scheduled for a bronchial challenge test (see Chapter 9), special instructions concerning medications to withhold are required. In addition, patients receiving bronchial challenge should not drink beverages that contain caffeine or theobromines (cola drinks) or eat chocolate.

Some patients may require special accommodations for pulmonary function tests to be performed safely and accurately. Patients, or those referring patients, should understand the requirements of the tests requested. Patients who are unable to sit or stand may require additional time or equipment for testing to be completed. Patients who have permanent tracheostomies may also require special devices to allow connection to standard pulmonary function circuits. Patients who do not speak the primary language used in the laboratory may require an interpreter to be present during testing. Asking appropriate questions before the patient's appointment can identify each of these special needs.

PHYSICAL MEASUREMENTS

Various physical measurements are required for estimating each patient's expected level of pulmonary function. Age, height, and weight are usually recorded in addition to the patient's sex. Race or ethnic origin should also be recorded. Basic physical assessment of the patient's respiratory status may be needed before and during testing.

The patient's age should be recorded as of the last birthday. Some computerized pulmonary function systems store the patient's birth date and calculate the age. This approach is helpful, especially when the patient returns periodically for serial testing. Care should be used when entering this type of data into a computerized system. Data entry errors can result in gross overestimation or underestimation of the patient's expected values.

Standing height, in either inches or centimeters, should be recorded with the patient barefoot or in stocking feet. A wall-mounted ruler allows the patient to stand with the back against the wall and the head close to the ruler. If the patient is unable to stand upright, the arm-span method should be used. Patients who have a history of kyphosis, scoliosis, or related problems should also have height estimated using their *arm span*. Arm span may be measured using a ruler or tape measure at least 4 ft long. The patient should extend the arms horizontally on either side, and the distance from the tip of the middle finger to the center of the vertebrum at the level of the scapula is measured. The measurement is repeated for the opposite side, and the two values obtained are added together. This length may be used in all calculations that require standing height.

The patient's weight in pounds or kilograms should be measured with an accurate scale. Because obesity is related to restrictive lung disease, a measurement of weight may be helpful for interpretation of reduced lung volumes. Body weight is used to calculate some reference values (see Appendix B). When weight is used to predict an expected value, the patient's ideal body weight should be used. Using actual weight in patients who are obese may overestimate expected values. Weight is also used to express oxygen consumption (i.e., ml/kg) for exercise and metabolic measurements. The patient's weight may also be required when lung volumes are determined with the body plethysmograph. Weight is used to estimate body volume in the plethysmograph (see Chapter 3).

PHYSICAL ASSESSMENT

Physical assessment of patients referred for pulmonary function studies may be needed to determine whether the individual can perform the test. Documentation concerning physical assessment of the patient can also assist with interpretation of test results. Physical assessment should focus on breathing pattern, breath sounds (if necessary), and respiratory symptoms (Table 1-10). These can be observed simply and noted as necessary. Commentary regarding the patient's signs or symptoms at the time of the test is a useful adjunct, especially when test performance is less than optimal.

PULMONARY HISTORY

Accurate interpretation of pulmonary function studies—from simple screening spirometry to complete cardiopulmonary evaluation—requires clinical information related to possible pulmonary disorders. An ordered array of questions that can be easily answered by the patient provides the most useful history. The interpreter of pulmonary function studies may have little clinical information other than that obtained at the time of testing. A pulmonary history should be taken routinely before pulmonary function testing and should include the following:

1. Age, sex, standing height, weight, race
2. Current diagnosis or reason for test

TABLE 1-10 Physical Assessment During Pulmonary Function Testing

A. Breathing pattern
1. Is there good chest expansion? Is it symmetric?
2. Is the breathing rate excessive?
3. Are there any complaints of chest tightness or chest discomfort?
4. Are accessory muscles being used for breathing?
5. Is the patient using pursed lips?

B. Breath sounds (with and without auscultation)
1. Are there audible breath sounds? Are breath sounds distant or absent?
2. Is there any wheezing? Over which lung fields?
3. Is there stridor, especially on inspiration?
4. Are there any other unusual breath sounds (e.g., crackles, rubs)?

C. Respiratory symptoms
1. Is there any cyanosis?
2. Is there obvious shortness of breath (mild, moderate, severe)?
3. Is the patient coughing? If so, is the cough productive?
4. Is the patient receiving supplemental oxygen? If so, how much?
5. What is the patient's oxygen saturation (pulse oximetry reading)?

3. Family history: Did anyone in your immediate family (mother, father, brother, or sister) ever have the following:
    Tuberculosis
    Emphysema
    Chronic bronchitis
    Asthma
    Hay fever or allergies
    Cancer
    Other lung disorders

4. Personal history: Have you ever had, or been told that you had, the following:
    Tuberculosis
    Emphysema
    Chronic bronchitis
    Asthma
    Recurrent lung infections
    Pneumonia or pleurisy
    Allergies or hay fever
    Chest injury (if so, what kind?) _____
    Chest surgery (if so, what kind?) _____

5. Occupation: Have you ever worked in the following situations:
    In a mine, quarry, or foundry
    Near gases or fumes (if so, what kind?)
    In a dusty place (if so, what kind?)
    What is, or was, your occupation? (_____)
    How many years? ( )

6. Smoking habits: Have you ever smoked the following:
    Cigarettes (how many per day?) _____
    Cigars (how many per day?) _____
    Pipe (how many bowls per day?) _____

How long? _____ years
Do you still smoke?   Y / N
Do you live with a smoker?   Y / N

7. Cough: Do you ever cough:
   In the morning   Y / N
   At night   Y / N
   Blood (when?) _____
   Phlegm (when?) _____
        (color?) _____
        (volume?) _____

8. Dyspnea: Do you get short of breath at the following times:
   At rest Y / N
   On exertion (when?) _____
   At night Y / N

9. Patient disposition at time of test
   Dyspneic Y / N
   Wheezing Y / N
   Coughing Y / N
   Cyanotic Y / N
   Apprehensive Y / N
   Cooperative Y / N

10. Current medications (for heart, lung, or blood pressure)

   _____
   _____
   _____

   Last taken:

   _____
   _____
   _____

Most of these questions can be answered by Yes or No, or by circling an appropriate response. Space should be provided so that the patient or history taker can enter comments. In instances in which the physician performs the test, such history may be redundant if a medical history is available.

PF Tips

Some patients may be unable to read and may become embarrassed when asked to complete a questionnaire. Take time to ask questions verbally. Even patients who can read may not understand all of the questions. Be sure to offer to help with any difficult questions or ones that are left blank.

Interpretation of pulmonary function tests is best made if the clinical question asked of the test is considered. The clinician requesting the test should indicate the reason for the test. Examples of clinical questions asked of pulmonary function studies include "Does the patient have airway obstruction?" or "Does the patient have hyperreactive airways?" The pulmonary history, including the reason for the test, should be used to decide what is normal or abnormal. Clinical information as provided by the history is especially important when the patient's pulmonary function tests are borderline. For example, an FEV_1 that is 80% of the expected value would be interpreted differently in a healthy young patient tested as part of a routine physical than it would be in a smoker who complained of increasing dyspnea.

Test Performance and Sequence

Pulmonary function laboratories should have written policies and procedures defining how each test is performed (see Chapter 11). Indications for performing a specific test should be related to the clinical question to be answered or to the patient's diagnosis. Testing protocols that can be modified for individual patients are usually the most cost-effective means of obtaining the required data. When the required tests are determined, the exact sequence of tests can be selected. The sequence in which to perform tests may vary according to patient need and the test method used.

TECHNOLOGIST-ADAPTED PROTOCOLS

As described previously, the basis for deciding appropriate pulmonary function testing is the patient's clinical question. The clinical question is often inappropriately stated as a diagnosis. In fact, many patients are referred for pulmonary function studies to establish a diagnosis. For example, a patient may be referred with a diagnosis listed as "asthma." The clinical question is "Does the patient have asthma?" Pulmonary function studies may be able to answer this question, but the exact tests to be performed may not be defined. In this example, spirometry is indicated. Using an adaptive protocol, the technologist performs spirometry and, based on the results, selects appropriate additional tests (Figure 1-3). Bronchial challenge tests may be performed if spirometry results are normal. Alternatively, additional tests such as lung volumes or DL_{CO} may be necessary.

The correct sequence for performing tests is important. Many laboratories use a fixed order for component pulmonary function tests. This may include spirometry, followed by lung volumes and DL_{CO}. In some instances, the order of tests may need to be altered. The methodology used for some tests has definite effects on the results of subsequent procedures. For example, the multiple-breath N_2 washout test to determine FRC has the patient inhale 100% O_2 for several minutes. If this test is performed immediately before a DL_{CO} test, the elevated O_2 level in the lungs (as well as in the blood and tissues) may reduce the measured DL_{CO}. Similarly, if the N_2 washout or He dilution methods of FRC determination are repeated, sufficient time should be allowed to wash out residual test gas.

PATIENT INSTRUCTION

Many pulmonary function tests are effort dependent. To obtain valid data, patients must be instructed and coached for each maneuver. Instruction and coaching are particularly important for the FVC maneuver. Instruction should include a description of what the patient is expected to do, such as "You will take a deep breath in, and then blow out as hard and as fast as possible." In addition to a description of the test, the maneuver should be demonstrated. During the actual test, vocal encouragement should be given so that the patient continues for an appropriate interval. Any problems that occur with the first few efforts should be explained before the patient attempts the test again. For example, "That was a very good effort, but you

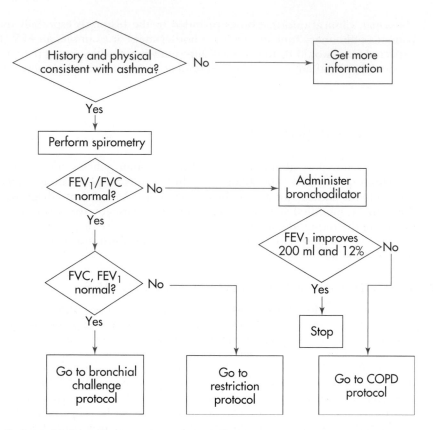

Figure 1-3 *Protocol-decision diagram used by a pulmonary function technologist to select appropriate testing.*
A patient with possible asthma is referred for evaluation. The diagram shows routes to appropriate tests based on the results of simple spirometry. Note that if the patient history and physical assessment suggest diagnoses other than hyperreactive airways, more information may be needed.

stopped before blowing out for 6 seconds. Let's try that again, and keep blowing out until I signal you to relax." This type of feedback is important for patients who may be uncertain of what is expected of them. Patients should be instructed that some maneuvers will be repeated so that their best effort can be obtained. They should be assured that repeating some tests is required and does not reflect a problem on their part.

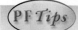

The most effective way to get good patient effort is to *demonstrate* each maneuver. For spirometry, this can be accomplished by using a mouthpiece and simulating the maneuver expected of the patient. Be sure to show what is meant by a maximal effort and how long the effort should last.

Patients should also be carefully instructed for tests that require quiet breathing, such as lung volume determinations. Instructions about maintaining a good seal on the mouthpiece and continuing normal breathing can help reduce leaks or interrupted tests. Some maneuvers are very complicated and may be difficult to describe to the patient. The $D_{L_{CO}}$ maneuver and panting in the body plethysmograph each consist of several steps. For these tests, a combination of demonstration and practice may be the most efficient means of instructing the patient.

Even after adequate instruction and demonstration, some patients may be unable to perform certain tests. This may be caused by lack of coordination related to illness, or inability to follow instructions. For example, a patient may experience uncontrollable coughing when asked to inspire deeply for an FVC maneuver. If the coughing prevents obtaining valid spirometry results, the fact should be noted in the technologist's comments (see Chapter 11). Suboptimal effort by the patient can usually be detected as poorly reproducible results on effort-dependent tests (e.g., the FVC). Care should be taken that adequate instructions are given and a sufficient number of efforts recorded before deciding that the patient did not give a maximal effort. If the patient cannot continue or refuses to continue a test, the exact reason should be documented in the technologist's comments.

Summary

This chapter serves as an introduction to pulmonary function testing. Categories of common pulmonary function tests are listed. This listing should acquaint the reader with the names of various tests, as well as their relationships to one another. Tests are categorized as airway function tests (spirometry), lung volume tests, diffusing capacity tests ($D_{L_{CO}}$), blood gases and gas exchange tests, cardiopulmonary exercise tests, and metabolic measurements. Within each of these groups are a wide variety of tests and techniques.

Indications for tests are also listed. Many indications overlap. For example, an indication for an airway function test may also be an indication for a lung volume, blood gases, or exercise test. Indications are extremely important because they help the practitioner select appropriate tests. For patients, the clinical question asked of the test must be related to a valid indication for the test.

This chapter also outlines patterns of impaired pulmonary function commonly encountered in the laboratory. This discussion assumes a basic knowledge of respiratory anatomy and physiology. The material presented aims to summarize the underlying pathology involved in common pulmonary diseases. The role of pulmonary function testing is discussed as it relates to diagnosis and assessment of these disease processes.

Patient preparation for pulmonary function studies is covered in general terms. More detailed information for specific tests is presented in subsequent chapters. Many of the physical measurements and assessments, as well as the pulmonary history, are similar regardless of the tests being performed. Technologist-adapted protocols are described. *Algorithms* for selecting only appropriate tests are becoming increasingly popular. Such tools improve the sensitivity of the tests to answer the clinical question, as well as make tests more cost-effective.

CASE STUDIES

This case should be evaluated in conjunction with the protocol described in Figure 1-3.

CASE 1-1

Reason for test: Does the patient have asthma?

HISTORY

J.C. is a 22-year-old physical therapy student referred by the student health center at her college. She complains of cough and shortness of breath after vigorous exercise such as playing soccer. She describes a history of "sinus problems" and allergies. No one in her family has a history of pulmonary disease. She has never smoked and has no history of unusual environmental exposure.

PULMONARY FUNCTION TESTING

Personal Data

Sex: Female
Age: 22
Height: 69 in
Weight: 122 lb

Spirometry

	Before Drug			After Drug		
	Actual	**Pred**	**%**	**Actual**	**%**	**Chg%**
FVC (L)	3.98	4.56	87	4.21	92	6
FEV_1 (L)	2.71	3.66	74	3.12	85	15
$FEV_{1\%}$ (%)	68	80		74		
$FEF_{25-75\%}$ (L/sec)	1.71	4.03	42	2.55	63	49

Technologist's Comments

All efforts met ATS criteria for acceptable spirometry. Patient had some coughing following prebronchodilator efforts.

QUESTIONS

1. What is the interpretation of:
   - Prebronchodilator spirometry?
   - Response to bronchodilator?
2. What is the cause of the patient's symptoms?
3. What other tests might be indicated?
4. What treatment might be recommended based on these findings?

DISCUSSION

Interpretation

All spirometric efforts were performed acceptably. Prebronchodilator spirometry reveals mild obstruction. There is a significant improvement following inhaled bronchodilator.

Impression: Reversible airway obstruction with significant response to bronchodilator.

Cause of symptoms

This patient's chief complaints of cough and shortness of breath following exertion are consistent with exercise-induced bronchospasm. The patient had mild obstruction that was evident using simple spirometry. Two puffs of a β-adrenergic inhaler produced a significant improvement in airflow. (The American Thoracic Society recommends a 12% *and* 200 ml improvement as evidence of significant response to bronchodilator.)

Other tests

Using the sample protocol in Figure 1-3, no additional tests are necessary to support the diagnosis of reversible airway obstruction. Bronchial challenge is not needed to document reversible obstruction.

Treatment

The patient was treated with a combination of long-acting β-adrenergic inhalers plus an inhaled steroid, which alleviated most of her symptoms. She was also given a fast-acting bronchodilator for premedication before vigorous exercise.

■ SELF-ASSESSMENT QUESTIONS

Entry-level

1. *Who popularized plotting flow versus volume to display a flow-volume loop?*

   a. Hutchinson
   b. Barach
   c. Severinghaus
   d. Hyatt

2. *Which of the following symptoms is an indication for performing spirometry?*

   a. Headache
   b. Shortness of breath
   c. Chest pain
   d. Daytime sleepiness

3. *Which of the following tests would be indicated to assess the severity of a restrictive pulmonary disease?*

   a. Blood gas analysis
   b. Simple spirometry
   c. Lung volume determination
   d. Cardiopulmonary exercise test

4. *Which of the following tests would be indicated in the evaluation of a patient exposed to dust, including asbestos?*

   a. Shunt study
   b. DL_{CO}
   c. Methacholine challenge
   d. Airway resistance

5. *A 17-year-old female complains of chest tightness and cough after soccer practice. These symptoms are most consistent with which of the following?*

   a. Emphysema
   b. Congestive heart failure
   c. Asthma
   d. Cystic fibrosis

6. *Which of the following diseases often results in an obstructive pattern when simple spirometry is performed?*

   a. Sarcoidosis
   b. Idiopathic pulmonary fibrosis
   c. Pleurisy
   d. Chronic bronchitis

7. *Lung volumes measured by closed-circuit He dilution may be expected to show a reduced FRC in which of the following?*

   a. Emphysema
   b. Asthma
   c. Pulmonary fibrosis
   d. Upper airway obstruction

8. *Which of the following should a pulmonary function technologist do before performing spirometry?*

   a. Limit feedback to the patient to reduce the placebo effect
   b. Explain the physiologic basis of the test
   c. Demonstrate how to correctly perform the test maneuver
   d. Explain the exact number of efforts that will be required for the test

Advanced

9. *Which of the following may be indications for exercise testing?*

   I. Airway hyperreactivity
   II. Guillain-Barré syndrome
   III. Myocardial ischemia
   IV. Exertional desaturation

   a. I and IV only
   b. II and III only
   c. I, II, and IV
   d. I, III, and IV

10. *In which of the following diseases is air-trapping likely to occur?*

    I. Acute exacerbation of asthma
    II. Sarcoidosis
    III. Asbestosis
    IV. Emphysema

    a. IV only
    b. I and III only

c. I and IV only
d. II, III, and IV

11. *Pulmonary function testing is usually contraindicated in which of the following conditions?*

    a. Untreated pneumothorax
    b. Congestive heart failure
    c. Cyanosis
    d. Tuberculosis

12. *Which of the following describe the appropriate physical measurements taken before pulmonary function testing?*

    I. Ideal body weight should be used to calculate predicted values in obese patients
    II. Standing height with patient barefooted should be measured
    III. Arm span instead of height should be measured in cystic fibrosis patients
    IV. Age should be recorded as of the last birthday

    a. I and II only
    b. III and IV only
    c. I, II, and IV
    d. I, II, III, and IV

13. *A patient referred for evaluation of possible asthma has simple spirometry performed. There is no obstruction present, but the FVC and FEV1 are abnormal. What would be the next appropriate step?*

    a. Perform a bronchial challenge
    b. Evaluate for possible restrictive disorder
    c. Evaluate for COPD
    d. Perform a cardiopulmonary exercise evaluation

14. *Spirometry, lung volumes by N_2 washout, DL_{CO}, and blood gases are to be performed on a patient with COPD. The most appropriate order for these tests is:*

    a. Blood gases, N_2 washout, DL_{CO}, spirometry
    b. Spirometry, N_2 washout, DL_{CO}, blood gases
    c. Blood gases, spirometry, DL_{CO}, N_2 washout
    d. N_2 washout, blood gases, spirometry, DL_{CO}

SELECTED BIBLIOGRAPHY

General References

Crapo RO: Pulmonary function testing, *N Engl J Med* 331:25-30, 1994.

Hess D: History of pulmonary function testing, *Respir Care* 34:427-445, 1989.

Spriggs EA: The history of spirometry, *Br J Dis Chest* 72:165-180, 1978.

Indications for Pulmonary Function Testing

American Association for Respiratory Care: Clinical practice guidelines: assessing response to bronchodilator therapy at the point of care, *Respir Care* 40:1300-1307, 1995.

American Association for Respiratory Care: Clinical practice guidelines: body plethysmography: 2001 revision and update, *Respir Care* 46(5):506-513, 2001.

American Association for Respiratory Care: Clinical practice guidelines: single-breath carbon monoxide diffusing capacity: 1999 update, *Respir Care* 44(5):539-546, 1999.

American Association for Respiratory Care: Clinical practice guidelines: spirometry: 1996 update, *Respir Care* 41(7):629-636, 1996.

American Association for Respiratory Care: Clinical practice guidelines: static lung volumes: 2001 revision and update, *Respir Care* 46(5):531-539, 2001.

American Thoracic Society: Single-breath carbon monoxide diffusing capacity (transfer factor); recommendations for a standard technique—1995 update, *Am J Respir Crit Care Med* 152:2185-2198, 1995.

American Thoracic Society: Standardization of spirometry: 1994 update, *Am J Respir Crit Care Med* 152:1107-1136, 1995.

American Thoracic Society: Standards for the diagnosis and care of patients with chronic obstructive pulmonary disease, *Am J Respir Crit Care Med* 152:S77-S120, 1995.

British Thoracic Society and the Association of Respiratory Technicians and Physiologists: Guidelines for the measurement of respiratory function, *Respir Med* 88:165-194, 1994.

Pauwels RA, Buist SA, Calverley PMA, et al: GOLD Scientific Committee: Global strategy for the diagnosis, management, and prevention of chronic obstructive pulmonary disease, *Am J Resp Crit Care Med* 163:1256-1276, 2001.

Raffin TA: Indications for arterial blood gas analysis, *Ann Intern Med* 105:390-398, 1986.

Ries AL: Measurement of lung volumes, *Clin Chest Med* 10:177-185, 1989.

Wasserman K, Hansen JE, Sue DY, et al: *Principles of exercise testing and interpretation*, ed 3, Philadelphia, 1999, Lippincott, Williams & Wilkins.

Zibrak JD, O'Donnell CR, Marton K: Indications for pulmonary function testing, *Ann Intern Med* 112:763-771, 1990.

Patterns of Impaired Pulmonary Function

American Thoracic Society: Lung transplantation: report of the ATS workshop on lung transplantation, *Am Rev Respir Dis* 147:772-776, 1993.

Bergofsky EH: Respiratory failure in disorders of the thoracic cage, *Am Rev Respir Dis* 119:643-669, 1979.

Burrows B: Airways obstructive diseases: pathogenetic mechanisms and natural histories of the disorders, *Med Clin North Am* 74:547-559, 1990.

Davis PB, Drumm M, Konstan MW: Cystic fibrosis, *Am J Respir Crit Care Med* 154:1229-1256, 1996.

Kelly BJ, Luce JM: The diagnosis and management of neuromuscular diseases causing respiratory failure, *Chest* 99:1485-1491, 1991.

Mitchell RS, Petty TL, Schwartz MI: *Synopsis of clinical pulmonary disease*, St Louis, 1989, Mosby.

Murphy DMF, Hall DR, Peterson MR, et al: The effect of diffuse pulmonary fibrosis on lung mechanics, *Bull Eur Physiopathol Respir* 17:27-41, 1981.

National Asthma Education and Prevention Program: *Expert panel report 2: guidelines for the diagnosis and management of asthma*, Bethesda, Md, 1997, Department of Health and Human Services (NIH Publication No. 97-4051).

Newman KB, Mason UG, Schmaling KB: Clinical features of vocal cord dysfunction, *Am J Respir Crit Care Med* 152:1382-1386, 1995.

Putnam MT, Wise RA: Myasthenia gravis and upper airway obstruction, *Chest* 109:400-404, 1996.

Snider GL: Emphysema: the first two centuries and beyond, *Am Rev Respir Dis* 146:1615-1623, 1992.

Trulock EP: Lung transplantation, *Am J Resp Crit Care Med* 155:789-818, 1997.

Preliminaries to Patient Testing

American Thoracic Society: Standards for the diagnosis and care of patients with chronic obstructive pulmonary disease, *Am J Respir Crit Care Med* 152:S77-S120, 1995.

NCCLS: A quality system model for health care. NCCLS document GP26-A, Wayne, PA, 1997.

Social Security Administration: *Guide to pulmonary function studies under the Social Security Disability Program*, U.S. Department of Health and Human Services, SSA Pub. No. 64-055, 1999.

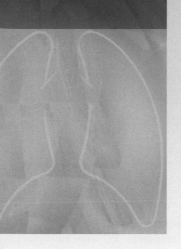

CHAPTER 2

SPIROMETRY AND RELATED TESTS

OBJECTIVES

After studying this chapter and reviewing the case studies, you should be able to do the following:

Entry-level

1. Determine whether spirometry is acceptable and reproducible
2. Identify airway obstruction using forced vital capacity (FVC) and forced expiratory volume (FEV_1)
3. Differentiate between obstruction and restriction as causes of reduced vital capacity
4. Distinguish between large and small airway obstruction by evaluating flow-volume curves
5. Determine whether there is a significant response to bronchodilators

Advanced

1. Select the appropriate FVC and FEV_1 for reporting from a series of spirometry maneuvers
2. Identify at least two pathophysiologic conditions in which maximal inspiratory or expiratory pressures might be abnormal
3. Recognize abnormal values for airway resistance and specific conductance
4. Describe the technique for measuring pulmonary compliance

This chapter begins with measurement of the vital capacity (VC) using simple spirometry. Then the most widely used pulmonary function tests, those based on the forced vital capacity (FVC) maneuver, are described. Special emphasis is placed on the performance of each test. Criteria for judging the acceptability and reproducibility of test data are provided. Volume-time and flow-volume curves are described as the two most common presentations of spirometric data. Other tests described include peak expiratory flow (PEF), maximal voluntary ventilation (MVV), maximal inspiratory pressure (MIP), maximal expiratory pressure (MEP), airway resistance (Raw) and its derivatives, and lung compliance (C_L). Bronchodilator studies to determine reversibility of airway obstruction are also presented. For each of these areas, interpretive strategies are suggested using questions that test interpreters might ask. Case studies and self-assessment questions are included at the end of the chapter.

Vital Capacity

■ DESCRIPTION

The vital capacity (VC) is the volume of gas measured from a slow, complete expiration after a *maximal inspiration,* without forced or rapid effort (Figure 2-1). Alternately, VC may be recorded as a maximal inspiration following a complete expiration. VC is normally recorded in either liters (L) or milliliters (ml), and reported at body temperature, pressure, and saturation (BTPS). VC is sometimes referred to as the slow vital capacity (SVC), distinguishing it from forced vital capacity (FVC). Inspiratory capacity (IC) and expiratory reserve volume (ERV) are subdivisions of the VC. IC is the largest volume of gas that can be inspired from the resting expiratory level (Figure 2-1). IC is sometimes further divided into the tidal volume (V_T) and inspiratory reserve volume (IRV). ERV is the largest volume of gas that can be expired from the resting end-expiratory level (Figure 2-1). Both the IC and ERV are recorded in liters or milliliters, corrected to body temperature, pressure, and saturation (BTPS).

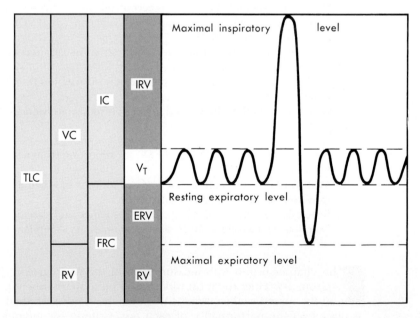

Figure 2-1 *Lung volumes and capacities.* Diagrammatic representation of lung volumes and capacities based on a simple spirogram. *TLC,* total lung capacity; *VC,* vital capacity; *RV,* residual volume; *FRC,* functional residual capacity; *IC,* inspiratory capacity; V_T, tidal volume; *IRV,* inspiratory reserve volume; *ERV,* expiratory reserve volume. Relationships between the subdivisions and relative sizes as compared with TLC are shown *(shaded areas).* Resting expiratory level is used as a starting point for FRC determinations because it remains more stable than other identifiable points during repeated measurements. (Modified from Comroe JH Jr, Forster RE, Dubois AB, et al: *The lung: clinical physiology and pulmonary function tests,* ed 2, St Louis, 1962, Mosby.)

SPIROMETRY 2-1   Criteria for Acceptability—Vital Capacity

1 End-expiratory volume varies by less than 100 ml for three preceding breaths.
2 Volume plateau observed at maximal inspiration and expiration.
3 Two acceptable VC maneuvers should be obtained; volumes within 200 ml.
4 VC should be within 200 ml of FVC value.

■ TECHNIQUE

VC is measured by having the patient inspire maximally and then exhale completely into a spirometer. (See Chapter 10 for a complete discussion of spirometers.) The patient is instructed to perform the maneuver slowly and completely. VC can also be measured from maximal expiration to maximal inspiration. The spirometer does not need to produce a graphic display if only VC is to be measured. However, if IC and ERV are to be determined (Figure 2-1), some means of recording volume change is required. The graphic display may be a computer screen or a recording device (see Chapter 10). A graphic display allows the technologist to determine that the test is performed correctly (Spirometry 2-1).

Obtaining a valid slow VC is important. The subdivisions of the VC (IC and ERV) are used in the calculation of residual volume (RV) and total lung capacity (TLC). An excessively large tidal volume or an irregular breathing pattern during the VC maneuver may alter ERV or IC. If either ERV or IC is erroneously recorded, other lung volumes may be incorrectly estimated (see Chapter 3).

IC is measured by having the patient breathe normally for three or four breaths and then inhale maximally. The volume inspired from the resting expiratory level is measured by the computer or from a spirogram. This is usually done as part of a slow VC maneuver. IC may also be calculated by subtracting the ERV from the VC. ERV is measured by having the patient breathe normally for three or four breaths and then exhale maximally. The change in volume from the end-expiratory level to the maximal expiratory level is the ERV. ERV may also be calculated by subtracting the IC from the VC. IC and ERV are usually measured from the same VC maneuver.

The accuracy of the IC and ERV measurements depends on the stability of the end-expiratory level. Three or more tidal breaths should be recorded before the VC maneuver is performed. The end-expiratory volume should vary by less than 100 ml. If the end-expiratory volume is not consistent, IC and/or ERV may be measured incorrectly (i.e., too large or too small). Even if the end-expiratory level is constant, the V_T usually increases when the patient breathes through a mouthpiece with a nose clip in place. This increase in V_T may change the IC or ERV, depending on the patient's breathing pattern. Erroneous estimates of ERV may affect the calculation of RV, as described in Chapter 3.

■ SIGNIFICANCE AND PATHOPHYSIOLOGY

Normal VC may vary as much as 20% above or below the predicted value in healthy individuals. VC also varies in individuals depending on body position or time of day. In adults, VC varies directly with height and inversely with age; tall patients have larger VCs than short patients. VC increases up to approximately age 20 and then decreases each year thereafter. It is usually smaller in women than in men, because of differences in body size. Recent evidence indicates that lung volumes may differ significantly according to ethnic origin. Interpretation of lung function should consider the factors of age, height, sex, and race (see Appendix B).

Decreased VC is often caused by loss of distensible lung tissue, as in lung cancer, pulmonary edema, pneumonias, atelectasis, pulmonary vascular congestion, or surgical removal of lung tissue. Other causes of decreased VC include tissue loss, space-occupying lesions, or changes in the lung tissue itself. Tissue loss may result from surgical removal, as in a *lobectomy.* In lung resection, the decrease in VC is roughly proportional to the tissue removed. A good example of a space-occupying lesion is a tumor, which directly displaces lung tissue. Fibrotic diseases such as silicosis often change the elastic properties of lung tissue, which usually results in loss of lung volume.

Normal values for lung function parameters are obtained by studying healthy subjects. The predicted or reference value for VC is computed using an equation like:

$$VC = xHeight - yAge - z$$

where:
x, y, and z are constants
Predicted values may be read from special diagrams called nomograms, but are usually calculated by computer. (See Appendix B.)

VC may also be reduced in obstructive lung diseases (e.g., emphysema). This occurs even when other lung compartments show increased volumes (see Chapter 3). As trapped gas volume increases, VC may become smaller. However, some patients have well-preserved VC even with increased air trapping.

Some decreases in VC are not caused by lung lesions. VC may be decreased from respiratory center depression or neuromuscular diseases. A low VC may also result from reduction of available thoracic space caused by pleural effusion, pneumothorax, hiatus hernia, or enlargement of the heart. Limited movement of the diaphragm may result from pregnancy, abdominal fluids, or tumors, causing decreased VC. Limitation of chest wall movement from scleroderma, kyphoscoliosis, or pain can also reduce the VC.

When the VC is reduced, additional pulmonary function measurements may be indicated. Forced expiratory maneuvers (see Forced Vital Capacity section) can reveal whether the reduced VC is caused by obstruction. Reduced VC without slowing of expiratory flow is a non-specific finding. Measurement of other lung volumes (see Chapter 3) may be indicated to determine whether a restrictive defect is present.

In adults, VC less than 80% of predicted or less than the 95% confidence limit (see Appendix B) may be considered abnormal. Interpretation of the measured VC in relation to the reference value should consider the clinical question to be answered (Spirometry 2-2). The clinical question is often revealed in the history and physical findings of the patient (see Chapter 1). The terms *mild, moderate,* and *severe* may be used to qualify the extent of reduction of the VC. Although these terms are relative, they should be based on a statistical comparison (i.e., confidence intervals) of the measured VC versus the predicted VC.

Artificially low estimates of the VC may result from poor patient effort. Similarly, inadequate patient instruction may affect performance of the test maneuver. These errors may be eliminated by applying appropriate criteria (Spirometry 2-1). Values for at least two maneuvers should be reproducible within 200 ml (see Chapter 11).

SPIROMETRY 2-2   Interpretive Strategies—Vital Capacity

1 Was the test performed acceptably? Is it reproducible?
2 Are reference values correct? Age? Sex? Height? Race?
3 Is VC less than predicted? If so, to what extent? Is it less than the lower limit of normal?
4 How does VC relate to the clinical question to be answered? Is VC correlated to the history and physical findings?
5 Are additional tests indicated? Lung volumes? FVC?

IC and ERV are approximately 75% and 25% of the VC, respectively. Changes in IC or ERV usually parallel increases or decreases in the VC. Increased V_T caused by exertion or acid-base disorders may reduce IRV or ERV. This occurs because end-inspiratory and end-expiratory levels (Figure 2-1) are altered. A similar pattern is commonly seen when patients breathe into a spirometer through a mouthpiece with a nose clips in place. Changes in IC or ERV are of minimal diagnostic significance when considered alone. Reduction of IC or ERV is consistent with restrictive defects. Some obese patients show a decrease in ERV, usually resulting in a low VC.

Forced Vital Capacity, Forced Expiratory Volume, and Forced Expiratory Flow

DESCRIPTION

Forced Vital Capacity (FVC) is the maximum volume of gas that can be expired when the patient exhales as forcefully and rapidly as possible after a maximal inspiration. This procedure is often referred to as the FVC maneuver. A similar maneuver, beginning at maximal expiration and inspiring as forcefully as possible, is called forced inspiratory vital capacity (FIVC). The FVC and FIVC maneuvers are often performed in sequence to provide a continuous flow-volume loop (see Flow-Volume Curve section).

The forced expiratory volume (FEV_T) is the volume of gas expired over a given time interval (T) from the beginning of the FVC maneuver. The time interval is stated as a subscript of FEV. The FEV_1 measurement is the most widely used. Other intervals in common use are $FEV_{0.5}$, FEV_3, and FEV_6. The FVC and FEV_T are both reported in liters corrected to BTPS. $FEV_{T\%}$ is the ratio of FEV_T to FVC expressed as a percentage, where T is the interval from the start of the FVC. The $FEV_{1\%}$ ($FEV_1/FVC \times 100$) is by far the most widely used of the various $FEV_{T\%}$ parameters. VC (slow vital capacity) may be used in place of FVC if the VC is significantly larger. Because a low value for the ratio of FEV_1 to FVC is used to detect obstruction, using the largest value obtained for vital capacity (either VC or FVC) for the denominator may be helpful.

Flows over specific intervals or at specific points in the FVC are expressed as FEF_X. The subscript X describes the point or interval in relation to the FVC maneuver. The $FEF_{25\%-75\%}$ is the average flow during the middle half (from the 25% to 75% points) of an FVC maneuver. FEF_X values are usually recorded in liters per second, BTPS. $FEF_{25\%-75\%}$ was formerly designated the maximum midexpiratory flow rate (MMFR). Other measures of average flow include the $FEF_{200-1200}$ (200 to 1200 ml portion of the FVC), and the $FEF_{75\%-85\%}$. FEF_X is also used to denote instantaneous flow at specific points in the FVC maneuver. Commonly reported flows are the $FEF_{25\%}$, $FEF_{50\%}$, and $FEF_{75\%}$. The subscript refers to the percentage of FVC that has been expired.

TECHNIQUE

FVC is measured by having the patient, after inspiring maximally, expire as forcefully and rapidly as possible into a spirometer (see Chapter 11). The patient should inspire completely. The inhalation should be rapid but not forced. There should be only a brief pause at maximal inspiration; a prolonged pause (4 to 6 seconds) may decrease flow during the subsequent expiration.

The volume expired may be read directly from a volume-time recording (Figure 2-2). This method is used by some small portable spirometers. More commonly, the maneuver is displayed on a computer monitor or LCD (liquid crystal display) screen. The computer analyzes the signal from the spirometer, then calculates and displays the FVC. A spirometer that produces a graphical tracing (either volume-time or flow-volume) is essential for clinical laboratory purposes to allow visual inspection of the maneuver (Figure 2-3). Devices providing only numerical data may be helpful for simple screening. Whether used for diagnosis or monitoring, all spirometers should meet the criteria proposed by the American Thoracic Society (see Chapter 11). The FVC maneuver depends on patient effort. Not all patients may be able to perform it acceptably (Spirometry 2-3).

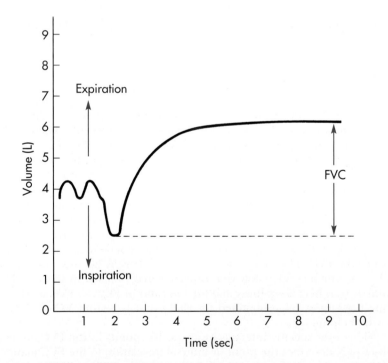

Figure 2-2 *Forced vital capacity (FVC).* Typical spirogram plotting volume against time as patient exhales forcefully. In this tracing, expiration causes an upward deflection; in some systems the tracing is inverted. The patient inspires to the maximal inspiratory level *(dashed line)* at which point lung volume is close to TLC. The patient then expires as forcefully and rapidly as possible to the maximal expiratory level, at which point the lungs contain only the RV (see text).

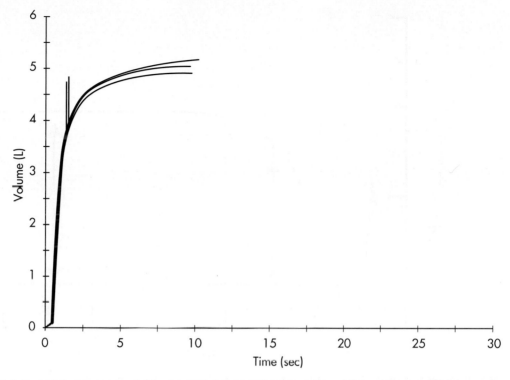

Figure 2-3 *Volume-time tracings of FVC maneuvers from a healthy patient.* Tracings show the forced expiratory portion of the FVC maneuver. Three FVC efforts are superimposed showing acceptable reproducibility of the maneuvers (see text). Tick marks indicate FEV_1.

SPIROMETRY 2-3 Criteria for Acceptability—FVC Maneuver

1 Maximal effort; no cough or glottic closure during the first second; no leaks or obstruction of the mouthpiece
2 Good start-of-test; back-extrapolated volume less than 5% of FVC or 150 ml
3 Tracing shows 6 seconds of exhalation or an obvious plateau; no early termination or cutoff; or subject cannot or should not continue to exhale
4 Three acceptable spirograms obtained; two largest FVC values within 200 ml; two largest FEV_1 values within 200 ml

From American Thoracic Society, 1994.

FEV_1 (and other FEV_T values) may be measured by timing the FVC maneuver over the described intervals. Historically this was done by recording the FVC spirogram on graph paper moving at a fixed speed. The FEV for any interval could then be read from the graph as shown in Figure 2-4. Most modern spirometers time the FVC maneuver using a computer. The computer then calculates and displays the FEV_1 or other FEV_T intervals. The spirometer should

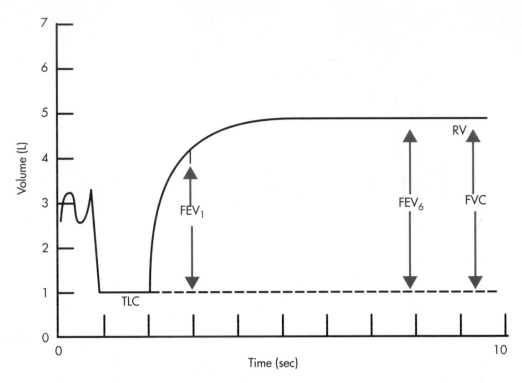

Figure 2–4 *Determination of FEV$_T$ values from an FVC maneuver.* Various FEV$_T$ values can be measured from the volume-time display of an FVC effort. FEV at intervals of 1 and 6 seconds, along with the FVC, are shown *(arrows)*. FEV$_1$ is the most commonly used index of airflow. FEV$_6$ is sometimes used as a surrogate for FVC in patients with airway obstruction. Precise timing and acceptable start-of-test are required to determine FEV$_T$ values accurately (Spirometry 2-3).

provide a volume-time display of each maneuver (Figure 2-5). A graphic representation allows monitoring of patient effort at the beginning of the test. Accurate measurement of FEV$_1$ (and other FEV$_T$ intervals) depends on determination of the *start-of-test* (Figure 2-6). Computerized spirometers detect the start-of-test as a change in flow or volume above a certain threshold. The computer then stores volume and flow data points in memory and calculates the FEV$_1$.

Some spirometers allow tidal breathing and record both inspiratory and expiratory flows, whereas others record forced expiratory flow only. If only the expiratory spirogram is presented, assessing the start-of-test may be difficult. Inaccurate FEV$_T$ values may result if the patient begins the FVC maneuver slowly, coughs, hesitates, or leaks at the mouthpiece. Most computerized spirometers correct for a slow start-of-test by *back-extrapolation* (Figure 2-6). Visualization of the volume-time spirogram is the best means of identifying poor initial effort. Some portable spirometers report FEV$_1$ without a spirogram. Such measurements should be used with caution because it may be difficult to determine whether the maneuver was performed acceptably.

The ratio of the FEV$_1$ to FVC is expressed as follows:

$$FEV_{1\%} = \frac{FEV_1}{FVC} \times 100$$

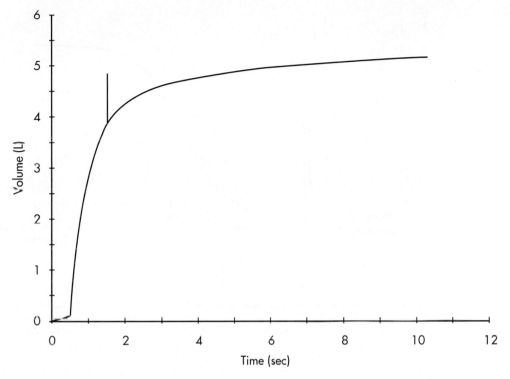

Figure 2-5 *Volume-time tracing from a healthy patient.* The graph shows an FVC tracing from a normal adult. The computer superimposes a tick mark on the curve to assist in identification of FEV_1.

$FEV_{1\%}$ is also commonly written as FEV_1/FVC. Both ratios are expressed as percentages. FEV_1 and FVC should be the maximal values obtained from at least three acceptable FVC maneuvers. The FEV_1/FVC ratio based on these values may be different from the ratio obtained from any single maneuver. If both VC and FVC maneuvers have been performed, it is preferable to use the largest VC in the calculation. Some computerized spirometers calculate only the ratio obtained from FVC maneuvers.

The $FEF_{25\%-75\%}$ is measured from an FVC maneuver. The time required for the patient to expire the middle 50% of the FVC is divided into 50% of the FVC. A computerized measurement of the $FEF_{25\%-75\%}$ requires storage of flow and volume data points for the entire maneuver. Calculation of the average flow over the middle portion of the exhalation is simply 50% of the volume expired divided by the time required to get from the 25% point to the 75% point. To calculate the $FEF_{25\%-75\%}$ manually, a volume-time spirogram is used. The points at which 25% and 75% of the vital capacity have been expired are marked on the curve (Figure 2-7). A straight line connecting these points can be extended to intersect two time-lines 1 second apart. The flow (in liters per second) can then be read directly as the vertical distance between the points of intersection. Instantaneous flows, such as the $FEF_{50\%}$ or $FEF_{75\%}$, cannot be read directly from a volume time display, but can be measured using a flow-volume curve (see Flow-Volume Curve section).

The $FEF_{25\%-75\%}$ depends on the FVC. Large $FEF_{25\%-75\%}$ values may be derived from maneuvers that produce small FVC measurements because the "middle half" of the volume is actually gas expired at the beginning of expiration. This effect may be particularly evident if

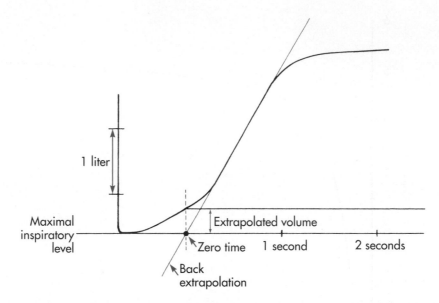

Figure 2-6 *Back-extrapolation of a volume-time spirogram.* Back-extrapolation is a method for correcting measurements made from a spirogram that does not show a sharp deflection from the maximal inspiratory level. This occurs when a patient does not begin forced exhalation rapidly enough or hesitates at the start-of-test. A straight line drawn through the steepest part of a volume-time tracing is extended to cross the volume baseline (maximum inspiration). The point of intersection is the back-extrapolated *time zero.* Timed volumes, such as FEV_1, are measured from this point rather than from the initial deflection from the baseline or from the point of maximal flow. The perpendicular distance from maximal inspiration to the volume-time tracing at time zero defines the *back-extrapolated volume.* To accurately determine FEV_1, the back-extrapolated volume should be less than 5% of the FVC or less than 150 ml, whichever is greater. FVC efforts with larger extrapolated volumes should be considered unacceptable. These measurements are commonly performed by computer.

the patient terminates the FVC maneuver before exhaling completely. When the $FEF_{25\%-75\%}$ is used for assessing the response to bronchodilator or bronchial challenge, the effect of changes in the absolute lung volumes should be considered. Measuring the $FEF_{25\%-75\%}$ at the same lung volumes in the comparison tests is called the isovolume technique. Isovolume corrections are usually applied when the FVC changes by more than 10% (indicating a change in TLC or RV). This technique requires that lung volumes (see Chapter 3) be measured in conjunction with flows. The isovolume technique may also be used with other flow measurements that are dependent on FVC.

The largest $FEF_{25\%-75\%}$ is not necessarily the value reported. The $FEF_{25\%-75\%}$ is recorded from the maneuver with the largest sum of FVC and FEV_1. Flows must be corrected to BTPS.

Criteria used to judge the acceptability of test results from the FVC maneuver include the following:

1. The volume-time tracing should show maximal effort with a smooth curve. There should be no coughing or hesitation during the first second. The tracing should show at least 6 seconds of forced effort. An obvious plateau with no volume change (30 ml or less) for at least 1 second should be achieved. Children, adolescents, and some restricted patients may plateau in less than 6 seconds. Patients with severe obstruction may continue

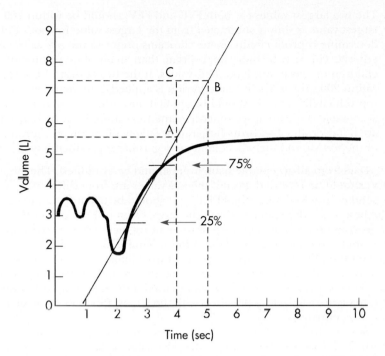

Figure 2-7 *FEF*$_{25\%-75\%}$. Short horizontal lines on an FVC spirogram show points at which 25% and 75% of the FVC have been expired; these points may be determined by multiplying the FVC by 0.25 and 0.75, respectively. The slope of the line connecting the 25% and 75% points can be determined by dividing one half of the FVC by the time interval between the points. This slope is the average flow over the middle half of the FVC maneuver. Alternatively, a line connecting these points may be drawn to intersect two timelines 1 second apart (points A and B). The flow in liters per second can be read as the vertical distance between the points of intersection (AC)—in this case, approximately 2 L/sec. These measurements are usually calculated by computer.

exhalation well past 15 seconds; therefore 6 seconds is simply a minimum. In severe obstruction, very low flows may be observed at the end of expiration. Continuation of the maneuver in these patients will not appreciably change the test results. The FVC maneuver may be stopped if the patient cannot continue for clinical reasons such as excessive coughing or dizziness. Multiple prolonged (longer than 6 seconds) exhalations are seldom necessary.

2. The start-of-test should be abrupt and unhesitating. Each maneuver should have the back-extrapolated volume calculated. FEV$_1$ and all other flows must be measured after back-extrapolation (Figure 2-6). If the volume of back-extrapolation is greater than 5% of the FVC or 150 ml (whichever is greater), the maneuver is unacceptable and should be repeated. The patient should be shown the correct technique for performing the maneuver. Demonstration by the technologist is often helpful.

3. A minimum of three acceptable efforts should be obtained. The test may be repeated any number of times. If reproducible values cannot be obtained after eight attempts, testing may be discontinued. The only criterion for eliminating a test completely is failure to obtain two acceptable maneuvers after at least eight attempts.

4. The two largest values for both FVC and FEV_1 should be within 200 ml. The second largest value is simply subtracted from the largest value for both FVC and FEV_1 to determine reproducibility. Some clinicians prefer to use 5% as the reproducibility criteria. This may be more appropriate than an absolute volume of 200 ml, particularly in children or those with large FVC values. If the two largest FVC or FEV_1 values are not within 200 ml (or 5%, if that criterion is applied), the maneuver should be repeated. The reproducibility criteria should be applied only after the maneuver has been judged acceptable. Individual spirometric maneuvers should not be rejected solely because they are not reproducible. Bronchospasm or fatigue often affects reproducibility. Interpretation of the test should include comments regarding reproducibility or lack of it.

Data from all acceptable maneuvers should be examined. The largest FVC and the largest FEV_1 should be reported, even if the two values are from different test maneuvers. Flows that depend on the FVC (e.g., the $FEF_{25\%-75\%}$) should be taken from the single best test maneuver. The best test is the maneuver with the largest sum of FVC and FEV_1 (Table 2-1).

A common problem may occur when using these criteria to produce a spirometry report. If a single volume-time or flow-volume tracing is included in the final report, it may not contain the FVC or FEV_1 that appears in the tabular data. It is advisable to maintain recordings, or raw data, for all acceptable maneuvers. Other methods of selecting the best test have been suggested and are sometimes used. PEF may be used to assess patient effort for an FVC maneuver. Selecting the effort with the largest PEF may cause errors if FVC and FEV_1 are not also evaluated.

Spirometry may be performed in either the sitting or standing position for adults and children. There is some evidence that FEV_1 may be larger in the standing position in adults and in children younger than 12 years of age. The position used for testing should be indicated on the final report. The use of nose clips is recommended for spirometric measurements that require rebreathing, even if just for a few breaths. Spirometers that record only expiratory flow may require the patient to place the mouthpiece into the mouth after maximal inspiration. If such is the case, nose clips are usually unnecessary. Care should be taken, however, that the patient places the mouthpiece into the mouth before beginning a forced expiration. Failure to do so may result in an undetectable loss of volume. It may be impossible to calculate the volume of back-extrapolation from a tracing that displays only expiratory flow. Spirometers that use mechanical recorders should have pen or paper moving at recording speed when the forced expiration begins. Recorders that trigger pen or paper

TABLE 2-1 Comparison of Spirometry Efforts

Test	Trial 1	Trial 2	Trial 3	Best Test
FVC (L)	5.20	5.30	5.35*	5.35
FEV_1 (L)	4.41*	4.35	4.36*	4.41
FEV_1/FVC (%)	85	82	82	82
$FEF_{25\%-75\%}$ (L/sec)	3.87	3.92	3.94	3.94
$FEF_{50\%}$ (L/sec)	3.99	3.95	3.41	3.41
$FEF_{25\%}$ (L/sec)	1.97	1.95	1.89	1.89
PEF (L/sec)	8.39	9.44	9.89	9.89

*These values are keys to selecting the best test results. The FEV_1 is taken from trial 1, even though the largest sum of FVC and FEV_1 occurs in trial 3. All FVC-dependent flows (average and instantaneous flows) come from trial 3. It should be noted that the $FEV_{1\%}$ (FEV_1/FVC) is calculated from the FEV_1 of trial 1 and the FVC of trial 3. The maximal expiratory flow-volume curve, if reported, would be the curve from trial 3 as well.

movement with exhalation may be unable to accurately record the start-of-test. Such spirometers often underestimate the FEV_1. Most spirometers use computer-generated graphics, avoiding the problems associated with mechanical recorders.

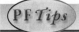

The largest FVC and FEV_1 are reported, even if they come from different efforts, as long as the efforts are acceptable. Peak flow (PEF) is always the largest value from an acceptable effort. All the other flows ($FEF_{27-75\%}$ etc.) are taken from the acceptable effort with the largest sum of FVC and FEV_1.

■ SIGNIFICANCE AND PATHOPHYSIOLOGY

Forced Vital Capacity

See Spirometry 2-4 for interpretive strategies. FVC equals VC in healthy individuals. In patients without obstruction, FVC and VC should be within 200 ml of each other. FVC and VC may differ if the patient's effort is variable or severe airway obstruction is present. FVC is often lower than VC in patients with obstructive diseases if forced expiration causes bronchiolar collapse. This pattern is seen in emphysema because of loss of support for the small airways (less than 2 mm in diameter). Large pressure gradients across the walls of the airways during forced expiration collapse the terminal portions of the airways. Gas is trapped in the alveoli and cannot be expired. This causes the FVC to appear smaller than the VC. The FVC can appear larger than the VC if the patient exerts greater effort on the forced maneuver.

FVC can be reduced by mucus plugging and bronchiolar narrowing, as is common in chronic bronchitis, chronic or acute asthma, bronchiectasis, and cystic fibrosis. Reduced FVC is also present in patients whose trachea or mainstem bronchi are obstructed. Tumors or diseases affecting the patency of the large airways produce this result.

SPIROMETRY 2-4   Interpretive Strategies—FVC Maneuver

1. Were at least three acceptable spirograms obtained? Are FVC and FEV_1 reproducible (within 200 ml)?
2. Are reference values appropriate? Age? Sex? Height? Race?
3. Is $FEV_{1\%}$ less than predicted? If so, obstruction is present.
   a. Is FVC also reduced? If so, is it caused by obstruction or restriction?
   b. If FVC is less than 80%, lung volumes may be indicated.
   c. Is the obstruction reversible? Bronchodilators may be indicated.
4. Is $FEV_{1\%}$ equal to or greater than expected?
   a. Are FVC and FEV_1 both reduced proportionately? If so, restriction may be present; lung volumes may be indicated.
   b. Are FVC and FEV_1 within normal limits? If so, spirometry is likely normal.
5. Is $FEF_{25\%-75\%}$ less than 65% of predicted? Is $FEV_{1\%}$ or FEV_1 borderline normal? If so, airway obstruction may be present.
6. Are the spirometric findings consistent with the patient history and physical findings? Is bronchial challenge indicated to reveal obstruction?

Some obstructed patients have a relatively normal FVC in relation to their predicted values. However, the time required to expire their FVC (forced expiratory time or FET) is usually prolonged. Healthy adults can expire their FVC within 4 to 6 seconds. Normal children and adolescents may exhale their FVC in less than 4 seconds. Patients with severe obstruction (e.g., those with emphysema) may require 20 seconds or more to exhale completely (Figure 2-8). Accurate measurement of FVC in such individuals may be limited by how long the spirometer can collect exhaled volume. Some spirometers allow only 15 seconds of volume recording. This is usually long enough to diagnose airway obstruction. However, the FVC and $FEV_{1\%}$ may be inaccurate if the patient continues to exhale for a longer time. The American Thoracic Society recommends that spirometers measure FVC for at least 15 seconds (see Chapter 11). An alternative to measuring FVC in severely obstructed patients is to use FEV_6. Since normal patients can exhale their FVC in 6 seconds, substituting FEV_6 for FVC allows the FEV_1/FEV_6 to be used as an index of obstruction. Using FEV_6 in place of FVC eliminates the necessity of having the patient try to exhale for a long interval. Predicted values for FEV_6 and FEV_1/FEV_6 may be calculated using coefficients in Appendix B.

Decreased FVC is also a common feature of restrictive diseases (Figure 2-9). Any disease that affects the bellows action of the chest or distensibility of lung tissue itself tends to reduce FVC. An FVC less than predicted may result from increased scar tissue as in pulmonary fibrosis. Fibrotic changes often result from inhalation of dust or other toxins that directly damage lung tissue. Fibrosis may also result from the toxic effects of drugs or radiation used in treating lung

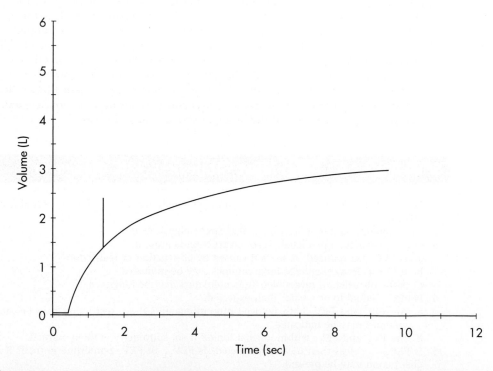

Figure 2-8 *FVC tracing from a patient with severe airway obstruction.* A tick mark notes the point at which the patient exhaled his FEV_1. A significant volume is exhaled after the first second, and the tracing does not show an obvious plateau.

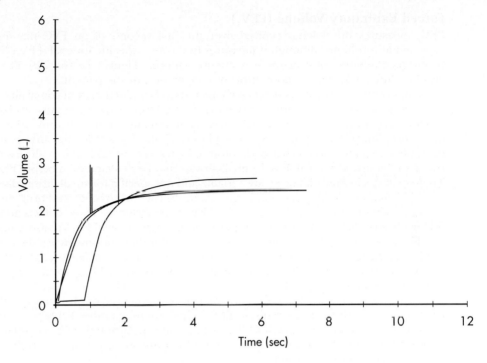

Figure 2-9 *Three FVC maneuvers from a patient with moderately severe restriction.* All three maneuvers show relatively normal flows; most of the FVC is expired in the first second. However, the FVC is much lower than the expected value of 3.5 L for this patient.

cancer. Congestion of pulmonary blood vessels, as in pneumonia, pulmonary hypertension, or pulmonary edema, can reduce FVC. Space-occupying lesions (e.g., tumors or pleural effusions) reduce FVC by compressing surrounding lung tissue. Neuromuscular disorders, (e.g., myasthenia gravis) or chest deformities (e.g., scoliosis) limit chest wall movement. Obesity and pregnancy are common causes of reduced FVC because they interfere with movement of the diaphragm and excursion of the chest wall.

Reduced FVC (or VC) is a nonspecific finding. Values lower than 80% of predicted or less than the 95% confidence limit are considered abnormal (see Appendix B). Low FVC may be caused by either obstruction or restriction. Interpretation of the FVC in obstructive diseases requires correlation with flows. An FVC that is significantly lower than VC suggests airway collapse. In restrictive patterns, low FVC may indicate the need to assess other lung volumes, particularly total lung capacity (see Chapter 3). Interpretation of FVC values close to the lower limit of normal depends on the clinical question to be answered. An FVC of 80% of predicted would be interpreted differently in a healthy patient with no symptoms than in a patient with a history of cough or wheezing. An FVC much lower than expected is often accompanied by the complaint of exertional dyspnea.

A low value for FVC may also occur if the patient's effort is suboptimal. Patients who stop exhaling before achieving an obvious plateau (on a volume-time display) typically have an underestimated FVC. These patients should be encouraged to exhale longer and continue testing until three acceptable maneuvers are obtained. Premature termination of the FVC effort may cause the $FEV_{1\%}$ to be overestimated, masking the presence of obstruction.

Forced Expiratory Volume (FEV_1)

FEV_1 measures the volume expired over the first second of an FVC maneuver. FEV_1 is reported as a volume, although it measures flow over a specific interval. FEV_1, like FVC, may be reduced in either obstructive or restrictive patterns (Figures 2-8 and 2-9). FEV_1 values may also be reduced because of poor effort or cooperation by the patient.

An obstructive ventilatory defect is characterized by reduction of maximal airflow at all lung volumes. Flow is limited by airway narrowing during forced expiration. Airway obstruction may be caused by mucus secretion, bronchospasm, and inflammation such as in asthma or bronchitis. Airflow limitation may also result from loss of elastic support for the airways themselves, as in emphysema. The earliest changes in obstructive patterns occur in the small airways (i.e., those less than 2 mm). Abnormal flows in small airways may be detected even before FEV_1 decreases. These changes in flows, however, are variable and not specific for small airway disease.

FEV_1 may also be decreased in large airway obstruction (trachea and bronchi). Tumors or foreign bodies that limit airflow cause the FEV_1 to be reduced. These defects are easily identified by flow reductions across the entire forced expiration (see Flow-Volume Curve section).

FEV_1 and FEV_1/FVC are the most standardized indices of obstructive disease. Reduction of FEV_1 along with a reduced FEV_1/FVC ratio defines an obstructive impairment. The severity of obstructive disease may be gauged by the extent to which FEV_1 is reduced. The ability to work and function in daily life is related to FEV_1 and FVC. *Mortality* (likelihood of dying) caused by respiratory disease is similarly related to the degree of obstruction as measured by FEV_1. Patients with markedly reduced FEV_1 values are much more likely to die from chronic obstructive pulmonary disease (COPD) or lung cancer. Although FEV_1 correlates with prognosis and severity of symptoms in obstructive lung disease, outcomes for individual patients cannot be accurately predicted.

Restrictive processes such as fibrosis, edema, space-occupying lesions, neuromuscular disorders, obesity, and chest wall deformities may all cause FEV_1 to be decreased. Reduction in FEV_1 occurs in much the same way as reduction in FVC. Unlike the pattern seen in obstructive disease in which FVC is preserved and FEV_1 reduced, in restriction FVC and FEV_1 values are proportionately decreased. Some patients with moderate or severe restriction have an FEV_1 nearly equal to the FVC. The entire FVC, because it is reduced, is exhaled in the first second. To distinguish between obstructive and restrictive causes of reduced FEV_1 values, the FEV_1/FVC ratio ($FEV_{1\%}$) and other flow measurements are useful. Further definition of obstruction versus restriction may require measurement of lung volumes (e.g., functional residual capacity or FRC, and TLC).

FEV_1 is the most widely used spirometric parameter, particularly for assessment of airway obstruction. FEV_1 is used in conjunction with FVC for simple screening, assessment of response to bronchodilators, inhalation challenge studies, and detection of exercise-induced bronchospasm (see Chapters 7 and 9).

Forced Expiratory Volume Ratio ($FEV_{T\%}$)

Normal $FEV_{T\%}$ ratios for healthy adults are as follows:
$FEV_{0.5\%} = 50\%\text{-}60\%$
$FEV_{1\%} = 75\%\text{-}85\%$
$FEV_{2\%} = 90\%\text{-}95\%$
$FEV_{3\%} = 95\%\text{-}98\%$
$FEV_{6\%} = 98\%\text{-}100\%$

These ratios may be derived by dividing predicted FEV_T by predicted FVC. Some studies of normal patients derive equations for the ratio itself. The FEV_1/FVC ratio decreases with increasing age, presumably because of changes in the elastic properties of the lung. Older healthy adults may have FEV_1/FVC ratios in the 65% to 70% range.

Patients with unobstructed airflow can usually exhale their entire FVC within 4 seconds. Conversely, patients with obstructive disease have reduced $FEV_{T\%}$ for each interval (i.e., 1 second, 2 seconds, etc.). The FEV_1/FVC ratio is the most important measurement for distinguishing an obstructive impairment. A decreased FEV_1/FVC ratio is the hallmark of obstructive disease. Because the FEV_1/FVC is a ratio, mild or moderate obstructive disease can be identified without reference to absolute predicted values. In young adults, if the ratio is less than 70%, some degree of obstruction is likely present. In older patients, the normal ratio is slightly lower (see Appendix B for predicted values). The $FEV_{1\%}$ may be as low as 30% in severe obstructive disease.

Diagnosis of an obstructive pattern based on spirometry should focus on three primary variables: FVC, FEV_1, and FEV_1/FVC. Measurements such as $FEF_{25\%-75\%}$ should be considered only after the presence and severity of obstruction has been determined using the primary variables. If the FEV_1/FVC is borderline abnormal, additional flow measurements may confirm the presence of an obstructive pattern. Care should be taken when interpreting the FEV_1/FVC ratio in patients who have FVC and FEV_1 values greater than predicted. The FEV_1/FVC ratio may appear to indicate an obstructive pattern because of the variability of the greater than normal FVC and FEV_1 values.

PF *Tips*

Look at the FEV_1/FVC ratio first if obstruction is suspected. If the FEV_1/FVC ratio is lower than expected, obstruction is present. If the ratio is normal or elevated, check the percent predicted for FVC and FEV_1. If FVC and FEV_1 are both reduced compared with the expected values, and FEV_1/FVC is normal or high, restriction may be present.

Patients who have restrictive disease, (e.g., pulmonary fibrosis) often have normal or increased $FEV_{T\%}$ values. Because airflow may be minimally affected in restrictive diseases, FEV_1 and FVC are usually reduced in equal proportion. If the restriction is severe, FEV_1 may approach the FVC value. As a result, $FEV_{1\%}$ appears to be higher than normal. The FEV_1/FVC ratio may be 100% if the FVC is severely reduced. The presence of a restrictive disorder may be suggested by a reduced FVC and a normal or increased FEV_1/FVC ratio. Further studies (e.g., measurement of TLC) should be used to confirm the diagnosis of restriction.

Forced Expiratory Flow 25%-75%

$FEF_{25\%-75\%}$ is measured from a segment of the FVC that includes flow from medium and small airways. Typical values for healthy young adults average 4 to 5 L/sec. These values decrease with age. $FEF_{25\%-75\%}$ is quite variable even in normal patients, with one standard deviation (**SD**) equal to approximately 1 L/sec. Values as low as 50% of the predicted may be statistically within normal limits. This variability requires guarded interpretation of the $FEF_{25\%-75\%}$.

The $FEF_{25\%-75\%}$ is indicative of the status of the medium to small airways. Decreased flows are common in the early stages of obstructive disease. Abnormalities in these measurements, however, are not specific for small airways disease. Although $FEF_{25\%-75\%}$ may suggest changes in the small airways, it should not be used to diagnose small airways disease in individual patients. In the presence of a borderline value for FEV_1/FVC, a low $FEF_{25\%-75\%}$ may help confirm airway obstruction. When FEV_1 and FEV_1/FVC are within normal limits, $FEF_{25\%-75\%}$ should not be graded as to severity. Assessment of $FEF_{25\%-75\%}$ after bronchodilator must consider changes in FVC as well. If FVC increases markedly, $FEF_{25\%-75\%}$ may actually decrease. Isovolume correction (as described previously) can be used to compare $FEF_{25\%-75\%}$ before and after bronchodilator therapy. The inherent variability of $FEF_{25\%-75\%}$ and its dependence on FVC make it less useful than the FEV_1 for assessing bronchodilator response.

Reduced $FEF_{25\%-75\%}$ values are sometimes seen in cases of moderate or severe restrictive patterns. This is assumed to be caused by a decrease in the cross-sectional area of the small airways. $FEF_{25\%-75\%}$ depends somewhat on patient effort because it depends on the FVC exhaled. Patients who perform the FVC maneuver inadequately often show widely varying midexpiratory flow rates.

Validity of FVC maneuvers depends largely on patient effort and cooperation. Equally important is the instruction and coaching supplied by the technologist. Many patients need several attempts before performing the maneuver acceptably. Demonstration of proper technique by the technologist helps the patient give maximal effort. Placement of the mouthpiece between the teeth and lips, maximal inspiration, a slight pause, and maximal expiration should all be demonstrated. Emphasis should be placed on the initial burst of air and on continuing expiration for at least 6 seconds. Acceptability of each FVC maneuver should be evaluated according to specific criteria (see Spirometry 2-3). The final report should include comments on the quality of the data obtained (see Chapter 11). These comments may be provided by the technologist, physician, or both.

Validity of the FEV_1 also depends on cooperation and effort. Adequate instruction and demonstration of the maneuver by the technologist is essential. Reproducibility of FEV_1 should be within 200 ml for the two best of at least three acceptable maneuvers. Accurate measurement of FEV_1 requires an acceptable spirometer (see Chapter 11), preferably one that allows inspection of the volume-time curve and back-extrapolation.

Validity of the $FEV_{1\%}$ also depends on patient effort and cooperation. Because the values used to derive the ratio may be taken from separate maneuvers, both FEV_1 and FVC should be reproducible. Poor effort on an FVC test may result in an overestimate of $FEV_{T\%}$. If the patient stops prematurely, the FVC (i.e., denominator of the ratio) will appear smaller than it actually is. The $FEV_{1\%}$ will then appear larger than it actually is. Some clinicians prefer to use the VC to calculate the $FEV_{1\%}$. This may be useful if the VC is significantly larger than FVC because of airway compression.

Patients who have moderate or severe obstruction may require longer than 10 seconds to completely exhale. Although continuing to exhale increases measured FVC, the diagnosis of obstruction can be made with less than complete expiration. The FEV_6 may be a useful surrogate measurement in obstructed patients who have difficulty with prolonged exhalation. In some cases, prolonged effort may be difficult for the patient. The large transpulmonary pressure generated by a forced expiratory maneuver often reduces cardiac output. Patients may complain of dizziness, seeing "spots," ringing in the ears, or numbness of extremities. A patient may occasionally faint as a result of decreased cerebral blood flow. This complication may be serious if it causes the patient to fall from a standing or sitting position.

Flow–Volume Curve

■ DESCRIPTION

The FVC graphs the flow generated during an FVC maneuver against volume change. The FVC may be followed by an FIVC maneuver, plotted similarly. Flow is usually recorded in liters per second, and the volume is recorded in liters, BTPS. The maximal expiratory flow-volume (MEFV) curve shows flow as the patient exhales from maximal inspiration (TLC) to maximal expiration (RV). The MIFV displays inspiratory flow plotted from RV to TLC. When MEFV and MIFV curves are plotted together, the resulting figure is called a flow-volume (F-V) loop (Figure 2-10).

TECHNIQUE

The patient performs an FVC maneuver, inspiring fully and then exhaling as rapidly as possible. To complete the loop, the patient inspires as rapidly as possible from the maximal expiratory level back to maximal inspiration. Volume is plotted on the horizontal X-axis, and flow is plotted on the vertical Y-axis. The F-V loop is usually displayed on a computer screen. It can also be printed or plotted. Expiratory flow is plotted upward. Expired volume is usually plotted from left to right. Airflow should be recorded at 2 L/sec/unit distance on the Y-axis. Volume should be recorded at 1 L/unit distance on the volume axis. Scale factors should be at least 5 mm/L/sec for flow and 10 mm/L for volume. These factors are required so that manual measurements can be made from a printed copy of the maneuver.

FVC, as well as PEF and peak inspiratory flow (PIF), can be read directly from the F-V loop. Instantaneous flow at any lung volume can be measured directly from the F-V loop. Maximal flow at 75%, 50%, and 25% of the FVC are commonly reported as the $\dot{V}_{max\ 75}$, $\dot{V}_{max\ 50}$, and $\dot{V}_{max\ 25}$. The subscript in these terms refers to the portion of the FVC remaining. The same flows are also reported as the $FEF_{25\%}$, $FEF_{50\%}$, and $FEF_{75\%}$ with the subscripts referring to the percentage of FVC exhaled. Most computerized spirometers superimpose timing marks (ticks) on the MEFV curve (Figure 2-11). These marks allow FEV_1 (or other FEV_T) values to be read from the F-V loop.

F-V loop data, stored in computer memory, can be easily manipulated. Multiple loops can be compared by superimposing them with contrasting colors. Bronchodilator or inhalation challenge F-V loops can be presented in a similar manner. A predicted MEFV curve can be plotted using points for PEF and maximal flows at 75%, 50%, and 25% of the FVC. A patient's flow-volume curve can then be superimposed directly over the expected values (Figure 2-11). Superimposing multiple FVC maneuvers as F-V loops can be used to assess reproducibility of the patient's effort (Figure 2-11). Positioning loops side by side or superimposing can also help detect decreasing flows with repeated efforts. This pattern may be seen because FVC maneuvers can induce bronchospasm. Storing tests in the order performed is recommended. This allows review of the test session and detection of bronchospasm or fatigue.

Reproducible MEFV curves, particularly the PEF, are good indicators of adequate patient effort (Spirometry 2-5). Assessing the start-of-test and determining whether exhalation lasted at least 6 seconds may be difficult if only the F-V loop is displayed. Simultaneous display of flow-volume and volume-time curves is useful (Figure 2-12). Although computerized systems calculate back-extrapolated volume, a volume-time tracing may be necessary to perform back-extrapolation manually (Figure 2-6).

SIGNIFICANCE AND PATHOPHYSIOLOGY

See Spirometry 2-6 for interpretive strategies. Maximal flow at any lung volume during forced expiration or forced inspiration can be easily measured from the F-V loop (Figure 2-13). Significant decreases in flow or volume are easily detected from a single graphic display. Many clinicians prefer to include the F-V loop or MEFV curve as part of the patient's medical record.

The shape of an MEFV curve from approximately 75% of FVC to maximal expiration is largely independent of patient effort. Flow over this segment is determined by two properties of the lung: elastic recoil and flow resistance. The lung is stretched by maximal inspiration.

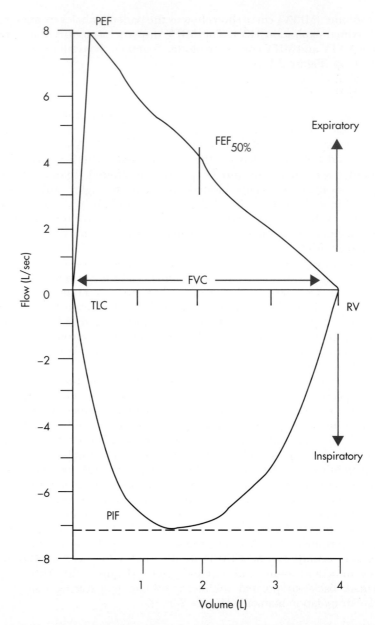

Figure 2-10 *Flow-volume loop.* A flow-volume recording in which an FVC and an FIVC maneuver are recorded in succession. Flow in liters per second is plotted on the *vertical axis* and volume, in liters, on the *horizontal axis*. By convention, *expiratory* flow is plotted upward (positive), and *inspiratory* flow is plotted downward (negative). The maximal exhalation begins with the patient at total lung capacity (TLC) and continues until residual volume (RV) is reached; a maximal inspiration then returns to TLC. The FVC can be read from the tracing as the maximal horizontal deflection along the zero flow line. Peak flows for expiration and inspiration (PEF and PIF) can be read directly from the tracing as the maximal deflections on the flow axis (positive and negative). The instantaneous flow (FEF) at any point in the FVC can also be measured directly. Phenomena, such as small or large airway obstruction, show up as characteristic changes in the maximal flow rates (Figure 2-12). The flow-volume loop is a graphic display of the MEFV and MIFV curves combined.

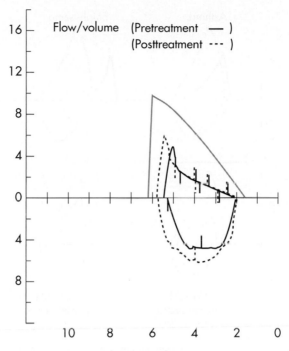

16

12

8

4

0

4

8

Flow/volume   (Pretreatment —)
(Posttreatment ---)

10   8   6   4   2   0

Figure 2-11 *Superimposed flow-volume loops.* Flow-volume curves from a patient with combined obstruction and restriction. Multiple F-V loops (in this case before and after bronchodilator therapy) are superimposed by the computer at RV. *Upward ticks* on the expiratory limb represent $FEV_{0.5}$, FEV_1, and FEV_3, respectively. *Downward ticks* on the expiratory curve represent the $FEF_{25\%}$, $FEF_{50\%}$, and $FEF_{75\%}$, respectively. *Upward ticks* on the inspiratory loop represent the $FIF_{50\%}$. The *large gray expiratory curve* is a computer-generated plot of the patient's predicted MEFV. As can be seen from the curves, expiratory flow is decreased at all lung volumes. The patient's FVC (horizontal axis) is also lower than predicted.

SPIROMETRY 2-5   Criteria for Acceptability—Flow-Volume Loop

1 Rapid rise from maximal inspiration to PEF
2 Maximal effort until flow returns to zero baseline; no glottic closure or abrupt end of flow
3 Maximal inspiratory effort with return of volume to point of maximal inspiration (Failure to close loop indicates that effort was not started from maximal inspiration, inspiratory effort was submaximal, or spirometer error.)
4 At least three acceptable loops recorded; superimposed or side-by-side loops should be reproducible, unless bronchospasm occurs

Elastic recoil determines the pressure applied to gas in the lung during a forced expiration. This pressure is determined by the recoil of the lung and chest wall and, to a certain extent, by the expiratory muscles. Resistance to flow in the airways is the second factor affecting the shape of the flow-volume curve. Flow limitation occurs in the large and medium airways during the early part of a forced expiration. The site of flow limitation migrates "upstream" rapidly during forced expiration. Resistance to flow in small (less than 2 mm) airways is

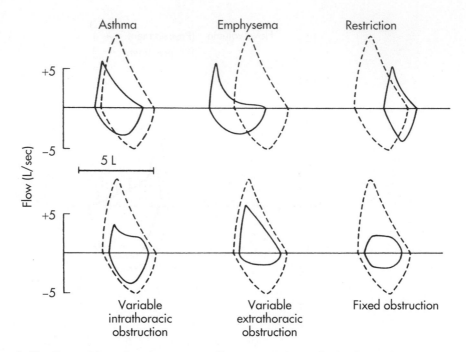

Figure 2-12 *Abnormal flow-volume loops patterns.* Six curves are shown plotting flow in liters per second against the FVC. In each example, the expected curve is shown *(dashed lines)*, while the curve illustrating the particular disease pattern is superimposed. In patients who have asthma and emphysema, the portion of the expiratory curve from the peak flow to residual volume (RV) is characteristically concave. Both the TLC and RV points are displaced toward higher lung volumes (to the left of the expected curves). These patterns are indicative of hyperinflation and/or air trapping. In restrictive patterns, the shape of the loop is preserved but the FVC is decreased. The TLC and RV displaced toward lower lung volume (to the right of the expected curves). The bottom three examples depict types of large airway obstruction. Variable intrathoracic obstruction shows reduced flows on expiration despite near-normal flows on inspiration resulting from flow limitation in the large airways during a forced expiration. Variable extrathoracic obstruction shows an opposite pattern. Inspiratory flow is reduced, while expiratory flow is relatively normal. Fixed large airway obstruction is characterized by equally reduced inspiratory and expiratory flows. Comparison of the $FEF_{50\%}$ with the $FIF_{50\%}$ may be helpful in differentiating large airway obstructive processes. Because the magnitude of inspiratory flow is effort dependent, low inspiratory flows should be carefully evaluated.

SPIROMETRY 2-6   Interpretive Strategies—Flow-Volume Loop

1 Were at least three acceptable F-V curves obtained? Does the beginning of the expiratory curve show a sharp rise to PEF? If not, suspect patient effort or large airway obstruction.
2 Are the PEF and PIF values consistent? Does PEF or other expiratory flows fall with repeated efforts? If so, suspect hyperreactive airways.
3 Does the expiratory curve from PEF to maximal exhalation appear concave? If so, suspect small airway obstruction.
4 Do either the expiratory or inspiratory portions of the curve show a "squared off" pattern? If so, suspect large airway obstruction. If both, suspect a fixed obstruction.
5 Is the inspiratory curve reproducible? If not, suspect variable effort or fatigue.
6 Does the F-V loop show any other unusual patterns (sudden changes in flow that are reproducible, or "sawtooth" pattern)?

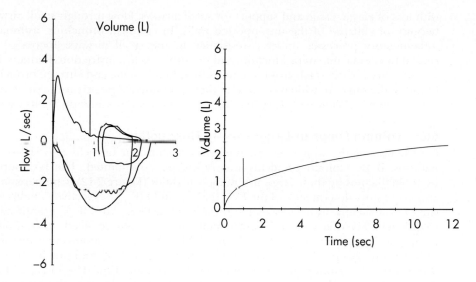

Figure 2-13 *MEFV and volume-time tracings from a patient with severe obstruction.* The expiratory flow-volume curve shows severely reduced flows at all lung volumes; inspiratory flows are also markedly reduced. Note that the tidal breathing loop (recorded immediately before the forced effort) shows higher flows than the MEFV curve. This is consistent with dynamic airway compression during forced exhalation. The expiratory volume-time tracing reveals reduced flow with no obvious plateau even after 12 seconds of exhalation.

determined primarily by the cross-sectional area. This cross-sectional area can be affected by a number of factors. Destruction of alveolar walls, as in emphysema, reduces support of the small airways. Bronchoconstriction and inflammation directly reduce the lumen of the small airways.

In healthy patients flow ($\dot{V}$max) over the effort-independent segment decreases linearly as lung volume decreases. Pressures around airways are balanced by gas pressures in the airways so that flow is limited at an "equal pressure point." As the lung empties, the equal pressure point moves upstream into increasingly smaller airways and continues until small airways begin to close, trapping some gas in the alveoli (the RV). This pattern of airflow limitation in healthy lungs causes the MEFV curve to have a *linear* or slightly concave appearance (Figure 2-10).

Flow-Volume Loops in Small Airway Obstruction

Maximal flow is decreased in patients who have obstruction in small airways, particularly at low lung volumes. The effort-independent segment of the MEFV curve appears more concave or "scooped out" (Figure 2-13). Values for $\dot{V}_{max\,50}$ and $\dot{V}_{max\,25}$ are characteristically decreased. Decreases in $\dot{V}_{max\,50}$ correlate well with the reduction in $FEF_{25\%-75\%}$ in patients with small airway obstructive disease.

Because elastic recoil *and* resistance in small airways determine the shape of the MEFV tracing, different lung diseases can cause similar F-V patterns. Emphysema destroys alveoli with loss of elastic tissue and support for small airways. Flow through small airways decreases because of collapse of the unsupported walls. In contrast, bronchitis, asthma, and similar inflammatory processes increase resistance in the small airways. Increased resistance is caused by edema, mucus production, and smooth muscle constriction. Reduction in the cross-sectional area of the small airways reduces flow. Emphysema and chronic bronchitis are often found in the same individual because of their common cause—cigarette smoking. The MEFV curve presents a picture of the extent of obstruction without identifying its cause.

Flow-Volume Loops in Large Airway Obstruction

Obstruction of the upper airway, trachea, or mainstem bronchi also shows characteristic patterns. Both expiratory and inspiratory flow may be limited. The F-V loop is extremely useful in diagnosing these large airway abnormalities (Figure 2-12). Comparison of expiratory and inspiratory flows at 50% of the FVC ($FEF_{50\%}$ and $FIF_{50\%}$, respectively) helps determine the site of obstruction. In healthy patients, the ratio of $FEF_{50\%}$ to $FIF_{50\%}$ is approximately 1.0 or slightly less. Fixed large airway obstruction causes equally reduced flows at 50% of the VC during inspiration and expiration (Figure 2-14). Obstructive lesions that vary with the phase of breathing also produce characteristic patterns. Variable extrathoracic obstruction usually shows normal expiratory flow but diminished inspiratory flow. The $FEF_{50\%}/FIF_{50\%}$ is greater than 1.0. Because the obstructive process is outside of the thorax, the MEFV portion of the curve appears as it would in a healthy individual. The inspiratory portion of the loop is flattened. Inspiratory flow depends on how much obstruction is present. In variable intrathoracic obstruction, PEF is reduced. Expiratory flow remains constant until the site of flow limitation reaches the smaller airways. This gives the expiratory limb a "squared-off" appearance (Figure 2-12). The inspiratory portion of the loop may be completely normal. The $FEF_{50\%}/FIF_{50\%}$ will be much less than 1.0, depending on the severity of obstruction.

Reduced peak expiratory flow (PEF) and/or peak inspiratory flow (PIF) as seen on the F-V loop may be due to disease or poor patient effort. Be sure to look at *ALL* maneuvers performed. If peak expiratory or peak inspiratory flows are uniformly reduced in all efforts, large airway obstruction may be present. An F-V loop performed with poor effort may mimic large airway obstruction.

Airway obstruction associated with abnormality of the muscular control of the posterior pharynx and larynx sometimes produces a "sawtooth" pattern visible on the inspiratory and expiratory limbs of the MEFV curve. This pattern is sometimes observed in patients suspected of having sleep apnea.

Peak inspiratory flow and the pattern of flow during inspiration are largely effort dependent. Poor patient effort may result in inspiratory flow patterns similar to variable extrathoracic obstruction. Instruction by the technologist should emphasize maximal effort during inspiration as well as expiration. If repeated efforts produce reduced inspiratory flows, an obstructive process should be suspected.

Restrictive disease processes may show normal or greater than normal peak flows with linear decreases in flow versus volume. The lung volume displayed on the X-axis is decreased. Moderate or severe restriction demonstrates equally reduced flows at all lung volumes. Reduced flows are primarily caused by the decreased cross-sectional area of the small airways

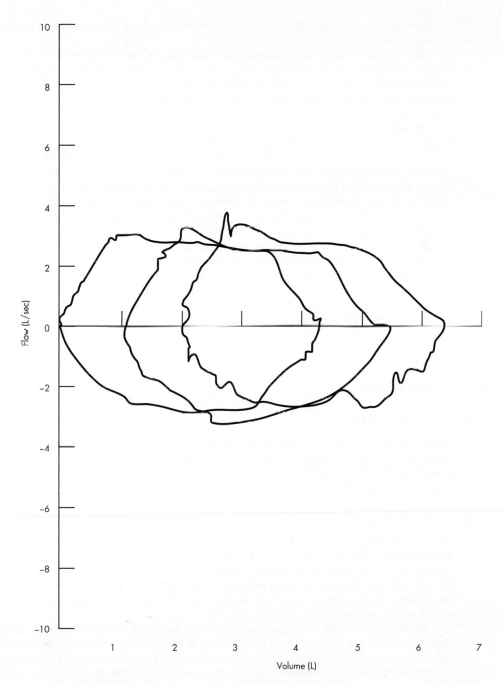

Figure 2-14 *MEFV tracings from a patient with a fixed upper airway obstruction.* Three flow-volume loops are displayed with the starting point (TLC) offset by 1 L. On each curve, the expiratory and inspiratory limbs show flattening consistent with a fixed obstruction. Note that maximal flow on both limbs is about 3 L/sec, much less than expected in a healthy patient.

at low lung volumes. Simple restriction causes the F-V loop to appear as a miniature of the normal curve (Figure 2-12).

Before- and after-bronchodilator F-V loops can be superimposed to measure changes in flow at specific lung volumes. The curves are usually positioned by superimposing at maximal inspiration. This method assumes that any increase in FVC occurs while TLC remains constant. If postbronchodilator lung volume tests are performed, the curves may be superimposed on an absolute volume scale (i.e., isovolume correction). This method shows bronchodilator-induced changes in lung volumes as well as flows. Inhalation challenge studies (see Chapter 9) can be displayed similarly to assess the reduction in flows at specific lung volumes.

Tidal breathing curves or MVV curves can also be superimposed on the F-V loop. The patient's *ventilatory reserve* can be assessed by comparing the areas enclosed under each of the curves. Patients who have obstructive lung disease may generate F-V loops only slightly larger than their tidal breathing curves. In severe obstruction, flow during tidal breathing may actually exceed flow during a forced expiration. Dynamic compression of small airways during forced expiration causes airway collapse, while tidal breathing may not. These patients have limited ventilatory reserve and shortness of breath with exertion.

F-V loops may also be measured during exercise (see Chapter 7). By superimposing a flow-volume curve during exercise over the maximal F-V loop, specific patterns of ventilatory response can be assessed. Patients who have airflow limitation are typically unable to increase ventilation during exercise when expiratory flow equals maximal flow. Exercise F-V curves can be used to demonstrate this phenomenon.

Peak Expiratory Flow

▇ DESCRIPTION

Peak expiratory flow (PEF) is the maximum flow attained during an FVC maneuver. When reported in conjunction with other spirometric variables, PEF is expressed in liters per second, BTPS. When performed alone using a peak flow meter, PEF is usually reported in liters per minute, BTPS.

▇ TECHNIQUE

PEF can be easily measured from a flow-volume curve (MEFV). PEF may also be measured by using devices that sense flow directly (see Chapter 10), or by using volume displacement spirometers and deriving the rate of volume change. Many portable devices (i.e., peak flow meters) are available to measure maximal flow during forced expiration. Most sense flow as movement of air against a turbine or through an orifice. PEF done in conjunction with spirometry is performed as described for F-V loops.

Measuring PEF with a peak flow meter may be done at the bedside, in the emergency department, in the clinic setting, or at home. In each setting, the individual performing the measurement must know how to operate the specific peak flow meter. The maneuver should be demonstrated to the patient. A return demonstration is essential when the patient is being trained to use the peak flow meter at home.

The peak flow meter should be set or zeroed, as required. The patient should sit or (preferably) stand up straight. The patient should inhale maximally; the inhalation should be rapid but not forced. The patient then exhales with maximal effort as soon as the teeth and lips are placed around the mouthpiece. As in the FVC maneuver, a long pause (4 to

SPIROMETRY 2-7   Criteria for Acceptability—Peak Flow

1 Patient was standing or sitting up straight.
2 Patient inhaled maximally (rapid, but not forced) and exhaled maximally without holding his or her breath.
3 At least three efforts were performed and recorded in order.
4 Largest PEF obtained is reported.

6 seconds) at maximal inspiration may decrease the PEF. The expiratory effort only needs to be 1 to 2 seconds to record PEF.

At least three maneuvers should be performed and recorded, along with the order in which the values were obtained. All readings are recorded in order to detect effort-induced bronchospasm. The largest PEF obtained should be reported. The PEF is effort dependent and variable. It may be particularly variable in patients with hyperreactive airways (Spirometry 2-7). There are no widely recognized criteria for reproducibility of PEF efforts.

When PEF is used to monitor asthmatic patients, it is important to establish each person's best PEF (i.e., the largest PEF achieved). Best values can be obtained over 2 to 3 weeks. PEF should be measured twice daily (morning and evening). The personal best is usually observed in the evening after a period of maximum therapy. Daily measurements are then compared with the personal best. The personal best PEF should be reevaluated annually. This allows PEF to be adjusted for growth in children or for progression of disease. PEF should be periodically compared with regular spirometry results (FEV_1).

Portable peak flow meters need to be precise (low variability in the same instrument). *Precision* is more important than accuracy for detecting changes from serial measurements. Peak flow meters should have ranges of 60 to 400 L/min for children and 100 to 850 L/min for adults. Standards for peak flow monitoring devices have been published by the American Thoracic Society (ATS) (see Chapters 10 and 11).

SIGNIFICANCE AND PATHOPHYSIOLOGY

See Spirometry 2-8 for interpretive strategies. The PEF attainable by healthy young adults may exceed 10 L/sec or 600 L/min, BTPS. Even when an accurate *pneumotachometer* is used, the value of PEF measurements may be limited. Peak flow is effort dependent. It primarily measures large airway function. Decreased PEF values should be evaluated for consistent patient effort. PEF values for patients without hyperreactive airways are usually similar with repeated efforts. Asthmatic patients often have a pattern of decreasing PEF with repeated trials. Widely varying peak flows without a pattern of induced bronchospasm suggest poor effort or cooperation. However, PEF measurements alone are not sufficient to make a diagnosis of asthma. Spirometry, lung volumes, diffusing capacity, and airway resistance measurements may be required to evaluate fully the associated physiologic impairment.

Effort dependence of PEF makes it a good indicator of patient effort during spirometry. Maximal transpulmonary pressures correlate well with maximal PEF. Patients who exert variable effort during FVC maneuvers are seldom able to reproduce their PEF. Some clinicians use PEF in addition to the FVC and FEV_1 to gauge maximal effort during spirometry. PEF measurements, when performed with a good effort, correlate well with the FEV_1 as measured by spirometry.

Patients with early small airways obstruction may initially develop high flows during an FVC maneuver. Despite obstruction, these individuals show relatively normal PEF values.

SPIROMETRY 2-8   Interpretive Strategies—Peak Flow

1 What is the patient's personal best PEF?
2 Is the current PEF the best of three trials? Was it obtained in the morning or evening? Was it obtained before or after inhaled bronchodilator therapy?
3 Zone system*:

Green   80%-100% personal best
         Routine treatment can be continued; consider reducing medications
Yellow   50%-80% of personal best
         Acute exacerbation may be present; temporary increase in medication may be indicated; maintenance therapy may need to be increased
Red   < 50% of personal best
         Bronchodilators should be taken immediately; clinician should be notified if PEF fails to return to yellow or green

*From National Asthma Education Program, NIH, 1991.

When small airway obstruction becomes severe, PEF also decreases. Reduction in PEF is often less than the decrease in $FEF_{50\%}$ or $FEF_{75\%}$ in patients with severe obstruction.

PEF measurements are particularly useful for monitoring asthma patients at home. Daily monitoring of PEF can provide early detection of asthmatic episodes. It can be used to detect day-night patterns (circadian rhythms) related to airway reactivity. PEF monitoring provides objective criteria for treatment. It can help determine specific triggers (e.g., allergens) or workplace exposures that cause symptoms. Daily morning and evening readings are recommended. For patients taking inhaled bronchodilators, PEF may be measured before and after treatment. Significant variation from their personal best or from one reading to the next should be emphasized.

The National Asthma Education Program suggests a "zone" system, based on the individual's personal best or predicted PEF. The zone system uses green, yellow, and red as indicators for maintaining or altering therapy. Green (80% to 100% of the personal best PEF) indicates continuation of routine therapy. Yellow (50% to 80% of the personal best PEF) indicates that an acute episode may be starting. Increased medication may be necessary. Red (less than 50% of the personal best PEF) indicates that an acute change has occurred. Immediate treatment is required, and the clinician should be notified. This approach dramatically improves the patient's ability to communicate symptomatic changes to the clinician.

Uniformly decreased PEF is often associated with upper airway obstruction but is nonspecific. PEF assessed from F-V loops (along with PIF) helps define both the severity and site of large airway obstruction.

Maximum Voluntary Ventilation

■ DESCRIPTION

MVV is the volume of air exhaled in a specific interval during rapid, forced breathing. The maneuver should last at least 12 seconds. It is recorded in liters per minute, BTPS, by extrapolating the volume to 1 minute.

■ TECHNIQUE

MVV is measured by having the patient breathe deeply and rapidly for a 12- or 15-second interval. Patients should set the rate, but breathe rapidly *and* deeply. The volume breathed should be greater than their V_T but less than their VC. Instruct the patient to move as much air as possible into and out of the spirometer. The technologist should encourage the patient throughout the maneuver.

MVV is continued for at least 12 seconds but no more than 15 seconds. The patient is hyperventilating. Efforts longer than 15 seconds exaggerate the sensation of lightheadedness. Even the 12-second interval may produce dizziness or syncope. The test may be performed with the patient in either a sitting or standing position. If done while standing, a chair should be available in case of dizziness. Some automated spirometers allow MVV to be terminated before 12 seconds. This accommodates patients who cannot continue because of coughing or lightheadedness. If MVV does not last 12 seconds, it should be noted in the technologist's comments (see Chapter 11). At least two MVV maneuvers should be performed. The two largest should be within 10% of each other. The largest value is reported (Spirometry 2-9).

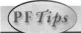

You can quickly check the validity of the MVV by comparing it with the patient's FEV_1 multiplied by 35. If the MVV is significantly lower than $FEV_1 \times 35$, patient effort may be the cause. Neuromuscular disease may also cause a reduced MVV in relation to FEV_1.

The volume expired is measured by a spirometer. The spirometer must have adequate frequency response over a wide range of flows (see Chapters 10 and 11). Historically, the volume of each breath was read from a volume-time spirogram or from a recording of accumulated volume (Figure 2-15). Now volume data from each breath are summed by computer for the interval measured. The MVV (for a 12-second test) is calculated as flow in liters per minute, as follows:

$$MVV = Vol_{12} \times \frac{60}{12}$$

where:
Vol_{12} = volume in liters expired in 12 seconds
60 = factor for extrapolation from seconds to minutes
For other intervals, the MVV is calculated similarly. The MVV must be corrected to BTPS.

SPIROMETRY 2-9 Criteria for Acceptability—MVV

1 Volume-time tracing shows continuous, rhythmic effort for at least 12 seconds.
2 End-expiratory lung volume is relatively constant.
3 Two acceptable maneuvers are obtained; MVV values are within 10%.
4 MVV is approximately equal to $35 \times FEV_1$.

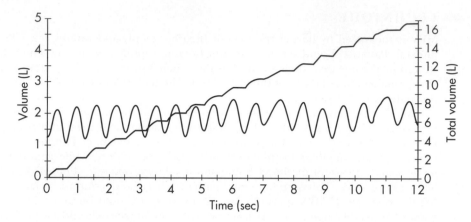

Figure 2-15 *Maximum voluntary ventilation (MVV).* A composite MVV spirogram on which breath-by-breath volume change and accumulated volume are plotted against time. The undulating line shows the tidal volume (approximately 1 L in this test) moved during each breath over a 12-second interval. The stair-step tracing depicts the accumulated (total) volume, in liters, exhaled during the 12-second maneuver. In this example, the volume is approximately 17 L, as read from the scale on the right. To calculate MVV, the volumes of individual breaths can be added and multiplied by a factor of 5 (i.e., 60 seconds/12 seconds = 5). Alternatively, the accumulated volume can be multiplied by 5. Because the MVV is reported in liters per minute, values for 12 seconds must be extrapolated to 1 minute. Healthy patients can maintain the same MVV flow throughout the maneuver. Patients who have pulmonary disease will show decreased absolute values. The MVV may decrease significantly as the maneuver progresses because of respiratory muscle fatigue, increased work of breathing, or air trapping.

◼ SIGNIFICANCE AND PATHOPHYSIOLOGY

See Spirometry 2-10 for interpretive strategies. MVV tests the overall function of the respiratory system. It is influenced by airway resistance, respiratory muscles, compliance of the lung and/or chest wall, and ventilatory control mechanisms. Values in healthy young men average between 150 and 200 L/min. Values are slightly lower in healthy women. MVV decreases with age in both men and women and varies considerably in healthy patients. Only large reductions in MVV (30% or more) are considered significant.

MVV is decreased in patients with moderate or severe obstructive disease. This may be the result of the increased airway resistance caused by bronchospasm or mucus secretion. Reduction of MVV may also occur because of airway collapse and hyperinflation, as in emphysema. The MVV maneuver exaggerates air trapping and airflow limitation. Volume-time MVV tracings may show a shift if gas trapping occurs during the test. A slight shift is usually noted during the first few breaths even in healthy patients. The patient adjusts to a lung volume that allows maximal airflow. These first few breaths are usually excluded from the MVV calculation.

The MVV maneuver also places a load on the respiratory muscles. Both inspiratory and expiratory muscles are used in the MVV maneuver. Weakness or decreased endurance of either system may result in low MVV values. Poor coordination of the respiratory muscles caused by a neurologic deficit may also cause a low MVV. Disorders such as paralysis or nerve damage reduce MVV as well.

A markedly reduced MVV correlates with postoperative risk for patients having abdominal or thoracic surgery. Patients who have low preoperative MVV values show an increased incidence of complications. Reduced strength or endurance of the respiratory muscles may be the factor that allows MVV to predict postoperative problems.

SPIROMETRY 2-10   Interpretive Strategies—MVV

1 Was MVV test performed acceptably? At least 12 seconds?
2 Does MVV approximate $FEV_1 \times 35$? If not, suspect subject effort.
3 Is MVV less than 70% of predicted? If so, correlate with obstruction ($FEV_{1\%}$).
4 If no obstruction, look for clinical correlation for reduced MVV. Consider testing maximal respiratory pressures, compliance.

The MVV value may be helpful in estimating ventilation during exercise. Airway-obstructed patients who have an MVV less than 50 L/min often have a ventilatory limitation to exercise. Maximal exercise ventilation in healthy patients is usually less than 70% of their MVV. In airway-obstructed patients, maximal ventilation during exercise approaches or even exceeds their MVV. This pattern occurs partly because the MVV itself is reduced in obstruction. Highly conditioned healthy patients may also reach their MVV during maximal exercise (see Chapter 7).

MVV may be normal in patients who have restrictive pulmonary disease. Diseases that limit lung or chest wall expansion may not interfere significantly with airflow. Patients who have restrictive disease can compensate by performing the MVV maneuver with low V_T and high breathing rates.

The MVV maneuver depends on patient effort and cooperation. Low MVV values may indicate obstruction, muscular weakness, defective ventilatory control, or poor patient performance. Patient effort during the MVV maneuver may be estimated by multiplying their FEV_1 by 35. For example, a patient with an FEV_1 of 2.0 L might be expected to ventilate approximately 70 L/min (35×2.0 L) during the MVV test. If the measured MVV is much less than 70 L/min, poor patient effort may be suspected. If the MVV exceeds 70 L/min by a large volume, the FEV_1 may be erroneous.

Before- and After-Bronchodilator Studies

■ DESCRIPTION

Spirometry can be performed before and after bronchodilator administration to determine the reversibility of airway obstruction. An $FEV_{1\%}$ less than predicted is a good indication for bronchodilator studies. In most patients, an $FEV_{1\%}$ less than 70% indicates obstruction. In older adults, the normal $FEV_{1\%}$ may be slightly less. Patients whose FEV_1 and FVC are within normal limits may have a low $FEV_{1\%}$. This happens when the FVC is greater than 100% of predicted while the FEV_1 is slightly reduced. Although any pulmonary function parameter may be measured before and after bronchodilator therapy, FEV_1 and specific airway conductance (SGaw) are usually evaluated.

■ TECHNIQUE

The patient may take an array of tests, including spirometry, lung volumes, and diffusing capacity (DL_{CO}). Lung volumes should be recorded before bronchodilator administration. This provides a baseline for comparing lung volume changes after bronchodilator therapy. Even though indices of flow (FEV_1, $FEF_{25\%-75\%}$, and SGaw) usually show the greatest change, lung volumes and DL_{CO} may also respond to bronchodilator therapy.

TABLE 2-2 Withholding Medications

Medication	Time to Withhold*
Regular β-agonists	8 hours
Sustained action β-agonists	12 hours
Methylxanthines (theophyllines)	12 hours
Slow-release methylxanthines	24 hours
Atropine-like preparations	8 hours
Cromolyn sodium	8-12 hours
Inhaled steroids	Maintain dosage

*Approximate times; may be adjusted for individual patients.

Patients referred for spirometry testing should withhold routine bronchodilator therapy before the procedure (Table 2-2). Some patients may be unable to manage their symptoms if bronchodilators are withheld. These patients should be instructed to take their bronchodilator medication as needed. In these instances, the time when the medication was last taken should be noted. Some patients who use bronchodilators shortly before testing (within 4 hours) still show significant improvement after a repeated dose.

Inhaled bronchodilators can be administered by a metered-dose inhaler (MDI) or a small-volume nebulizer. An MDI provides a reproducible means of administering the bronchodilator. Some patients are unable to coordinate activation of the MDI with slow, deep inspiration. For these patients, use of an aerosol reservoir, or spacer, may provide a more consistent delivery of medication. If the patient is unfamiliar with the MDI, the technologist may need to activate the device (Spirometry 2-11). Small-volume, jet-powered nebulizers may be used to administer more bronchodilator over a longer interval. Nebulizers, if reused, must be carefully disinfected between patients.

β_2-Adrenergic aerosols, such as albuterol, are most commonly used. Each of these drugs has a rapid onset of action, usually within 5 minutes. Maximum bronchodilatation usually takes longer. A minimum interval of 15 minutes between administration and repeat testing is recommended. Even with this delay, peak bronchodilator response may not be observed. Response to atropine-like drugs (ipratropium bromide) may require a delay of 45 to 60 minutes after inhalation.

Bronchodilator administration often causes side effects. The most common side effect of β-agonist use is tachycardia. Increased blood pressure, flushing, dizziness, or lightheadedness is not unusual. Monitoring pulse rate and blood pressure is recommended for susceptible patients. This includes patients with known cardiac arrhythmias or elevated blood pressure.

SPIROMETRY 2-11   Using an MDI

- Shake the MDI; activate once to prime and check contents. If empty, replace.
- Hold the MDI mouthpiece slightly away from the patient's open mouth; *or, if a spacer is used* Place the spacer mouthpiece between the lips, per manufacturer's instructions.
- As the patient inspires slowly from the resting expiratory level, activate the MDI.
- Have the patient continue slowly inhaling to maximal inspiration.
- Have patient hold the breath for 3 to 5 seconds, followed by a slow exhalation.
- Repeat inhalations as indicated.

Marked changes in heart rate, rhythm, or blood pressure, or symptoms like chest pain indicate a need to stabilize the patient. The referring physician or laboratory medical director should be notified immediately. Management of the patient's symptoms and continuation of testing are the decision of the physician.

Measurements of FEV_1, FVC, $FEF_{25\%-75\%}$, PEF, and SGaw are commonly made before and after bronchodilator administration. In each case, the percentage of change is calculated as follows:

$$\% \text{ Change} = \frac{\text{Postdrug} - \text{Predrug}}{\text{Predrug}} \times 100$$

where:

Postdrug = test parameter after administration

Predrug = test parameter before administration

If the test value improves, the percentage of change will be positive. If the parameter worsens, a negative percentage results. Small prebronchodilator values (e.g., an FEV_1 of 0.5 L) may show large changes even though the improvement is minimal.

FEV_1 is the most commonly used test for quantifying bronchodilator response. If $FEF_{25\%-75\%}$ or flows such as $\dot{V}_{max\,50}$ are used, they should be isovolume-corrected for changes in the FVC. If FVC increases more than FEV_1 after bronchodilator therapy, $FEV_{1\%}$ may actually decrease. $FEV_{1\%}$ should not be used to judge bronchodilator response. SGaw may show a marked increase after bronchodilator therapy. Improved conductance may occur despite minimal change in FEV_1 or conventional measures of flow. Spirometry or plethysmography after bronchodilator therapy should meet the usual criteria for acceptability and reproducibility.

PF *Tips*

Patients who have a normal FEV_1/FVC ratio may be candidates for a bronchodilator study, even if they have taken their own medication within 4 hours. Many patients with a history of asthma or COPD may show a significant improvement if they have been using their MDI incorrectly (see Spirometry 2-11, Using an MDI).

■ SIGNIFICANCE AND PATHOPHYSIOLOGY

See Spirometry 2-12 for interpretive strategies. Reversibility of airway obstruction is considered significant for increases of greater than 12% *and* 200 ml for either the FEV_1 or FVC. If the SGaw is assessed, an increase of 30% to 40% is usually considered significant. Some patients may show little or no improvement in FEV_1 but have a significant improvement in SGaw. Changes in $FEF_{25\%-75\%}$ of 20% to 30% are sometimes considered significant. However, flows that depend on the FVC should be volume-corrected (Case 2-2). If not corrected, $FEF_{25\%-75\%}$ may appear to decrease although FEV_1 and FVC improve.

Diseases involving the bronchial (and bronchiolar) smooth muscle usually improve most from "before" to "after." Increases greater than 50% in the FEV_1 may occur in patients with asthma. Patients with chronic obstructive diseases may show little improvement in flows. Poor bronchodilator response may be related to inadequate deposition of the inhaled drug because of poor inspiratory effort. Failure to show a significant improvement after inhaled bronchodilator therapy does not exclude a response. Some patients have a significant

---

SPIROMETRY 2-12 Interpretive Strategies—Bronchodilator Studies

1 Are the prebronchodilator and postbronchodilator measurements acceptable? Reproducible within 200 ml? If not, postbronchodilator changes may be erroneous.

2 Is there a 12% or greater improvement in FEV_1 or FVC? Is there also a 200 ml increase? If so, there is a significant improvement.

3 Is there an increase in SGaw (if done) greater than 35%? If so, there is a significant improvement.

4 No significant improvement observed? Trial of bronchodilator therapy may be recommended, if clinically indicated.

---

response to one drug but little or no response to another. Efficacy of a specific drug may require repeat testing after a trial on the medication. Long-acting bronchodilators or inhaled corticosteroids may significantly improve a patient's lung function, even if there is no acute response to an inhaled β_2-adrenergic.

Some patients show a paradoxical response to bronchodilator therapy. In these individuals, flows may actually decrease after the bronchodilator therapy. Decreased flows after bronchodilator therapy may also be related to fatigue from multiple FVC efforts. Changes of less than 8% or 150 ml are within the variability of measurement of FEV_1. Such small changes may occur just with testing and are unlikely to be significant.

Maximal Inspiratory Pressure and Maximal Expiratory Pressure

■ DESCRIPTION

Maximal inspiratory pressure (MIP) is the lowest pressure developed during a forceful inspiration against an occluded airway. It is usually measured at maximal expiration (near residual volume). It is recorded as a negative number in either cm H_2O or mm Hg. Maximal expiratory pressure (MEP) is the highest pressure that can be developed during a forceful expiratory effort against an occluded airway. It is usually measured at maximal inspiration and reported as a positive number in either cm H_2O or mm Hg. MIP and MEP are sometimes measured at the resting end-expiratory level (FRC).

■ TECHNIQUE

The patient is connected to a valve or shutter apparatus, with a flanged mouthpiece and nose clip in place. The mouthpiece can be placed in the mouth with teeth resting on bite blocks, or the lips pressed against the mouthpiece opening, as would be done with a bugle. With either technique, there should be a tight fit so that the patient can exert maximal pressure. The airway is occluded by blocking a port in the valve or by closing a shutter. In either system, a small, fixed leak is introduced between the occlusion and the patient's mouth. The leak can be created using a large-bore needle or similar small opening (~1 mm). The leak eliminates pressures generated by the cheek muscles by allowing a small amount of gas to enter the oral cavity. This does not significantly change lung volume or the pressure measurement.

Pressure may be measured using a manometer, an aneroid-type gauge, or a pressure transducer. The pressure-monitoring device should be linear over its range. It should be able to record pressures from −200 to approximately +200 cm H_2O. If a pressure transducer is used,

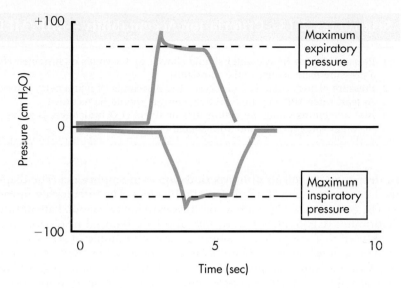

Figure 2-16 *Maximal inspiratory and maximal expiratory pressures (MIP, MEP).* These tracings plot the respective pressures recorded in cm H_2O against time on a single graph. Maximal inspiratory pressure shows a downward or negative deflection. Maximal inspiratory pressure shows a positive or upward deflection. Each maneuver is conducted with the airway occluded (see text). The occlusion is maintained for a short interval (1 to 3 seconds), and any initial transient tracings are discarded.

its signal can be directed to a recorder or computer display. If a manometer or aneroid gauge is used, the technologist observes the pressure and records it. Devices that use a "trip" indicator can be misleading. The highest pressure recorded may be a transient pressure that occurs at the very beginning of the maneuver (Figure 2-16). The technologist should record the plateau pressure that the patient can maintain for 1 to 3 seconds.

For the MIP test, the patient is instructed to expire maximally. Monitoring expiratory flow or having the patient signal helps determine when maximal expiration has been achieved. Then the airway is occluded as described. The patient inspires maximally and maintains the inspiration for 1 to 3 seconds. The first portion of each maneuver is disregarded because it may include transient pressure changes that occur initially (Figure 2-16). The most negative value from at least three efforts is recorded.

MEP is recorded similarly. The patient inhales as much as possible, then exhales maximally against the occluded airway for 1 to 3 seconds. Longer efforts should be avoided. Cardiac output can be reduced by the high thoracic pressures (i.e., *Valsalva maneuvers*) that are sometimes developed. MEP is usually larger than MIP in healthy patients. The pressure-monitoring device should be able to withstand the higher pressure without damage. The best of at least three MEP efforts is reported. As for MIP, initial pressure transients during the MEP are disregarded. Both MIP and MEP require patient cooperation and effort (Spirometry 2-13). Low values may reflect lack of understanding or insufficient effort.

■ SIGNIFICANCE AND PATHOPHYSIOLOGY

MIP primarily measures inspiratory muscle *strength*. Healthy adults can generate inspiratory pressures greater than −60 cm H_2O. Decreased MIP is seen in patients with neuromuscular disease or diseases involving the diaphragm, intercostals, or accessory muscles. MIP may also

SPIROMETRY 2-13   Criteria for Acceptability—MIP/MEP

1 Pressure tracing (if available) should show 1 to 3 seconds of sustained effort; there should be a pressure plateau after initial transients.
2 Pressure plateau should be observed, 1 to 3 seconds (if manometer is used).
3 At least three MIP and three MEP maneuvers should be recorded.
4 Best two efforts should be within 10% or 10 cm H_2O, whichever is greater.
5 Maximal value for MIP and MEP should be reported.

be decreased in patients with hyperinflation as in emphysema. The diaphragm is flattened by the increased volume of trapped gas in the lungs. The intercostals and accessory muscles may also be compromised by injury to or diseases of the chest wall. Patients with chest wall or spinal deformities (e.g., kyphoscoliosis) may also have reduced inspiratory pressures. MIP is sometimes used to assess patient response to strength training of respiratory muscles. MIP is often used in the assessment of respiratory muscle function in patients who need ventilatory support.

MEP measures the pressure generated during maximal expiration. It depends on the function of the abdominal muscles and accessory muscles of respiration and the elastic recoil of the lungs and thorax. Healthy adults can generate MEP values more than 80 to 100 cm H_2O. Adult males may develop pressures greater than 200 cm H_2O. MEP may be decreased in neuromuscular disorders, particularly those resulting in generalized muscle weakness. Another common disorder that results in reduction of MEP is high cervical spine fracture. Damage to nerves controlling abdominal and accessory muscles of expiration can dramatically reduce MEP. However, MIP may be preserved in these patients.

Reduced MEP often accompanies increased RV, as seen in emphysema. A low MEP is associated with inability to cough effectively. Inability to generate an adequate cough may complicate chronic bronchitis, cystic fibrosis, or other diseases that result in excessive mucus secretion.

Accurate measurement of MIP and MEP depends largely on patient effort. The technologist should carefully instruct the patient how to do the maneuver. Low values may result if the patient fails to inhale or exhale completely before the airway is occluded. At least three maximal efforts should be recorded. Some patients may show increased MIP or MEP with repeated efforts (training effect). Others may demonstrate decreasing pressures with repeated efforts (muscle fatigue). The best efforts should be reproducible within 10% or 10 cm H_2O, whichever is greater. Widely varying pressures for either MIP or MEP should be assessed carefully before interpretation.

Airway Resistance and Conductance

DESCRIPTION

Airway resistance (Raw) is the pressure difference per unit flow as gas flows into or out of the lungs. Raw is the difference between mouth pressure and alveolar pressure, divided by flow at the mouth. This pressure difference is caused primarily by the friction of gas molecules in contact with the airways. Raw is recorded in centimeters of water per liter per second (cm H_2O/L/sec).

Airway conductance (Gaw) is the flow generated per unit of pressure drop across the airways. It is the reciprocal of Raw (1/Raw) and is recorded in liters per second per centimeter of water (L/sec/cm H_2O). Gaw is not commonly reported because it changes with lung volume. Specific airway conductance (SGaw) is usually reported. SGaw is Gaw divided by the lung volume (in liters) at which the measurement was made. It is reported in liters per second per centimeter of water per liter of lung volume (L/sec/cm H_2O/L).

▥ TECHNIQUE

Raw can be measured as the ratio of alveolar pressure (P_A) to airflow ($\dot{V}$). Gas flow at the mouth is measured with a pneumotachometer (see Chapter 10). P_A is measured in the body plethysmograph (Figure 2-17, *A*). For gas to flow into the lungs during inspiration, P_A must fall below atmospheric pressure (mouth pressure). During expiration, P_A rises above atmospheric pressure. Changes in $\dot{V}$ are plotted against plethysmograph pressure changes. Changes in plethysmograph pressure are proportional to alveolar volume changes. The patient pants with a small V_T at a rate of 1.5 to 3 breaths/sec (1.5 to 3 Hz). Shallow, rapid breathing produces an S-shaped pressure-flow curve (Figure 2-17, *B*). A *tangent* (the *slope*) is measured from this curve. The tangent passes through zero flow and connects the +0.5 L/sec and –0.5 L/sec flow points. The slope of this line is the ratio of $\dot{V}/P_{BOX}$. $\dot{V}$ is flow at the mouth, and P_{BOX} is plethysmograph pressure.

Immediately after this measurement, a shutter at the mouthpiece is closed and the patient continues panting. Changes in P_{BOX} are then plotted against airway pressure at the mouth (P_{MOUTH}). Because there is no flow into or out of the lungs, P_{MOUTH} equals P_A. A second tangent is measured from this curve. The slope of this line is P_A/P_{BOX}, where P_A equals alveolar pressure. Computerized plethysmographs usually calculate a "best fit" line to measure the open-shutter and closed-shutter tangents. The technologist should visually inspect all computer-fitted lines. The system should allow the technologist to adjust computer-generated tangents manually.

Raw is then calculated by taking the ratio of these two slopes, as follows:

$$\text{Raw} = \frac{P_A/P_{BOX}}{\dot{V}/P_{BOX}} \times \frac{\text{Mouth cal}}{\text{Flow cal}}$$

where:
$\dot{V}$ = airflow
P_A = alveolar pressure
P_{BOX} = plethysmographic pressure, measured with the shutter open and closed
Mouth cal = calibration factor for the mouth pressure transducer
Flow cal = calibration factor for the pneumotachometer

Calibration factors for the flow and mouth pressure transducers are included in the previous equation. (See sample calculations in Appendix F.)

Panting eliminates a number of artifacts from the tracing. Small rapid breaths (2 to 3 per second) reduce thermal drift, both in the box and in the pneumotachometer. Panting helps keep the glottis open, allowing measurement of alveolar pressure. Panting also allows measurements to be made near FRC. The resistances of the mouthpiece and pneumotachometer are subtracted from the patient's Raw.

Airway conductance (Gaw) can be calculated as the reciprocal of Raw. Specific conductance is calculated by dividing Gaw by the lung volume at which it was measured. Lung volume is measured at the same time, using the plethysmographic method (see Chapter 3). SGaw should be calculated separately for each maneuver because the lung volume at which measurements are made influences Raw and Gaw. After three to five acceptable trials are obtained, calculated Raw and SGaw are averaged. Individual values should be within approximately 10% of the mean (Spirometry 2-14).

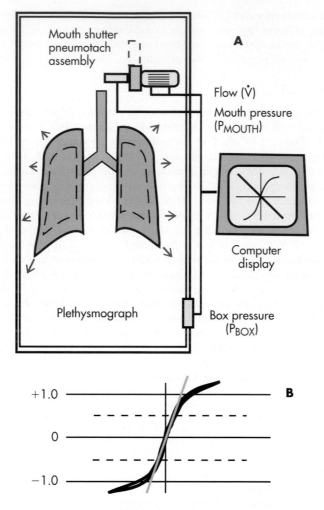

Figure 2-17 *Measurement of airway resistance (Raw) using the body plethysmograph.* **A**, Diagrammatic representation of airway resistance measurement:

$$Raw = \frac{Atmospheric\ pressure - Alveolar\ pressure}{Flow}$$

Flow ($\dot{V}$) is measured directly by means of the pneumotachometer. As the patient pants with the shutter open, flow is plotted against box pressure ($\dot{V}/P_{BOX}$) as an **S**-shaped curve on the computer display. A shutter occludes the airway momentarily, usually at end-expiration, and a sloping line representing the ratio of mouth pressure to box pressure (P_{MOUTH}/P_{BOX}) is recorded in a manner similar to that used for measurement of V_{TG} (see Chapter 3). In this example, the flow tracing (shutter open) and volume tracing (shutter closed) are superimposed on the computer display. The Pmouth/Pbox tangent is measured as for the V_{TG}. **B**, The flow tangent is measured from the steep portion of the flow tracing, from −0.5 to +0.5 L/sec. Airway resistance is then calculated as the ratio of these two tangents using appropriate calibration factors (see text and Appendix F).

SPIROMETRY 2-14   Criteria for Acceptability—Raw and SGaw

1 Pressure-flow loops should be closed; pressure and flow should be within the calibrated range of the respective transducers.
2 Thermal equilibrium should be established; no drift during recording.
3 Panting frequency should be 1.5 to 3.0 Hz for each maneuver.
4 Raw and SGaw should be calculated for each maneuver; do not average tangents.
5 Mean of three or more acceptable efforts should be reported; individual values should be within 10% of mean.

Computerized plethysmographs permit thoracic gas volume (V_{TC}), Raw, and SGaw to be measured from a combined maneuver. The patient breathes through the pneumotachometer with the plethysmograph sealed. Tidal breathing is recorded with the patient breathing near FRC. The computer stores this end-expiratory volume as a reference point. Then the patient pants, and the open-shutter slope of $\dot{V}/P_{BOX}$ is recorded. The mouth shutter is then closed and P_{MOUTH}/P_{BOX} is recorded as described previously. The V_{TG} in this maneuver does not equal the FRC because the shutter is closed at a volume different from the FRC. However, the change in volume from the tidal breathing level was stored at the beginning of the maneuver. This volume can be added to or subtracted from the V_{TG} to determine FRC. Most patients pant above their FRC, so the V_{TG} in this method is usually slightly greater. The combined maneuver allows V_{TG}, Raw, and SGaw to be determined at the same time. However, optimal panting frequencies are slightly different for V_{TG} and Raw maneuvers. The tests may need to be done separately for some patients.

Raw and Gaw may be expressed per liter of lung volume as specific airway resistance and specific airway conductance (SRaw and SGaw, respectively). Expressing Raw and Gaw in this way allows comparisons to be made between patients with different lung volumes or in the same patient when lung volume changes.

■ SIGNIFICANCE AND PATHOPHYSIOLOGY

See Spirometry 2-15 for interpretive strategies. Normal values of Raw in adults range from 0.6 to 2.4 cm H_2O/L/sec. Gaw in healthy adults is between 0.42 and 1.67 L/sec/cm H_2O. SGaw varies in a manner similar to Gaw. SGaw values less than 0.15 to 0.20 L/sec/cm H_2O/L are consistent with airway obstruction. Measurements are standardized at flow rates of ±0.5 L/sec, as described previously.

SPIROMETRY 2-15   Interpretive Strategies—Raw and SGaw

1 Were all maneuvers performed acceptably? Pressure-flow curves closed? Thermal equilibrium established?
2 Are individual Raw and SGaw values reproducible? Within 10%?
3 Is Raw greater than 2.4 cm H_2O/L/sec? Is SGaw less than lower limit of normal? If so, suspect obstruction. Correlate with PEF, FEV_1 to distinguish large versus small airway obstruction.
4 If large airway obstruction indicated, check clinical history. Extrathoracic or intrathoracic?

Raw in healthy adults is divided across the airway as follows:

Nose, mouth, upper airway	50%
Trachea and bronchi	30%
Small airways	20%

Small airways (less than 2 mm in diameter) contribute only approximately one fifth of the total resistance to flow. Significant obstruction can develop in the small airways with little increase in Raw or decrease in SGaw. Early or mild obstructive processes are not usually identified by abnormal Raw or SGaw. Raw may be increased in an acute asthmatic episode by as much as three times the normal values. Inflammation, mucus secretion, and bronchospasm all increase Raw in the small and medium airways. Raw is increased in advanced emphysema because of airway narrowing and collapse, especially in the bronchioles. Other obstructive diseases (e.g., bronchitis) may cause increases in Raw proportionate to the degree of obstruction in medium and small airways.

PF Tips

SGaw measurements are easy to evaluate in adult patients. Healthy subjects have an SGaw of 0.20 or greater. Values much lower than 0.20 are usually associated with increased airway resistance and are commonly found in patients who have obstructive lung disease.

Lesions obstructing the larger airways (e.g., tumors, traumatic injuries, or foreign bodies) may also cause a significant increase in Raw. Large airway obstruction is often accompanied by increased work of breathing and dyspnea on exertion. Airflow in the trachea and mainstem bronchi is predominately turbulent. Any large airway obstruction can exaggerate this turbulent flow. Breathing low-density gas mixtures (e.g., helium + oxygen) reduces Raw and hence the work of breathing.

Raw is decreased at increased lung volume. The airways (particularly large and medium airways) are distended slightly, and their cross-sectional area increases. For this reason, the V_{TG} is always obtained with Raw measurements. Raw and Gaw are often expressed per liter of lung volume. This allows comparison of values in different patients, or in the same patient after treatment. SGaw is particularly useful for assessing changes in airway caliber after bronchodilator therapy or inhalation challenge. SGaw may change significantly after bronchodilator or inhalation challenge, even though other measures of flow (i.e., FEV_1) vary only slightly. The primary site of airway obstruction (i.e., large versus small airways) may determine which parameters reflect changes in airway caliber.

Raw and SGaw measurements are not influenced by the degree of patient effort. Raw and SGaw measurements may be useful for determining airway status in patients who are unable or unwilling to exert maximum effort. Acceptable panting maneuvers in the plethysmograph require a certain degree of patient coordination. Not all patients may be able to perform these maneuvers. Patients with severe obstruction may produce pressure-flow curves during panting that are difficult to measure. Such curves may be flat (Figure 2-18) or show hysteresis. Inspiratory and expiratory flows may produce different resistances, causing the curve to appear as a loop. In these cases, inspiratory flow resistance is usually reported.

In addition to resistance caused by flow through conducting airways, some frictional resistance is caused by the displacement of the lungs, rib cage, and diaphragm. In healthy patients, this tissue resistance is only approximately one fifth of the total

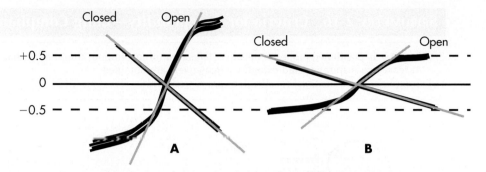

Figure 2-18 *Airway resistance tracings.* **A**, Tracing from a normal patient. **B**, Tracing from a patient with increased airway resistance caused by obstructive lung disease. Note that the open shutter loop (flow) is flattened because a greater change in alveolar pressure is required to generate flow at the mouth. The closed shutter loop also shows a reduction in mouth pressure (*y-axis*) in relation to box pressure (*x-axis*). This is consistent with increased lung volume.

resistance, and therefore total pulmonary resistance is approximately 20% greater than the measured Raw.

Pulmonary Compliance

■ DESCRIPTION

Pulmonary compliance (C_L) is volume change per unit of pressure change for the lungs. Lung compliance is recorded in liters (or milliliters) per centimeter of water. Elastic recoil pressure is usually measured with C_L. Elastic recoil pressure is the force generated by the lungs, usually at maximal volume. Elastic recoil pressure is reported in centimeters of water.

■ TECHNIQUE

C_L is measured by passing a catheter into the esophagus. The catheter has a 10-cm-long balloon near its end. The catheter is inserted through the nose. The patient is then asked to swallow the catheter. The catheter is advanced to mid-thorax level and connected to a pressure transducer. Proper positioning of the catheter is verified by noting negative pressure deflections on inspiration. If the catheter is advanced too far, the balloon may enter the stomach. This causes positive pressure changes with inspiration. If the balloon is positioned at the level of the heart, cardiac systole may cause an unwanted artifact (Spirometry 2-16).

The pressure transducer is set at zero with a small volume (0.5 to 1.0 ml) of air in the balloon. Pressures are then recorded at different lung volumes. These pressures are plotted to produce a compliance curve (Figure 2-19). The patient inhales maximally before the test to standardize the measurements. C_L increases slightly after a full inspiration. Then the patient inhales again. Pressure and volume are measured during the inhalation. Static compliance measurements must be made at zero flow. The patient may hold his or her breath with the glottis open, or flow may be interrupted with a shutter. If the latter technique is used, mouth pressure is subtracted from esophageal pressure to obtain the recoil pressure of the lungs. Similar measurements are recorded during the subsequent expiration.

SPIROMETRY 2-16   Criteria for Acceptability—Lung Compliance

1 Catheter is positioned properly; negative deflection on inspiration; minimal cardiac artifact.
2 At least two inspiratory and expiratory maneuvers are obtained.
3 Compliance and maximal recoil values are reproducible.

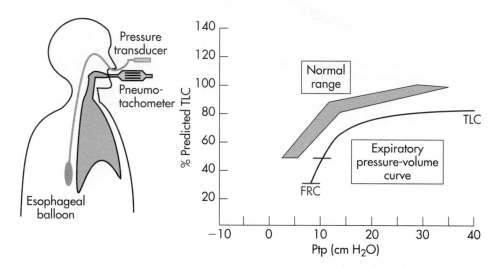

Figure 2-19 *Measurement of pulmonary compliance (C_L) using esophageal balloon technique.* Determination of C_L requires measurement of intrapleural pressure (ΔP) during periods of no flow at various lung volumes. A pressure transducer is connected to an esophageal balloon containing a small amount of air and located in the mid-thorax. The balloon reflects ΔP as the patient inspires to TLC and then expires back to FRC. A pneumotachometer is used to measure lung volumes (ΔV). Static C_L is the slope of the line defined by:

$$\frac{\Delta V \text{ (Liters)}}{\Delta P \text{ (cm } H_2O)}$$

C_L is usually recorded from the breathing range of FRC + 500 ml (*horizontal lines*). Static elastic recoil (Pst) pressure is usually measured at TLC. In the graph shown, the expiratory pressure volume is plotted. Transpulmonary pressure (Ptp) is plotted on the *x*-axis, and percentage of predicted TLC on the *y*-axis. The normal range is represented by the *shaded area*. The pressure-volume curve in this example is displaced down and to the right, consistent with lungs that are stiffer than normal.

    C_L is usually recorded as the slope of the pressure-volume curve from FRC to FRC + 0.5 L (Figure 2-19). Because the deep inspiration increases compliance, measurements are usually recorded from the exhalation curve. Maximum static elastic recoil pressure (P_{ST}) is the most negative pressure recorded at maximal inspiration. The optimal method of presenting compliance data is to plot the entire pressure curve (inflation and deflation) versus lung volume. The C_L curve can then be plotted along with normal ranges.

    Compliance is sometimes measured in patients supported by positive pressure mechanical ventilation. The ventilator inflates the lungs-thorax system with a fixed volume. By recording pressure when flow is zero (by occlusion of the exhalation valve), a compliance measurement can be obtained. Pressure may be measured from the ventilator circuit. A more sophisticated technique uses an esophageal balloon like the laboratory method. In each case, the volume of gas compressed in the patient's lungs is divided by the observed pressure. This compliance measure differs slightly from true C_L. It measures the distensibility of the chest wall as well as the lungs. This technique may be influenced by the patient's position or by any contribution from the respiratory muscles.

SIGNIFICANCE AND PATHOPHYSIOLOGY

See Spirometry 2-17 for interpretive strategies. C_L measures the distensibility of the lungs. The average C_L in a healthy adult is approximately 0.2 L/cm H_2O. The lungs are distended in series with the chest wall. The compliance of the thorax (C_T) is also approximately 0.2 L/cm H_2O in healthy patients. In series, the total compliance (C_{LT}) is calculated using the following equation:

$$\frac{1}{C_{LT}} = \frac{1}{C_T} + \frac{1}{C_L}$$

or substituting the normal values:

$$10 = \frac{1}{0.2} + \frac{1}{0.2}$$

where the reciprocal of 10 is the C_{LT}:

$$\frac{1}{10} = 0.1 \, L/cmH_2O$$

It should be noted that C_{LT} is less than (approximately half) C_L or C_T alone. The elastic forces act in series, counterbalancing the lung tissue and the chest wall. C_L varies with the lung volume at the end-expiratory level (i.e., FRC). To compare the C_L of diseased and normal lungs, the FRC in each case should be known. Plotting the entire C_L curve against lung volume helps relate the two factors.

Lung compliance is decreased in diseases such as edema. Congestion of the pulmonary blood vessels makes the lung stiff. The same is true for diseases in which airways become filled with fluid. Such disorders include atelectasis, pneumonia, or loss of surfactant. Diseases that alter elasticity of lung tissue also lower compliance. Examples include pulmonary fibrosis resulting from silicosis, asbestosis, or sarcoidosis. Decreased C_L may also result when lung volume is reduced as a result of space-occupying lesions such as tumors. When C_L is severely reduced from any cause, symptoms such as dyspnea on exertion are usually present. C_L decreases with age, presumably because of changes in the connective tissues of the lung.

SPIROMETRY 2-17   Interpretive Strategies—Lung Compliance

1 Were the data obtained reproducible? C_L? Pst?
2 Is C_L less than the lower limit of normal? If so, check for clinical correlation. Are lung volumes also reduced?
3 Is C_L greater than the upper limit of normal? Check for findings consistent with obstruction (e.g., $FEV_{1\%}$). Is maximal static recoil decreased?

Emphysema is often accompanied by an increase in C_L. Emphysema destroys alveolar septa with loss of elastic tissue. As a result, the balance between the lungs and chest wall is upset. The chest wall tends to spring outward. The highly compliant lungs exert less pressure to cause recoil. Hyperinflation results as thoracic volume increases. Patients with severe air trapping typically have abnormal breathing patterns and markedly increased work of breathing.

Measurement of C_L requires cooperation by the patient. Some patients may be unable to swallow the esophageal balloon easily. If a mouth shutter is not used to interrupt flow, the patient must hold his or her breath with the glottis open. The C_L and elastic recoil pressure measurements are largely independent of effort, provided the patient is cooperative.

Summary

This chapter describes spirometry—the most commonly performed pulmonary function study. Various spirometry tests are identified. Techniques for performing the tests and criteria for acceptability are enumerated. Simple spirometry, F-V loops, and bronchodilator studies are discussed. Differentiation between obstructive and restrictive disorders is made by explaining the pathophysiologies involved.

Other tests of respiratory mechanics are also discussed. Maximum voluntary ventilation, maximal respiratory pressures, airway resistance and conductance, and pulmonary compliance are related to diagnosis of various lung diseases. Interpretive strategies are presented. These strategies, in the form of questions, provide a systematic approach to understanding the implications of the test results. Case studies, with representative data and graphics, are included to help relate the tests to real pulmonary disorders. Multiple-choice self-assessment questions and selected references follow.

CASE STUDIES

CASE 2-1

HISTORY

L.L. is a 21-year-old male in good health who plays college football. His chief complaint is shortness of breath after wind sprints and similar vigorous exercises. L.L. denies any other symptoms, including cough or sputum production. He has never smoked. His grandfather had lung problems, but there is no other history of pulmonary disease involving the family. He states that his brothers and sisters have hay fever. There is no history of exposure to environmental pollutants.

PULMONARY FUNCTION TESTING

Personal Data

Sex: Male
Age: 21 yr
Height: 73 in
Weight: 180 lb

Spirometry and Airway Resistance

	Predrug	Pred	% Pred	Postdrug	% Pred	Δ (%)
FVC (L)	6.85	6.04	111	6.73	111	−2
FEV_1(L)	4.65	4.78	97	5.45	114	17
$FEV_{1\%}$(%)	70	79	—	81	—	
$FEF_{25\%-75\%}$(L/sec)	3.9	5	78	4.88	97	25
MVV (L/min)	218	166	131	215	130	−1
Raw (cm H_2O/L/sec)	2.1	0.6-2.4	—	1.6	—	−24
SGaw (L/sec/cm H_2O/L)	0.14	0.20	—	0.22	—	57

TECHNOLOGIST'S COMMENTS

All FVC efforts performed acceptably. All tests meet ATS criteria. Body plethysmograph efforts were reproducible.

QUESTIONS

1. What is the interpretation of:
   - Prebronchodilator spirometry?
   - Response to bronchodilator?
   - Airway resistance and conductance?
2. What is the cause of the patient's symptoms?
3. What other tests might be indicated?
4. What treatment might be recommended based on these findings?

DISCUSSION

Interpretation

All spirometry efforts before and after bronchodilator therapy were performed acceptably. All body box maneuvers were acceptable. Spirometry results are within normal limits except for a decrease in the $FEV_{1\%}$. There is a significant increase in the FEV_1, $FEV_{1\%}$, and $FEF_{25\%-75\%}$ after administration of the bronchodilator. MVV is normal, as are Raw and SGaw. Raw and SGaw also show significant improvement after bronchodilator therapy.

Impression: Mild obstructive defect with significant response to bronchodilator. Evaluation for exercise-induced bronchospasm may be indicated.

Cause of Symptoms

This patient has normal or slightly above average values for most of his lung function parameters. The exception is his $FEV_{1\%}$. It is below the expected value, consistent with mild obstruction. Simply evaluating FVC and FEV_1 compared with predicted values might give the impression that he is normal. The $FEV_{1\%}$ indicates that the patient, whose FVC is slightly larger than normal, expired a disproportionately small FEV_1. This pattern of supranormal volumes with lower than normal $FEV_{1\%}$ is sometimes seen in healthy young adults. The slightly decreased values for $FEF_{25\%-75\%}$ suggest an obstructive process (Figure 2-20). There is a 17% increase (0.8 L) in FEV_1 after administration of a bronchodilator. This response is significant in view of the patient's complaint of shortness of breath after exercise. He appears to have reversible airway obstruction triggered by exercise.

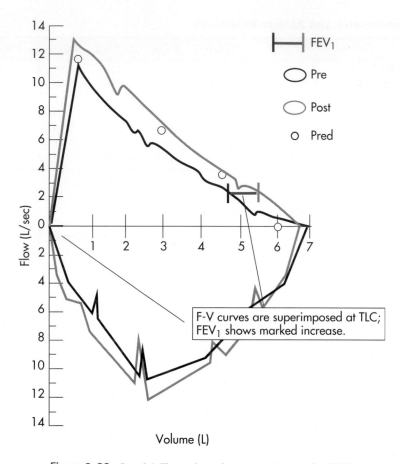

Figure 2–20   *Case 2-1.* Flow-volume loops superimposed at TLC.

Other Tests

Further evaluation of L.L. included an exercise test to demonstrate exercise-induced asthma (EIA). He jogged for 6 minutes on a treadmill at 85% of his predicted maximal heart rate. Upon completing the exercise, L.L.'s FEV_1 began to decrease. Five minutes after stopping the test, his FEV_1 decreased to 4.1 L. Scattered wheezes were heard on auscultation. The obstruction was readily reversed by inhaled bronchodilator. Inhalation-challenge testing was deferred because the obstructive defect was obvious after the exercise test.

Treatment

The patient was given a regimen of inhaled bronchodilators plus cromolyn sodium. He was given a portable peak flow meter to monitor his lung function. He reported marked decrease in symptoms by pretreating himself with the inhaled medication before athletic activities.

CASE 2-2

HISTORY

R.Z. is a 47-year-old carpenter whose chief complaint is shortness of breath on exertion. His dyspnea, although worse recently, has been present for several years. He smoked $1\frac{1}{2}$ packs of cigarettes per day for 32 years (48 pack years). He has a cough in the morning. He says that he produces a "small amount of grayish sputum." R.Z.'s father had tuberculosis. A sister had asthma as a child and now as an adult. He denies any extraordinary exposure to environmental dusts or fumes.

PULMONARY FUNCTION TESTING

Personal Data

Sex: Male
Age: 47 yr
Height: 70 in
Weight: 190 lb

Spirometry and Airway Resistance

	Predrug	Pred	% Pred	Postdrug	% Pred	% Chg
FVC (L)	4.01	4.97	81	4.49	90	12%
FEV_1 (L)	2.05	3.67	56	2.20	6	7%
$FEV_{1\%}$ (%)	51	74	—	49	—	−4%
$FEF_{25\%-75\%}$ (L/sec)	1.2	3.69	33	1.3	35	8%
$\dot{V}max_{50}$ (L/sec)	1.35	5.54	24	2.67	30	98%
$\dot{V}max_{25}$ (L/sec)	0.55	2.58	21	1.02	40	85%
MVV (L/min)	71	136	52	85	63	20%
Raw (cm H_2O/L/sec)	3.1	0.6-2.4	—	2.9	—	−6%
SGaw (L/sec/cm H_2O/L)	0.07	0.20	—	0.11	—	57%

TECHNOLOGIST'S COMMENTS

All tests met ATS criteria. All body plethysmograph efforts were performed acceptably.

QUESTIONS

1. What is the interpretation of:
   - Prebronchodilator spirometry?
   - Response to bronchodilator?
   - Airway resistance and conductance?

2. What is the cause of the patient's symptoms?
3. What other tests might be indicated?
4. What treatment might be recommended based on these findings?

DISCUSSION

Interpretation

All spirometry efforts were acceptable. All body-box efforts were reproducible. The patient has a reduced FEV_1, but his FVC is only slightly decreased. $FEF_{25\%-75\%}$ is decreased, as are $\dot{V}_{max\ 50}$ and $\dot{V}_{max\ 25}$. MVV is reduced in proportion to the patient's FEV_1. Raw is greater than the reference value, and SGaw is below the lower limit of normal. Little or no change occurs in FEV_1 after inhaled bronchodilator therapy. FVC does improve significantly. SGaw is significantly better after bronchodilator.

Impression: Moderately severe airway obstruction with significant improvement in vital capacity and airway conductance after inhaled bronchodilator.

Cause of symptoms

R.Z. is a smoker who has developed moderate airway obstruction. His spirometry results reveal the extent of the obstruction: FEV_1, 56% of predicted; $FEF_{25\%-75\%}$, 33% of predicted; and MVV, 52% of predicted. The FVC, however, is relatively well preserved. It even increases by more than 200 ml and 12% after bronchodilator therapy. The $FEF_{25\%-75\%}$ must always be interpreted cautiously because it is variable even in normal patients. The 95% confidence limits for this patient include values from 1.45 to 5.93 L/sec. (See Appendix B for predicted values and the standard error of estimate.) His $FEF_{25\%-75\%}$ is well below the lower limit. MVV is reduced as might be expected, almost exactly 35 times his FEV_1. This indicates that the patient made a consistent effort on both the FEV_1 and MVV.

Raw is above the upper normal limit of 2.4 cm H_2O/L/sec. This is consistent with moderate airway obstruction and a productive cough. Specific conductance is quite low, consistent with increased Raw and increased lung volumes.

FEV_1 does not improve significantly after bronchodilator therapy. The $FEV_{1\%}$ actually decreases as a result of the greater increase in FVC. This pattern is not unusual in patients with obstructive airway disease. Airway resistance falls slightly with inhaled bronchodilator therapy. Most notably, SGaw improves by 57%. The large increase in conductance with only marginal change in flow suggests a shift in lung volumes. Figure 2-21 shows F-V curves plotted at absolute lung volumes (measured in the body-box). Improvement in flow is evident by noting the curves at any particular lung volume.

Other postbronchodilator changes are also important. MVV improves by 20%. This may be related to a change in lung volume. The $FEF_{25\%-75\%}$ is hardly changed after bronchodilator therapy. This pattern is often seen when the FVC improves. A larger FVC means the time required to exhale the middle half of the breath may be longer. Because the $FEF_{25\%-75\%}$ depends on the FVC, the calculated flow may not improve; it may even go down.

Other tests

The lung function of this patient is common in both emphysema and chronic bronchitis. Air trapping is consistent with emphysematous changes but may be present in bronchitis and asthma during acute exacerbations. Further evaluation of R.Z. included measurement of lung volumes, DL_{CO}, and blood gas analysis. The findings from each of these additional tests were consistent with the results of his spirometry. He had some air trapping, which might explain the improved FVC after bronchodilator therapy. Blood gases and diffusing capacity were relatively normal.

Treatment

A combination of bronchodilators and inhaled steroids was prescribed. The patient was also referred to a counselor for smoking cessation and successfully quit smoking. His cough gradually subsided during a 6-month period. The patient noted a marked improvement in his dyspnea.

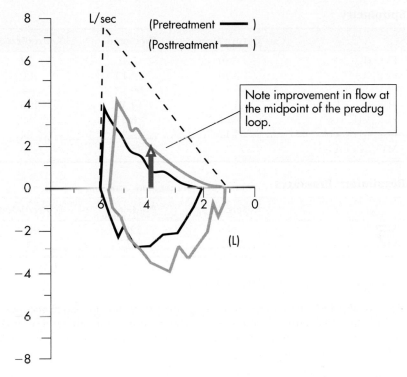

Figure 2–21 *Case 2-2.* Isovolume flow-volume loops. Each loop is plotted at the absolute lung volume at which it was measured. The increase in $FEF_{50\%}$ accurately describes the degree of bronchodilator response.

CASE 2-3

HISTORY

P.W. is a 27-year-old auto mechanic referred to the pulmonary function laboratory by his private physician. His chief complaint is "breathing problems." He describes breathlessness that occurs suddenly and then subsides. He has no other symptoms and no history of lung disease. None of his immediate family has any lung disease. He has smoked one pack of cigarettes per day for the past 10 years (10 pack years). He has no unusual environmental exposure. He claims that gasoline fumes sometimes bring on the episodes of shortness of breath.

PULMONARY FUNCTION TESTS

Personal Data

Sex: Male
Age: 27 yr
Height: 68 in
Weight: 150 lb

Spirometry

	Before Drug	Predicted	% Predicted
FVC (L)	3.80	5.15	74
FEV_1 (L)	3.70	4.13	90
$FEV_{1\%}$ (%)	97	80	—
$FEF_{25\%-75\%}$ (L/sec)	4.62	4.49	103
$FEF_{50\%}$ (L/sec)	4.81	6.01	80
$FEF_{75\%}$ (L/sec)	3.12	3.33	94
MVV (L/min)	77	146	53

Respiratory Pressures

	Before Drug	Predicted	% Predicted
MIP cm H_2O	118	128	92
MEP cm H_2O	57	240	24

TECHNOLOGIST'S COMMENTS

None of the FVC maneuvers were acceptable; they did not last 6 seconds or show an obvious plateau. Best FVC values were not within 200 ml. Inspiratory efforts were variable. A total of eight maneuvers were attempted. Respiratory pressure measurements were variable. The patient had difficulty completing all maneuvers.

QUESTIONS

1. What is the interpretation of:
   - Spirometry
   - Low value for MEP
   - Variability of the patient's efforts
2. What is the cause of the patient's symptoms?
3. What other tests might be indicated?
4. What treatment might be recommended based on these findings?

DISCUSSION

Interpretation

All spirometry maneuvers and respiratory pressures are unacceptable because of poor patient effort or technical errors. The patient's best effort shows a reduced FVC. The FEV_1 is normal, and the $FEV_{1\%}$ is above the expected range. All other flows and the MVV are within normal limits.

Impression: Spirometry results are inconsistent. The FVC and FEV_1 are not reproducible. Inadequate patient effort or technical errors are present.

Cause of symptoms

This test shows poor reproducibility, especially for effort-dependent measurements. Figure 2-22 shows the variability for three FVC maneuvers. The tracings show incomplete exhalations, as well as variability.

The low FVC seems to be consistent with a mild restrictive process. The FEV_1, however, is close to normal. If simple restriction were present, both FVC and FEV_1 should be reduced similarly. The

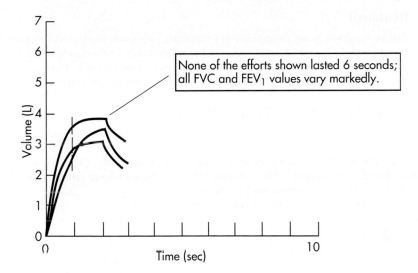

Figure 2-22 *Case 2-3.* Multiple FVC maneuvers are superimposed. None of the recorded efforts are acceptable.

patient's other flows are normal. Flows that depend on the FVC (e.g., the $FEF_{25\%-75\%}$) might also be in error if the FVC is incorrect. The FEV_1 and MVV do not depend on the FVC. The MVV is much less than 35 times the FEV_1, so the MVV is probably not accurate.

Because of the low MVV, respiratory pressures were measured. MIP appears to be normal but was variable. MEP was also performed variably. The best effort was only 24% of expected. Both MEP and MIP depend largely on patient effort.

Examination of the volume-time spirograms reveals that the patient terminated each FVC maneuver after approximately 2 seconds. The FVC values all varied by more than 200 ml, confirming poor patient cooperation. Lack of reproducibility of the FVC maneuvers is not sufficient reason for discarding the test results. This patient's FVC maneuvers lasted only 2 seconds, despite repeated coaching by the technologist. The efforts did not meet the criteria of continuing for at least 6 seconds or showing an obvious plateau. Failure to exhale completely is one of the most common errors in spirometry. This error may be caused by lack of cooperation on the part of the patient or inability to continue exhalation due to cough. It may also occur if the technologist does not adequately explain or demonstrate the maneuver.

The technologist performing this test repeated the FVC maneuver eight times. Only the three best efforts were recorded. Appropriate comments were added at the end of the test data. The poor quality of the data makes it impossible to determine whether the patient's symptoms are real. The patient appears to be malingering; that is, not giving maximal effort on tests that are effort dependent. Poor reproducibility in a patient who is free of symptoms at the time of the test suggests poor effort or lack of cooperation.

Other tests

Alternative tests for this patient should be independent of patient effort. A simple blood gas analysis was performed. The results indicated normal oxygenation and acid-base status. Testing of lung volumes and diffusing capacity was postponed because both of these depend on patient effort and cooperation. A *bronchial challenge* test (see Chapter 9) might have been indicated because the patient had asthma-like symptoms. However, bronchial challenge tests use spirometry, which this patient was unable or unwilling to perform acceptably.

Treatment

Before suggesting any treatment, the referring physician contacted the patient's employer to ask about possible environmental hazards that might cause the symptoms. He learned that the patient was facing possible termination for excessive absence from work. The patient's supervisor revealed that the patient claimed to have asthma, which caused his excessive absenteeism.

▨ SELF-ASSESSMENT QUESTIONS

Entry-level

1. *A patient performs three FVC maneuvers using a computerized spirometer. The spirometer reports that the third maneuver had a "back-extrapolated volume of 6%." The technologist should:*

   a. Report only the first two maneuvers
   b. Correct the volume of the last maneuver by 6%
   c. Perform at least one more maneuver
   d. Report the largest FVC value

2. *A 44-year-old woman who complains of shortness of breath has the following spirometry results:*

	Measured	Predicted
FVC (L BTPS)	4.11	4.01
FEV$_1$ (L BTPS)	2.23	3.33

   These results are consistent with which of the following?

   a. Restrictive lung disease
   b. Obstructive lung disease
   c. Normal lung function
   d. Erroneously reported FVC

3. *A 75-year-old man performs three acceptable spirometry efforts, and records these results:*

	Measured	Predicted
FVC (L BTPS)	2.75	4.58
FEV$_1$ (L BTPS)	2.42	3.44

   Which of the following do these values suggest?

   a. Normal spirometry for an elderly man
   b. A restrictive pattern
   c. Severe obstruction
   d. Incorrect predicted values

4. *Which of the following best describes the flow-volume curve shown?*

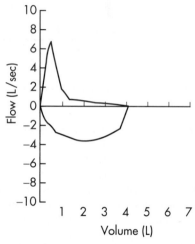

   a. Normal forced expiratory flow pattern
   b. Variable intrathoracic obstruction
   c. Small airway obstruction
   d. Fixed large airway obstruction

5. *An adult patient has spirometry before and after inhaled bronchodilators. The following data are obtained:*

	Predicted	Before Drug	After Drug
FVC	4.10	4.12	4.72
FEV$_1$	3.60	2.68	3.03
PEF	8.84	7.77	7.89

   Which of the following statements best describes these findings?

   a. There is a paradoxical response to bronchodilators
   b. Spirometry is within normal limits

c. There is mild obstruction with significant response to bronchodilators

d. There is mild obstruction without significant response to bronchodilators

6. *A patient with a history of asbestos exposure performs spirometry and records these values:*

	Predicted	Before Drug	% Pred
FVC	4.54	4.44	98
FEV₁	3.22	3.12	97
PEF	9.04	9.46	105
MVV	125	86	69

Based on these results, the technologist should:

a. Question the accuracy of the PEF

b. Question the accuracy of the MVV

c. Perform a bronchodilator study

d. Measure MIP and MEP

7. *How long before bronchodilator studies should slow-release methylxanthines be withheld?*

a. 4 hours

b. 8 hours

c. 12 hours

d. 24 hours

Advanced

8. *A 14-year-old male with cystic fibrosis performs three spirometry trials:*

	Trial 1	Trial 2	Trial 3
FVC (L BTPS)	3.01	2.99	3.12
FEV₁ (L BTPS)	1.99	2.01	1.95

The pulmonary function technologist should do which of the following?

a. Report the trial with the largest sum of FVC and FEV₁

b. Perform at least one more maneuver

c. Report the largest FVC and FEV₁

d. Report the values from trial three

9. *In which of the following conditions would an abnormal MIP and MEP be expected?*

I. Severe emphysema

II. Myasthenia gravis

III. Asthma

IV. Kyphoscoliosis

a. I and IV only

b. II and III only

c. I, II, and IV

d. II, III, and IV

10. *A patient with asthma has her Raw and SGaw measured in a plethysmograph. Which of the following values is most consistent with her disease?*

	Raw	SGaw
a.	1.1	0.23
b.	2.8	0.09
c.	2.1	0.24
d.	2.9	0.19

11. *A patient with pulmonary fibrosis has a compliance study performed. Which of the following indicate that the esophageal balloon is placed correctly?*

a. Only 0.5 ml of air is needed to inflate the catheter balloon

b. Inspiration causes a negative pressure deflection

c. Cardiac pulsations are recorded by the pressure transducer

d. No pressure change occurs during inspiration

12. *A patient performs an airway resistance maneuver in a body plethysmograph. His Raw is measured as 0.89 cm H_2O/L/sec at a thoracic gas volume of 3.65 L. The SGaw for this effort would be:*

a. 0.27 cm H_2O/L/sec/L

b. 0.31 cm H_2O/L/sec/L

c. 1.12 cm H_2O/L/sec/L

d. 4.10 cm H_2O/L/sec/L

13. *A healthy, physically fit patient performs spirometry, and the following values are recorded:*

	Trial 1	Trial 2	Trial 3
FVC (L BTPS)	6.52	6.23	6.34
FEV₁ (L BTPS)	5.01	5.22	5.19

What FEV1% should be reported for this patient?

a. 77%
b. 80%
c. 82%
d. 84%

14. *A patient, whose chief complaints are cough and hoarseness, performs a series of FVC efforts, and flow-volume curves are recorded. The following data are reported:*

	Trials				
	1	2	3	4	5
FVC (L)	4.10	4.12	4.20	4.18	3.99
PEF (L/sec)	9.2	9.0	9.5	9.1	8.9
$FEF_{50\%}/FIF_{50\%}$	1.55	1.45	1.60	1.57	1.49

From these data, the pulmonary function technologist should conclude that

a. Severe small airway obstruction is present
b. The patient was malingering
c. Variable intrathoracic obstruction is present
d. Variable extrathoracic obstruction is present

SELECTED BIBLIOGRAPHY

General References

Crapo RO: Pulmonary function testing, *N Engl J Med* 331:25-30, 1994.

Ferguson GT, Enright PL, Buist SA, et al: Office spirometry for lung health assessment in adults: a consensus statement from the National Lung Health Education Program, *Chest* 117:1146-1161, 2000.

Forster RE: *The lung: clinical physiology and pulmonary function tests,* ed 3, St Louis, 1986, Mosby.

West JB: *Pulmonary physiology and pathophysiology: an integrated, case-based approach,* Baltimore, 2001, Lippincott, Williams & Wilkins.

Spirometry

Aaron SD, Dales RE, Cardinal P: How accurate is spirometry at predicting restrictive pulmonary impairment? *Chest* 115:869-873, 1999.

Dillard TA, Hnatiuk OW, McCumber TR: Maximum voluntary ventilation: spirometric determinants in chronic obstructive pulmonary disease patients and normal subjects, *Am Rev Respir Dis* 147:870-875, 1993.

Eaton T, Withy S, Garrett JE, et al: Spirometry in primary care practice: the importance of quality assurance and the impact of spirometry workshops, *Chest* 116:416-423, 1999.

Enright PL, Linn WS, Avol EL, et al: Quality of spirometry test performance in children and adolescents: experience in a large field study, *Chest* 118:665-671, 2000.

Knudson, RJ, Lebowitz MD: Maximal mid-expiratory flow ($FEF_{25\%-75\%}$): normal limits and assessment of sensitivity, *Am Rev Respir Dis* 117:609, 1978.

Krowka MJ, Enright PL, Rodarte JR, et al: Effect of effort on measurement of forced expiratory volume in one second, *Am Rev Respir Dis* 136:829, 1987.

Leuallen EC, Fowler WS: Maximal midexpiratory flow, *Am Rev Tuberculosis* 72:783, 1955.

Peak Expiratory Flow

Godfrey S: Monitoring asthma severity and response to treatment, *Respiration* 68:637-648, 2001.

Hankinson JL: Beyond the peak flow meter: newer technologies for determining and documenting changes in lung function in the workplace, *Occup Med* 15:411-420, 2000.

Kennedy DT: Selection of peak flowmeters in ambulatory asthma patients: a review of the literature, *Chest* 114:587-592, 1998.

Lebowitz MD: The use of peak expiratory flow rate measurements in respiratory disease, *Pediatr Pulmonol* 11:166-174, 1991.

Before- and After-Bronchodilator Studies

Brocklebank D, Ram F, Wright J, et al: Comparison of the effectiveness of inhaler devices in asthma and chronic obstructive airways disease: a systematic review of the literature *Health Technol Assess* 5:1-149, 2001.

Casaburi R, Adame D, Hong CK: Comparison of albuterol to isoproterenol as a bronchodilator for use in pulmonary function testing, *Chest* 100:1597-1600, 1991.

Dales RE, Spitzer WO, Tousignant P, et al: Clinical interpretation of airway response to a bronchodilator: epidemiologic considerations, *Am Rev Respir Dis* 138:317, 1988.

Guyatt GH, Townsend M, Nogradi S, et al: Acute response to bronchodilator, an imperfect guide for bronchodilator therapy in chronic airflow limitation, *Arch Intern Med* 148:1949, 1988.

Light RW, Conrad SA, George RB: The one best test for evaluating the effects of bronchodilator therapy, *Chest* 72:512, 1977.

Smith HR, Irvin CG, Cherniack RM: The utility of spirometry in the diagnosis of reversible airways obstruction, *Chest* 101:1577-1581, 1992.

Flow–Volume Curves

Acres J, Kryger M: Clinical significance of pulmonary function tests: upper airway obstruction, *Chest* 80:207, 1981.

Bass H: The flow volume loop: normal standards and abnormalities in chronic obstructive pulmonary disease, *Chest* 63:171, 1973.

Chan ED, Irvin CG: The detection of collapsible airways contributing to airflow limitation, *Chest* 107:856-859, 1995.

Haponik FF, Blecker ER, Allen RP, et al: Abnormal inspiratory flow-volume curves in patients with sleep disordered breathing, *Am Rev Respir Dis* 124:571, 1981.

Hyatt RE, Black LF: The flow volume curve, *Am Rev Respir Dis* 107:191, 1973.

Knudson RJ, Lebowitz MD, Holberg CJ, et al: Changes in the normal maximal expiratory flow-volume curve with growth and aging, *Am Rev Respir Dis* 127:725, 1983.

Knudson RJ, Slatin RC, Lebowitz MD, et al: The maximal expiratory flow-volume curve: normal standards, variability and effects of age, *Am Rev Respir Dis* 113:587, 1976.

Lunn WW, Sheller JR: Flow volume loops in the evaluation of upper airway obstruction, *Otolaryngol Clin North Am* 28:721-729, 1995.

Miller RD, Hyatt RE: Evaluation of obstructing lesions of the trachea and larynx by flow volume loops, *Am Rev Respir Dis* 108:475, 1973.

Maximal Respiratory Pressures

Aldrick TK, Spiro P: Maximal inspiratory pressure: does reproducibility indicate full effort? *Thorax* 50:40-43, 1995.

Black LF, Hyatt RE: Maximal static respiratory pressure in generalized neuromuscular disease, *Am Rev Respir Dis* 103:641, 1971.

Karvonen J, Soarelainen S, Nieminen MM: Measurement of respiratory muscle forces based on maximal inspiratory and expiratory pressures, *Respiration* 61:28-31, 1994.

Vincken GH, Cosio MG: Maximal static respiratory pressures in adults: normal values and their relationship to determinants of respiratory function, *Bull Eur Physiopathol Respir* 23:435, 1987.

Compliance and Airways Resistance

Baydur A, Behrakis PK, Zin WA, et al: A simple method for assessing the validity of the esophageal balloon technique, *Am Rev Respir Dis* 126:788, 1982.

Behrakis PK, Baydur A, Jaeger MJ, et al: Lung mechanics in sitting and horizontal body positions, *Chest* 83:643, 1983.

Dubois AB, Bothello SV, Comroe JH: A new method for measuring airway resistance in man using a body plethysmograph: values in normal subjects and in patients with respiratory disease, *J Clin Invest* 35:327, 1956.

National Heart and Lung Institute, Division of Lung Diseases: *Procedures for standardized measurements of lung mechanics: principles of body plethysmography*, Bethesda, Md, 1974, National Heart and Lung Institute, pp 1-21.

Standards and Guidelines

American Association for Respiratory Care: Clinical practice guidelines: assessing response to bronchodilator therapy at the point of care, *Respir Care* 40:1300-1307, 1995.

American Association for Respiratory Care: Clinical practice guidelines: body plethysmography, *Respir Care* 46:506-513, 2001.

American Association for Respiratory Care: Clinical practice guidelines: spirometry, *Respir Care* 41:629-636, 1996.

American Association for Respiratory Care: Clinical practice guidelines: static lung volumes, *Respir Care* 46:531-539, 2001.

American Thoracic Society: Lung function testing: selection of reference values and interpretative strategies, *Am Rev Respir Dis* 144:1202, 1991.

American Thoracic Society: Standardization of spirometry: 1994 update, *Am J Respir Crit Care Med* 152:1107-1136, 1995.

British Thoracic Society and the Association of Respiratory Technicians and Physiologists: Guidelines for the measurement of respiratory function, *Respir Med* 88:165-194, 1994.

National Asthma Education Program: *Expert panel report 2: guidelines for the diagnosis and management of asthma*, Bethesda, Md, 1997, Department of Health and Human Services (NIH Publication No. 97-4051).

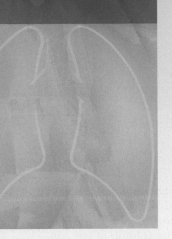

CHAPTER 3

LUNG VOLUMES AND GAS DISTRIBUTION TESTS

OBJECTIVES

After studying this chapter and reviewing its tables and case studies, you should be able to do the following:

Entry-level

1. Describe the measurement of lung volumes using open-circuit and closed-circuit methods
2. Explain two advantages of measuring lung volumes using the body plethysmograph
3. Calculate residual volume and total lung capacity from FRC and the subdivisions of VC
4. Identify restriction from measured lung volumes

Advanced

1. Calculate FRC using open circuit and closed-circuit methods
2. Describe the correct technique for measuring V_{TG}
3. Identify air trapping and hyperinflation using measured lung volumes
4. Identify uneven distribution of gas in the lungs by either single- or multiple-breath techniques.

This chapter introduces the measurement of lung volumes. Some gas remains in the lungs even after the vital capacity (VC) has been exhaled. This gas volume must be measured indirectly. Several methods can accomplish this. Each method has its own advantages and disadvantages. Two methods involve having the patient breathe gases not normally present in the lungs: helium (closed-circuit) or 100% oxygen (open-circuit). These techniques are sometimes referred to as dilutional lung volumes. A third method uses the body plethysmograph to measure the volume of thoracic gas (V_{TG}). The gas dilution techniques can also provide information about the distribution of gas in the lungs. Nuclear medicine imaging of the lungs, computerized tomography (CT), and *magnetic resonance imaging (MRI)* all provide a direct view of the distribution of ventilation in the lungs. Nonetheless, gas distribution indices obtained during lung volume determination are often helpful.

LUNG VOLUMES

Functional Residual Capacity, Residual Volume, Total Lung Capacity, and Residual Volume/Total Lung Capacity Ratio

■ DESCRIPTION

Functional residual capacity (FRC) is the volume of gas remaining in the lungs at the end of a quiet breath. On a simple spirogram, this point is termed the end-expiratory level (see Figure 2-1). Residual volume (RV) is the volume of gas remaining in the lungs at the end of a maximal expiration (see Figure 2-1). Total lung capacity (TLC) is the volume of gas contained in the lungs after maximal inspiration. FRC, TLC, and RV are reported in liters or milliliters, corrected to BTPS. The RV/TLC ratio defines the fraction of TLC that cannot be exhaled (RV), expressed as a percentage.

■ TECHNIQUE

Various methods of measuring lung volumes are available (Table 3-1). Although some methods estimate TLC directly, FRC is usually measured. RV, which is a component of the FRC, is also measured indirectly. RV cannot be exhaled; it is the volume remaining in the lungs after the airways have closed. Once FRC has been measured, RV can be calculated by subtracting expiratory reserve volume (ERV) obtained from simple spirometry. The end-expiratory level is the point in the breathing cycle to which the lungs and chest wall recoil after a quiet breath.

TABLE 3-1 Methods for Measurement of Lung Volumes

Method	Lung Volume	Advantages/Disadvantages
Closed-circuit (He dilution; multiple-breath)	FRC	Simple, relatively inexpensive; affected by distribution of ventilation in moderate or severe obstruction; requires IC, ERV to calculate other lung volumes
Open-circuit (multiple-breath N_2 washout)	FRC	Simple, relatively inexpensive; affected by distribution of ventilation in moderate or severe obstruction; requires IC, ERV to calculate other lung volumes
Single-breath N_2 washout	TLC	Calculated from single-breath N_2 distribution test; may underestimate lung volume in the presence of obstruction
Single-breath He dilution	TLC	Calculated as part of DL_{CO} (V_A); may underestimate lung volume in the presence of obstruction
Plethysmograph	V_{TG} (FRC)	Plethysmographic method somewhat complex; not affected by degree of airway obstruction
Chest x-ray	TLC	Requires posterior-anterior and lateral chest films; not accurate in the presence of diffuse, space-occupying diseases

N_2, Nitrogen; *IC,* inspiratory capacity; DL_{CO}, diffusing capacity; V_A, alveolar volume.

This point can be easily identified by recording tidal breathing using a spirometer. Measurements of FRC are usually started with the patient at the end-expiratory level.

Two methods of measuring FRC use gases not normally present in the lungs. These methods are sometimes referred to as gas dilution techniques. The open-circuit or nitrogen (N_2) washout method uses 100% O_2. The closed-circuit or helium dilution technique uses a low concentration of He in air.

Open-Circuit Method (Multiple-Breath Nitrogen Washout)

The concentration of N_2 in the lungs is presumed to be between 75% and 80%. After the patient breathes 100% O_2 for several minutes, the N_2 in the lungs is gradually washed out. Because not all N_2 can be washed out, the test is usually continued until the alveolar N_2 concentration is approximately 1%. Historically, all exhaled gas was collected in a spirometer or bag that had been flushed with O_2. The concentration of collected N_2 was then measured. The volume that was in the lungs at the end-expiratory level was then computed using the following formula:

$$FRC = \frac{F_E N_{2final} \times Expired\ volume - N_{2tissue}}{F_A N_{2alveolar1} - F_A N_{2alveolar2}}$$

where:

$F_E N_{2final}$ = fraction of N_2 in volume expired
$F_A N_{2alveolar1}$ = fraction of N_2 in alveolar gas initially
$F_A N_{2alveolar2}$ = fraction of N_2 in alveolar gas at end (from an alveolar sample)
$N_{2tissue}$ = volume of N_2 washed out of blood/tissues

Corrections must be made for N_2 washed out of the blood and tissue. For each minute of O_2 breathing, approximately 30 to 40 ml of N_2 are removed from blood and tissue. $N_{2tissue} = 0.04 \times T$ (where T is time of the test). This value is subtracted from the total volume of N_2 washed out. Not all of the N_2 in the lungs may be washed out, even after 7 minutes of O_2 breathing. The $F_A N_{2alveolar2}$ is measured by taking an alveolar sample near the end of the test. This value is subtracted from alveolar N_2 present at the beginning of the test. The final FRC is then corrected to BTPS (see Appendix F for a sample calculation).

To obtain RV, the ERV determined from a slow vital capacity maneuver (see Chapter 2) is subtracted from the FRC:

$$RV = FRC - ERV$$

Alternatively, the total lung capacity (TLC) can be calculated, and RV determined by subtracting the largest VC (see Total Lung Capacity and Residual Volume/Total Lung Capacity Ratio section).

A common method currently used for open-circuit FRC measurement uses a rapid N_2 analyzer in combination with a spirometer to provide a "breath-by-breath" analysis of expired N_2 (Figure 3-1, *A*). An alternate approach is to use fast-response O_2 and CO_2 analyzers to calculate the concentration of N_2 in expired gas during the washout:

$$N_2 = 1 - F_E O_2 - F_E CO_2$$

where:

$F_E O_2$ = fraction of O_2 in expired gas (dry)
$F_E CO_2$ = fraction of CO_2 in expired gas (dry)

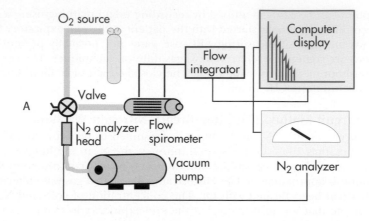

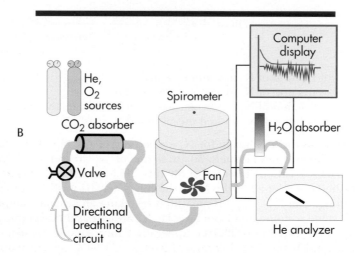

Figure 3-1 *Open-circuit and closed-circuit FRC systems.* **A,** Open-circuit equipment used for N_2 washout determination of FRC. The patient inspires O_2 from a regulated source and exhales past a rapidly responding N_2 analyzer into a pneumotachometer. Flow and gas concentration are integrated and displayed on a computer screen. FRC is calculated from the total volume of N_2 exhaled and the change in alveolar N_2 from the beginning to the end of the test (Figure 3-2 and Open-Circuit Method). **B,** Closed-circuit equipment used for He dilution FRC determination includes a volume-based spirometer with He analyzer, CO_2 absorber, and a directional breathing circuit. A fan or blower promotes gas mixing within the rebreathing system. A breathing valve near the mouth allows the patient to be "switched in" to the system after He has been added and the system volume determined. The O_2 source allows the addition of O_2 during the test to replenish that taken up by the patient and to maintain a constant system volume. The CO_2 absorber permits rebreathing without accumulation of CO_2. Water vapor is removed by a chemical absorber before the gas is sampled by the He analyzer. Tidal breathing and the He dilution curve are displayed on the computer.

The patient breathes through a mouthpiece-valve system. Precisely at end-expiration, a valve is opened to allow O_2 breathing to begin. Each breath of pure O_2 washes out some of the residual N_2 in the lungs. *Analog signals* proportional to N_2 concentration and volume (or flow) are integrated to derive the volume of N_2 exhaled for each breath. Values for each breath are summed to provide a total volume of N_2 washed out (Figure 3-2). The test is

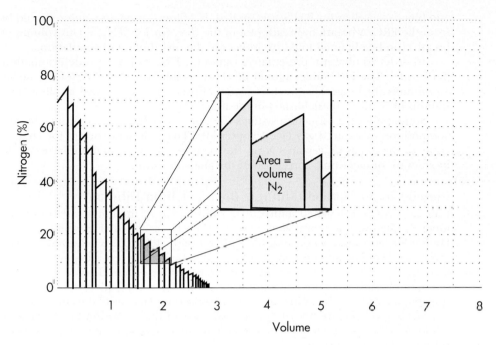

Figure 3-2 *Open-circuit (N$_2$ washout) determination of FRC.* The concentration (or log concentration) of N$_2$ is plotted against time or against the volume expired as the patient breathes through a circuit (Figure 3-1, *A*). The volume of N$_2$ expired with each breath is measured by integrating flow and N$_2$ concentration to determine the area under each curve (see *inset*). The volume of N$_2$ expired for each breath is summed. The test continues until most of the N$_2$ in the lung has been washed out (usually 1.5% or less). FRC is determined by dividing the volume of N$_2$ expired by the change in alveolar N$_2$ from the beginning to the end of the test, with corrections, as described in the text.

LUNG VOLUMES 3-1   Criteria for Acceptability—N$_2$ Washout FRC

1 The washout tracing or display should indicate a continually falling concentration of alveolar N$_2$.
2 The test should be continued until the N$_2$ concentration falls to 1.0%.
3 Washout times should be appropriate for the type of subject tested. Healthy subjects should wash out N$_2$ completely in 3 to 4 minutes.
4 The washout time should be reported. Failure to wash out N$_2$ within 7 minutes should be noted.
5 Multiple measurements should agree within 10%; the average FRC from acceptable trials should be used to calculate lung volumes. At least 15 minutes of room-air breathing should elapse between repeated trials.

---

continued until the N$_2$ in alveolar gas has been reduced to approximately 1% (Lung Volumes 3-1). Some older systems terminate the test at 7 minutes. Ideally, oxygen breathing should be continued until alveolar N$_2$ falls to less than 1.0%.

FRC is calculated by dividing the volume of N$_2$ washed out by the difference in N$_2$ concentration from the beginning to the end of the test. Corrections for N$_2$ excretion from tissue and blood, as well as for BTPS, are applied. If a filter is used, its volume should be subtracted from the FRC. A breath-by-breath plot of the $\%N_2$ (or log $\%N_2$) versus volume or number of breaths can be obtained to derive indices of the distribution of ventilation.

In order to obtain representative values for FRC, at least two determinations should be performed. The FRC values should be reproducible to within 10% of the mean. A delay of 15 minutes (or longer) between repeated efforts is recommended to allow normal concentrations of N_2 to be reestablished in the lungs, blood, and tissues.

Some pulmonary function systems use pneumotachometers that may be sensitive to the composition of expired gas (see Chapter 10). These devices correct for changes in the viscosity of the gas as O_2 replaces N_2 in the expirate. Such corrections are easily accomplished by software or electronic correction of the analyzer output.

Closed-Circuit Method (Multiple-Breath Helium Dilution)

FRC can also be calculated indirectly by diluting gas in the lungs with an inert gas. A spirometer is filled with a known volume of air, then He is added (Figure 3-1, *B*). The volume of He is adjusted so that a concentration of approximately 10% is achieved. The exact concentration and volume are measured and recorded before the test is begun. The patient respires through a valve that allows connection to a rebreathing system. The valve is opened at the end of a quiet breath (i.e., the end-expiratory level). Then the patient rebreathes the gas in the spirometer, with a carbon dioxide (CO_2) absorber in place, until the concentration of He falls to a stable level (Figure 3-3). A fan or blower mixes the gas within the spirometer system. O_2 is added to the spirometer system to maintain the FIO_2 near or above 0.21 and to keep system volume relatively constant.

An older closed-circuit method (i.e., the *bolus* method) added a large volume of O_2 to the spirometer at the beginning of the test. The patient then rebreathed and gradually consumed the O_2. Because of the possibility of equilibrium not being attained before the added O_2 was depleted, this method is no longer used.

Equilibration between normal lungs and the rebreathing system takes place in approximately 3 minutes when a 10% He mixture in a system volume of 6 to 8 L is used (Figure 3-4). The final concentration of He is then recorded. The system volume is computed first. System volume is the volume of the spirometer, breathing circuitry, and valves before the patient is connected. It can be calculated as follows:

$$\text{System volume (L)} = \frac{\text{He}_{\text{added}}(\text{L})}{F_{\text{He initial}}}$$

where:
He_{added} = volume of He placed in the spirometer
$F_{\text{He initial}}$ = %He converted to a fraction (%He/100)
When the system volume is known, FRC can be computed as follows:

$$\text{FRC} = \frac{(\%\text{He}_{\text{initial}} - \%\text{He}_{\text{final}})}{\%\text{He}_{\text{final}}} \times \text{System volume}$$

Either percent or *fractional* concentration of He may be used because the term is a ratio.

Some automated systems use a similar method to calculate the system volume; a small amount of He is added to the closed system, followed by a known volume of air. The change in He concentration after the addition of the air is used to determine the system volume.

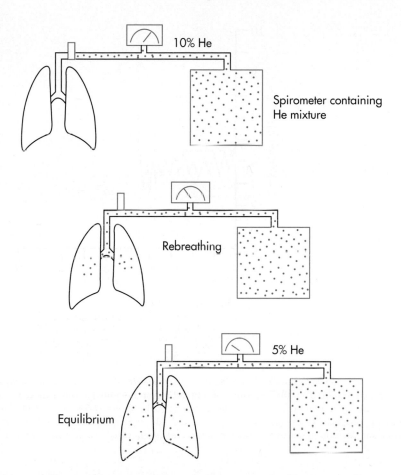

Figure 3-3 *Closed-circuit (He dilution) determination of FRC.* At the beginning of the test, the patient's lungs contain no He. The spirometer contains a known concentration of He in a known volume (see text). The patient then rebreathes the He mixture from this system (Figure 3-1, *B*). He is diluted until equilibrium is reached. At the end of the test, the known volume of He has been diluted in the rebreathing system and the lungs. FRC is calculated from the change in He concentration and the known system volume. The patient must be switched from breathing air to the He mixture at the end-expiratory level for accurate measurement of FRC. RV is derived by subtracting the ERV. (Modified from Comroe JH Jr, Forster RE, Dubois AB, et al: *The lung: clinical physiology and pulmonary function tests,* ed 2, St Louis, 1962, Mosby.)

Rebreathing is continued until the He concentration changes by no more than 0.02% in 30 seconds (Lung Volumes 3-2).

Several corrections are often made to the FRC value obtained by He dilution. A small volume of He dissolves in the patient's blood during the test. The final He reading is less than it would be due solely to dilution by the patient's FRC. Loss of He to the blood results in a negligible increase in the apparent FRC. A volume of 100 ml is sometimes subtracted from the FRC to correct for this effect. The dead space volume of the breathing valve should also be subtracted from the measured FRC. If a filter is used, its volume must also be subtracted.

Most manufacturers provide "switch-in" error correction when the patient begins the test at a point either above or below the actual end-expiratory level (FRC). This type of correction

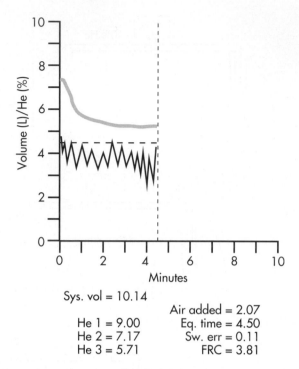

Sys. vol = 10.14

	Air added = 2.07
He 1 = 9.00	Eq. time = 4.50
He 2 = 7.17	Sw. err = 0.11
He 3 = 5.71	FRC = 3.81

Figure 3-4 *Computer-generated recording of closed-circuit FRC determination in a healthy patient.* Graph shows He concentration from the beginning of rebreathing until equilibrium is achieved *(upper line)*. System volume of the spirometer and the patient's tidal breathing is also shown *(lower line)*. A CO_2 absorber removes carbon dioxide produced by the patient. A computerized valve system replaces O_2 to keep the system volume constant. Measurements of He concentrations and system variables are also displayed.

LUNG VOLUMES 3-2   Criteria for Acceptability—He Dilution FRC

1 A tracing or display of spirometer volume should indicate that no leaks are present (system baseline flat). He concentration should be stable before testing.
2 The rebreathing pattern should be regular. If recorded, successive tidal breaths should show a gradually falling end-tidal level as O_2 is consumed. Addition of O_2 should return breathing to close to the system baseline.
3 The test should be continued until the He readings change by less than 0.02% in 30 seconds or until 10 minutes has elapsed.
4 Addition of O_2 should be appropriate for quiet tidal breathing (i.e., 200-400 ml/min).
5 The He equilibration curve, if plotted or displayed, should show a smooth and regular fall of He concentration until equilibrium is achieved.
6 Multiple measurements of FRC should agree within 10%; the average of acceptable multiple measurements should be reported.

is used for both open-circuit and closed-circuit systems. Depending on the patient's breathing pattern, a volume difference of several hundred milliliters may result. The effect of the switch-in error may be insignificant, especially with the closed-circuit method. Equilibrium does not occur instantaneously at switch-in. The total volume of spirometer and lungs is constantly changing with tidal breathing, removal of CO_2, and addition of O_2. If the switch-in error is large or the end-expiratory level appears to change during the maneuver, the test may need to be repeated.

In the gas dilution techniques, RV is measured indirectly as a subdivision of the FRC. This method is preferred because the resting end-expiratory level depends less on patient effort than on maximal inspiration or expiration. The end-expiratory level (and the ERV) must be accurately measured. If tidal breathing is irregular, ERV may be overestimated or underestimated. Subtraction of an ERV value that is too large from the FRC will cause the RV to appear smaller than it actually is. Similarly, a small ERV will produce a larger than actual RV. The patient's tidal breathing pattern must be carefully monitored during the vital capacity (VC) measurement (see Chapter 2).

The accuracy of the gas dilution techniques depends on all parts of the lung being well ventilated. In patients who have obstructive disease, some lung units are poorly ventilated. In these patients, it is often difficult to wash N_2 out or mix He to a stable level in poorly ventilated parts of the lungs. FRC, RV, and TLC may all be underestimated, usually in proportion to the degree of obstruction. Extending the time of these tests improves their accuracy. However, prolonging the test may not measure completely trapped gas, as found in *bullous* emphysema. As for the open-circuit method, two or more closed-circuit FRC measurements should be averaged. Repeat determinations should be reproducible to within 10% of the mean. For He dilution, at least 5 minutes should elapse between repeated tests.

The graphic method of displaying breath-by-breath N_2 washout provides a means of quantifying the evenness of ventilation. Some systems plot the logarithm of the N_2 concentration against time or volume exhaled. The slope of the washout curve is determined by the FRC, tidal volume, dead space volume, and frequency of breathing. If N_2 is washed out of the lungs evenly, the log N_2 plot appears as a straight line. Because the lung is not perfectly symmetric, the washout curve is slightly concave. The deviation from the expected curve indicates the extent to which ventilation is uneven. Washout should be complete within 3 to 4 minutes in healthy patients. The time to reach He equilibrium during the closed-circuit FRC determination can also be used as an index of distribution of ventilation. By simply recording the time to reach equilibrium and plotting the dilution curve, an estimate of the evenness of ventilation is obtained. In healthy patients, either type of gas dilution should be complete in 3 to 4 minutes. Use of gas dilution techniques to assess distribution has been replaced by ventilation scans using radioisotopes, as well as by CT scanning.

The gas dilution techniques of measuring lung volumes usually *underestimate* lung volumes in the presence of moderate or severe obstruction. Both methods (open and closed) are also subject to leaks in their respective breathing circuits. Leaks usually cause the measured lung volume to be *overestimated.*

In either of the gas dilution techniques, a leak will cause erroneous estimates of FRC. Leaks may occur in breathing valves or circuitry, or at the patient connection. Some patients have difficulty maintaining an adequate seal at the mouthpiece throughout the test. Failure to properly apply nose clips can also result in a leak. Leaks usually result in an overestimate

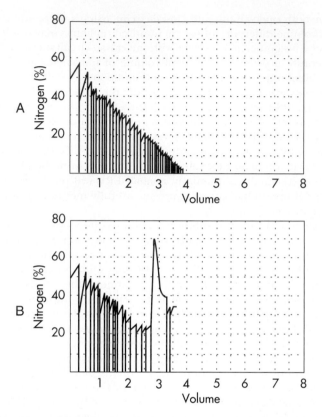

Figure 3-5 *Open-circuit N_2 washout tracings*. **A,** A computer-generated recording of an N_2 washout test in a healthy patient. The tracings show a continuous decrease in end-tidal N_2 concentration with successive breaths. The test is continued until the N_2 concentration falls to less than 1%. **B,** A similar plot of N_2 washout from a healthy patient, but in this instance a leak develops during the test. Leaks may occur if the patient does not maintain a tight seal at the mouthpiece. Leaks are usually easy to detect because room air enters the system and indicates an abrupt increase in N_2 concentration.

of lung volume. A leak in an open-circuit system allows room air to enter, increasing the volume of N_2 to be washed out. A leak in a closed-circuit system allows air to dilute the He concentration or He to escape. Each situation causes the test gas concentration to change more than it should. Leaks can usually be identified by inspection of the graphic display or recording (Figure 3-5). Inaccuracy or malfunction of the gas analyzers in either method often causes errors. Leaks or analyzer problems should be considered whenever FRC values are inconsistent with spirometry results.

Total Lung Capacity and Residual Volume/Total Lung Capacity Ratio

TLC is calculated combining other lung volume measurements. The two most common are as follows:

$$TLC = RV + VC$$

$$TLC = FRC + IC$$

Each method requires accurate measurement of the subdivisions of the VC. TLC can also be calculated using single-breath techniques (i.e., single-breath He dilution or single-breath N_2 washout). Single-breath measurements of lung volumes are usually done as part of other tests, such as the diffusing capacity (DL_{CO}) test (see Chapter 5). Single-breath lung volumes correlate well with multiple-breath techniques in healthy patients. However, single-breath lung volumes tend to underestimate true values in moderate to severe obstruction. TLC can also be measured from standard chest x-ray films, as well as from CT scans of the thorax.

The RV/TLC ratio is calculated by dividing the RV by the TLC. This ratio is expressed as a percentage. Either ATPS (ambient temperature, pressure, saturation) or BTPS values may be used in the ratio, but both RV and TLC must be expressed in the same units.

The FRC, RV, and TLC should be reported in liters or milliliters, BTPS. Barrier filters may be used during lung volume determinations, particularly in rebreathing systems. If a filter is used, its volume must be subtracted from the lung volume measured. Sample calculations of both the open-circuit and closed-circuit techniques can be found in Appendix F.

■ SIGNIFICANCE AND PATHOPHYSIOLOGY

See Lung Volumes 3-3 for interpretive strategies. FRC varies with body size, with change in body position, and with time of day (i.e., diurnal variation). As with other lung volumes, normal FRC may be affected by racial or ethnic background. Equations for calculating predicted FRC are found in Appendix B.

Increased FRC is considered pathologic. FRC values greater than approximately 120% of predicted values represent air trapping. Air trapping may result from emphysematous changes or from obstruction caused by asthma or bronchitis (see Chapter 1). Compensation for surgical removal of lung tissue or thoracic deformity can also cause increased FRC. Elevated FRC usually results in muscular and mechanical inefficiency of the respiratory apparatus. As lung volume increases, the chest wall and lungs themselves become "stiffer." This causes an increase in the work of breathing. FRC can increase dynamically; patients with airway obstruction may increase their end-expiratory lung volume (EELV) during exercise (see Chapter 7). This change in lung volume with increased ventilatory demand often results in a sensation of breathlessness.

The RV is the volume left in the lungs after the VC is exhaled. An increased RV indicates that despite maximal expiratory effort, the lungs contain a larger volume of gas than normal. Increased RV often results in an equivalent decrease in VC (Figure 3-6). Elevated RV may occur during an acute asthmatic episode but is usually reversible. Increased RV is characteristic of emphysema and bronchial obstruction; both may cause chronic air trapping. RV and FRC usually increase together. As RV becomes larger, increased ventilation is needed to adequately exchange O_2 and CO_2 in the lung. This requires an increase in tidal volume, respiratory rate, or both. Because of altered pressure-volume characteristics of the lung, work of breathing is also increased. Patients with increased RV often display gas exchange abnormalities such as hypoxemia or CO_2 retention.

FRC, RV, and TLC are typically decreased in restrictive diseases (see Chapter 1). Decreased lung volumes are seen in interstitial diseases associated with extensive fibrosis (e.g., sarcoidosis, asbestosis, and complicated silicosis). Restrictive disorders affecting the chest wall include kyphoscoliosis, neuromuscular disorders, and obesity. Diseases that impair the diaphragm often result in reduced lung volumes, particularly TLC. Lung volumes may also be decreased in diseases that occlude many alveoli, such as pneumonia. Congestive heart failure causes pulmonary congestion, which can also reduce lung volume. Any disease process that occupies volume in the thorax can reduce lung volume. Examples include tumors and pleural effusions.

LUNG VOLUMES 3-3   Interpretive Strategies—He Dilution FRC

1 Was the FRC determination performed acceptably? Were multiple trials performed? If so, were they within 10%?
2 Was the VC maneuver acceptable? Were the ERV and inspiratory capacity (IC) measurements within 5% or 60 ml?
3 Were other lung volumes calculated appropriately (TLC, RV)?
4 Are the reference values appropriate? Age, height, sex, race?
5 Is the TLC less than the lower limit of normal? If so, restriction is present. Are other lung volumes (FRC, RV) reduced in similar proportion?
6 Is the TLC greater than the upper limit of normal? If so, suspect hyperinflation.
7 Is the RV/TLC ratio greater than predicted ($\approx$35%)? Is the TLC normal or increased? If both are true, suspect air trapping.
8 Are lung volumes consistent with spirometric findings in regard to obstruction or restriction? Are they consistent with the history and physical findings?
9 Are additional tests indicated (plethysmographic lung volumes)?

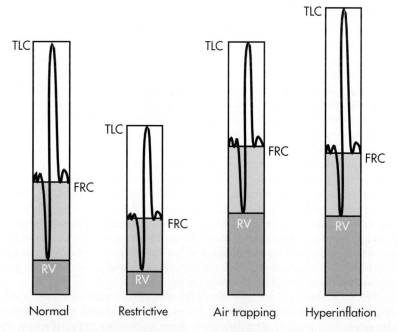

Figure 3-6 *Lung volumes in normal, restrictive, and obstructive patterns.* A comparison of changes in lung volume compartments and VC *(superimposed)* shows the following: in restrictive patterns FRC, RV, and VC are all decreased proportionately, resulting in a decrease in the TLC, which defines restriction (see text). In obstruction (with air trapping) FRC and RV are both increased at the expense of the VC, and hence TLC remains relatively unchanged. Similar increases in RV and FRC may occur without reduction of VC, in which case the TLC increases (hyperinflation).

TABLE 3-2 Comparative Lung Volumes for a Healthy Adult Male and Patients with Air Trapping, Hyperinflation, and Restriction

Value	Normal	Air Trapping	Hyperinflation	Restriction
VC (L)	4.80	3.00	4.80	3.00
FRC (L)	2.40	3.60	3.60	1.50
RV (L)	1.20	3.00	3.00	0.75
TLC (L)	6.00	6.00	7.80	3.75
RV/TLC (%)	20	50	38	20

Table 3-2 lists comparative lung volumes for a healthy adult male and for patients with air trapping (as in emphysema), hyperinflation, and restriction (as in sarcoidosis). Restrictive processes usually cause lung volumes to be reduced equally. Proportional relationships between lung volume compartments, such as the RV/TLC ratio, may be relatively normal in restrictive diseases.

In obstruction, two different patterns may be observed. RV is usually increased. This increase may be at the expense of a reduction in VC (Figure 3-6), with TLC remaining close to normal. In other cases, RV may increase while VC is preserved, so TLC is greater than predicted. The term *air trapping* is sometimes used to describe an increase in FRC and RV, and the term *hyperinflation* is used to describe the absolute increase in TLC. TLC may be either normal or increased in obstructive processes such as asthma, chronic bronchitis, bronchiectasis, cystic fibrosis, and emphysema. TLC does not appear to change dynamically, even though FRC may increase acutely during exercise.

PF *Tips*

Total lung capacity (TLC) is an important diagnostic tool in both obstructive and restrictive lung diseases. In restriction, the TLC is usually less than 80% of the predicted value, or below the lower limit of normal (LLN). In obstruction, the TLC is either normal or increased (hyperinflation).

Processes that occupy space in the lungs such as edema, atelectasis, neoplasms, or fibrotic lesions may decrease TLC. Other diseases that commonly result in decreased TLC include pulmonary congestion, pleural effusions, pneumothorax, or thoracic deformities. Pure restrictive defects show proportional decreases in most lung compartments as described for FRC and RV. When the TLC value is less than 80% of predicted, or less than the 95% confidence limit, a restrictive process is present. Reduced VC along with a normal or increased FEV_1/FVC ratio (see Chapter 2) is suggestive of restriction, but a measurement of TLC is needed to confirm the diagnosis of a restrictive defect.

The RV/TLC ratio describes the percentage of total lung volume that must be ventilated by tidal breathing. In healthy adults, the RV/TLC ratio may vary from 20% in young adults to 35% in older patients. Values greater than 35% may result from absolute increases of RV (as in emphysema) or from a decrease in TLC because of a loss of VC. A large RV/TLC in the presence of increased TLC is often indicative of hyperinflation. An increased RV/TLC with a normal TLC indicates that air trapping is present.

Thoracic Gas Volume

■ DESCRIPTION

The thoracic gas volume (V_{TG}) is the gas contained in the thorax whether in communication with patent airways or trapped in any compartment of the thorax. V_{TG} is usually measured at the end-expiratory level and is then equal to FRC. It may also be measured at other lung volumes and then corrected to relate to FRC. The V_{TG} is reported in liters or milliliters, BTPS.

■ TECHNIQUE

V_{TG} is measured using the body plethysmograph (Figure 3-7). The technique is based on Boyle's law relating pressure to volume. A volume of gas varies in inverse proportion to the pressure to which it is subjected if the temperature remains constant. The patient has an unknown volume of gas in the thorax (i.e., the FRC). The airway is occluded momentarily, allowing the patient to compress and decompress gas in the chest by breathing in and out against the occlusion. This causes a change in volume and pressure. The changes in pressure are easily measured at the airway with a pressure transducer. Mouth pressure theoretically equals alveolar pressure when there is no airflow. Changes in pulmonary gas volume are estimated by measuring pressure changes in the plethysmograph (see Chapter 10). The pressure in the plethysmograph (sometimes called a body box) is measured by a sensitive transducer. This transducer is calibrated by introducing a small, known volume of gas into the sealed box and relating the pressure change to the known volume. The calibration factor is then applied to measurements made on human patients.

In the plethysmograph, the patient pants while an electrical or pneumatic shutter briefly occludes the airway. Gas within the chest is alternately compressed and decompressed by the action of the ventilatory muscles. When the shutter blocks flow, mouth pressure is presumed to equal alveolar pressure. Mouth pressure (P_{MOUTH}) is plotted on the vertical axis of a computer display. At the same time, box pressure (P_{BOX}) is plotted on the horizontal axis (Figure 3-7). Pressure changes on each axis are graphed continuously. The resulting figure appears as a sloping line equal to $\Delta P / \Delta V$, where ΔP equals change in alveolar pressure and ΔV equals change in alveolar volume. Change in alveolar volume is measured indirectly by noting the reciprocal change in plethysmograph volume.

The V_{TG} can then be obtained from the slope of the tracing by applying a derivation of Boyle's law:

$$V_{TG} = \frac{P_B}{\lambda V_{TG}} \times \frac{P_{BOX}cal}{P_{MOUTH}cal} \times K$$

where:

V_{TG} = thoracic gas volume
P_B = barometric pressure minus water vapor pressure
λV_{TG} = slope of the displayed line equal to $\Delta P / \Delta V$
$P_{BOX}cal$ = box pressure transducer calibration factor
$P_{MOUTH}cal$ = mouth pressure transducer calibration factor
K = correction factor for volume displaced by the patient

For the complete derivation of the equation and sample calculations, see Appendices E and F.

These measurements are usually made with the patient panting gently at a rate of approximately 1 breath/sec (1 Hz) with an open *glottis*. Panting allows small pressure changes to be

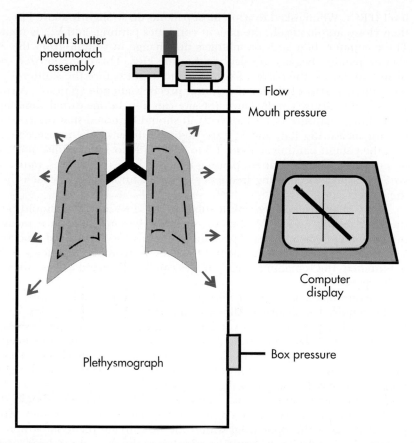

Figure 3-7 *Components of the body plethysmograph used to measure thoracic gas volume (V_{TG}).* Boyle's law states that volume varies inversely with pressure if temperature is held constant. A pressure-type (constant volume) plethysmograph, with pressure transducers for measurements of box pressure and mouth (alveolar) pressure, is shown. A pneumotachometer measures flow to track lung volumes. The mouth shutter occludes the airway momentarily so alveolar pressure can be estimated. The patient pants gently against the closed shutter. Gas in the lungs is alternately compressed and decompressed. Changes in lung volume are reflected by changes in box pressure. These changes are displayed as a sloping line on a computer display. When the original pressure (P), the new pressure (P′), and the new volume (V′ or V + ΔV) are known, the original volume (V or V_{TG}) can be computed from Boyle's law (see Thoracic Gas Volume—Technique and Appendix E).

recorded near FRC. It also eliminates some artifact related to gas temperature and saturation. Some plethysmograph systems allow V_{TG} measurements by occluding the airway during normal breathing without panting. If the mouth shutter is closed at precisely end-expiration, V_{TG} equals FRC. Several panting efforts are recorded to obtain an average for the slope of ΔP/ΔV. The averaged slope is then used in the previous equation to derive the V_{TG}.

Computerized plethysmograph systems permit monitoring of tidal breathing in conjunction with the V_{TG} maneuver. Instantaneous changes in lung volume can be monitored by continuously integrating the flow through the plethysmograph's pneumotachometer. The end-expiratory level can be determined from tidal breathing. The patient then pants with the shutter open. The computer records the change in lung volume above or below the resting level (FRC). When asked to pant, most patients do so slightly above FRC. The mouth shutter then closes automatically, the patient continues panting, and V_{TG} is measured as described. The computer then adds or subtracts the change in volume from the end-expiratory level (before panting began) to calculate the true FRC. This computerized technique allows the patient to pant at the correct frequency and depth before the shutter is closed. It also eliminates the necessity of closing the shutter precisely at end-expiration. Airway resistance (Raw) and specific airway conductance (SGaw) can also be measured simultaneously during the open-shutter panting (see Chapter 2). It should be noted that the correct panting frequencies for measuring Raw and V_{TG} are slightly different. Raw measurements should be made with the patient panting at about 1.5 to 2.5 Hz (90 to 150 breaths/min), whereas V_{TG} should be measured with the patient panting at about 1 Hz (60 breaths/min). Many computerized systems display the panting frequency so the technologist can coach the patient to achieve the correct rate.

A VC maneuver along with it subdivisions (ERV and IC) should be performed during the same testing session. Most plethysmograph systems allow these measurements using the built-in pneumotachometer. The same standards for accuracy should be applied to a slow VC measured in the plethysmograph as for any other spirometer. When FRC has been determined, the remaining lung volumes can be calculated as described for the gas dilution techniques.

Measurement of V_{TG} is a complex procedure. Each patient must be carefully instructed in the required maneuvers. Allowing the patient to sit in the box with the door open is helpful. A few patients may experience *claustrophobia* in the plethysmograph. The panting maneuver should be demonstrated by the technologist and then practiced by the patient. The patient should be instructed to place both hands against the cheeks. This prevents unwanted pressure changes in the mouth when the patient pants against the closed shutter. If practical, the shutter may be closed so that the patient knows what to expect during the test. The door of the plethysmograph can then be closed. The patient should understand that the plethysmograph can be opened if he or she becomes uncomfortable. Most systems allow the patient to open the door from within the box. If the plethysmograph is equipped with a communication device, it should be adjusted so the patient can hear instructions.

Depending on the construction of the plethysmograph, venting to the atmosphere is usually required to establish thermal equilibrium. Equilibrium can be presumed when the flow-volume recording stabilizes (i.e., does not drift). The patient is then instructed to pant at a frequency of approximately 1 Hz (i.e., once per second). When the correct panting frequency and depth have been established, the shutter may be closed. Some plethysmograph systems require tidal breathing prior to shutter closure to establish the patient's end-expiratory level. In either type of system, the patient should pant against the closed shutter until a stable tracing is produced. Two to four pants are usually sufficient. If the patient pants too hard, the tracing may drift or appear as an "open" loop (Figure 3-8). The recorded pressure changes should be within the range over which the transducers were calibrated. The entire tracing should be visible on the display. If the tracing goes off-screen, the pressure changes probably exceed the calibration ranges.

The tangents (slopes) from three or more maneuvers should be recorded (Lung Volumes 3-4). These tangents should agree within 10% of their mean. Most computerized plethysmographs automatically measure the slope of the $\Delta P/\Delta V$ tracings. This is done by using the least-squares method to calculate a "best-fit" line through the recorded data points. The technologist may need to correct computer-generated tangents, depending on data quality from the panting maneuvers. If the shutter is closed at volumes other than FRC, the tangents may vary by more than 10%. However, derived lung volumes (i.e., the FRC) should be within 10%.

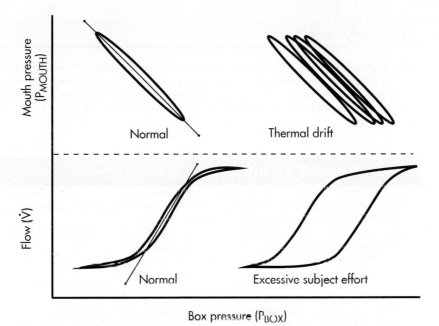

Figure 3-8 *Normal and abnormal plethysmograph recordings.* *Top,* Normal closed-shutter maneuver in which mouth pressure is plotted against box pressure. The loop should be closed, or nearly so. If thermal equilibrium has not been achieved, the loop tends to be open and to drift across the screen. *Bottom,* Normal open-shutter measurement in which flow is plotted against box pressure. If the patient pants near FRC, the loop takes on a nearly closed S-shaped appearance. If the patient pants too rapidly or too deeply, the tracing becomes open and flattened. Thermal drift can also cause the open-shutter tracing to resemble excessive patient effort.

Lung Volumes 3-4   Criteria for Acceptability—V_{TG}

1 The planting maneuver shows a closed loop without drift or other artifact.
2 Pressure changes are within calibration ranges; the tracing does not go off-screen.
3 Panting frequency is approximately 1 Hz, preferably recorded.
4 Tangents or angles should agree within 10%; if the shutter was closed at a volume other than FRC, calculated FRC values should be within 10%.
5 Reported V_{TG} is averaged from three to five acceptable panting maneuvers.

The technologist's comments should note the acceptability of the maneuvers. V_{TG} should be determined from three or more acceptable maneuvers. If the tangents or volumes vary by more than 10%, this too should be noted. Comparing lung volumes determined by two or more methods is sometimes useful. The difference between lung volumes (FRC) measured using the plethysmograph and a gas dilution method may be used as an index of gas trapping. This difference can be significant in patients with airway obstruction. Plethysmographic lung volumes are usually larger in these patients.

Plethysmography offers several advantages over other methods of measuring lung volumes. V_{TG} is not affected by the distribution of ventilation. Multiple measurements can be made quickly and averaged. It provides a more accurate estimate of lung volumes in patients who have airway obstruction. In addition, Raw and SGaw can be measured in the same testing session.

LUNG VOLUMES 3-5   Interpretive Strategies—V_{TG}

1 Were the panting maneuvers performed acceptably? Was the panting frequency appropriate (1 Hz)? If not, interpret results cautiously.
2 Were at least three maneuvers averaged to obtain V_{TG} or FRC? Were individual values reproducible (within 10%)? If not, interpret cautiously.
3 Are reference values appropriate? Age, height, weight, race? Were they obtained plethysmographically?
4 Were other lung volumes (TLC) calculated appropriately? Were VC, ERV, and IC acceptable? IF not, evaluate only FRC.
5 If the TLC is less than the lower limit of normal, suspect restriction.
6 If the TLC is greater than the upper limit of normal, suspect hyperinflation.
7 Are lung volumes consistent with spirometric findings? If not, evaluate carefully for combined obstruction and restriction.

■ SIGNIFICANCE AND PATHOPHYSIOLOGY

See Lung Volumes 3-5 for interpretive strategies. The V_{TG} is a quick and accurate means of measuring lung volumes. It can be used in combination with simple spirometry to derive all lung volume compartments. The plethysmograph's primary advantage is that it measures all gas in the thorax, whether in ventilatory communication with the atmosphere or not. The plethysmographic measurement of FRC is often larger than that measured by He dilution or N_2 washout. This is the case in emphysema and other diseases characterized by air trapping, as well as in the presence of uneven distribution of ventilation. When gas dilution tests are continued for more than 7 minutes, the results for FRC determinations approach the V_{TG} value.

It is often useful to compare FRC values obtained by plethysmography with values obtained by gas dilution methods, particularly in patients with obstructive disease. The ratio of FRC_{BOX}/FRC_{GAS} can be used as an index of gas trapping. This ratio is usually near 1.0 in patients with normal lungs, or even with restriction. Values greater than 1 indicate gas volumes detectable by the plethysmograph but hidden to the gas techniques. Care must be taken that lung volumes determined by the two separate methods are reliable before the values can be expressed as a ratio. This ratio has been used to evaluate candidates for lung volume reduction surgery (LVRS). Lung volume reduction attempts to directly reduce gas trapping by removal of unperfused lung tissue. Patients with bullous emphysema may have a liter or more difference in TLC when the methods are compared.

Some evidence suggests that in severe airways obstruction, FRC may actually be overestimated when the plethysmographic technique is used. This occurs primarily because P_{MOUTH} (measured when the shutter is closed) may not equal alveolar pressure if the airways are severely obstructed. Rapid panting rates aggravate this inaccuracy. Care should be taken that patients with spirometric evidence of obstruction pant at a rate of 1 Hz or less.

Spirometry (e.g., FVC, FEV_1, and VC) may be performed with the patient in the plethysmograph. The pneumotachometer must be capable of accurately measuring the entire range of gas flows required (i.e., up to 12 L/sec). Two varieties of body boxes are commonly used: constant-volume and flow-based (see Chapter 10). For constant-volume plethysmographs, spirometry is done with the door open. Flow-based plethysmographs have the advantage of allowing forced spirometry with the door closed. Flow boxes also allow a slightly different type of flow-volume curve to be recorded. Normal spirometry plots airflow at the mouth against volume at the mouth (as detected by the spirometer). With the patient in a flow box, flow at the mouth can be plotted against actual lung volume changes as detected by the box. This may be particularly useful in patients with severe airway obstruction. It is possible to detect a significant compression volume during forced expiration and plot it against the flow generated. Spirometry, lung volumes, and airway resistance (see Chapter 2) can all be obtained in a single sitting using either type of plethysmograph.

GAS DISTRIBUTION TESTS

Single–Breath Nitrogen Washout, Closing Volume, and Closing Capacity

■ DESCRIPTION

The single-breath nitrogen washout test (SBN_2) measures the distribution of ventilation. Distribution is analyzed by measuring the change in N_2 concentration during expiration of the VC after a single breath of 100% O_2. Evenness of distribution is assessed by two parameters: the change in percentage of N_2 between the 750 to 1250 ml portion of the SBN_2 test ($\Delta\%N_{2\ 750\text{-}1250}$) and the slope of phase III of the expiratory tracing. Each of these indices is recorded as a percent. Closing volume (**CV**) is the portion of the VC that can be exhaled from the lungs after the onset of airway closure. CV is also measured from the SBN_2 maneuver and is usually expressed as a percentage of the VC. A related measurement, *closing capacity (CC)*, is the sum of the CV and RV. CC is expressed as a percentage of the TLC.

■ TECHNIQUE

The test is performed with equipment similar to that used for the open-circuit FRC determination (Figure 3-1, *A*). The patient exhales to RV, then inspires a VC breath of 100% O_2 from a reservoir or demand valve. Without holding the breath, the patient exhales slowly and evenly at a flow of 0.3 to 0.5 L/sec. The N_2 analyzer monitors the N_2 concentration of the expired gas, while the exhaled volume is measured by the spirometer. Volume expired is plotted against N_2 concentration on a graph (Figure 3-9). This washout curve can be divided into four phases:

Phase I: upper airway gas from the anatomic dead space (V_{Danat}), consisting of 100% O_2
Phase II: mixed dead space gas in which the relative concentrations of O_2 and N_2 change abruptly as the V_{Danat} volume is expired
Phase III: a plateau caused by the exhalation of alveolar gas in which relative O_2 and N_2 concentrations change slowly and evenly
Phase IV: an abrupt increase in the concentration of N_2 that continues until RV is reached

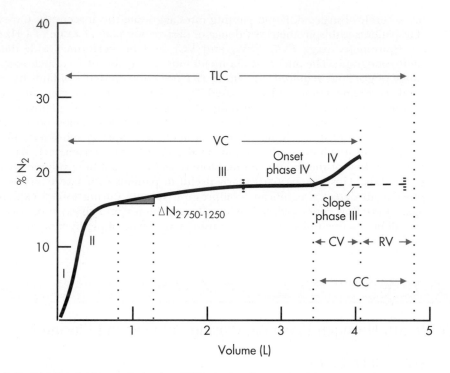

Figure 3-9 *Single-breath nitrogen elimination (SBN$_2$).* A plot of increasing N$_2$ concentration on expiration after a single VC breath of 100% O$_2$. The curve is divided into four phases. *Phase I* is the extreme beginning of the expiration, when only O$_2$ is being exhaled. *Phase II* shows an abrupt rise in N$_2$ concentration as mixed bronchial and alveolar air is expired. *Phase III* is the alveolar gas plateau. N$_2$ concentration changes slowly as long as ventilation is uniformly distributed. *Phase IV* is an abrupt increase in N$_2$ concentration as basal airways close and a larger proportion of gas comes from the N$_2$-rich lung apices. Several useful parameters are derived from the SBN$_2$ tracing. The ΔN$_{2\ 750\text{-}1250}$ and slope of phase III are indices of the evenness of ventilation distribution. CV can be read directly from the onset of phase IV until RV is reached; VC can also be read directly. RV, TLC, and CC can be calculated if the area under the curve is determined either by planimetry or electronic integration (see text).

The initial 750 ml of expired gas contains dead space gas from phases I and II and is not used to assess distribution of ventilation. The difference in N$_2$ concentration between the 750 ml and 1250 ml points is called the delta N$_2$ ($\Delta\%$N$_{2\ 750\text{-}1250}$).

The slope of phase III is the change in N$_2$ concentration from the point at which 30% of the VC remains up to the onset of phase IV. It is recorded as $\Delta\%$N$_2$ per liter of lung volume.

The volume expired after the onset of phase IV is the CV. CV may be added to the RV, if the RV has been determined, and expressed as the CC. CV is reported as a percentage of VC:

$$\frac{CV}{VC} \times 100$$

CC is recorded as a percentage of TLC:

$$\frac{CC}{TLC} \times 100$$

Lung Volumes 3-6   Criteria for Acceptability—SBN₂

1 Inspired and expired VC should be within 5% or 200 ml.
2 The VC during SBN₂ should be within 200 ml of a previously determined VC.
3 Expiratory flow should be maintained between 0.3 and 0.5 L/sec.
4 The N₂ tracing should show minimal cardiac oscillations.

TLC can be determined from the SBN₂ test by integrating the area of the washout curve. When the volume of N_2 is known, a dilution equation can be used to calculate RV. RV is then added to the measured VC to derive TLC. RV is calculated as follows:

$$RV = VC \times \frac{F_{\bar{E}}N_2}{F_A N_2 - F_{\bar{E}}N_2}$$

where:
$F_{\bar{E}}N_2$ = mean expired N_2 concentration determined by integration of the area under the curve
$F_A N_2$ = N_2 concentration in the lungs at the beginning of inspiration, approximately 0.75 to 0.79

This method is accurate only in patients who do not have significant obstruction or dead space–producing disease. CV and CC measurements may be in error if the patient does not perform an acceptable VC maneuver (Lung Volumes 3-6). The inspired and expired VC should be within 5%. The VC during the SBN₂ should match the FVC or VC within 5% or 200 ml. Expiratory flow should be maintained between 0.3 and 0.5 L/sec.

■ SIGNIFICANCE AND PATHOPHYSIOLOGY

See Lung Volumes 3-7 for interpretive strategies.

Δ%N₂ 750-1250
The normal $\Delta\%N_{2\ 750\text{-}1250}$ is 1.5% or less for healthy young adults and slightly higher for healthy older adults (up to approximately 3%). Increased $\Delta\%N_{2\ 750\text{-}1250}$ is found in diseases characterized by uneven distribution of gas during inspiration or unequal emptying rates during expiration. In patients with severe emphysema, $\Delta\%N_{2\ 750\text{-}1250}$ may exceed 10%.

Slope of Phase III
A best-fit line is drawn through the phase III segment of the tracing from the point where 30% of the VC remains above RV to the onset of phase IV. The slope of this line is an index of gas distribution, similar to the $\Delta\%N_{2\ 750\text{-}1250}$. Values in healthy young adults range from 0.5% to 1.0% N_2/L of lung volume, with wide variability. Very slow expiratory flow rates may cause oscillations in the tracing of phase III, making the accurate measurement of $\Delta\%N_2$ difficult. These oscillations are attributed to changes in alveolar N_2 concentrations as blood pulses through the pulmonary capillaries during cardiac systole. Increasing the expiratory flow rate slightly eliminates this artifact. Patients who have small VC values may have difficulty exhaling enough gas to make the $\Delta\%N_2$ or slope of phase III meaningful.

Other gases, such as He or sulfur hexafluoride (SF_6), may also be used to assess the distribution of ventilation. The slope of the alveolar phase using these gases may be useful in

Lung Volumes 3-7   Interpretive—SBN$_2$

1. Was the test performed acceptably? VC reproducible within 5% or 200 ml? Expiratory flow appropriate?
2. Are reference values appropriate? Age, height, sex, race?
3. Is $\Delta\%N_{2\ 750\text{-}1250}$ greater than 1.5%? If so, suspect uneven distribution of ventilation.
4. Is slope of Phase III greater than 1.0% to 1.5%? If so, there is uneven distribution of ventilation.
5. Is CV/VC% greater than 20% (or age-related expected value)? If so, suspect small airway abnormalities. Correlate with clinical findings.

detecting early changes in the small airways. Detecting these changes may identify bronchiolitis obliterans in double–lung transplant recipients.

Closing Volume and Closing Capacity

After maximal expiration by an upright patient, more RV remains at the apices of the lungs than at the bases. Gravity causes this difference. When the test gas (O_2) is inspired, the apices receive the gas occupying the patient's dead space, which consists mostly of N_2. O_2 then goes preferentially to the bases of the lungs. Gas concentrations in the lungs become widely different. The apices contain RV gas plus dead space gas rich in N_2. The bases of the lungs contain a higher concentration of the test gas O_2. Compression of the airways during the subsequent expiration causes airways to narrow and then close, as lung volume approaches RV. Airways at the bases close first because of gravity and the weight of the lung in patients sitting upright. As airways at the bases close, proportionately more gas comes from the apices. This appears as an abrupt rise in the concentration of N_2—the onset of phase IV.

The onset of phase IV marks the lung volume at which airway closure begins. The point at which this occurs in the VC depends on the caliber of the small airways. In healthy young adults, airways begin closing after 80% to 90% of the VC has been expired. This equates to a CC in healthy young adults of approximately 30% of the TLC, with wide variations. CV and CC may be increased, indicating earlier onset of airway closure in:

- Elderly patients
- Restrictive disease patterns in which the FRC becomes less than the CV
- Smokers and other patients with early obstructive disease of small airways
- Congestive heart failure when the caliber of the small airways is compromised by edema

Patients with moderate or severe obstructive disease may have no sharp inflection separating phases III and IV of the SBN$_2$. This lack of a clear point of airway closure is the result of grossly uneven distribution of gas in the lungs. Patients who have airway obstruction typically show greater than normal values for the $\Delta\%N_{2\ 750\text{-}1250}$ and slope of phase III.

In some patients with no pulmonary disease, the onset of phase IV cannot be accurately determined. Because of the variability in both the CV and CC, the mean of three tests is usually reported. Because of its poor reproducibility, the CV test is not widely used. Although it appears to be a sensitive indicator of abnormalities in the small airways, particularly in smokers, an increased CV/VC ratio is not highly predictive of which individuals will develop chronic airway obstruction. To calculate normal values for CV/VC and CC/TLC according to age and sex, see Appendix B.

Summary

This chapter describes the various methods of measuring lung volumes, particularly total lung capacity (TLC). In order to measure TLC, the functional residual capacity (FRC) is measured first. FRC can be measured using either an open-circuit or closed-circuit gas dilution technique. The open-circuit technique uses an N_2 washout of gas in the lungs, whereas the closed-circuit technique utilizes equilibration of He between the lungs and a spirometer. FRC may also be determined by measuring the volume of thoracic gas (V_{TG}) in a body plethysmograph. TLC is then calculated by adding the inspiratory capacity (IC, measured from simple spirometry) to the FRC. Alternatively, the expiratory reserve volume (ERV, also measured by simple spirometry) may be subtracted from FRC to derive RV. The addition of RV and VC (from spirometry) also provides an estimate of TLC. The plethysmographic technique is the preferred method because it is largely independent of gas distribution in the lungs. Gas dilution techniques may underestimate lung volumes in the presence of significant airway obstruction. Gas dilution techniques, along with analysis of N_2 after a single breath of oxygen (SBN_2), provide a qualitative means of assessing gas distribution in the lungs.

CASE STUDIES

CASE 3-1

HISTORY

M.B. is a 27-year-old male high school teacher whose chief complaint is dyspnea on exertion. He states that his breathlessness has worsened over the past several months. He has smoked one pack of cigarettes per day for 10 years (10 pack years). He denies a cough or sputum production. No one in his family ever had emphysema, asthma, chronic bronchitis, carcinoma, or tuberculosis. There is no history of exposure to extraordinary environmental pollutants.

PULMONARY FUNCTION TESTING

Personal Data

Sex:	Male
Age:	27 yr
Height:	65 in
Weight:	297 lb
Body surface area (BSA):	2.28 M^2

Spirometry and Airway Resistance

	Before Drug	Predicted	%
FVC (L)	2.9	4.7	62
FEV_1 (L)	2.47	3.86	64
$FEV_{1\%}$ (%)	85	82	—
$FEF_{25\%-75\%}$ (L/sec)	4.62	4.35	106
$FEF_{50\%}$ (L/sec)	4.94	5.82	85
MVV (L/min)	178	130	137
Raw (cm H_2O/L/sec)	2.33	0.6-2.4	—
SGaw (L/sec/cm H_2O/L)	0.23	0.12-0.50	—

Lung Volumes (by Plethysmograph)

	Before Drug	Predicted	%
VC (L)	2.9	4.7	62
IC (L)	1.96	2.91	67
ERV (L)	0.94	1.8	59
FRC (L)	1.87	3.29	57
RV (L)	0.93	1.49	57
TLC (L)	3.83	6.2	62
RV/TLC (%)	25	24	—

QUESTIONS

1. What is the interpretation of:
   - Spirometry?
   - Lung volumes?
   - Airway resistance?
2. What is the cause of the patient's symptoms?
3. What other tests might be indicated?
4. What treatment might be recommended based on these findings?

DISCUSSION

Interpretation

All data from spirometry and lung volumes are acceptable. Spirometry shows a decreased FVC and FEV_1. The $FEV_{1\%}$ is normal. Flows are within normal limits, as is the maximal voluntary ventilation (MVV). Raw is near the upper limit of normal, but SGaw is normal. Lung volumes are decreased, with the RV/TLC ratio preserved.

Impression: Moderate restrictive lung disease without evidence of obstruction. The restrictive pattern may be related to the patient's weight. Recommend arterial blood gas testing to evaluate gas exchange abnormalities.

Cause of symptoms

This case is a good example of what might be considered a pure restrictive defect. A proportional decrease in all lung volumes, including FVC and FEV_1, is characteristic of a restrictive process. Flows such as $FEF_{25\%-75\%}$ or $FEF_{50\%}$ show little or no decrease (Figure 3-10). In addition, characteristic of simple restriction is the well-preserved ratio of FEV_1 to FVC. The volume expired in the first second was in correct proportion to the VC, despite decreases in their absolute volumes. The MVV demonstrates the patient's ability to move a normal maximal volume. This may be accomplished despite moderately severe restriction by an increase in the rate rather than the tidal volume.

The explanation for the restrictive pattern lies in the patient's weight of 297 pounds. His actual weight is approximately 200% of his ideal weight. Obesity commonly causes restrictive patterns.

Other tests

The patient returned for analysis of arterial blood gases, which revealed resting hypoxemia and slightly elevated $PaCO_2$. Blood gas measurements confirmed the degree of impairment caused by the moderately severe restrictive pattern. Other tests that might be considered include ventilatory response tests for hypoxemia or hypercapnia (see Chapter 4). Studies to diagnose *sleep apnea* might

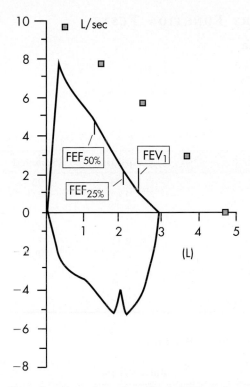

Figure 3-10 *Case 3-1.* Flow-volume loop from the patient. Upward tick mark superimposed on the loop denotes the FEV_1, whereas downward tick marks show $FEF_{50\%}$ and $FEF_{25\%}$, respectively. Small, shaded boxes represent the patient's reference values.

be indicated if the patient had symptoms of disordered breathing during sleep or excessive daytime sleepiness. This patient's borderline Raw suggests upper airway involvement, which might predispose him to obstructive sleep apnea.

Treatment

The patient was referred to a dietician for counseling in weight management.

CASE 3-2

HISTORY

R.B. is a 37-year-old pipe fitter whose chief complaint is shortness of breath at rest and with exertion. His dyspnea has worsened in the past 6 months, so much so that he is no longer able to work. Additional symptoms include a dry cough. He admits some sputum production when he has a chest cold. He has smoked one pack of cigarettes per day for 19 years (19 pack years). He quit smoking approximately 3 weeks before the tests. His father died of emphysema, and his mother of lung cancer. His brother is in good health. His occupational exposure includes working for the past 13 years in the assembly room of a boiler plant. He admits to seldom using the respirators provided at work despite a dusty environment.

PULMONARY FUNCTION TESTS

Personal Data

Sex: Male
Age: 37 yr
Height: 69 in
Weight: 143 lb

Spirometry

	Before Drug	Predicted	%	After Drug	%
FVC (L)	3.04	5.05	10	3.1	61
FEV_1 (L)	2.03	3.90	52	2.26	58
$FEV_{1\%}$ (%)	67	77	—	73	—
$FEF_{25\%-75\%}$ (L/sec)	1.3	4.09	32	1.60	39
$FEF_{50\%}$ (L/sec)	2.12	5.78	37	2.42	42
$FEF_{25\%}$ (L/sec)	0.78	2.95	26	1.2	41
MVV (L/min)	83	141	59	91	65
Raw (cm H_2O)/L/sec)	2.51	0.6-2.4	—	2.47	—
SGaw (L/sec/cm H_2O/L)	0.14	0.11-0.44	—	0.15	—

Lung Volumes (by N_2 Washout)

	Before Drug	Predicted	%
VC (L)	3.04	5.05	60
IC (L)	1.62	3.18	51
ERV (L)	1.42	1.87	76
FRC (L)	2.75	3.81	72
RV (L)	0.33	1.94	69
TLC (L)	4.37	6.99	63
RV/TLC (%)	30	28	—

Technologist's Comments

Spirometry results met all American Thoracic Society (ATS) recommendations, prebronchodilator and postbronchodilator. Lung volumes by N_2 washout: all maneuvers were performed acceptably. Duplicate measurements were averaged. Raw and SGaw efforts were performed appropriately.

QUESTIONS

1. What is the interpretation of:
   - Prebronchodilator spirometry?
   - Response to bronchodilator?
   - Airway resistance and conductance?
   - Lung volumes?
2. What is the cause of the patient's symptoms?
3. What other tests might be indicated?
4. What treatment might be recommended based on these findings?

DISCUSSION

Interpretation

All data from spirometry and lung volumes are acceptable. Spirometry shows a reduced FVC and FEV_1. The $FEF_{25\%-75\%}$, $FEF_{50\%}$, and $FEF_{25\%}$ are all reduced. The MVV is low. Raw and SGaw are close to their respective limits of normal. Response to bronchodilators is borderline, with an increase in the FEV_1 of 230 ml (11%). The $FEF_{25\%}$ improved somewhat more than the other flows. The patient's lung volumes are all decreased. His RV/TLC ratio is normal.

Impression: There is moderate airway obstruction combined with a restrictive pattern. The response to inhaled bronchodilator medication is borderline. A trial of bronchodilators should be considered. Recommend arterial blood gas testing to evaluate possible hypoxemia.

Cause of symptoms

R.B. typifies a patient who has combined obstructive and restrictive disease. His spirometry results indicate that a serious obstructive component is present, as revealed by his FEV_1 (52% of predicted) and the other flows. His $FEV_{1\%}$, however, is close to normal because his FVC is also reduced. Airway narrowing as a result of restriction is sometimes responsible for decreased flows. This is particularly evident when restriction is severe. R.B.'s symptoms of cough and sputum suggest a genuine obstructive process. His smoking and family history place him at risk. Because FVC can be reduced in either obstructive or restrictive processes, spirometry alone would not have adequately defined the patient's disease.

Lung volume measurements (Figure 3-11) confirm the presence of a restrictive component (Figure 3-6). All lung volumes are reduced in similar proportions. The reduction in VC matches decreases in FRC, RV, and TLC. The patient's history and symptoms suggest the possibility of restrictive or obstructive disease, or both. The obstructive component may be related to the patient's

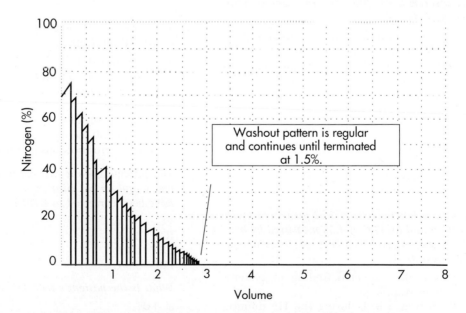

Washout pattern is regular
and continues until terminated
at 1.5%.

Figure 3-11 *Case 3-2.* Open-circuit N_2 washout from the patient. Tracing shows a normal pattern of washout with N_2 concentration plotted against lung volume (FRC). The test was terminated when N_2 concentration fell to less than 1.5%.

smoking history, but the etiology of the restrictive component is less clear. On further inquiry, it was learned that the patient's occupation involved exposure to asbestos, which can cause fibrosis and/or carcinoma. Chest x-rays revealed linear calcifications of the diaphragmatic pleura and pleural thickening, as well as fibrotic changes. These findings are all consistent with asbestos exposure.

Other tests

A sputum examination was performed, and asbestos bodies were identified from the patient's sputum. Open-lung biopsy was deferred because both the obstructive and restrictive components seemed to be appropriately identified. Measurement of pulmonary compliance (C_L) could be used to document the severity of the fibrosis. Analysis of resting arterial blood gases is probably indicated because the patient has a significant degree of restriction. Diffusing capacity (DL_{CO}) could also be used to identify possible gas exchange abnormalities.

Because of his dyspnea on exertion, the patient returned for an exercise evaluation. He walked on a treadmill with an arterial catheter in place. His PaO_2 fell from 65 mm Hg (rest) to 55 mm Hg after only 2 minutes of walking at 2 miles per hour. The desaturation was corrected when the patient breathed O_2 by nasal cannula at 1 L/min.

Treatment

The patient was given a trial of bronchodilators and reported significant symptomatic improvement. He began using supplemental O_2 via a portable system and was able to return to work in a position modified to accommodate his abilities.

■ SELF-ASSESSMENT QUESTIONS

Entry-level

1. *Which of the following correctly describes the measurement of FRC by the open-circuit method?*

  I.   The system volume of spirometer and circuitry must be calculated
  II. The test is continued until alveolar N_2 is less than 1.5%
  III. A correction for N_2 washed out of blood and tissues is required
  IV. A CO_2 absorber is required

  a. I and IV only
  b. II and III only
  c. I, II, and III
  d. II, III, and IV

2. *A patient has an FRC of 3.62 measured by He dilution and an FRC of 4.55 measured by body plethysmography. The best explanation for these results is:*

  a. This is the expected finding in patients with air trapping.
  b. There was a leak during the He dilution measurement.
  c. There was a leak during the plethysmographic measurement.

  d. The body box may overestimate FRC in patients with restriction.

3. *The closed-circuit method of measuring FRC is continued until the:*

  a. N_2 concentration has decreased to less than 2.5% or 7 minutes
  b. He concentration has decreased to less than 1.5%
  c. He concentration changes by less than 0.02% in 30 seconds
  d. N_2 concentration has reached equilibrium

4. *The following data are obtained from spirometry and an He dilution FRC test (all values have been corrected to BTPS):*

  VC   5.0 L
  IC   3.9 L
  ERV 1.1 L
  FRC 3.5 L

  What is the patient's RV/TLC ratio?

  a. 11%
  b. 22%
  c. 32%
  d. 60%

5. *A 43-year-old man has the following lung volumes measured using a body plethysmograph:*

	Measured	Predicted
VC	4.80	4.90
FRC	3.66	3.71
RV	1.25	1.35
TLC	6.05	6.25

These values are consistent with which of the following?

a. Normal lung volumes
b. A restrictive pattern as in pulmonary fibrosis
c. An obstructive pattern such as emphysema
d. A malfunction in the body plethysmograph

6. *Which of the following patterns of lung volumes are characteristic of restriction?*

a. Reduced FRC with an elevated V_{TG}
b. Increased RV, increased TLC, increased RV/TLC
c. Decreased FRC, increased TLC, normal RV/TLC
d. Decreased VC, decreased TLC, normal RV/TLC

Advanced

7. *The following data are obtained during a closed-circuit FRC determination:*

He added:	0.5 L
%He initial:	10.0%
%He final:	7.5%
Temperature:	22°C
He absorption correction:	0.1 L

Which of the following is the FRC? (See sample calculation in Appendix F.)

a. 1.57 L BTPS
b. 1.67 L BTPS
c. 1.71 L BTPS
d. 2.11 L BTPS

8. *A 53-year-old woman has the following measurements obtained during pulmonary function testing:*

FVC	2.95 L
FEV_1	1.10 L
FRC (He)	2.62 L
V_{TG}	3.59 L

Which of the following best explains these findings?

a. Normal pulmonary function
b. A leak during the FRC determination
c. Poor patient effort
d. Severe obstruction with air trapping

9. *Which of the following describe the correct technique for measuring V_{TG}?*

I. Patient should pant at about 1 Hz
II. Patient should pant at about 90 breaths/minute
III. The largest of three acceptable tests is reported
IV. The average of three acceptable tests is reported

a. I and III only
b. II and IV only
c. I and IV only
d. I, II, and III

10. *A 25-year-old patient performs an SBN_2 test and records a slope of phase III of 2.9%. This value is:*

a. Consistent with increased physiologic dead space
b. Indicative of uneven distribution of gas within the lungs
c. Within normal limits
d. Consistent with a gas analyzer malfunction

11. *A patient with pulmonary fibrosis has lung volumes measured using the open-circuit method and by plethysmography with the following results:*

FRC (N_2)	2.99 L
V_{TG}	8.98 L
FRC predicted	3.67 L

Which of the following best explains these results?

a. This is a normal pattern for the patient's diagnosis.
b. FRC by N_2 washout is consistent with air trapping.
c. A technical problem occurred with the V_{TG} measurement.
d. The predicted FRC was calculated incorrectly.

12. *A patient with an FEV$_1$/FVC ratio of 33%*
performs a closed-circuit measurement of
FRC. After 6.5 minutes, equilibration has not
occurred. The most likely explanation is:

a. This is consistent with severe airway obstruction
b. The N$_2$ analyzer has malfunctioned
c. The CO$_2$ absorber is contaminated
d. The patient is malingering

SELECTED BIBLIOGRAPHY

General References

Crapo RO, Morris AH, Clayton PD, et al: Lung volumes in healthy nonsmoking adults, *Bull Eur Physiopathol Respir* 18:419, 1982.

Forster RE: *The lung: clinical physiology and pulmonary function tests*, ed 3, St Louis, 1988, Mosby.

Goldman HI, Becklake MR: Respiratory function tests: normal values at median altitudes and the prediction of normal results, *Am Rev TB Pulm Dis* 79:457, 1959.

Hibbert ME, Lanigan A, Raven J, et al: Relation of armspan to height and the prediction of lung function, *Thorax* 43:657, 1988.

Ries A: Measurement of lung volumes, *Clin Chest Med* 10:177-186, 1989.

Thoracic Gas Volume

Begin P, Peslin R: Influence of panting frequency on thoracic gas volume measurements in chronic obstructive pulmonary disease, *Am Rev Respir Dis* 130:121, 1984.

Dubois AB, Bothelo SY, Bedell GH, et al: A rapid plethysmographic method for measuring thoracic gas volume: a comparison with a nitrogen washout method for measuring functional residual capacity, *J Clin Invest* 35:322, 1956.

Habib MP, Engel LA: Influence of the panting technique on the plethysmographic measurement of thoracic gas volume, *Am Rev Respir Dis* 117:265, 1978.

Lourenco RV, Chung SYK: Calibration of a body plethysmograph for measurement of lung volume, *Am Rev Respir Dis* 95:687, 1967.

Rodenstein DO, Stanescu DC, Francis C: Demonstration of failure of body plethysmography in airway obstruction, *J Appl Physiol* 52:949, 1982.

Gas Dilution Lung Volumes

Hathirat S, Renzetti AD, Mitchell M: Measurement of the total lung capacity by helium dilution in a constant volume system, *Am Rev Respir Dis* 102:760, 1970.

McMichael J: A rapid method of determining lung capacity, *Clin Sci* 4:167, 1939.

Meneely GR, Ball CO, Kory RC, et al: A simplified closed-circuit helium dilution method for the determination of the residual volume of the lungs, *Am J Med* 28:824, 1960.

Rodenstein DO, Stanescu DC: Reassessment of lung volume measurements by helium dilution and by body plethysmography in chronic airflow obstruction, *Am Rev Respir Dis* 126:1040, 1982.

Schaaning CG, Gulsvik A: Accuracy and precision of helium dilution technique and body plethysmography in measuring lung volume, *Scand J Clin Invest* 32:271, 1973.

Gas Distribution

Berend N, Glanville AR, Grunstein MM: Determinants of the slope of phase III of the single-breath nitrogen test, *Bull Eur Physiopathol Respir* 20:521, 1984.

Buist AS, Ross BB: Quantitative analysis of the alveolar plateau in the diagnosis of early airway obstruction, *Am Rev Respir Dis* 108:1078-1087, 1973.

Estenne M, Van Muylem A, Knoop C, et al: Detection of obliterative bronchiolitis after lung transplantation by indexes of ventilation distribution, *Am J Respir Crit Care Med* 162:1047-1051, 2000.

Fowler WS: Lung function studies. III. Uneven pulmonary ventilation in normal subjects and in patients with pulmonary disease, *J Appl Physiol* 2:283, 1949.

Hathirat S, Renzetti AD, Mitchell M: Intrapulmonary gas distribution: a comparison of the helium mixing time and nitrogen single-breath test in normal and diseased subjects, *Am Rev Respir Dis* 102:750, 1970.

Standards and Guidelines

American Association for Respiratory Care: Clinical practice guidelines: body plethysmography: 2001 revision and update, *Respir Care* 46:506-513, 2001.

American Association for Respiratory Care: Clinical practice guidelines: static lung volumes: 2001 revision and update, *Respir Care* 46:531-539, 2001.

American Thoracic Society: Lung function testing: selection of reference values and interpretive strategies, *Am Rev Respir Dis* 144:1202, 1991.

British Thoracic Society and Association of Respiratory Technicians and Physiologists: Guidelines for the measurement of respiratory function, *Respir Med* 88:165-194, 1994.

Martin R, Macklem PT: Suggested standardization procedures for closing volume determinations (nitrogen method), *DHD-NHLBI*, 1973.

Quanjer PH, ed: Lung volumes and ventilatory flows. Report of the Working Party, Standardization of Lung Function Tests, European Community for Steel and Coal, *Bull Eur Physiopathol Respir* 16(suppl 6):5-40, 1993.

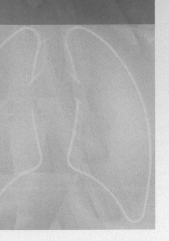

CHAPTER 4

VENTILATION AND VENTILATORY CONTROL TESTS

OBJECTIVES

After studying this chapter and reviewing its tables and case studies, you should be able to do the following:

Entry-level

1. Calculate tidal volume and minute ventilation when given appropriate data
2. Describe two causes of increased ventilation
3. Identify an abnormal V_D/V_T ratio

Advanced

1. Calculate dead space and alveolar ventilation
2. Describe two methods for measuring the breathing response to oxygen
3. Identify the normal ventilatory response to carbon dioxide

This chapter discusses the measurement of ventilation and its components: tidal volume (V_T), respiratory frequency (f) and minute ventilation ($\dot{V}_E$). Wasted or dead space ventilation is also defined. Techniques for estimating dead space (V_D) and alveolar ventilation ($\dot{V}_A$) are described. Because a variety of diseases can affect dead space, measurements of V_D and V_D/V_T are used to evaluate many disorders. Ventilation and V_D measurements are used in several different clinical situations. These parameters may be measured in the critical care unit as well as in the pulmonary function laboratory.

Assessment of ventilatory responses is closely related to measurement of resting ventilation. The responses to two stimuli, carbon dioxide (CO_2) and oxygen (O_2), are commonly evaluated. Ventilatory response is usually assessed by measuring the change in ventilation that occurs with elevated CO_2 or decreased O_2. The output of the respiratory centers is also sometimes measured as the pressure developed during the first tenth of a second when the airway is blocked (P_{100}).

Tidal Volume, Rate, and Minute Ventilation

■ DESCRIPTION

V_T is the volume of gas inspired or expired during each respiratory cycle (see Figure 2-1). It is usually measured in liters or milliliters, corrected to BTPS. Conventionally, the volume expired is expressed as V_T. The respiratory rate is the number of breaths per unit of time, usually per minute. The total volume of gas expired per minute is $\dot{V}_E$, or minute ventilation. $\dot{V}_E$ includes alveolar and dead space ventilation, and is recorded in liters per minute, BTPS.

■ TECHNIQUE

V_T can be measured directly by simple spirometry (see Figure 2-1). The patient breathes into a volume-displacement or flow-sensing spirometer (see Chapter 10). Volume change may be measured directly from the excursions of a volume spirometer. V_T may also be measured from an integrated flow signal (see Chapter 10). V_T can be recorded on either paper or a computer screen. Because no two breaths are the same, inhaled or exhaled tidal breaths should be measured for at least 1 minute and then divided by the rate to determine an average volume:

$$V_T = \frac{\dot{V}}{f_B}$$

where:

$\dot{V}$ = volume expired or inspired over a given interval, usually the $\dot{V}_E$

f_B = number of breaths for same interval (i.e., the respiratory rate)

The inspired volume $\dot{V}_I$ and V_T are normally slightly greater than the $\dot{V}_E$ because the body at rest produces a slightly lower volume of CO_2 than the volume of O_2 consumed. This exchange difference is termed the *respiratory exchange ratio* (*RER*). It is calculated as the $\dot{V}CO_2/\dot{V}O_2$, where $\dot{V}CO_2$ is the volume of CO_2 produced and $\dot{V}O_2$ is the volume of O_2 consumed per minute. It is assumed that RER is approximately 0.8 in resting patients. For most clinical purposes, expired volume is measured to calculate V_T.

V_T may also be estimated by means of a respiratory inductive plethysmography (RIP). The RIP uses coils of wire as transducers that respond to changes in the cross-sectional area of the rib cage and abdominal compartments. With appropriate calibration, RIP can be used to measure V_T without connections to the airway.

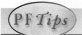

Not all spirometers allow bidirectional breathing (i.e., breathing in and out of the spirometer). For flow-based spirometers that do not measure flow in both directions, a one-way breathing circuit may be used. In order to measure ventilation with a volume-based spirometer, the subject rebreathes; CO_2 must be removed and O_2 added for prolonged measurements.

Respiratory frequency (f_B) may be determined by counting chest movements or the excursions of a spirometer (Ventilation 4-1). Counting the rate for several minutes and taking an average produces a more accurate value than shorter measurements. Prolonged measurements of V_T and rate using a volume-displacement spirometer require a means of removing CO_2. This is called a rebreathing system and uses a chemical CO_2 absorber

---

VENTILATION 4-1   Criteria for Acceptability—Tidal Volume, Rate, Minute Ventilation

1 V_T averaged from at least 60 seconds of ventilatory data; either accumulated volume divided by respiratory rate or multiple breaths summed and averaged.
2 $\dot{V}_E$ measured for at least 60 seconds; one-way breathing circuit or appropriate rebreathing system used. Repeated measurements should be within 10%.
3 Respiratory rate measured for at least 15 seconds; longer intervals may be necessary for patients with disordered breathing patterns.

(see Figure 3-1, *B*). Sodium hydroxide crystals (Sodasorb) or barium hydroxide crystals (Baralyme) are commonly used to scrub CO_2 from rebreathing systems. Flow-sensing spirometers usually do not require a chemical absorber.

The $\dot{V}_E$ may be measured by allowing the patient to breathe into or out of a volume-displacement or flow-sensing spirometer for at least 1 minute. If a rebreathing system is used, a CO_2 absorber must be included, as well as a means of replenishing O_2. Measuring expired gas volume for several minutes and dividing by the time gives an average $\dot{V}_E$. $\dot{V}_E$, measured from expired gas, is usually slightly smaller than the $\dot{V}_I$ because of the RER as described previously. For most clinical purposes, this difference is negligible. BTPS corrections should be made.

■ SIGNIFICANCE AND PATHOPHYSIOLOGY

See Ventilation 4-2 for interpretive strategies. Average V_T for healthy adults ranges between 400 and 700 ml, but there is considerable variation. Decreased V_T occurs in many types of pulmonary disorders, particularly those that cause severe restrictive patterns. Pulmonary fibrosis and neuromuscular diseases (e.g., myasthenia gravis) often cause reduced V_T. Decreased tidal breathing is usually caused by changes in the mechanical properties of the lungs or chest wall (i.e., compliance and resistance). These changes are usually accompanied by increased respiratory rate (f_B) required to maintain $\dot{V}_A$. Decreases in both V_T and respiratory rate are often associated with respiratory center depression. Low V_I and rate usually result in alveolar hypoventilation. Rapid breathing rates and small V_T may suggest increased V_D or hypoventilation but must be correlated with arterial pH and P_{CO_2} values to be definitive.

VENTILATION 4-2   Interpretive Strategies—Tidal Volume, Rate, Minute Ventilation

1 Were V_T, respiratory rate, and $\dot{V}_E$ measured appropriately? Were adequate data collected? Did the ventilatory pattern change during the measurements? If so, suspect breathing circuit problems.
2 Were repeated measurements made? If so, were they reproducible within 10%?
3 Is the pattern of ventilation consistent with the patient's clinical status?
4 Is V_T, respiratory rate, or $\dot{V}_E$ excessive? If so, suspect hyperventilation. Arterial blood gas testing may be necessary.
5 Is V_T, respiratory rate, or $\dot{V}_E$ decreased? If so, suspect hypoventilation. Arterial blood gas testing is indicated.

Some patients who have pulmonary disease may exhibit increased V_T, particularly at rest. The V_T alone is not a good indicator of the adequacy of alveolar ventilation ($\dot{V}_A$). Tidal volume should always be considered in conjunction with respiratory rate and $\dot{V}_E$. Many healthy patients display increased V_T simply because of breathing into the pulmonary function apparatus with the nose occluded. Estimates of resting ventilation may be artifactually increased when measured during pulmonary function testing.

The normal respiratory rate (f_B) ranges from 10 to 20 breaths/min. Increased demand for ventilation, such as during exercise, usually results in increases in both the rate and depth of breathing (i.e., the tidal volume). Increases or decreases in the respiratory rate are indications of a change in the ventilatory status. Breathing frequency, when evaluated with the V_T, may be used as an index of ventilation. Hypoxia, hypercapnia, metabolic acidosis, decreased lung compliance, and exercise can all result in increased respiratory rate. Rapid breathing rates and small tidal volumes may suggest increased V_D or hypoventilation but must be correlated with arterial pH and P_{CO_2} values to confirm those conditions. Decreased breathing frequency is common in central nervous system depression and in CO_2 narcosis. As with measurement of V_T, respiratory rate may be falsely elevated in patients connected to unfamiliar breathing circuits, with or without a nose clip.

Normal $\dot{V}_E$ ranges from 5 to 10 L/min, with wide variations in normal patients. The $\dot{V}_E$, when used in conjunction with blood gas values, indicates the adequacy of ventilation. $\dot{V}_E$ is the sum of the $\dot{V}_D$ (dead space ventilation per minute) and $\dot{V}_A$. Because the relative proportions of these components can change, absolute values for $\dot{V}_E$ do not necessarily indicate either hypoventilation or hyperventilation. In other words, low minute ventilation does not necessarily indicate hypoventilation. Similarly, elevated $\dot{V}_E$ does not indicate hyperventilation. To make these diagnoses, arterial pH and P_{CO_2} must be measured.

A large $\dot{V}_E$ at rest (greater than 20 L/min) may result from an enlarged V_D, because an increase in total ventilation is required to maintain adequate $\dot{V}_A$. $\dot{V}_E$ increases in response to hypoxia, hypercapnia, metabolic acidosis, anxiety, and exercise. Hyperventilation is ventilation in excess of that needed to adequately remove CO_2, resulting in respiratory alkalosis.

Decreased ventilation may result from hypocapnia, metabolic alkalosis, respiratory center depression, or neuromuscular disorders that involve the ventilatory muscles. Hypoventilation is defined as inadequate ventilation to maintain a normal arterial P_{CO_2}, with respiratory acidosis as the result. The diagnosis of either hyperventilation or hypoventilation requires blood gas analysis (see Chapter 6).

Respiratory Dead Space and Alveolar Ventilation

■ DESCRIPTION

Respiratory dead space (V_D) is the lung volume that is ventilated but not perfused by pulmonary capillary blood flow. V_D can be divided into the conducting airways, or anatomic dead space, and the nonperfused alveoli, or alveolar dead space. The combination of alveolar and anatomic dead space is respiratory (or physiologic) dead space. V_D is recorded in milliliters or liters, BTPS.

$\dot{V}_A$ is the volume of gas that participates in gas exchange in the lungs. It can be expressed as:

$$\dot{V}_A = \dot{V}_E - \dot{V}_D$$

where:

$\dot{V}_A$ = alveolar ventilation

$\dot{V}_E$ = minute ventilation

$\dot{V}_D$ = dead space ventilation per minute

For a single breath, the V_A equals the V_T minus the V_D. $\dot{V}_A$ is usually expressed in liters per minute, BTPS.

■ TECHNIQUE

Dead Space

Anatomic dead space is sometimes estimated from an individual's body size as 1 ml/lb of ideal body weight. The actual respiratory dead space, however, is of greater clinical importance. V_D can be calculated in two ways. The first uses Bohr's equation defining V_D:

$$V_D = \frac{F_A CO_2 - F_{\bar{E}} CO_2}{F_A CO_2} \times V_T$$

where:

V_T = tidal volume

$F_A CO_2$ = fraction of CO_2 in alveolar gas

$F_{\bar{E}} CO_2$ = fraction of CO_2 in mixed expired gas

Because the fractional concentration of alveolar CO_2 is difficult to measure, partial pressure may be substituted and the equation written as follows:

$$V_D = \frac{(Pa CO_2 - P_{\bar{E}} CO_2)}{Pa CO_2} \times V_T$$

where:

$Pa CO_2$ = arterial $P CO_2$

$P_{\bar{E}} CO_2$ = $P CO_2$ of mixed expired gas sample

Note that the $Pa CO_2$ is substituted for the alveolar $P CO_2$. This substitution presumes perfect equilibration between alveoli and pulmonary capillaries. This may not be true in certain diseases. The test also assumes that little CO_2 is in the atmosphere. Therefore, the $P CO_2$ in expired gas is inversely proportional to the V_D. Exhaled gas is collected over a short interval, and arterial blood is obtained simultaneously to measure $Pa CO_2$. V_D is calculated by applying the previous equation. The estimate becomes more accurate as more expired gas is collected. Accuracy depends on measurement of $\dot{V}_E$, as well as on the partial pressures of CO_2 measured in expired gas and arterial blood. The mixed expired gas sample is usually collected in a bag or balloon after filling and emptying it several times with expired gas to wash out room air from the valves, tubing, and bag itself. The volume of gas in the bag can be measured during collection by including a flow-sensing spirometer in the circuit. If $\dot{V}_E$ and respiratory rate are recorded, the volumes of V_D and V_T can be determined. If expired volume is not measured, only a dilution ratio can be determined; this is called the V_D/V_T ratio.

The V_D/V_T ratio can be calculated if arterial and mixed-expired $P CO_2$ values are known. It can also be estimated noninvasively. End-tidal $P CO_2$ can be used to estimate $Pa CO_2$. The main advantage is that it is not necessary to obtain an arterial blood sample. This technique is often used in systems that monitor expired CO_2 continuously, and in breath-by-breath metabolic measurement devices. V_D/V_T is calculated as follows:

$$\frac{V_D}{V_T} = \frac{(PetCO_2 - P_{\bar{E}}CO_2)}{PetCO_2}$$

where:
$PetCO_2$ = end-tidal PCO_2
$P_{\bar{E}}CO_2$ = PCO_2 of mixed-expired gas sample

Dead space consists of anatomic and alveolar components. Anatomic dead space is usually estimated from body weight. Respiratory dead space, measured using mixed expired and arterial CO_2, measures both components.

In some patients, particularly those with severe obstruction, $PetCO_2$ may not accurately reflect $PaCO_2$. Consequently, the V_D/V_T ratio may be estimated incorrectly. $PaCO_2$ should be used in the $\dot{V}_D$ calculation whenever possible.

Alveolar Ventilation
$\dot{V}_A$ can be calculated in two ways:

$$\dot{V}_A = f_B(V_T - V_D)$$

where:
V_T = tidal volume
V_D = respiratory dead space
f_B = respiratory rate

For convenience, V_D is often estimated as equal to anatomic dead space. This method is valid only when there is little or no alveolar dead space, as in individuals who do not have pulmonary disease.

Because atmospheric gas contains almost no CO_2, $\dot{V}_A$ can be calculated based on CO_2 elimination from the lungs. A volume of expired gas is collected in a bag, balloon, or spirometer, and analyzed to determine the volume of CO_2 (see Chapter 7). The following equation can then be used:

$$\dot{V}_A = \frac{\dot{V}CO_2}{F_ACO_2}$$

where:
$\dot{V}CO_2$ = volume of CO_2 produced in liters per minute (STPD)
F_ACO_2 = fractional concentration of CO_2 in alveolar gas

If an end-tidal CO_2 monitor is used, a close approximation of the concentration of alveolar CO_2 is easily obtained and the equation simplified as follows:

$$\dot{V}_A = \frac{\dot{V}CO_2}{\% \text{ alveolar } CO_2} \times 100$$

End-tidal CO_2 may not equal alveolar CO_2 in patients with grossly abnormal patterns of ventilation-perfusion (see Chapter 6).

The same equation can be used with a substitution of the $PaCO_2$ for the alveolar PCO_2 (i.e., $PaCO_2$), again presuming that arterial blood and alveolar gas are in equilibrium. The equation is then as follows:

$$\dot{V}_A = \frac{\dot{V}CO_2}{PaCO_2} \times 0.863$$

where:
$\dot{V}CO_2$ = CO_2 production in ml/min (STPD)
$PaCO_2$ = partial pressure of arterial CO_2
0.863 = conversion factor (concentration to partial pressure, correcting $\dot{V}CO_2$ to BTPS)

SIGNIFICANCE AND PATHOPHYSIOLOGY

See Ventilation 4-3 for interpretive strategies. Measurement of V_D yields important information regarding the ventilation-perfusion characteristics of the lungs. Anatomic dead space is larger in men than in women because of differences in body size. It increases along with the V_T during exercise, as well as in certain forms of pulmonary disease (e.g., bronchiectasis). It may be decreased in asthma or in diseases characterized by bronchial obstruction or mucus plugging. Because of the difficulty in measuring the anatomic dead space, estimates based on age, sex, functional residual capacity, or body size may be used. For clinical purposes, anatomic dead space in milliliters is sometimes considered equal to the patient's ideal body weight in pounds.

Of greater clinical significance is the measurement of respiratory dead space, which is accomplished reasonably well by applying the Bohr equation. The portion of ventilation wasted on the conducting airways and poorly perfused alveoli is usually expressed as the V_D/V_T ratio. The normal value for V_D/V_T in adults is about 0.3 (with a range of 0.2 to 0.4). V_D/V_T is also commonly expressed as a percentage, with a value of 30% considered normal. Expressing dead space in this way eliminates the need to measure the volume of expired gas in the Bohr equation. However, if V_T or $\dot{V}_E$ is known, dead space volume can be easily

VENTILATION 4-3   Interpretive Strategies—V_D and $\dot{V}_A$

1 Was dead space determination based on $PaCO_2$? If not, interpret cautiously.
2 Was $\dot{V}_E$ or V_T measured? If not, then interpret only V_D/V_T.
3 Is the V_D/V_T ratio greater than 0.40? If so, elevated dead space is likely. Consider clinical correlation, especially pulmonary embolism or pulmonary hypertension.
4 Is the V_D/V_T ratio less than 0.20 with the patient at rest? Is there an elevated level of ventilation? Consider technical problems.
5 Is $\dot{V}_A$ (if measured) consistent with the patient's clinical signs and symptoms?

calculated. Physiologic dead space measurements are a good index of ventilation-blood flow ratios because all CO_2 in expired gas comes from perfused alveoli (see Chapter 6). If there were no dead space in the lung, arterial and mixed-expired CO_2 would be equal. The greater the difference between arterial and mixed-expired CO_2, the larger the volume of "wasted" ventilation.

The V_D/V_T ratio decreases in normal patients during exercise. As cardiac output increases, perfusion of alveoli at the lung apices also increases. This increased perfusion is referred to as *recruitment*. Alveoli at the apices are poorly perfused at rest, accounting for some of the normal resting dead space. Both V_D and V_T increase with exercise. In healthy patients, the V_T increases more than V_D, hence the ratio decreases.

Increased dead space, and V_D/V_T ratio, may be observed in *pulmonary embolism* and in pulmonary hypertension. In pulmonary embolism, large numbers of arterioles may be blocked, resulting in little or no CO_2 removal in the associated alveoli. In pulmonary hypertension, increased pulmonary arterial pressure causes most alveoli to be perfused, so there is little or no recruitment of underperfused gas exchange units. This is most notable during exercise when the V_D/V_T ratio normally decreases. In both pulmonary embolism and hypertension, the patient may be very short of breath (i.e., dyspneic) because of the increased dead space.

The $\dot{V}_A$ at rest is approximately 4 to 5 L/min with wide variations in healthy individuals. The adequacy of $\dot{V}_A$ can be determined only by arterial blood gas studies. Low $\dot{V}_A$ associated with acute respiratory acidosis ($Paco_2$ greater than 45 and pH less than 7.35 in normal patients) defines hypoventilation. Excessive $\dot{V}_A$ ($Paco_2$ less than 35 and pH greater than 7.45 in normal patients) defines hyperventilation. Chronic hypoventilation and hyperventilation are associated with abnormal $Paco_2$ values but near-normal pH values (see Chapter 6). Decreased $\dot{V}_A$ can result from absolute increases in dead space as well as decreases in $\dot{V}_E$.

Ventilatory Response Tests for Carbon Dioxide and Oxygen

■ DESCRIPTION

Ventilatory response to CO_2 is a measurement of the increase or decrease in $\dot{V}_E$ caused by breathing various concentrations of CO_2 under normoxic conditions ($Pao_2 = 90$ to 100 mm Hg). It is recorded as L/min/mm Hg Pco_2.

Ventilatory response to O_2 is a measurement of the increase or decrease in $\dot{V}_E$ caused by breathing various concentrations of O_2 under isocapnic conditions ($Paco_2 \cong 40$ mm Hg). The change in ventilation (in liters per minute) may be recorded in relation to changes in Pao_2 or saturation as monitored by oximetry.

Occlusion pressure (P_{100} or $P_{0.1}$) is the pressure generated at the mouth during the first 100 milliseconds of an inspiratory effort against an occluded airway. Changes in P_{100} are related to changes in the ventilatory stimulant (hypercapnia or hypoxemia). It is usually measured in centimeters of water (cm H_2O).

■ TECHNIQUE

CO_2 response can be measured in two ways:

1. *Open-circuit technique.* The patient breathes various concentrations (1% to 7%) of CO_2 in air or O_2 from a *demand valve* or reservoir until a steady state is reached. Measurements of $Petco_2$, $Paco_2$, P_{100}, and $\dot{V}_E$ may be made at each concentration.

2. *Closed-circuit or rebreathing technique.* The patient rebreathes from a reservoir (usually an anesthesia bag) of 7% CO_2 in O_2. The breathing circuit usually includes ports for pressure monitoring (P_{100}), and for extracting gas samples ($PetCO_2$). A pneumotachometer (see Chapter 10) is placed in the rebreathing circuit to record $\dot{V}_E$. Alternatively, the gas reservoir bag may be placed in a rigid container or box, and volume change measured by connecting a spirometer to the container (i.e., "bag-in-box" setup). The patient rebreathes until the concentration of $PetCO_2$ exceeds 9% or until 4 minutes have elapsed. The rebreathed gas may be analyzed to ensure that the FIO_2 remains above 0.21. The patient's SpO_2 may also be monitored by means of a pulse oximeter (see Chapter 10). Changes in $\dot{V}_E$ are monitored and plotted against $PetCO_2$ to obtain a response curve. A plot of $\dot{V}_E$ versus $PetCO_2$ may be used to determine a slope or response curve. The CO_2 response curve may be extrapolated backward to determine the PCO_2 at which ventilation would be zero. This PCO_2 is termed the *threshold* and is sometimes used as a measure of sensitivity to the ventilatory stimulant.

O_2 response can be measured by either open-circuit or closed-circuit techniques:

1. *Open-circuit technique.* The patient breathes gas mixtures containing O_2 concentrations from 20% to 12%, to which CO_2 is added to maintain alveolar PCO_2 ($PaCO_2$) at a constant level. When a steady state is reached, PaO_2, $\dot{V}_E$, and P_{100} can be measured. This procedure, often called a step test, is repeated with decreasing O_2 concentrations to produce the response curve. Continuous monitoring of $PetCO_2$ is necessary to titrate the addition of CO_2 to the system to maintain *isocapnia* (Figure 4-1). Pulse oximetry may be used to monitor changes in saturation. CO_2 response curves are sometimes measured at widely varying PaO_2 levels, and the subsequent difference in ventilation or P_{100} at any particular PCO_2 is attributed to the response to hypoxemia.

2. *Closed-circuit technique (progressive hypoxemia).* The patient rebreathes from a system similar to that used for the closed-circuit CO_2 response, but the system contains a CO_2 *scrubber*. CO_2 can be added to the inspired gas to maintain isocapnia, or an adjustable blower may be used to direct a portion of the rebreathed gas through the scrubber to maintain isocapnia (Figure 4-1). Response to decreasing inspired PO_2 is monitored by recording $\dot{V}_E$ or P_{100}, and the PaO_2 or saturation is measured either directly by indwelling catheter or by pulse oximetry.

PF Tips

To measure response to hypoxemia, it is necessary to maintain a constant level of CO_2 (isocapnia). To measure response to hypercapnia, it is necessary to maintain normoxia (PaO_2 of 80-100 mm Hg).

P_{100} is measured using a system similar to that in Figure 4-1. A port at the mouth records pressure changes versus time, via computer or high-speed recorder. A large-bore stopcock or electronic shutter mechanism is included in the inspiratory line so that inspiratory flow can be randomly occluded. The stopcock or shutter can be closed so that inspiration occurs against a complete occlusion near functional residual capacity. The entire apparatus is usually hidden so that the patient is unaware of the impending airway occlusion. A pressure-time curve is recorded. P_{100} is usually measured at varying $PetCO_2$ values or levels of desaturation to assess the effect of changing stimuli to ventilation. P_{100} and $\dot{V}_E$ are usually graphed against $PetCO_2$ (Figure 4-2) or versus O_2 saturation (for O_2 response tests). See Ventilation 4-4 for acceptability criteria for ventilatory response measurements.

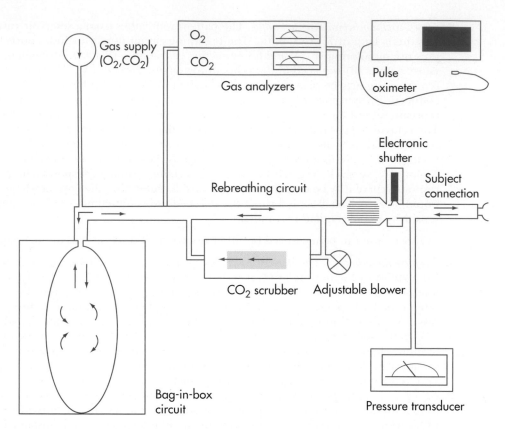

Figure 4–1 *Closed-circuit system for the rebreathing O_2 response test.* The circuit allows the patient to rebreathe into a bag to which CO_2 or O_2 can be added. Gas analyzers allow continuous monitoring of gas concentrations in the circuit during testing. Ventilation is measured by integrating flow from the pneumotachometer or attaching a spirometer to the bag-in-box setup. A pressure transducer and mouth shutter allow the measurement of P_{100}, and a pulse oximeter provides data on the patient's saturation. A CO_2 scrubber with an adjustable blower allows the level of CO_2 in the system to be maintained at baseline levels (isocapnia). Increases in ventilation caused by the gradual consumption of O_2 in the circuit can be measured by scrubbing just enough of the exhaled CO_2 to maintain a near-normal alveolar P_{CO_2}. The same circuit can be used to measure response to CO_2 by rebreathing. The bag is filled with 5% to 7% CO_2 in O_2, and the scrubber is removed from the circuit.

■ SIGNIFICANCE AND PATHOPHYSIOLOGY

See Ventilation 4-5 for interpretive strategies. The response to an increase in Pa_{CO_2} in a normal individual is a linear increase in $\dot{V}_E$ of approximately 3 L/min/mm Hg (P_{CO_2}). The normal range of response varies from 1 to 6 L/min/mm Hg P_{CO_2}. Some variation is present in repeated testing of the same individual. The response to CO_2 in patients who have obstructive disease may be reduced. This is partially attributable to increased airway resistance, which has been shown to reduce ventilatory drive in healthy individuals. It is unclear why some patients who have obstructive disease increase ventilation to maintain a normal Pa_{CO_2}, whereas others tolerate an increased Pa_{CO_2}. Genetic variation in drive may explain some of the differences in blood gas tensions in patients with chronic obstructive pulmonary disease (COPD). Lesions in the central nervous system may also cause a decreased sensitivity to CO_2.

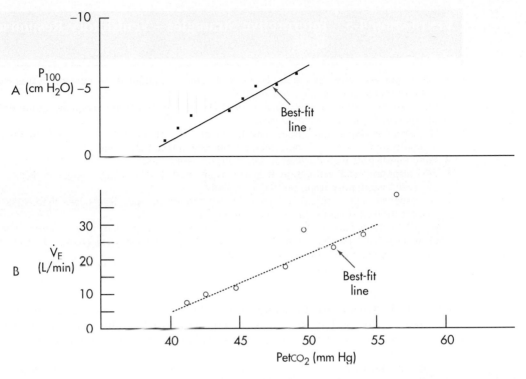

Figure 4–2 A, P_{100} plotted against end-tidal CO_2 ($PetCO_2$), as might be obtained during a CO_2 rebreathing study. **B,** Minute ventilation plotted against $PetCO_2$ during the same study. Individual points may be plotted and a "best-fit" line constructed by statistical methods. The slope of the best-fit line is the rate at which ventilation or occlusion pressure increases with increasing stimulation from the rebreathed CO_2.

VENTILATION 4-4   Criteria For Acceptability—Ventilatory Response Tests

1 CO_2 response—Appropriate concentrations of CO_2 (i.e., 7% CO_2 in O_2 for rebreathing studies) must be used.
2 CO_2 response—**Normoxia** maintained; subject's SpO_2 should remain >95% during testing.
3 O_2 response—FIO_2 appropriate to induce hypoxic response; isocapnia demonstrated by monitoring $PetCO_2$.
4 P_{100}—Pressure transducer and monitor capable of recording up to 50 cm H_2O at 50 to 100 mm/sec. Occlusion device should be hidden from the patient.
5 Ventilatory responses (O_2, CO_2) should be reproducible within 10%; average of two trials should be reported if clinically practical.
6 Reported P_{100} should be the average of three or more occlusions at each level of challenge.

VENTILATION 4-5   Interpretive Strategies—Ventilatory Response Tests

1 CO_2 response—Were appropriate levels of elevated CO_2 attained? If rebreathing was used, was test terminated at 4 minutes or 9% CO_2?

2 CO_2 response—Was normoxia maintained? Did Spo_2 demonstrate adequate saturation? If not, interpretation may be compromised.

3 O_2 response—Were appropriate low levels of Fio_2 attained? Was isocapnia maintained as demonstrated by $Petco_2$? If not, interpretation may be compromised.

4 Were repeat tests reproducible? If not, interpret cautiously.

5 CO_2 response—Did ventilation increase by at least 1 L/mm Hg change in $Petco_2$? If not, decreased ventilatory response to CO_2 is likely.

6 O_2 response—Did ventilation increase exponentially at Spo_2 levels less than 90%? If not, suspect decreased ventilatory response to hypoxia.

7 P_{100}—Was the occlusion pressure appropriate for the baseline $Paco_2$ (1.5-5.0 cm H_2O at a $Paco_2$ of 40 mm Hg)? Did P_{100} increase by at least 0.5 cm H_2O/mm Hg change in $Petco_2$? If not, a decreased central ventilatory drive is likely.

Some individuals who have no respiratory muscle weakness, mechanical ventilatory problems, or neurologic disease have a decreased sensitivity to CO_2. This condition is described as primary alveolar hypoventilation. These patients can lower their Pco_2 by voluntary hyperventilation.

The normal response to a decrease in $Paco_2$ varies depending on the level of Pco_2 at which the measurement is made. There is little change in ventilation until the Pao_2 falls to less than 60 mm Hg. The response appears to be exponential once the Pao_2 has fallen to the range of 40 to 60 mm Hg, and it varies widely between individuals on a genetically determined basis. The hypoxic response is increased in the presence of hypercapnia and decreased in hypocapnia. Patients who have severe COPD with CO_2 retention receive their primary respiratory stimulus from the hypoxemic response. This group of patients may experience severe or even fatal respiratory depression if that response is obliterated by uncontrolled O_2 therapy.

Some patients with minimal intrinsic lung disease show markedly decreased response to hypoxemia or hypercapnia. These include patients with *myxedema,* obesity-hypoventilation syndrome, obstructive sleep apnea, and idiopathic hypoventilation. CO_2 and O_2 response measurements, along with tests of pulmonary mechanics, may be particularly valuable in the evaluation and treatment of these types of patients.

The P_{100} ($P_{0.1}$) has been suggested as a measurement of ventilatory drive independent of the mechanical properties of the lungs. Because no airflow occurs during occlusion of the airway, significant interference from mechanical abnormalities (e.g., increased resistance or decreased compliance) is omitted. Reflexes from the airways and chest wall are also of little influence during the first 100 millisec of the occluded breath. Therefore, the pressure generated can be viewed as proportional to the neural output of the *medullary centers* that drive the rate and depth of breathing. This proportionality may be influenced by other factors, however, such as body position and the contractile properties of the respiratory muscles.

Individuals with normal $Paco_2$ values have P_{100} values in the range of 1.5 to 5 cm H_2O. P_{100} has been shown to increase in hypercapnia and hypoxia and appears to correlate well with the observed ventilatory responses. Increasing Pco_2, and thereby inducing hypercapnia, in healthy patients typically results in an increase in the occlusion pressure of 0.5 to 0.6 cm H_2O/mm Hg Pco_2, with as much as 20% variability. Some patients who have chronic airway obstruction demonstrate no increase in P_{100} in response to an increase in their P_{CO_2}, even with increased airway resistance. Normal patients increase their P_{100} when breathing through artificial resistance on challenge with high P_{CO_2} or low P_{O_2}. This failure to respond to increased resistance in the airways may predispose individuals with COPD to respiratory failure when lung infections occur. Similarly, patients on mechanical ventilation may have trouble in weaning if their ventilatory drive is compromised, as demonstrated by failure to increase P_{100} when challenged with increased P_{CO_2}. Determination of P_{100} may prove helpful in determining the effects of treatment in patients who have abnormal ventilatory responses.

Summary

This chapter discusses measurement of $\dot{V}_E$, V_T, and respiratory rate. Resting ventilatory measurements can be used in conjunction with blood gases to evaluate respiratory status. One of the most important parameters is the respiratory or physiologic dead space. An estimate of wasted ventilation can be made by comparing expired CO_2 with arterial P_{CO_2}. Dead space and reduced $\dot{V}_A$ are common in many pulmonary disorders. When dead space increases, ventilation must increase to maintain a normal acid-base status.

Disorders of ventilatory control are also common to many diseases. Evaluation of responses to hypoxemia and hypercapnia are often useful in characterizing types of ventilatory response disorders. Different techniques of assessing responses have been described. The rebreathing techniques for O_2 and CO_2 are used most often. P_{100} can discriminate central ventilatory drive problems from other causes of abnormal responses.

CASE STUDIES

CASE 4-1

HISTORY

T.J. is a 45-year-old man admitted to the hospital for acute shortness of breath. He has never smoked but has a family history of heart disease. His lungs are clear during auscultation. He becomes breathless just moving around his hospital room. He denies any recent respiratory infections. Because of his rapid respiratory rate, his attending physician requested an arterial blood gas test using room air and a V_D/V_T ratio determination.

PULMONARY FUNCTION STUDIES

Personal Data

Age:	45
Height:	67 in
Weight:	175 lb
Race:	White

Blood Gas Analysis

pH	7.49
P_{CO_2} (mm Hg)	29
P_{O_2} (mm Hg)	102
HCO_3^- (mEq/L)	21
Hb (g/dl)	14.2
Sa_{O_2} (%)	98

Exhaled Gas Analysis

$\dot{V}_E$ (L/min)	24.20
f_B (breaths/min)	20
$P_{\bar{E}}CO_2$ (mm Hg)	14

QUESTIONS

1. Determine the following for this patient:
   - V_T
   - V_D/V_T
   - $\dot{V}_A$
2. What is the interpretation of the patient's ventilation?
3. What other tests might be indicated?
4. What treatment might be recommended based on these findings?

DISCUSSION

Calculations

a.
$$V_T = \frac{\dot{V}_E}{f_B}$$
$$= \frac{24.2}{20}$$
$$V_T = 1.21\,L$$

b.
$$\frac{V_D}{V_T} = \frac{(P_{aCO_2} - P_{\bar{E}}CO_2)}{P_{aCO_2}}$$
$$= \frac{(29 - 14)}{29}$$
$$\frac{V_D}{V_T} = 0.517$$

c.
$$\dot{V}_A = f_B(V_T - V_D)$$

where:

$$V_D = \frac{V_D}{V_T}(V_T)$$
$$= 0.517(1.21)$$
$$V_D = 0.626$$

Substituting this value in the alveolar ventilation equation:

$$\dot{V}_A = 20(1.21 - 0.626)$$
$$= 20(0.584)$$
$$\dot{V}_A = 11.68$$

Ventilation

This patient has a rapid respiratory rate and a large V_T. The result of this is a large $\dot{V}_E$ (i.e., 24.2 L/min). The blood gas analysis shows hyperventilation (respiratory alkalosis; see Chapter 6) consistent with excessive ventilation. The V_D/V_T ratio is increased at 52% (0.517 as a fraction). Healthy patients have V_D/V_T ratios of 30% to 40% at rest. In effect, this patient is wasting more than half of each breath. Calculation of the $\dot{V}_A$ similarly reveals that less than half of his $\dot{V}_E$ is actually available for gas exchange. To maintain a normal $PaCO_2$ (or in this case, to hyperventilate), patients who have increased dead space must increase their total ventilation. Large increases in dead space can occur as a result of obstruction of pulmonary arterial vessels by blood clots or similar lesions. Congestion of pulmonary vessels (resulting from pulmonary hypertension) can also cause imbalances in ventilation-perfusion ratios, especially during exercise.

Other Tests

Other diagnostic procedures that might be indicated include perfusion or ventilation-perfusion scanning of the lungs. Perfusion scans can identify areas of the lung in which there is little or no blood flow. $\dot{V}/\dot{Q}$ scans can detect which areas of the lungs have decreased blood flow in relation to their ventilation. These imaging tests are often used when pulmonary *emboli* are suspected. Ventilation-perfusion scans of T.J. indicated multiple areas of decreased perfusion in both lower lobes, consistent with multiple pulmonary emboli.

Treatment

The patient was given O_2 therapy after the blood gas test results were obtained. Because there was adequate oxygenation on room air, the O_2 therapy was inappropriate and discontinued. After the lung scans, the patient was started on anticoagulant therapy (*heparin*). During the next week, the pattern of pulmonary embolization gradually resolved. His ventilation and V_D/V_T ratio returned to normal.

CASE 4-2

HISTORY

T.B. is a 37-year-old white man who weighs 275 lb. He was referred to the pulmonary function laboratory after an evaluation in the sleep laboratory revealed obstructive sleep apnea (OSA). He admits to daytime somnolence. Baseline pulmonary function studies revealed the following:

	Actual	% Predicted
FVC (L)	3.2	72%
FEV$_1$ (L)	2.7	81%
TLC (L)	4.1	71%
RV/TLC	22 %	

Baseline blood gas results were as follows:

pH	7.36
P_{CO_2} (mm Hg)	47
P_{O_2} (mm Hg)	77
HCO_3^- (mEq/L)	28
$S_{a_{O_2}}$ (%)	93

A CO_2 response test was performed to assess T.B.'s respiratory drive. The rebreathing method was used. T.B. rebreathed a mixture of 7% CO_2 in O_2 for 4 minutes. Triplicate measurements of P_{100} were made at intervals throughout the test using a pneumatically operated occlusion valve. The following data were obtained:

PET_{CO_2} (mm Hg)	$\dot{V}_E$ (L/min)	P_{100} (cm H_2O)
43	4.5	2.2
46	4.4	—
50	5.9	—
54	7.9	7.8
57	15.1	—
59	17.1	12.0

QUESTIONS

1. What is the interpretation of:
   - Ventilatory response to CO_2 stimulation?
   - Respiratory drive response to CO_2 stimulation?
2. What is the cause of the patient's daytime somnolence?
3. What treatment might be recommended based on these findings?

DISCUSSION

Interpretation

All data obtained during the CO_2 rebreathing test were acceptable. The PET_{CO_2} increased appropriately, and the test was terminated after 4 minutes of rebreathing. P_{100} was obtained at baseline, after 2 minutes, and near the end of the test. All pressures were reproducible, and the average values were reported. Ventilatory response was diminished at 0.8 L/mm Hg P_{CO_2}. P_{100} appeared to increase appropriately.

Impression: Markedly reduced ventilatory response to CO_2, with a normal occlusion pressure.

Cause of Symptoms

This patient, who has documented sleep apnea, also displays a reduced sensitivity to increasing levels of CO_2. His spirometry and total lung capacity show a restrictive pattern. His baseline blood gases indicate mild CO_2 retention. His slightly elevated HCO_3^- suggests that this is a chronic condition. The P_{O_2} is mildly reduced as a result of hypoventilation.

The CO_2 rebreathing test documents that the patient does not increase his ventilation appropriately in response to an increasing load of CO_2 (Figure 4-3). At the same time, the patient's P_{100} shows a relatively normal response to hypercapnia. This pattern suggests that the patient does not increase ventilation, although his respiratory center is signaling otherwise. These findings are consistent with his obstructive sleep apnea. Patients who retain CO_2 because of large airway or

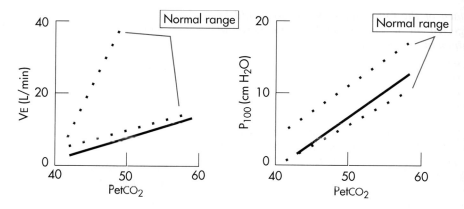

Figure 4-3 *Plot of data from Case 4-2.*

small airway obstruction often have reduced sensitivity to elevated CO_2. This patient might be suspected of having obesity-hypoventilation syndrome. However, patients with obesity-hypoventilation typically have a decreased central drive to ventilation along with their daytime hypercapnia. Obesity-hypoventilation is often associated with OSA or central apnea and usually involves severe hypoxemia and hypercapnia. T.B. has less severe blood gas abnormalities and a normal respiratory drive (P_{100}), suggesting a different cause for the reduced ventilatory response to CO_2.

Treatment

This patient was given nasal continuous positive airway pressure (CPAP) at night. Nasal CPAP alleviates much of the obstruction occurring in the upper airway. The patient reported a marked decrease in daytime hypersomnolence. He was also referred for weight-loss counseling, because his increased weight and reduced ventilatory response placed him at increased risk for pulmonary and cardiac complications.

■ SELF-ASSESSMENT QUESTIONS

Entry Level

1. *A patient with asthma has the following data recorded:*

   $\dot{V}_E$: 5.7 L/min (BTPS)
   f_B: 15/min

   What is this patient's V_T?
   a. 0.15 L (BTPS)
   b. 0.32 L (BTPS)
   c. 0.38 L (BTPS)
   d. 0.44 L (BTPS)

2. *In which of the following conditions would increased minute ventilation be expected?*

   I. Metabolic acidosis
   II. Hypoxemia
   III. Central nervous system depression
   IV. CO_2 narcosis

   a. I and II only
   b. III and IV only
   c. I, II, and III
   d. II, III, and IV

3. *In addition to Pa_{CO_2}, what other measurement is needed to calculate the V_D/V_T ratio?*

   a. Tidal volume
   b. Minute ventilation
   c. Mixed expired CO_2
   d. Pa_{O_2}

4. Wh
   exp.
   pul:
   a. (
   b. (
   c. (
   d. (

5. A (
   as (
   16/.
   his
   a.]
   b. (
   c.]
   d.]

Adva

6. Exh
   mix
   are
   tior

   $P_{\bar{E}}$(
   pH
   Pac
   Pac

   Wh
   a. (
   b. (
   c. (
   d. (

7. Wh
   ope
   me(
   a.]

S E

Gener;
Forster
   fun
West JI
   199
West J
   inte
   Lip

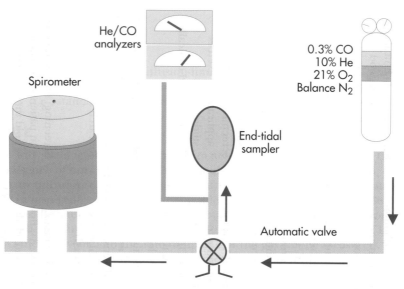

Figure 5-1 *DL$_{CO}$ apparatus.* Basic equipment for performing the DL$_{CO}$ test (specifically the DL$_{CO}$sb). The test gas contains 0.3% CO, 10% He, 21% O$_2$, and the balance N$_2$. Gas is delivered to the automated valve from a large-volume bag *(not shown)*, the spirometer, or a demand valve *(not shown)*. The automatic valve allows the patient to inhale the test gas rapidly. The valve then closes, assisting the breath-hold maneuver. After 10 seconds, the valve opens, allowing exhalation to the spirometer to measure dead space (washout). It then directs exhaled gas to the alveolar sampling device. Gas analyzers for CO and the tracer gas (usually He) then measure concentrations of gas from the alveolar sample. Some systems measure exhaled gas continuously with rapid responding analyzers *(see text)*. In these systems, gas is sampled directly at the mouth without an alveolar sample bag. A computer records a volume-time display of the entire maneuver *(not shown)* (Figure 5-2). Timing of the maneuver may be accomplished automatically by the computer or from a recording device such as a kymograph.

determined as well. It is calculated as follows (assuming He is the tracer gas used):

$$F_A CO_0 = F_I CO \times \frac{F_A He}{F_I He}$$

where:
$F_A CO_0$ = fraction of CO in alveolar gas at beginning of breath hold (time = 0)
$F_I CO$ = fraction of CO in reservoir (usually 0.003)
$F_A He$ = fraction of He in alveolar gas in end-tidal sample
$F_I He$ = fraction of He in inspired gas (usually 0.10)
(Other tracer gases may be used in place of He, in different concentrations)

The change in tracer gas concentration reflects dilution by the gas remaining in the lungs (i.e., RV). This change is used to determine the initial CO concentration, before diffusion from the alveoli into the pulmonary capillaries. The DL$_{CO}$sb (single-breath) is then calculated as follows:

$$DL_{CO}sb = \frac{V_A \times 60}{(P_B - 47) \times (T)} \times Ln \frac{F_A CO_0}{F_A CO_T}$$

where:
V_A = alveolar volume, ml (STPD)
60 = correction from seconds to minutes

P_B = barometric pressure, mm Hg
47   = water vapor pressure at 37° C, mm Hg
T   = breath-hold interval, seconds
Ln   = natural logarithm
F_ACO_0 = fraction of CO in alveolar gas at beginning of breath hold
F_ACO_T = fraction of CO in alveolar gas at end of breath hold

V_A may be calculated from the single-breath dilution of the tracer gas (He in this example):

$$V_A = (V_I - V_D) \times \frac{F_I He}{F_A He} \times STPD \text{ correction factor}$$

where:

V_I = volume of test gas inspired, ml (Figure 5-2)
V_D = dead space volume (anatomic and instrumental), ml
$F_A He$ = fraction of He in alveolar gas
$F_I He$ = fraction of He in inspired gas (usually 0.10)

The dilution of tracer gas is used twice: to determine the CO concentration at the beginning of the breath hold and to determine the lung volume at which the breath hold occurred.

A simplification of the above single-breath method is widely used. The tracer gas and CO analyzers may be calibrated to read full scale (100% or 1.000) when sampling the diffusion

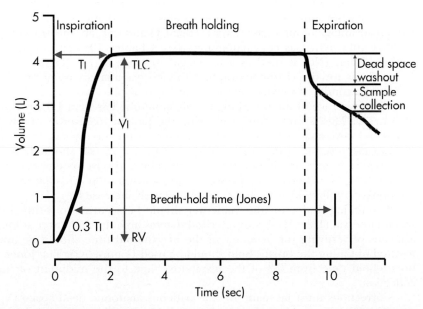

Figure 5-2 *Dl$_{CO}$sb maneuver tracing.* Tracing of single-breath Dl$_{CO}$ maneuver proceeding from left to right (*heavy line*). Inspiration is up. After exhaling to RV, the patient rapidly inspires a vital capacity breath (V$_I$) of the test gas, then holds the breath at TLC for approximately 10 seconds. At the end of the breath hold, the patient exhales the dead space washout volume (usually 0.750 to 1.0 L). Then a sample of the alveolar gas is collected (usually 0.5 to 1.0 L). Any remaining volume is exhaled. The recommended timing method is illustrated. The Jones method measures from 0.3 of the inspiratory time (T$_I$) to the midpoint of the alveolar sample.

mixture and to read zero when sampling air (no tracer or CO). If the analyzers have a linear response to each other, the fractional concentration of the tracer gas in the end-tidal sample is equal to the F_ACO_0. This technique assumes that both the tracer gas and CO are diluted equally during inspiration. Because no tracer gas leaves the lung during the breath hold, its concentration in the alveolar sample must equal that of the CO before any diffusion occurred. The exponential rate of CO diffusion from the alveoli can then be expressed as follows (assuming He is the tracer gas):

$$Ln \left(\frac{F_A He}{F_A CO_T} \right)$$

where:

$F_A He$ = fraction of He in alveolar gas, equal to $F_A CO_0$
$F_A CO_T$ = fraction of CO in alveolar gas at end of breath hold
Ln = natural logarithm of the ratio

This technique avoids the necessity of analyzing the absolute concentrations of the two gases. However, it requires that the analyzers be linear with respect to each other. Analysis of CO is often done using infrared analyzers (see Chapter 10), and their output is nonlinear. Care must be taken to ensure that corrected CO readings are used in the computation. This correction is easily accomplished either electronically or via software in computerized systems. The linearity of the system should be within 1% of full scale. This means that any drift or non-linearity should cause no more than a 1% error when analyzing a known gas concentration.

Other approaches to DL_{CO} gas analysis include rapidly responding multigas analyzers and gas chromatography. Multigas analyzers are specialized infrared analyzers capable of detecting several gases simultaneously. These systems use methane (CH_4) as a tracer gas in place of He. An advantage of multigas analysis is that CO and CH_4 are measured rapidly and continuously (Figure 5-3). Gas chromatography (see Chapter 10) can also be used for DL_{CO} gas analysis. Neon (Ne) is used as a tracer gas in place of He (Figure 5-4). He is used as a "carrier" gas for the chromatograph. Although gas analysis using chromatography is slow (60 to 90 seconds), it is extremely accurate.

The resistance of the breathing circuit should be less than 1.5 cm H_2O/L/sec, at a flow of 6 L/sec. This is important in allowing the patient to inspire rapidly from RV to TLC. A demand valve may be used instead of a reservoir for the test gas. In a demand-flow system, the maximal inspiratory pressure to maintain a flow of 6 L/sec should be less than 10 cm H_2O. Increased resistance, in either a reservoir or a demand valve system, may cause the patient to produce large subatmospheric pressures during inspiration. This has the effect of increasing pulmonary capillary blood volume, and may falsely increase DL_{CO}.

The timing device for the maneuver should be accurate to within 100 msec over a 10-second interval (1%). Most computerized systems time the maneuver automatically. However, a means of verifying the accuracy of the breath-hold time should be available. The Jones method of timing the breath hold should be used (Figure 5-2). The Jones method measures breath-hold time from 0.3 of the inspiratory time to the midpoint of the alveolar sample collection.

Corrections must be made for the patient's anatomic dead space (V_D) as well as dead space in the valve and sample bag. Anatomic V_D should be calculated as 2.2 ml/kg of ideal body weight. The equipment manufacturer should specify instrument V_D. Instrument V_D should not exceed 100 ml, including any filters that might be used. Anatomic and instrument V_D are subtracted from inspired volume (V_I) before the alveolar volume (V_A) is calculated.

All gas volumes must be corrected from ATPS to STPD for the DL_{CO} calculations. However, when the V_A is used to calculate the ratio of DL_{CO} to lung volume (DL/V_A), it is normally

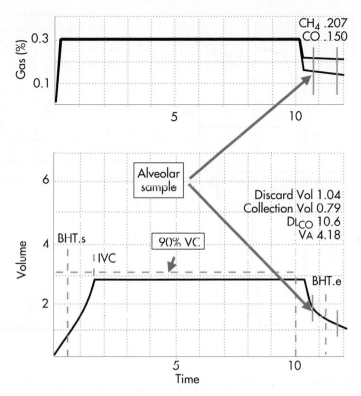

Figure 5-3 *DL_{CO}sb maneuver using continuous gas analysis.* Changes in gas concentrations are shown *(top)*. Test gases (CO and CH_4) rise rapidly to their initial values of 0.3% during the breath hold. During exhalation, both gas concentrations fall with dead space wash out. CH_4 shows a plateau as alveolar gas is exhaled. CO shows a similar pattern, but with a lower concentration because of diffusion during the breath hold. Gas concentration measurements are made from an alveolar window *(gray lines)* that can be adjusted. Changes in lung volumes are shown *(bottom)*. IVC indicates inspiratory volume. In this test, the patient failed to inspire at least 90% of vital capacity (VC) *(dashed gray line)*. BHTs indicates start of breath-hold timing; BHTe indicates end of breath hold at midpoint of the alveolar sample "window." Calculated DL_{CO} and related measurements are displayed *(computer screen)*, allowing inspection of changes as the alveolar sample "window" is adjusted. *(Courtesy VIASYS Healthcare Critical Care Division, Palm Springs, Calif.)*

expressed in BTPS units. Accurate measurement of lung volumes requires that the spirometer have an accuracy of 3% over a range of 8 L. Volume-based spirometer systems must also be free from leaks.

Gas analyzers that are affected by carbon dioxide (CO_2) or water vapor require appropriate absorbers. Absorption of CO_2 is usually accomplished with a chemical absorber using $Ba(OH)_2$ (baralyme) or NaOH (soda lyme). Each of these reactions produces water vapor. Therefore, CO_2 absorbers should be placed upstream of an H_2O absorber. Anhydrous $CaSO_4$ is commonly used to remove water vapor. Selectively permeable tubing (PERMAPURE) can also be used to establish a known water vapor content. Gas-conditioning devices must be routinely checked to ensure accurate gas analysis. Chemical absorbers typically add an indicator that changes color as the absorber becomes exhausted.

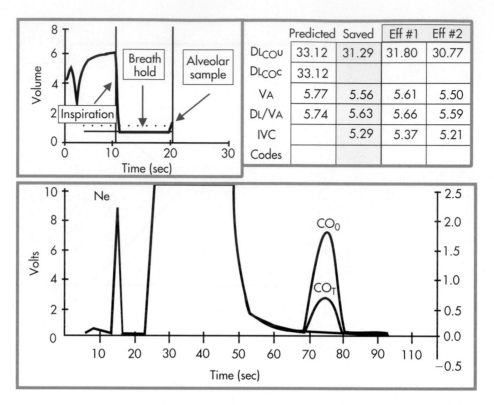

	Predicted	Saved	Eff #1	Eff #2
$DL_{CO}u$	33.12	31.29	31.80	30.77
$DL_{CO}c$	33.12			
VA	5.77	5.56	5.61	5.50
DL/VA	5.74	5.63	5.66	5.59
IVC		5.29	5.37	5.21
Codes				

Figure 5-4 *DL_{CO}sb test using gas chromatography.* Volume-time tracing with inspiration, breath-hold, and alveolar sampling is shown *(top left)*. In this scheme, inspiration causes a downward deflection. Output of the gas chromatograph is shown *(lower graph)*. Neon (Ne) (the tracer gas) and CO show distinct peaks. CO concentrations from the beginning (CO_0) and end (CO_T) of the breath hold are superimposed. Calculated DL_{CO} and related values for multiple efforts are shown *(top right)*. *(Courtesy Medical Graphics, Inc., St. Paul, Minn.)*

PF Tips

Watch the patient carefully during the DL_{CO} effort in order to detect either a Valsalva or Müller maneuver. Widely varying results in two or more DL_{CO} measurements are often caused by the patient failing to relax during the breath hold. Some systems provide a pressure monitor to detect large positive or negative pressures during the breath hold.

DL_{CO}sb maneuvers should be performed after the patient has been seated for at least 5 minutes. The patient should refrain from exertion immediately before the test; exercise increases cardiac output, which increases DL_{CO}. The patient should be instructed about the requirements of the maneuver. After expiration to RV, inspiration should be rapid but not forced. Healthy patients should be able to inspire at least 90% of their VC within 2.5 seconds (DL_{CO} 5-1). Patients with moderate or severe airway obstruction should inspire the same volume within 4.0 seconds. The breath hold should be relaxed, against either the closed glottis or a closed valve. The patient should avoid excessive positive intrathoracic pressure (Valsalva maneuver) or excessive negative intrathoracic pressure (Müller maneuver). A Valsalva maneuver reduces pulmonary capillary blood volume and may produce a falsely low DL_{CO}. A Müller maneuver increases pulmonary capillary blood volume and may falsely increase DL_{CO}. Expiration after the breath hold should be smooth and uninterrupted. A sample volume of 0.5 to 1.0 L should be collected within 4 seconds. In $DL_{CO}sb$ systems that analyze expired gas continuously (Figure 5-3), inspection of the washout of the tracer gas may be used to select an appropriate alveolar sample.

DL_{CO} is affected by both Hb and COHb levels in the patient's blood. A low Hb (anemia) or high COHb reduces the measured DL_{CO}. A high Hb (polycythemia) causes the DL_{CO} to appear elevated. If the DL_{CO} is corrected for Hb or COHb, both corrected and uncorrected values should be reported.

Two or more acceptable $DL_{CO}sb$ maneuvers are usually averaged (see DL_{CO} 5-1). Duplicate determinations should be within 10% or 3 ml CO/min/mm Hg, whichever is greater. The difference between two tests may be calculated as follows:

$$\frac{\text{Test 1} - \text{Test 2}}{\text{Average}} \times 100$$

Note that two tests should not differ by more than 10% or 3 ml CO from the average, nor from each other. There should be a 4-minute delay between repeated maneuvers to allow for washout of the test gas from the lungs.

Corrections for abnormal hemoglobin (Hb) concentrations should be applied using a current Hb value. DL_{CO} should be corrected so that it is standardized to an Hb value of 14.6 g% for adult men and adolescent boys. DL_{CO} should be corrected to an Hb value of

DL_{CO} 5-1   Criteria for Acceptability—$DL_{CO}sb$

1 Volume-time tracing should show smooth, rapid inspiration from RV to TLC.
2 Inspiration should be rapid but not forced; less than 2.5 seconds in healthy patients and less than 4 seconds in patients with obstruction.
3 Dead space washout should be 0.75 to 1.00 L (0.5 L if VC is less than 2.0 L). If continuous analysis of expired gas is used, visual inspection of dead space washout should be made.
4 Alveolar sample volume should be 0.5 to 1.0 L, unless continuous analysis is used.
5 V_1 should be at least 90% of previously recorded best VC.
6 Breath-hold time should be between 9 and 11 seconds, using the Jones method.
7 The average of two or more acceptable tests should be reported. Duplicate determinations should be within 10% of 3 ml CO/min/mm Hg.

13.4 g% for women, and children of either sex less than 15 years of age. The correction factor for men may be calculated as follows:

$$Hb\ correction = \frac{(10.22 + Hb)}{1.7 \times Hb}$$

Similarly, the correction factor for women and children less than 15 years of age is calculated as follows:

$$Hb\ correction = \frac{(9.38 + Hb)}{1.7 \times Hb}$$

DL_{CO} may then be corrected:

$$Hb\ adjusted\ DL_{CO} = Hb\ correction \times Observed\ DL_{CO}$$

Both uncorrected and corrected DL_{CO} values should be reported, along with the Hb value.

Correction for the presence of carboxyhemoglobin (COHb) in the patient's blood is also recommended. The DL_{CO} may be adjusted as follows:

$$COHb - Adjusted\ DL_{CO} = Measured\ DL_{CO} \times \left(1.00 + \frac{\%\ COHb}{100}\right)$$

The %COHb is the fraction of carboxyhemoglobin determined by a spectrophotometer (co-oximeter) expressed as a percentage. Patients should be asked to refrain from smoking for 24 hours before the test to reduce the CO back pressure in the blood.

DL_{CO} varies inversely with changes in alveolar oxygen pressure (P_AO_2). P_AO_2 changes as a function of altitude, as well as with the partial pressure of oxygen in the test gas. DL_{CO} increases approximately 0.35% for each mm Hg decrease in P_AO_2. When test gas mixtures that produce an inspired O_2 pressure of 150 mm Hg (i.e., 21% at sea level) are used, DL_{CO} values will be equivalent to those measured at sea level. Alternatively, standard test gas ($F_IO_2 = 0.21$) can be used and DL_{CO} corrected by adjusting either P_AO_2 or P_IO_2. For a standard P_AO_2 of 120 mm Hg, the equation is as follows:

$$Altitude - Adjusted\ DL_{CO} = Measured\ DL_{CO} \times (1.0 + 0.0035[P_AO_2 - 120])$$

where:

P_AO_2 = Measured or estimated alveolar oxygen partial pressure

For a P_IO_2 of 150 mm Hg (sea level), the equation is as follows:

$$Altitude - Adjusted\ DL_{CO} = Measured\ DL_{CO} \times (1.0 + 0.0031[P_IO_2 - 120])$$

where:

$P_IO_2 = 0.21(P_B - 47)$

Steady State–Filey Technique

The patient breathes a gas mixture of 0.1% to 0.2% CO in air for 5 to 6 minutes. During the final 2 minutes, expired gas is collected in a bag or balloon, and an arterial blood sample is drawn. Exhaled volume is measured. Expired gas is analyzed for CO, CO_2, and O_2. The arterial blood is analyzed for P_{CO_2}. Steady-state diffusing capacity is calculated as follows:

$$DL_{CO}ss1 = \frac{\dot{V}_{CO}}{P_A CO}$$

where:

$\dot{V}_{CO}$ = volume of CO transferred, milliliters/minute (STPD)

$P_A CO$ = mean alveolar partial pressure of CO

CO is determined by analyzing inspired and expired CO ($F_I CO$ and $F_E CO$, respectively); $\dot{V}_E$, inspired N_2 ($F_I N_2$), and expired N_2 ($F_E N_2$) are determined indirectly from the fractions of O_2, CO_2, and H_2O vapor in the exhaled gas as follows:

$$\dot{V}_{CO} = \dot{V}_E \left(F_I CO \frac{F_E N_2}{F_I N_2} - F_E CO \right)$$

$P_A CO$ is calculated as follows using a form of Bohr's equation:

$$P_A CO = P_B - 47 \left(\frac{F_E CO - r F_I CO}{1 - r} \right)$$

where:

$$r = \frac{PaCO_2 - P_{\bar{E}}CO_2}{P_{\bar{E}}CO_2}$$

where:

$PaCO_2$ = partial pressure of arterial CO_2

$P_{\bar{E}}CO_2$ = partial pressure of mixed expired CO_2

Estimating $P_A CO$ in this way avoids the necessity of obtaining a direct alveolar sample.

End-Tidal CO Determination

The end-tidal CO determination ($DL_{CO}ss2$) method resembles the $DL_{CO}ss1$ in CO and is derived similarly. $P_A CO$, however, is determined by taking the average end-tidal CO tension (PetCO) from instantaneous analysis of multiple breaths. The end-tidal value is assumed to be equal to the mean $P_A CO$.

Assumed V_D Technique

The assumed V_D technique ($DL_{CO}ss3$) is also similar to the $DL_{CO}ss1$. CO is determined as in $DL_{CO}ss1$, but $P_A CO$ is measured differently. The fraction of CO in alveolar gas ($F_A CO$), which is used to derive $P_A CO$ when P_B is known, is calculated as follows:

$$F_A CO = \frac{V_T(F_E CO) - V_D(F_I CO)}{V_T - V_D}$$

where:

V_T = tidal volume

V_D = dead space volume

$F_E CO$ = fraction of expired CO
$F_I CO$ = fraction of inspired CO

V_T is measured by averaging multiple breaths. V_D is often assumed to be equal to 2.2 ml/kg of ideal body weight. The mechanical V_D of the breathing circuit is subtracted.

Mixed Venous Pco₂ Technique

$\dot{V}CO$ is obtained as in DL_{CO}ss1. $P_A CO$ is calculated by estimating the mixed venous Pco_2 from an equilibration technique. $P_A CO_2$ is then determined from the $P_V CO_2$ and the normal gradient. When $P_A CO_2$ is derived, an equation similar to that used to determine $P_A CO$ in the DL_{CO}ss1 technique can be used. Using mixed venous Pco_2 avoids the necessity of arterial puncture.

DL_{CO} is most often measured using the single-breath (breath-hold) technique. The equipment and procedures used for the DL_{CO}sb have been standardized by several professional organizations.

Rebreathing Technique

The patient rebreathes from a reservoir containing a mixture of 0.3% CO, 10% He, and air for 30 to 60 seconds at a rate of approximately 30 breaths/min. The final CO, He, and O_2 concentrations in the reservoir are measured after this interval. An equation similar to that used for the single-breath technique is used (see DL_{CO}sb):

$$DL_{CO}rb = \frac{V_S \times 60}{(P_B - 47)(T2 - T1)} \times Ln\left(\frac{F_A CO_{T1}}{F_A CO_{T2}}\right)$$

where:
V_S	= volume of lung reservoir system (initial volume $\times F_I He/F_A He$)
60	= correction from seconds to minutes
P_B	= barometric pressure, mm Hg
47	= water vapor pressure, mm Hg
T2 − T1	= rebreathing interval, seconds
Ln	= natural logarithm
$F_A CO_{T1}$	= fraction of CO in alveolar gas at beginning of the rebreathing
$F_A CO_{T2}$	= fraction of CO in alveolar gas at the end of the rebreathing

Equilibration-Washout Method

The patient rebreathes from a reservoir containing 0.3% CO and 10% He in air until equilibrium is reached. Then the patient again breathes room air, and the washouts of both CO and He are recorded by a rapid gas analyzer. During the washout, CO is removed at a rapid rate by diffusion as well as by ventilation, whereas He is removed more slowly by ventilation alone. The difference in washout rates is caused by the rate of CO diffusion. An equation similar to the DL_{CO}sb equation is used to calculate DL_{CO}ssHe. A logarithmic expression of the ratio of final He concentration to initial He concentration is included as a factor with the CO concentration ratio.

Slow Exhalation Single Breath–Intrabreath Method

The patient inspires a vital capacity (VC) breath of test gas containing 0.3% CO, 0.3% CH_4, 21% O_2, and the balance N_2. Then the patient exhales slowly and evenly at approximately 0.5 L/sec from TLC to RV. A rapidly responding infrared analyzer monitors gas concentrations. The rate of disappearance of CO can be calculated in a manner similar to the equilibration–wash out method. Change in V_A is calculated from the change in concentration of the CH_4 tracer gas. CH_4 is used in place of He because it can be rapidly measured using an infrared analyzer. Multiple estimates of DL_{CO} can be made during a single exhalation, recording DL_{CO} as a function of lung volume. This is done using an equation similar to that used for the single-breath method. Instead of one estimate of V_A (equal to the lung volume at breath hold), multiple increments of V_A are made, and DL_{CO} is plotted against lung volume. A single estimate of overall DL_{CO} can also be obtained.

Fractional CO Uptake

The patient first inspires a mixture of 0.1% CO in air from a reservoir to establish a steady-state breathing pattern. Then the patient exhales into a spirometer or reservoir, from which an average expired CO sample is analyzed. The $F_U CO$ is expressed as follows:

$$F_U CO = \frac{F_I CO - F_E CO}{F_I CO}$$

where:
$F_I CO$ = fraction of inspired CO
$F_E CO$ = fraction of expired CO

The resulting fraction may be multiplied by 100 and expressed as a percentage. A consistent level of $\dot{V}_E$ is critical for a valid determination of $F_U CO$ and should be monitored closely.

Membrane Diffusion Coefficient and Capillary Blood Volume

The patient performs two DL_{CO}sb tests, each at a different level of alveolar PO_2. The first DL_{CO}sb is performed as described previously. The patient then breathes an elevated concentration of O_2 (balance N_2) for approximately 5 minutes, exhales to RV, and performs the second DL_{CO}sb maneuver. DL_{CO} values are calculated for both the air- and oxygen-breathing maneuvers. The total resistance caused by the alveolocapillary membrane (Dm) and the resistance caused by the rate of chemical combination with Hb and transfer into the red blood cell (θQc) is calculated as follows:

$$\frac{1}{DL_{CO}} = \frac{1}{Dm} + \frac{1}{\theta Qc}$$

where:
$1/DL_{CO}$ = reciprocal of diffusing capacity, or resistance
$1/Dm$ = alveolocapillary membrane resistance
$1/\theta Qc$ = resistance of red blood cell membrane and rate of reaction with Hb
θ = transfer rate of CO/milliliter of capillary blood
Qc = capillary blood volume

Because CO and O_2 compete for binding sites on Hb, measurement of diffusion of CO at different levels of alveolar PO_2 can be used to distinguish resistance caused by the alveolocapillary membrane from resistance caused by the red blood cell membrane and Hb reaction rate. Qc is presumed to remain the same for both tests, but θ varies in response to changes in PO_2. Resistance caused by the alveolocapillary membrane can be calculated by plotting θ at two points against $1/DL_{CO}$ and extrapolating back to zero (as if no O_2 were present).

Significance and Pathophysiology

See DL_{CO} 5-2 for interpretive strategies. The average DL_{CO} value for resting adult patients by the single-breath method is 25 ml CO/min/mm Hg (STPD). The expected DL_{CO} value in a healthy patient varies directly with the patient's lung volume. Values derived using one of the steady-state methods are usually slightly less than those derived using the single-breath method in healthy patients, but they may vary by as much as 30%. Women have slightly lower normal values, presumably in correlation with smaller normal lung volumes. DL_{CO} values can increase two to three times in healthy individuals during exercise.

Most reference equations use height, sex, and age to predict DL_{CO}. Some equations use V_A or body surface area (BSA) to calculate expected values. If the patient's weight is used (i.e., to calculate BSA), the ideal body weight is recommended. Using the actual body weight in obese patients can result in erroneously large predicted values. Significant differences exist among reference equations. These discrepancies result from different methods used to measure DL_{CO} in various laboratories. Laboratories should check the appropriateness of their reference equations by comparing the results obtained from normal patients. They should measure DL_{CO} of 15 to 20 healthy patients of each sex. If the reference equations used are appropriate, the differences between the measured and expected values for the healthy patients should be minimal. Regression equations for calculation of expected DL_{CO} values are included in Appendix B.

DL_{CO} is often decreased in restrictive lung diseases, particularly those associated with pulmonary fibrosis. Fibrotic changes in the lung parenchyma are associated with asbestosis, berylliosis, and silicosis. Many other diseases with causes related to inhalation of dusts also cause fibrotic changes in lung tissue. Idiopathic pulmonary fibrosis, sarcoidosis, systemic lupus erythematosus, and scleroderma are also commonly associated with reduction in DL_{CO}.

DL_{CO} 5-2   Interpretive Strategies—DL_{CO}

1 Were the test maneuvers performed acceptably? Were the tests reproducible within 10% or 3 ml CO/min/mm Hg of the mean?
2 Were all appropriate corrections made? Hb? COHb? Altitude?
3 Are reference values appropriate? Age? Height? Sex? Weight?
4 Is DL_{CO} less than the lower limit of normal? If not explained by abnormal Hb or COHb, check DL/V_A.
5 Is the DL/V_A ratio within normal limits? If so, suspect reduced diffusing capacity related to decreased lung volumes or parenchymal changes. Consider clinical correlation.
6 Is the DL/V_A ratio reduced? If so, suspect reduced diffusing capacity related to obstruction or increased dead space. Look for clinical correlation.
7 Is DL_{CO} increased? If not explained by abnormal Hb, consider increased pulmonary blood volume or hemorrhage. Look for clinical correlation.
8 Is DL_{CO} less than 50% of predicted? If so, consider addtional tests (blood gases, exercise desaturation study).

Inhalation of toxic gases or organic agents may cause inflammation of the alveoli (alveolitis) and decrease DL_{CO}. These disease states are sometimes categorized as *diffusion defects*. The decrease in DL_{CO} is probably more closely related to the loss of lung volume, alveolar surface area, or capillary bed than to thickening of the alveolocapillary membranes. DL_{CO} also decreases when there is loss of lung tissue or replacement of normal parenchyma by space-occupying lesions such as tumors.

DL_{CO} may also be reduced in the presence of pulmonary edema. Disruption of alveolar ventilation and reduction of lung volume as well as congestion of the alveoli cause the reduction in DL_{CO} in edema. In the early stages of congestive heart failure (CHF), DL_{CO} may actually be increased. As the left ventricle decompensates, pulmonary vessels become engorged. The increased blood volume causes the DL_{CO} to increase, until the congestion becomes advanced. In most patients with heart failure, DL_{CO} is decreased because of the restrictive ventilatory pattern. DL_{CO} in patients who receive a heart transplant for chronic heart failure does not return to normal, as might be expected.

DL_{CO} may also be decreased as a result of medical or surgical intervention for cardiopulmonary disease. Lung resection for cancer or other reasons typically results in decreased DL_{CO}. The extent of reduction is usually directly proportional to the volume of lung removed. An exception to this pattern occurs in lung volume reduction surgery (LVRS) or in bullectomy. These surgical procedures resect areas of the lung that have little or no blood flow. Lack of perfusion is documented by a lung scan. Excision of tissue in such areas reduces lung volume without necessarily reducing the surface area available for diffusion. Improved ventilation-perfusion matching in the remaining lung often results in increased DL_{CO}.

Radiation therapy that involves the lungs usually causes a loss of DL_{CO}. Radiation causes pneumonitis that commonly results in fibrotic changes. Drugs used in chemotherapy (e.g., bleomycin) and those used to suppress rejection in organ transplantation may cause reductions in DL_{CO}. These drugs appear to directly affect the alveolocapillary membranes. Some drugs used in the treatment of cardiac arrhythmias (e.g., amiodarone) have been shown to decrease DL_{CO}. DL_{CO} is commonly used to monitor drug toxicity. DL_{CO} may also be helpful in evaluating disorders such as hepatopulmonary syndrome, in which gas exchange and pulmonary vascular defects coexist.

DL_{CO} may also be decreased in both acute and chronic obstructive lung disease. DL_{CO} is decreased in emphysema for several reasons. Emphysematous lungs have a reduced surface area, with the loss of both alveolar walls and their associated capillary beds. As a result of the decreased surface area, less gas can be transferred per minute even if the remaining gas exchange units are structurally normal. In addition to loss of surface area for gas exchange, the distance from the terminal bronchiole to the alveolocapillary membrane increases in emphysema. As alveoli break down, terminal lung units become larger. Gas must diffuse farther just to reach the alveolocapillary surface. There is also mismatching of ventilation and pulmonary capillary blood flow in emphysema. Disruption of alveolar structures causes loss of support for terminal airways. Airway collapse and gas trapping result in ventilation-perfusion (V/Q) abnormalities.

Other obstructive diseases (e.g., chronic bronchitis, asthma) may not reduce DL_{CO} unless they result in markedly abnormal V/Q patterns. DL_{CO} is sometimes used to differentiate among these obstructive patterns. Low DL_{CO} in the presence of obstruction is sometimes assumed to be evidence of emphysema. However, V/Q mismatching can cause DL_{CO} to appear to be decreased in asthma, chronic bronchitis, or emphysema. Some asthmatic patients may have an increased DL_{CO}, but the cause is not completely understood.

DL_{CO} measurements at rest have been suggested to estimate the probability of O_2 desaturation during exercise. Not all clinicians agree that a decrease in DL_{CO} can predict desaturation. However, there does appear to be a correlation between resting DL_{CO} and gas exchange during exercise. In patients who have chronic obstructive pulmonary disease (COPD), DL_{CO} less than 50% of predicted is accompanied by O_2 desaturation during exercise. Patients with restrictive lung disease and a low resting DL_{CO} are at risk of O_2 desaturation, even with low levels of exercise. Low resting DL_{CO} (i.e., less than 50% to 60% of predicted) may indicate the need for assessment of oxygenation during exercise.

DL_{CO} is directly related to lung volume (V_A) in healthy individuals. DL_{CO} may be divided by the lung volume at which the measurement was obtained to express DL_{CO} per unit of V_A. This ratio is reported as DL/V_L or DL/V_A. This calculation is simple because V_A must be measured to derive DL_{CO} (Figure 5-4). Analysis of this relationship can be useful to differentiate whether decreased DL_{CO} resulted from loss of lung volume (as in restriction) or from another cause. In healthy individuals, alveolar volume and DL_{CO} are proportional to body size (height). Two patients of different height will have different DL_{CO} and V_A values, but their DL/V_A ratios will be similar. In healthy adults, DL/V_A is approximately 4 to 5 ml CO transferred/minute/liter of lung volume.

In the presence of pulmonary disease, both DL_{CO} and V_A may be affected. In obstruction, low DL_{CO} without reduction in V_A results in a low ratio. In a purely restrictive process, loss of DL_{CO} reflects loss of V_A and the ratio is preserved. For example, a patient who has a DL_{CO} of 12 ml CO/min/mm Hg (50% of predicted) and a V_A of 3.0 L would have a DL/V_A ratio of 4. This reduction in DL_{CO} is roughly proportional to loss of lung volume. Other pulmonary conditions (such as pneumonectomy) may result in an increased DL/V_A, where gas exchange is preserved and lung volume is decreased.

DL_{CO} and DL/V_A may also be affected if the patient performs the breath-hold maneuver at a lung volume less than TLC. Some clinicians suggest correcting the predicted DL_{CO} for the reduced V_A, or comparing the DL/V_A to the predicted value that would be derived using the actual TLC at which the measurement was made. There are important implications for interpretation of diffusing capacity in the complex relationship between DL_{CO} and DL/V_A. Patients who fail to inspire fully during the maneuver will have a decreased DL_{CO}, but the DL/V_A may appear to increase. Correcting for V_A does not correct for poor inspiratory effort (less than 90% of VC). In patients who have a low DL_{CO}, a "normal" DL/V_A should not be confused with normal gas exchange.

The $DL_{CO}sb$ is the most widely used method because of its relative simplicity and noninvasive nature. The rapidity with which repeated maneuvers can be performed also lends to its popularity. Many automated systems use the $DL_{CO}sb$, contributing a certain degree of standardization to the methodology. Large differences in reported DL_{CO} values exist between laboratories. This variability has been attributed to different testing techniques, problems in the gas analysis involved in the test, and differences in computations. Breath holding at TLC is not a physiologic maneuver. This and the fact that DL_{CO} varies with lung volume cause some concerns about $DL_{CO}sb$ as an accurate description of diffusing capacity. $DL_{CO}sb$ is not practical for use during exercise. Some patients have difficulty expiring fully, inspiring fully, or holding their breath. The American Thoracic Society (ATS) has provided guidelines to improve standardization of the single-breath maneuver (Table 5-2).

The steady-state methods ($DL_{CO}ss_{1-4}$) use various techniques to estimate the mean alveolar PCO. $DL_{CO}ss_1$ has the broadest application of the steady-state methods. Availability of arterial blood gas analysis is a primary requirement for $DL_{CO}ss_1$. $DL_{CO}ss_2$ has gained popularity because of the availability of fast-response CO analyzers (see Chapter 10). $DL_{CO}ss_3$ may be used to measure DL_{CO} during exercise because small differences in the assumed V_D become less significant as V_T increases. All steady-state methods can be applied to exercise testing, but $DL_{CO}ss_1$ and $DL_{CO}ss_4$ are most commonly used.

The rebreathing method ($DL_{CO}rb$) requires somewhat complicated calculations but offers the advantages of a normal breathing pattern without arterial puncture. $DL_{CO}rb$ is less

TABLE 5-2   DL$_{CO}$sb Recommendations

A. Equipment

1. Volume accuracy same as for spirometry (±3% over 8-L range, all gases).
2. Documented analyzer linearity from 0 to full span ± 1%.
3. Circuit resistance less than 1.5 cm H_2O at 6 L/sec.
4. Demand valve sensitivity less than 10 cm H_2O to generate 6 L/sec flow.
5. Timing mechanism accurate to ±1% over 10 sec; checked quarterly.
6. Documented instrument dead space (inspiratory/expiratory) less than 0.1 L.
7. Check for leaks and volume accuracy (3 L calibration) daily.
8. Validate system by testing healthy nonsmokers (biologic controls) quarterly.

B. Technique

1. Subject should refrain from smoking for 24 hr before test.
2. Subject should be instructed carefully before procedure.
3. Subject should inspire rapidly; 2.5 sec or less for healthy subjects, 4 seconds or less in obstruction.
4. Subject should achieve an inspired volume greater than 90% of VC.
5. Subject should perform breath hold for 9-11 sec, relaxing against closed glottis or closed valve (no Valsalva or Müller maneuver).
6. VD washout should be 0.75-1.0 L (0.5 L if VC less than 2.0 L).
7. Alveolar sample volume should be 0.5-1.0 L collected in less than 4 sec.
8. Visual inspection of VD washout and alveolar sampling should be used for system that continuously analyzes expired gas.
9. Test gas should contain 21% O_2 at sea level; supplemented O_2 should be discontinued 5 min before testing if possible.
10. Four min should elapse between repeat tests.

C. Calculations

1. Average at least two acceptable tests; duplicate determinations should be within 10% or 3 ml CO/min/mm Hg.
2. Use Jones method of timing breath hold.
3. Alveolar volume should be determined by single-breath dilution of tracer gas.
4. Adjust for V_D volumes (instrument and patient).
5. Determine inspired gas conditions (ATPS or ATPD).
6. Correct for CO_2 and H_2O absorption.
7. Report DL/V_A in ml CO (STPD)/min/mmHg per L (BTPS).
8. Correct for Hb concentration (see text).
9. Adjust for COHb (recommended).
10. Adjust for altitude (recommended).
11. Use reference equations appropriate to the laboratory method and patient population.

Summarized from American Thoracic Society: Single-breath carbon monoxide diffusing capacity (transfer factor): recommendations for a standard technique—1995 update, *Am J Respir Crit Care Med* 152:2185–2198, 1995.

sensitive to $\dot{V}/\dot{Q}$ abnormalities and uneven ventilation distribution than either the DL$_{CO}$sb or the steady-state methods. The rebreathing method and the steady-state methods may have some inaccuracy from accumulation of COHb in the capillary blood and the resultant back-pressure. Capillary PCO is routinely assumed to be zero. The actual alveolocapillary CO gradient at the time of testing can be estimated, although with some difficulty. DL$_{CO}$ss$_{He}$ is the most sophisticated technique. It is relatively insensitive to $\dot{V}/\dot{Q}$ and ventilation abnormalities. However, it is probably limited to research applications.

Measurement of DL_{CO} by the intrabreath method ($DL_{CO}ib$) offers the advantage of not requiring a breath hold at TLC. However, the patient must inspire a large enough volume of test gas so that the subsequent exhalation will clear the instrument and anatomic V_D. In addition, the single-breath exhalation must be slow and even. In some systems, a flow restrictor may be necessary to limit expiratory flow. The single-breath slow-exhalation method produces values similar to those obtained by the breath-hold method in healthy patients when flow is maintained at 0.5 L/sec. Uneven distribution of ventilation may produce intrabreath DL_{CO} values that are artificially elevated. Because the evenness of ventilation distribution can be assessed from the washout of CH_4, unacceptable DL_{CO} values can be detected. Table 5-1 compares some advantages and disadvantages of DL_{CO} testing methods.

Measurement of membrane (Dm) and red blood cell components (θVc) of diffusion resistance in healthy patients reveals that each factor accounts for approximately half of the total resistance. Difficulty in quantifying the partial pressure of O_2 in the lungs (pulmonary capillaries) restricts the use of the membrane diffusing capacity determination.

Numerous other factors can influence the observed DL_{CO}:

1. *Hemoglobin and hematocrit (Hct).* Decreased Hb or Hct reduces DL_{CO}, whereas increased Hb and Hct elevate DL_{CO}. DL_{CO} may be corrected if the patient's Hb is known. CO uptake varies approximately 7% for each gram of Hb. The measured DL_{CO} may be corrected so that the value reported is standardized to Hb levels of 14.6 g% for men, and 13.4 g% for women and children younger than 15 years of age. When this correction is applied, DL_{CO} will be reduced if the patient's Hb is greater than the standard value (14.6 g% or 13.4 g%, respectively). Conversely, DL_{CO} increases if the Hb is less than the standard value. Both corrected and uncorrected DL_{CO} values should be reported, along with the Hb value used for adjustment. Care should be taken to use Hb values that are representative of the patient's actual Hb level at the time of the DL_{CO} test.

2. *COHb.* Increased COHb levels, as found in smokers, reduce DL_{CO}. Smokers may have COHb levels of 10% or even greater, causing significant CO back-pressure. The diffusion gradient for CO across alveolocapillary membranes is assumed to equal the alveolar pressure of CO. In healthy nonsmoking patients, very little CO is present in pulmonary capillary blood. When there is carboxyhemoglobinemia, diffusion of CO is reduced because the gradient across the membrane is reduced. COHb also shifts the oxyhemoglobin dissociation curve, further altering gas transfer. Each 1% increase in COHb causes an approximate 1% decrease in the measured DL_{CO}. CO back-pressure corrections can also be made by estimating the partial pressure of CO in the pulmonary capillaries. This pressure can be used to correct the F_ACO_0 and the F_ACO_T.

3. *Alveolar PCO_2.* Increased PCO_2 elevates DL_{CO} because the alveolar PO_2 is necessarily decreased. Significant increases in alveolar PCO_2 reduce the alveolar PO_2 (i.e., hypoventilation).

4. *Pulmonary capillary blood volume.* Increased blood volume in the lungs (Qc) causes increased DL_{CO}. Increases in pulmonary capillary blood volume may result from increased cardiac output as occurs during exercise. Patients should be seated and resting for several minutes before DL_{CO} testing is performed. Pulmonary hemorrhage may also cause an increase in blood volume in the lungs. In each of these cases, the increase in DL_{CO} is related to the increased volume of Hb available for gas transfer. Excessive negative intrathoracic pressure during breath holding can increase pulmonary capillary volume and elevate the DL_{CO}. Conversely, excessive positive intrathoracic pressure (Valsalva maneuver) can reduce pulmonary blood flow and decrease DL_{CO}.

5. *Body position.* The supine position increases DL_{CO}. Changes in body position affect the distribution of capillary blood flow.
6. *Altitude above sea level.* DL_{CO} varies inversely with changes in alveolar oxygen pressure (P_AO_2). At altitudes significantly greater than sea level, DL_{CO} increases unless corrections are made (see Technique section).

Several additional technical considerations may affect the measurement of DL_{CO} (particularly $DL_{CO}sb$). V_A is calculated from He dilution during the single-breath maneuver. This technique may underestimate lung volume in patients who have moderate or severe obstruction. Low estimated V_A results in low DL_{CO} values. Some clinicians prefer to use a separately determined lung volume to estimate V_A. RV, measured independently by one of the gas techniques or by plethysmography, can be added to the inspired volume (V_I) to derive V_A. V_A calculated by this method is usually larger in patients with airway obstruction than V_A calculated from the single-breath dilution method. The resulting estimate of DL_{CO} is larger. This approach may be questionable because the single-breath He dilution value (F_AHe) is also used in the exponential ratio that describes transfer of CO from the alveoli. Some laboratories report DL_{CO} calculated by both methods. The ATS recommends calculation of V_A using the single-breath method.

The method of timing of breath hold also influences the calculation of DL_{CO} (Figure 5-2). Most systems measure breath-hold time by one of three methods:

1. *Ogilvie method:* from the beginning of inspiration (V_I) to the beginning of alveolar sampling
2. *Epidemiology Standardization Project (ESP) method:* from the midpoint of inspiration (half of the V_I) to the beginning of alveolar sampling
3. *Jones method:* includes 0.7 of the inspiratory time to the midpoint of the alveolar sample

Theoretically, breath-hold time is considered the time during which diffusion occurs. However, because some gas transfer takes place during inspiration, DL_{CO} will be greater if timing starts at the midpoint of V_I, as is the case when the ESP method is used. Similarly, some diffusion occurs during washout and alveolar sampling. If the timing period is extended into the alveolar sampling phase, as is done in the Jones method, the actual time of breath holding is increased and the additional diffusion accounted for. The timing method may become significant if the reference values used for comparison were generated by one of the other methods. The Jones method is the recommended method (Table 5-2). Rapid inspiration from RV to TLC, and rapid expiration to the alveolar sampling phase reduce differences resulting from the timing methods (Table 5-2).

The volume of gas discarded before collecting the alveolar sample may affect the measured DL_{CO}. Most automated systems allow the washout volume to be adjusted, with 0.75 to 1.0 L most commonly used. Washout volume may need to be reduced to 0.5 L if the patient's VC is less than 2.0 L. In patients who have obstructive disease, reducing the washout volume may result in increased dead-space gas being added to the alveolar sample. Because dead-space gas resembles the diffusion mixture, DL_{CO} may be underestimated.

Alveolar sampling technique also affects DL_{CO} measurement. Alveolar samples should be collected within 4 seconds, including washout and alveolar sampling. A sample volume of 0.5 to 1.0 L is recommended. Patients with a small VC (i.e., less than 2.0 L) may require a smaller volume, just as with the washout. When only a small sample is obtained, the gas may not accurately reflect alveolar concentrations of CO and tracer gas, particularly in the presence of V/Q abnormalities. Continuous analysis of the expirate using rapidly responding analyzers allows identification of alveolar gas. Infrared analyzers that can simultaneously analyze the tracer gas and CO will allow the entire breath to be analyzed. These instruments permit adjustment of the alveolar sampling window so that a representative gas sample can be obtained (Figure 5-3).

Summary

This chapter addresses the measurement of DL_{CO}. DL_{CO} can be measured by various techniques. These techniques include the single-breath method and steady-state methods, as well as others. The single-breath method, or $DL_{CO}sb$, is the most commonly used. $DL_{CO}sb$ is noninvasive and can be repeated easily to obtain multiple measurements. Many automated $DL_{CO}sb$ systems are available. The ATS and others have published standardization guidelines for $DL_{CO}sb$. DL_{CO} measurements may be affected by a variety of factors, such Hb level or altitude. Careful attention to standards and clinical practice guidelines can reduce the variance in $DL_{CO}sb$ measurements in different laboratories. The steady-state DL_{CO} and other methods, although not used as widely, have advantages for measuring diffusing capacity in special situations (e.g., exercise).

DL_{CO} measurements are used diagnostically for a variety of diseases. Because DL_{CO} assesses gas exchange, it is useful in both obstructive and restrictive disease patterns. DL_{CO} and DL/V_A are commonly used to assess the course of diseases such as idiopathic pulmonary fibrosis and sarcoidosis. DL_{CO} is often measured in patients with obstructive breathing patterns to characterize the physiology of the obstructive process. In both obstructive and restrictive disorders, DL_{CO} is used to measure response to surgical or medical interventions.

CASE STUDIES

CASE 5-1

HISTORY

P.M. is a 55-year-old woman referred to the pulmonary function laboratory because of shortness of breath on exertion. She has a 38-pack-year smoking history, but stopped smoking 6 months ago. She still coughs each morning, but her sputum volume has decreased since she stopped smoking. She has no significant environmental or family history of pulmonary disease. She had been using an inhaled β-agonist but withheld it for 12 hours before the test.

PULMONARY FUNCTION TESTING

Personal Data

Age: 55
Height: 65 in
Weight: 137 lb
Race: African American

Spirometry

	Predicted	Before Drug Actual	Before Drug % Predicted	After Drug Actual	After Drug % Predicted	% Change
FVC (L)	2.81	2.77	99	2.82	100	2
FEV_1 (L)	2.11	1.91	91	2.01	95	5
$FEV_{1\%}$ (%)	75	69		71		
$FEF_{25\%-75\%}$ (L/sec)	2.80	1.44	51	1.51	54	5
PEF (L/min)	5.99	4.01	67	5.13	86	28
$FEF_{25\%}$ (L/sec)	5.59	3.31	59	3.60	64	9
$FEF_{50\%}$ (L/sec)	4.19	2.27	54	2.60	62	15
$FEF_{75\%}$ (L/sec)	1.79	0.69	39	1.01	56	46

Lung Volumes

	Predicted	Actual	% Predicted
TLC (L)	4.39	4.97	113
FRC (L)	2.45	3.10	127
RV (L)	1.58	2.20	139
VC (L)	2.81	2.77	99
IC (L)	1.94	1.87	96
ERV (L)	0.87	0.90	103
RV/TLC (%)	36	44	

Diffusing Capacity

	Predicted	Actual	% Predicted
DL_{CO}sb (ml CO/min/mm Hg)	19.7	10.0	51
DL_{CO}sb, adjusted (ml CO/min/mm Hg)	19.7	10.3	52
V_A (L)	4.39	4.81	109
DL/V_A	4.49	2.08	46

TECHNOLOGIST'S COMMENTS

All spirometry maneuvers met ATS criteria. Lung volumes by body plethysmography were performed acceptably. All DL_{CO} maneuvers exceeded 11 seconds for breath hold; otherwise they were acceptable (two tests were averaged). DL_{CO} was corrected for Hb.

QUESTIONS

1. What is the interpretation of:
   a. Prebronchodilator and postbronchodilator spirometry?
   b. Lung volumes?
   c. DL_{CO}?
2. What is the cause of the patient's symptoms?
3. What other tests might be indicated?
4. What treatment might be recommended based on these findings?

DISCUSSION

Interpretation

All maneuvers were performed acceptably except for the breath-hold time during the DL_{CO}sb. Spirometry is normal, but there is a mild decrease in $FEV_{1\%}$. There is also a decrease in $FEF_{50\%}$ and $FEF_{75\%}$. After bronchodilator therapy, there is only a 100-ml improvement (5%) in FEV_1. Lung volumes reveal a slightly increased functional residual capacity and moderately increased RV. The RV/TLC ratio is increased, consistent with air trapping. DL_{CO} is markedly decreased, even after correction for Hb. DL/V_A is decreased, consistent with an obstructive process.

Impression: Mild obstruction with minimal response to bronchodilator; this should not preclude a therapeutic trial if clinically indicated. Lung volumes suggest air trapping. DL_{CO} is severely decreased even when corrected for Hb.

Cause of Symptoms

This patient has symptoms characteristic of airway obstruction that has progressed to the point where dyspnea on exertion prompted a visit to the physician. Her obstruction appears mild. Low flows, particularly $FEF_{50\%}$ and $FEF_{75\%}$, suggest peripheral airway involvement. Her response to bronchodilator therapy seems to indicate obstruction caused by inflammation rather than reversible bronchospasm. Lung volume testing confirms that the obstruction appears to have caused some air trapping. This pattern is not unusual for patients with chronic bronchitis and emphysema.

Her gas exchange, as measured by DL_{CO}, is markedly impaired. Emphysema reduces DL_{CO} by reducing the alveolocapillary surface area available for diffusion. Chronic bronchitis can reduce DL_{CO} by causing a ventilation-perfusion mismatch. The patient appears to have both of these diseases disrupting gas transfer. Patients who have reduced DL_{CO} values seldom have normal blood gases. Exertion or exercise often aggravates the gas-exchange impairment. Many patients with markedly reduced DL_{CO} (less than 50% to 60% of predicted) display exercise desaturation. That is, their PaO_2 falls to levels of 55 mm Hg or less with exercise. The decrease in DL_{CO} does not, however, accurately predict the degree of desaturation that will occur.

Other Tests

An obvious additional test for this patient would be measuring resting arterial blood gases while she breathes room air. Resting hypoxemia would explain dyspnea on exertion. P.M. had blood gas samples drawn. Her PaO_2 while breathing air was 63 mm Hg, with a saturation of 91%. Because this value did not qualify her for supplemental O_2, an exercise test was performed with an arterial catheter in place (see Chapter 7). At a low workload, her PaO_2 decreased to 51 mm Hg. She was then retested while breathing O_2 via nasal cannula at 1 L/min. She then tolerated more exercise, and her PaO_2 never decreased below 68 mm Hg.

Treatment

Based on the results of the exercise evaluation, supplemental O_2 was prescribed for the patient to use during exertion. She was given a portable liquid O_2 system. Because she showed little response to bronchodilators, she was told to stop using the inhaled β-agonist. However, a trial of inhaled steroids (beclamethasone) resulted in noticeable improvement in symptoms.

CASE 5-2

HISTORY

B.C. is a 63-year-old woman with a history of cardiomyopathy, hypertension, and pernicious anemia. She has had episodes of ventricular tachycardia that have been managed by means of an automatic implantable cardiac defibrillator (AICD). She has never smoked and denies cough or sputum production. She experiences shortness of breath with exertion. Her family history includes a sister who had asthma and chronic bronchitis. She has no history of environmental toxin exposure. To manage her arrhythmias, her physician prescribed amiodarone. To monitor the effects of this medication, she was referred for tests before starting the drug and again after 3 months of therapy.

PULMONARY FUNCTION TESTING

Personal Data

Sex: Female
Age: 63

Height: 62 in
Weight: 131 lb
Race: White

Spirometry

	Predicted	Pretreatment Actual	% Predicted	3 Months Actual	% Predicted
FVC (L)	2.77	2.50	90	1.97	70
FEV$_1$ (L)	2.01	2.09	104	1.81	90
FEV$_{1\%}$ (%)	72	84		92	
FEF$_{25\%-75\%}$ (L/sec)	2.38	2.82	118	2.77	116

Lung Volumes (He Dilution)

	Predicted	Pretreatment Actual	% Predicted	3 Months Actual	% Predicted
TLC (L)	4.88	3.92	87	3.50	78
FRC (L)	2.54	2.26	89	2.23	88
RV (L)	1.71	1.50	87	1.52	89
VC (L)	2.77	2.42	87	1.97	71
IC (L)	1.94	1.66	85	1.26	65
ERV (L)	0.83	0.76	91	0.71	85
RV/TLC (%)	38	38		44	

Diffusing Capacity (DL$_{CO}$sb)

	Predicted	Pretreatment Actual	% Predicted	3 Months Actual	% Predicted
DL$_{CO}$ (ml/min/mm Hg)	18.0	12.6	69	9.7	54
DL$_{CO}$, adjusted (ml/min/mm Hg)	18.0	15.5	86	10.9	60
V$_A$sb (L)	4.48	3.26	72	3.25	72
DL/V$_A$	4.0	3.9	96	3.0	74

Technologist's Comments

Pretreatment	3 Months
Spirometry: All ATS criteria are met. Lung volumes: Maneuver was performed acceptably. DL$_{CO}$: Inspired volume was less than 90% of best VC (83%, 83%); DL$_{CO}$ was corrected for Hb of 10.7 g%.	Spirometry: All ATS criteria are met. Lung volumes: Maneuver was performed acceptably. DL$_{CO}$: Inspired volume was less than 90% of best VC (81%, 76%); DL$_{CO}$ was corrected for Hb of 11.3 g%.

QUESTIONS

1. What is the interpretation of:
   a. Pretreatment spirometry, lung volumes?
   b. DL_{CO} before treatment?
   c. DL_{CO} after 3 months of treatment?
2. What is the cause of change in the patient's DL_{CO}?
3. What technical problems might have affected the interpretation of the DL_{CO} both before and after treatment?

DISCUSSION

Interpretation

Pretreatment, FVC is normal, as are FEV_1 and $FEV_{1\%}$. Lung volumes by He dilution are normal. The diffusing capacity was substandard in performance because the patient could not inspire fully. The best efforts show mildly reduced DL_{CO} that becomes normal when corrected for the patient's Hb of 10.7.

    After 3 months, FVC is decreased, but FEV_1 is normal. This makes the $FEV_{1\%}$ appear greater than expected. Lung volumes by He dilution show a TLC that is mildly decreased but with a normal FRC and RV. The DL_{CO} maneuver is again substandard because of poor inspiratory volume. DL_{CO} is moderately decreased, even when corrected for an Hb of 11.3 g%. Since the previous test, the patient's VC has decreased slightly, and the DL_{CO} has decreased significantly.

CAUSE OF CHANGES IN DIFFUSING CAPACITY

This case presents a good example of one application of DL_{CO}: monitoring drug therapy. B.C. had normal lung function. Initially, her DL_{CO} was slightly reduced. However, because she had a history of anemia, her Hb level was checked. The Hb-adjusted DL_{CO} was within normal limits. Because amiodarone has been shown to cause changes to the lung parenchyma, her cardiologist requested pulmonary function studies, including DL_{CO}.

    On her return visit after 3 months of antiarrhythmic therapy, some significant changes had occurred. As pointed out in the interpretation of the 3-month follow-up, her FVC and FEV_1 had decreased slightly. TLC also decreased by a similar volume (400 to 500 ml). Her other lung volumes (FRC, RV) remained largely unchanged. These changes suggest that something happened that primarily affected her VC.

    B.C.'s DL_{CO} showed the greatest decrease during the 3-month period. Her Hb-adjusted DL_{CO} decreased by approximately 30%. This marked decrease occurred although the measured V_A did not change. Consequently, DL/V_A was reduced. The DL/V_A ratio is usually preserved when DL_{CO} decreases, simply because of loss of lung volume. When the DL/V_A ratio decreases in conjunction with a low DL_{CO}, factors other than loss of lung volume are assumed responsible for the change. In this patient, it appears that drug therapy did affect DL_{CO}. However, a pattern of pneumonitis and fibrosis causing reduced lung volumes is not clearly evident. Because of the changes in DL_{CO}, amiodarone therapy was discontinued.

TECHNICAL FACTORS INFLUENCING DL_{CO}

Two noteworthy technical factors are illustrated by this case. Correction of DL_{CO} for the effects of abnormal levels of Hb is very important. In this mildly anemic patient, correction for Hb resulted in a significant difference in DL_{CO} in both tests. Her pretreatment DL_{CO} appears mildly decreased until corrected for Hb. After 3 months of amiodarone therapy, both the uncorrected and corrected

DL_{CO} values are below normal. Comparison of serial DL_{CO} measurements can be compromised if one test is Hb-adjusted and the other is not.

A second factor is that none of the patient's DL_{CO} tests met established criteria for acceptability. She was unable to inspire at least 90% of her VC in any of the maneuvers. This information is documented in the technologist's comments for each test. When the patient fails to inspire maximally, the breath hold does not occur at TLC. Therefore, DL_{CO} may appear low compared with predicted values. This technical difficulty may have influenced these test results. However, because a similar pattern was seen on both the initial and follow-up tests, the data can be cautiously interpreted.

■ SELF-ASSESSMENT QUESTIONS

Entry-level

1. *In which DL_{CO} method does the patient perform a breath-hold maneuver?*

   a. $DL_{CO}ss1$
   b. $DL_{CO}ss3$
   c. $DL_{CO}sb$
   d. $DL_{CO}rb$

2. *A patient performing a $DL_{CO}sb$ should inspire at least:*

   a. 90% of the TLC
   b. 90% of the VC
   c. 80% of the IC
   d. 2 to 3 times the V_T

3. *Pulmonary function studies are performed on a patient with an FVC of 4.4 L and a TLC of 6.0 L. The patient then performs a $DL_{CO}sb$ maneuver with these results:*

Volume inspired	3.99 L
Breath-hold time	12.4 seconds
DL_{CO}	14.2 ml CO/min/mm Hg

   The pulmonary function technologist should:

   a. Accept the maneuver and perform another test
   b. Discard the effort because the volume inspired is too low
   c. Discard the effort because breath hold time is too long
   d. Report the DL_{CO} as 14.2 ml CO/min/mm Hg

4. *In which of the following conditions would a reduction in DL_{CO} be expected?*

   I. Polycythemia
   II. Emphysema
   III. After pneumonectomy
   IV. During exercise

   a. I and III
   b. II and IV
   c. II and III
   d. I, II, and III

5. *The function of the tracer gas (e.g., He, Ne) in the $DL_{CO}sb$ method is to:*

   I. Calculate breath-hold time
   II. Estimate CO at the beginning of breath hold
   III. Enhance distribution of CO in the lung
   IV. Measure alveolar volume (V_A)

   a. I and III
   b. II and IV
   c. I, II, and III
   d. II, III, and IV

Advanced

6. *A 12-year-old patient has a DL_{CO} of 16.5 ml CO/min/mm Hg and an Hb of 9.0. What is the patient's corrected diffusing capacity?*

   a. 15.3 ml CO/min/mm Hg
   b. 18.4 ml CO/min/mm Hg
   c. 19.8 ml CO/min/mm Hg
   d. 20.7 ml CO/min/mm Hg

7. *A patient who smokes has a DL_{CO} of 20.2 ml CO/min/mm Hg and a COHb of 9.5%. What is the patient's approximate actual diffusing capacity?*

   a. 17.7 ml CO/min/mm Hg
   b. 19.5 ml CO/min/mm Hg
   c. 20.0 ml CO/min/mm Hg
   d. 22.1 ml CO/min/mm Hg

8. *A patient performs $DL_{CO}sb$ and records the following data:*

   $DL_{CO}sb$ 10.7 ml CO/min/mmHg
   V_A 6.5 L

   Which of the following is most consistent with these values?

   a. Normal lung function
   b. Sarcoidosis
   c. Idiopathic pulmonary fibrosis
   d. Emphysema

9. *Which of the following DL_{CO} methods requires an arterial blood sample to be drawn during the test?*

   a. $DL_{CO}ss1$
   b. $DL_{CO}ss3$
   c. Rebreathing DL_{CO}
   d. Intrabreath DL_{CO}

10. *A patient has a $DL_{CO}sb$ of 11.6 ml CO/min/mm Hg (STPD), which is 47% of her predicted value. Her DL/V_A ratio is 4.0. Which of the following is most consistent with these values?*

    a. Pulmonary emphysema
    b. Pneumonectomy
    c. Cystic fibrosis
    d. Pulmonary hemorrhage

SELECTED BIBLIOGRAPHY

General References

Crapo RO, Forster RE: Carbon monoxide diffusing capacity, *Clin Chest Med* 10:187, 1989.

Ferris BG, ed: Epidemiology standardization project: recommended standardized procedure for pulmonary function testing, *Am Rev Respir Dis* 118(suppl 2:55):1, 1978.

Forster RE: Diffusion of gases across the alveolar membrane. In Farhi LE, Tenney SM, eds: *Handbook of physiology*, vol 4, Bethesda, Md, 1987, Physiologic Society.

Hadeli KO, Siegel EM, Sherrill DL, et al: Predictors of oxygen desaturation during submaximal exercise in 8,000 patients, *Chest* 120:88-92, 2001.

West JB: *Pulmonary physiology and pathophysiology: an integrated, case-based approach*, Baltimore: Lippincott, Williams & Wilkins, 2001.

$DL_{CO}sb$

Crapo RO, Morris AH: Standardized single breath normal values for carbon monoxide diffusing capacity, *Am Rev Respir Dis* 123:185, 1981.

Dinakara P, Blumenthal WS, Johnston RF, et al: The effect of anemia on pulmonary diffusing capacity with derivation of a correction equation, *Am Rev Respir Dis* 102:965, 1970.

Gaensler EA, Smith AA: Attachment for automated single breath diffusing capacity measurement, *Chest* 63:136, 1973.

Graham BL, Mink JT, Cotton DJ: Effect of breath hold time on $DL_{CO}sb$ in patients with airway obstruction, *J Appl Physiol* 58:1319-1325, 1985.

Graham BL, Mink JT, Cotton DJ: Overestimation of the single breath carbon monoxide diffusing capacity in patients with air-flow obstruction, *Am Rev Respir Dis* 129:403, 1984.

Huang Y-C, MacIntyre NR: Real-time gas analysis improves the measurement of single-breath diffusing capacity, *Am Rev Respir Dis* 146:946-950, 1992.

Johnson DC: Importance of adjusting carbon monoxide diffusing capacity (DL_{CO}) and carbon monoxide transfer coefficient (K_{CO}) for alveolar volume, *Respir Med* 94:28-37, 2000.

Kanner RE, Crapo RO: The relationship between alveolar oxygen tension and the single breath carbon monoxide diffusing capacity, *Am Rev Respir Dis* 133:676, 1986.

Leech JA, Martz L, Liben A, et al: Diffusing capacity for carbon monoxide: the effects of different durations of breath hold time and alveolar volume and of carbon monoxide back pressure on calculated results, *Am Rev Respir Dis* 132:1127, 1985.

Mohsenifar Z, Tashkin DP: Effect of carboxyhemoglobin on the single breath diffusing capacity: derivation of an empirical correction factor, *Respiration* 37:185, 1979.

Ogilvie CM, Forster RE, Blakemore WS, et al: A standardized breath holding technique for the clinical measurement of the diffusing capacity of the lung for carbon monoxide, *J Clin Invest,* 36:1, 1957.

Stam H, Splinter TAW, Versprille A: Evaluation of diffusing capacity in patients with a restrictive lung disease, *Chest* 117:752-757, 2000.

DL_{CO}ss

Davies NJH: Does the lung work? What does the transfer of carbon monoxide mean? *Br J Dis Chest* 76:105, 1982.

Filey GF, Macintosh DJ, Wright GW: Carbon monoxide uptake and pulmonary diffusing capacity in normal patients at rest and during exercise, *J Clin Invest* 33:530, 1954.

DL_{CO}ib

Newth CJL, Cotton DJ, Nadel JA: Pulmonary diffusing capacity measured at multiple intervals during a single exhalation in man, *J Appl Physiol Respir Environ Physiol* 43:617, 1977.

Wilson AF, Hearne J, Brennan M, et al: Measurement of transfer factor during constant exhalation, *Thorax* 49:1121-1126, 1994.

Standards and Guidelines

Abboud RT, Sansores R: ATS recommendations for DL_{CO}. *Am J Respir Crit Care Med* 154:265-268, 1996.

American Association for Respiratory Care: Single-breath carbon monoxide diffusing capacity: 1999 Update, *Respir Care* 44:539-546, 1999.

American Thoracic Society: Single-breath carbon monoxide diffusing capacity (transfer factor): recommendations for a standard technique: 1995 update, *Am J Respir Crit Care Med,* 152:2185-2198, 1995.

British Thoracic Society and the Association of Respiratory Technicians and Physiologists: Guidelines for the measurement of respiratory function, *Respir Med* 88:165-194, 1994.

European Respiratory Society: Standardization of transfer factor (diffusing capacity), *Eur Respir J* 6(suppl 16): 41-52, 1993.

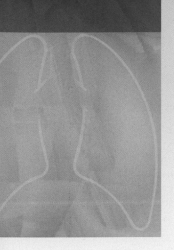

CHAPTER 6

BLOOD GASES AND RELATED TESTS

OBJECTIVES

After studying this chapter and reviewing its tables and case studies, you should be able to do the following:

Entry-level

1. Describe how pH and P_{CO_2} are used to assess acid-base status
2. Interpret P_{O_2} and oxygen saturation to assess oxygenation
3. Identify the correct procedure for obtaining an arterial blood gas specimen
4. List situations in which pulse oximetry can be used to evaluate a patient's oxygenation

Advanced

1. Describe at least two limitations of pulse oximetry
2. Describe the use of capnography to assess changes in ventilation-perfusion patterns of the lung
3. Assess oxygenation using arterial oxygen content
4. Calculate the shunt fraction using appropriate laboratory data

Blood gas analysis is the most basic test of lung function. Evaluation of the acid-base and oxygenation status of the body provides information about the function of the lungs themselves. Sampling of arterial blood is required. Other measures of gas exchange (e.g., pulse oximetry and capnography) have the advantage of monitoring patients noninvasively. Understanding the limitations of noninvasive techniques allows them to be used to provide appropriate patient care. Calculating the shunt fraction uses blood gas measurements to assess gas exchange as it applies to oxygenation.

This chapter addresses how blood gas measurements are used in the pulmonary function laboratory. A complete description of blood gas electrodes is included in Chapter 10. The use of pulse oximetry and capnography as adjuncts to traditional invasive measures is discussed. Two methods of calculating shunt fraction are detailed so that the most appropriate method may be used.

BLOOD GAS ANALYSIS

pH

pH is the negative logarithm of the hydrogen ion [H⁺] concentration in the blood, used as a positive number. The pH scale has no units. It is derived by converting the [H⁺] to a negative exponent of 10 and calculating its logarithm. The [H⁺] of water is 1×10^{-7} mol/L. The negative logarithm of 1×10^{-7} is 7. The pH of water (7) represents the midpoint of the pH scale. The physiologic range of pH in blood in clinical practice is from approximately 6.90 to 7.80.

Carbon Dioxide Tension

P_{CO_2} is a measurement of the partial pressure exerted by CO_2 in solution in the blood. The measurement is expressed in millimeters of mercury (mm Hg or torr) or in *kilopascals* (kPa) used in the International System of Units (1 mm Hg = 0.133 kPa). The normal range for P_{CO_2} in arterial blood is 35 to 45 mm Hg (4.66 to 5.99 kPa). In mixed venous blood, P_{CO_2} varies from 40 to 46 mm Hg (5.32 to 6.12 kPa).

Oxygen Tension

P_{O_2} measures the partial pressure exerted by oxygen (O_2) dissolved in the blood. Like P_{CO_2}, it is recorded in millimeters of mercury or in kilopascals. The normal range for arterial P_{O_2} is 80 to 100 mm Hg (10.64 to 13.30 kPa) for healthy young adults breathing air at sea level. Mixed venous P_{O_2} averages 40 mm Hg (5.32 kPa) in healthy patients.

■ TECHNIQUE

pH

Blood pH is measured by exposing the specimen to a glass electrode (see Figure 10-24) under *anaerobic* conditions. pH measurements are made at 37° C. The pH of arterial blood is related to the Pa_{CO_2} by the Henderson-Hasselbalch equation:

$$pH = pK + \log \frac{[HCO_3^-]}{[CO_2]}$$

where:
pK   = negative log of dissociation constant for carbonic acid (6.1)
$[HCO_3^-]$ = molar concentration of serum bicarbonate
$[CO_2]$ = molar concentration of CO_2

Paco$_2$ (measured directly by a CO$_2$ electrode) may be multiplied by 0.03 (the solubility coefficient for CO$_2$) to express Paco$_2$ in mEq/L. The equation then may be expressed as follows:

$$pH = pK + \log \frac{[HCO_3^-]}{[0.03(Paco_2)]}$$

Carbon Dioxide Tension

Pco$_2$ is measured by exposing whole blood to a modified pH electrode (i.e., a Severinghaus electrode) contained in a jacket with a Teflon membrane at its tip (see Chapter 10). Inside the jacket is a bicarbonate buffer. As CO$_2$ diffuses through the membrane, it combines with water to form carbonic acid (H$_2$CO$_3$). The H$_2$CO$_3$ dissociates into H$^+$ and HCO$_3^-$ thereby changing the pH of the bicarbonate buffer. The change in pH is measured by the electrode and is proportional to the Pco$_2$. The blood must be anticoagulated and kept in an anaerobic state (usually in an ice-water bath) until analysis. Pco$_2$ may also be estimated using a transcutaneous electrode. Measurement of end-tidal CO$_2$ (Petco$_2$) is sometimes used to track Pco$_2$ (see Capnography section).

pH and Pco$_2$ are usually measured from the same sample, so bicarbonate can be easily calculated. Automated blood gas analyzers perform this calculation along with others to derive values such as total CO$_2$ (dissolved CO$_2$ plus HCO$_3^-$) and standard bicarbonate (i.e., HCO$_3^-$ corrected to a Paco$_2$ of 40 mm Hg). If the hemoglobin (Hb) is measured or estimated, the base excess (BE) can be calculated. The normal buffer base at a pH of 7.40 is approximately 48 mEq/L. BE is the difference between the actual buffering capacity of the blood and the expected value ($\cong$ 48 mEq/L). When the buffering capacity is less than the expected value, the difference is a negative value. This is sometimes referred to as a base deficit rather than a negative base excess. The main buffers that affect the BE are HCO$_3^-$ and Hb.

Oxygen Tension

The Po$_2$ (arterial or mixed venous) is measured by exposing whole blood, obtained anaerobically, to a platinum electrode covered with a thin polypropylene membrane. This type of electrode is called a *polarographic electrode* or *Clark electrode*. Oxygen molecules are reduced at the platinum cathode after diffusing through the membrane (see Chapter 10). Po$_2$ may also be measured using a transcutaneous electrode (see Chapter 10).

Blood gas analyzers usually report blood gas values at 37° C. If the patient has an extreme body temperature (hypothermia or hyperthermia), correction may be useful. At low body temperatures, more gas dissolves in the blood; so Po$_2$ and Pco$_2$ show lower values when exposed to electrodes that measure their activity. At elevated temperatures, the opposite occurs; less gas dissolves and partial pressures appear higher. pH changes in relation to Pco$_2$.

Blood gas values depend on the patient's temperature. Alteration of body temperature affects the partial pressure of dissolved CO$_2$, which influences pH as described in the previous equations (Table 6-1). Although blood gas measurements are made at 37° C, the value reported may be corrected to the patient's temperature.

TABLE 6-1 Effects of Body Temperature on Blood Gas Values*

Temperature (°C)	34°	37°	40°
pH	7.44	7.40	7.36
P_{CO_2}	35	40	46
P_{O_2}	79	95	114

*Temperature corrections based on algorithms from *NCCLS: definitions of quantities and conventions related to blood pH and gas analysis*, ed 2, (Tentative Standard), vol 12, No 11, 1991.

Technical problems with blood gas electrodes include contamination by protein or blood products. Depletion of the potassium chloride (KCl) bridge between the pH measuring and reference electrodes (see Chapter 10) is also a common problem. Depletion of the bicarbonate buffer in the P_{CO_2} electrode may reduce accuracy and cause unacceptable drift. Oxidation-reduction reactions in the P_{O_2} electrode cause metal ions to deposit on the platinum cathode. After a period of use, the tip of the O_2 electrode must be abraded to expose the platinum wire. This is usually accomplished by brushing the tip with a mild abrasive. Tears or ruptures of the membranes used to cover the P_{CO_2} and P_{O_2} electrodes are also common malfunctions.

Specimen Collection for Blood Gases

Arterial samples are usually obtained from either the radial or the brachial artery. Arterial specimens may also be drawn from the femoral or dorsalis pedis arteries. The radial artery is the preferred site. Before a radial artery puncture, the adequacy of collateral circulation to the hand via the ulnar artery should be established using the modified Allen's test. The technologist occludes both the radial and ulnar arteries by pressing down over the wrist. The patient is instructed to make a fist, then open the hand and relax the fingers. The palm of the hand is pale and bloodless because both arteries are occluded. The ulnar artery is released while the radial remains occluded. The hand should be reperfused rapidly (5 to 10 seconds) if the ulnar supply is adequate. If perfusion is inadequate, an alternate site should be used.

Arterial puncture should not be performed through any type of lesion. Similarly, puncture distal to a surgical shunt (e.g., shunts used for dialysis) should be avoided. Infection or evidence of peripheral vascular disease should prompt selection of an alternative site. Many patients may be using anticoagulant drugs such as heparin, coumadin, or streptokinase. High dosages of these drugs or a history of prolonged clotting times may be relative contraindications to arterial puncture. Table 6-2 lists some of the potential hazards associated with arterial puncture.

Success in obtaining an arterial specimen by radial puncture requires careful positioning of the patient's wrist. The hand should be hyperextended with good support under the wrist. A topical anesthetic may be useful for some patients, but is usually unnecessary. The person drawing the sample should be in a comfortable position to maximize control of the needle during insertion. A vented syringe or similar device allows the blood to "pulse" into the syringe, ensuring that the needle is in the lumen of the artery.

TABLE 6–2   Complications of Arterial Puncture for Blood Gas Testing

Pain and discomfort
Hematoma
Air or blood emboli
Infection or contamination
Inadvertent needle stick
Vascular trauma or occlusion
Vasovagal response
Arterial spasm

Mixed venous samples are drawn from a pulmonary artery (Swan-Ganz) catheter. Contamination of the mixed venous specimen with flush solution is a common problem. Withdrawing a small volume of blood into a "waste" syringe ensures that the sample is not diluted by flush solution in the catheter. Care should be taken to limit the volume of blood removed in this process. Significant blood loss can occur with repetitive measurements. Another common problem with mixed venous specimen collection is displacement of the catheter tip. If the catheter is advanced too far, it may "wedge" into a pulmonary arteriole. Specimens drawn from this position often reflect arterialized pulmonary capillary blood. Similarly, if the catheter tip is withdrawn or "loops back," it may be in the right ventricle or atrium rather than the pulmonary artery. Specimens obtained from this location may not represent true mixed venous blood.

Venous samples from peripheral veins are not useful for assessing oxygenation. Venous blood only reflects the metabolism of the area drained by that particular vein. Venous samples may be used for measurement of pH or blood lactate during exercise.

Blood is usually collected in a heparinized syringe and sealed from the atmosphere immediately (Blood Gases 6-1). Care must be taken that heparin solution (if used) does not dilute the sample. Heparin solution (sodium heparin) has a Po_2 of approximately 150 mm Hg and a Pco_2 near 0. If the volume of heparin solution is large in relation to the blood sample, Po_2 and Pco_2 will be altered. The Po_2 will increase, if it is less than 150 mm Hg, and the Pco_2 will decrease. Although liquid heparin is slightly acidic compared with blood, pH is usually not directly affected. The large buffering capacity of whole blood prevents large changes in pH. To prevent dilution effects when a heparin solution is used, the following guidelines are helpful:

1. Draw up a small volume of sterile heparin in the syringe. Typically, 0.25 ml of 1000 units/ml concentration is sufficient for a 3-ml syringe.
2. Hold the syringe with the needle pointed up. Pull back the plunger so that the heparin solution coats the interior walls of the syringe.
3. Expel all of the heparin solution through the needle, leaving liquid only in the hub and lumen of the needle.
4. Obtain a blood sample volume of 2 to 4 ml, if possible.

Blood gas kits that feature dry (lyophilyzed) heparin are available. Dry heparin is applied to the lumen of the needle and the interior of the syringe. A small heparin pellet is often placed in the syringe to provide additional anticoagulation. Use of a kit with dry heparin avoids the problems of dilution that sometimes occur when liquid heparin is used.

After the syringe has been capped (see Chapter 11), the sample should be thoroughly mixed by rolling or gently shaking. Mixing helps prevent the sample from clotting, whether dry or liquid heparin is used. Lithium heparin or a similar preparation should be used for specimens that will also be used for electrolyte analysis.

BLOOD GASES 6-1   Criteria for Acceptability—Blood Gases

1 Blood should be collected anaerobically. Syringe body and plunger should be tight-fitting. Commercially available blood gas kits should be used according to manufacturers' specifications. Air bubbles should be expelled immediately.

2 The specimen must be adequately anticoagulated; sodium or lithium heparin is preferred. If liquid heparin is used, all excess should be expelled. Choice of anticoagulant should be determined by analyses to be performed (e.g., electrolytes).

3 A sample volume of 2 to 4 ml is recommended.

4 The specimen should be analyzed as soon as possible. If immediate analysis is not available, the specimen should be stored in an ice-water slurry at $0°$ C and analyzed within 1 hour.

5 The specimen should be adequately identified, including patient name and/or number, date/time, ordering physician, and accession number. Information provided with the specimen should be the site from which it was obtained, F_{IO_2} (if applicable), and ventilator settings (if applicable).

6 Analysis should be performed on an instrument that has been recently calibrated and whose function is documented by appropriate controls.

TABLE 6-3 Air Contamination of Blood Gas Samples

	In Vivo Values	Air Contamination*
pH	7.40	7.45
P_{CO_2}	40	30
P_{O_2}	95	110

*Typical values that might occur when a blood gas specimen is exposed to air, either directly or by mixing with a solution that has been exposed to air (e.g., heparinized flush solution). The change in pH occurs because of the change in P_{CO_2}.

Air contamination of arterial or mixed venous blood specimens can seriously alter blood gas values. Room air at sea level has a P_{O_2} of approximately 150 mm Hg, and a P_{CO_2} near 0. If air bubbles are present in a blood gas specimen, equilibration of gases between the sample and air occurs (Table 6-3). Contamination commonly occurs during sampling when air is left in the syringe after the sample is collected. Small bubbles may also be introduced if the needle does not connect tightly to the syringe. Other sources of air contamination include poorly fitting plungers and failure to properly cap the syringe. Use of a vented syringe or one in which the pulse pressure of the blood displaces the plunger can help prevent air bubble contamination.

Sample storage depends on the type of syringe used. If a glass syringe is used, the sample may be stored in ice-water slush if analysis is not done within a few minutes. Ice water reduces the metabolism of red and white blood cells in the sample. Specimens with O_2 tensions in the normal physiologic range (50 to 150 mm Hg) show minimal changes over 1 to 2 hours if kept in ice water. Changes in specimens held at room temperature are related to cellular metabolism in the blood, particularly in white blood cells and platelets. Specimens with P_{O_2} values above 150 mm Hg are most susceptible to alterations resulting from gas leakage or cell metabolism. When the P_{O_2} is 150 mm Hg or more, Hb is almost completely bound with O_2. In such cases, a small change in O_2 content results in a large change in P_{O_2}.

If a plastic syringe is used, blood gas specimens should be analyzed within 15 minutes. Plastic syringes are not completely gas tight, so room air can contaminate the sample. The influx of O_2 may be counterbalanced by the consumption of O_2 if the sample is not iced. When a blood gas specimen is placed in an ice-water bath, the solubility of O_2 increases, along with the affinity of hemoglobin for oxygen. This lowers the partial pressure of O_2 in the sample and increases the gradient between the sample and the environment. This gradient exaggerates the leakage of O_2 into the specimen (as occurs with plastic syringes). When the sample is introduced into the analyzer at 37° C, solubility and Hb affinity return to their normal values, the oxygen that leaked in is released, and the Po_2 is falsely increased. If specimens cannot be routinely analyzed within about 15 minutes, glass syringes with ice-water storage may be preferable.

Capillary samples are useful in infants when arterial puncture is impractical. The area for collection (the heel is commonly chosen) should be heated by a warm compress and lanced. Blood is then allowed to fill the required volume of heparinized glass capillary tubes. Squeezing the tissue should be avoided because predominately venous blood will be obtained. The capillary tubes should be carefully sealed to avoid air bubbles. Guidelines for quality control of blood gas analyzers and for the safe handling of blood specimens are included in Chapter 11.

■ SIGNIFICANCE AND PATHOPHYSIOLOGY

See Blood Gases 6-2 for interpretive strategies.

pH

The pH of arterial blood in healthy adults averages 7.40 with a range of 7.35 to 7.45. Arterial pH below 7.35 constitutes acidemia. A pH above 7.45 constitutes alkalemia. Because of the logarithmic scale, a change of 0.3 pH units represents a twofold change in $[H^+]$ concentration. If the pH decreases from 7.40 to 7.10 with no change in Pco_2, the concentration of hydrogen ions has doubled. Conversely, if the concentration of $[H^+]$ is halved, the pH increases from 7.40 to 7.70, assuming the Pco_2 remains at 40 mm Hg. Changes of this magnitude represent marked abnormalities in the acid-base status of the blood and are almost always accompanied by clinical symptoms such as cardiac arrhythmias.

Acid-base disorders arising from lung disease are often related to Pco_2 and its transport as carbonic acid. If the pH is outside of its normal range (i.e., acidemia or alkalemia) but Pco_2 is normal, the condition is termed *nonrespiratory* or *metabolic* (Table 6-4). The calculated HCO_3^- is a useful indicator of the relationship between pH and Pco_2. In the presence of acidemia (pH less than 7.35) and normal CO_2 (Pco_2 35 to 45 mm Hg), HCO_3^- will be low and a nonrespiratory acidosis is present. A Pco_2 of less than 35 mm Hg in the presence of acidosis indicates that ventilatory compensation for acidemia is occurring. The acid-base status would be considered partially compensated nonrespiratory (i.e., metabolic) acidosis. Complete compensation occurs if pH returns to the normal range. This happens when ventilation reduces Pco_2 to match the HCO_3^-.

In the presence of alkalemia (pH above 7.45) and normal Pco_2 (35 to 45 mm Hg), calculated bicarbonate will be increased and nonrespiratory (i.e., metabolic) alkalosis is present. If ventilatory compensation occurs, Pco_2 will be slightly increased. However, decreased ventilation is required so that the CO_2 can increase. Reduced minute ventilation may interfere with oxygenation. For this reason, $Paco_2$ seldom increases above 50 to 55 mm Hg to compensate for nonrespiratory (i.e., metabolic) alkalosis. Compensation may be incomplete if the alkalosis is severe.

Abnormal Pco_2 and HCO_3^- characterize combined respiratory and nonrespiratory acid-base disorders. In combined acidosis, Pco_2 is elevated (more than 45 mm Hg) and HCO_3^- is

BLOOD GASES 6-2   Interpretive Strategies—Blood Gases

1 Was the blood gas specimen obtained acceptably? Free of air bubbles and clots? Analyzed promptly and/or iced appropriately?

2 Did the blood gas analyzer function properly? Was there a recent acceptable calibration of all electrodes? Was analyzer function validated by appropriate quality controls?

3 Is pH within normal limits (7.35 to 7.45)? If so, go to Step 4. If below 7.35, acidosis is present; if above 7.45, alkalosis is present. Otherwise, look for compensatory changes or combined disorders.

4 Is Pco_2 within normal limits (35 to 45 mm Hg)? If so, go to Step 5.
   If Pco_2 >45 and pH <7.35, then respiratory acidosis is present.
   If Pco_2 >45 and pH >7.35, then compensated respiratory acidosis is present.
   If Pco_2 <35 and pH >7.45, then respiratory alkalosis is present.
   If Pco_2 <35 and pH <7.45, then compensated respiratory alkalosis is present.

5 Is calculated HCO_3^- within normal limits (22 to 27 mEq/L)? If so, acid-base status is probably normal; go to Step 6.
   If HCO_3^- <22 and pH <7.35, then metabolic* acidosis is present.
   If HCO_3^- <22 and pH >7.35, then compensated metabolic* acidosis is present.
   If HCO_3^- >27 and pH >7.45, then metabolic* alkalosis is present.
   If HCO_3^- >27 and pH <7.45, then compensated metabolic* alkalosis is present.

6 Is Po_2 within normal limits (80 to 100 mm Hg)? If so, oxygenation status is probably normal; check O_2Hb saturation via co-oximetry. Is Po_2 appropriate for Fio_2? Is A-a gradient increased? If Po_2 <55, significant hypoxemia is present.

7 Are blood gas results consistent with patient's clinical history and status? Are additional tests indicated (co-oximetry, shunt study)?

*Metabolic = nonrespiratory.

TABLE 6-4   Acid–Base Disorders

Status	pH	Pco_2	Hco_3^-
Simple disorders			
Metabolic acidosis	Low	Normal	Low
Metabolic alkalosis	High	Normal	High
Respiratory acidosis	Low	High	Normal
Respiratory alkalosis	High	Low	Normal
Compensated disorders			
Compensated respiratory acidosis, or metabolic alkalosis	Normal*	High	High
Compensated metabolic acidosis, or respiratory alkalosis	Normal*	Low	Low a
Combined disorders			
Metabolic/respiratory acidosis	Low	High	Low
Metabolic/respiratory alkalosis	High	Low	High

*Compensation cannot return values to within normal limits in severe acid-base disturbances. In addition, a normal pH may result in instances of respiratory and metabolic disturbances that occur together but are not compensatory.

low (less than 22 mEq/L). In combined alkalosis, HCO_3^- is elevated (more than 26 mEq/L) and PCO_2 is low (less than 35 mm Hg). pH is more severely deranged than if just one disorder were present.

Carbon Dioxide Tension

The arterial carbon dioxide tension ($PaCO_2$) in a healthy adult is approximately 40 mm Hg; it may range from 35 to 45 mm Hg. The PCO_2 of venous or mixed venous blood is seldom used clinically. Body temperature affects $PaCO_2$ as described in Table 6-1.

$PaCO_2$ is inversely proportional to alveolar ventilation ($\dot{V}_A$) (see Chapter 4). When $\dot{V}_A$ decreases, CO_2 is not removed by the lungs as fast as it is produced. This causes $PaCO_2$ to increase. The pH falls as CO_2 is hydrated to form carbonic acid:

$$CO_2 + H_2O \leftrightarrow H_2CO_3 \leftrightarrow H^+ + HCO_3^-$$

Increasing levels of CO_2 in the blood drive this reaction to the right. The patient develops respiratory acidosis resulting from hypoventilation. Conversely, when alveolar ventilation removes CO_2 more rapidly than it is produced, $PaCO_2$ decreases. The pH increases as the patient becomes alkalotic. This condition is called hyperventilation, or respiratory alkalosis.

If dead space increases, high minute ventilation ($\dot{V}_E$) may be required to adequately ventilate alveoli and keep $PaCO_2$ within normal limits. Respiratory dead space occurs because some lung units are ventilated but not perfused by pulmonary capillary blood. Pulmonary embolization is an example of dead-space–producing disease. Emboli may block pulmonary arterioles, causing ventilation of the affected lung units to be "wasted." To maintain normal $PaCO_2$, total ventilation must be increased to compensate for wasted ventilation.

$PaCO_2$ may be normal, or even decreased, when significant pulmonary disease is present. Patients who have disorders such as lobar pneumonia may increase their $\dot{V}_E$ to produce more alveolar ventilation of functioning lung units. This mechanism compensates for lung units that do not participate in gas exchange. Hypoxemia is a common cause of hyperventilation (i.e., respiratory alkalosis). Hyperventilation may be seen in patients with asthma, emphysema, bronchitis, or foreign body obstruction. Anxiety or central nervous system disorders may also cause hyperventilation.

Increased $PaCO_2$ (i.e., hypercapnia) is commonly found in patients who have advanced obstructive or restrictive disease. These individuals are characterized by markedly abnormal ventilation-perfusion ($\dot{V}/\dot{Q}$) patterns. They are unable to maintain adequate alveolar ventilation. Not all patients with advanced pulmonary disease retain CO_2. Those who do become hypercapnic often have a low ventilatory response to CO_2 (see Chapter 4). Their response to the increased work of breathing caused by obstruction or restriction is to allow CO_2 to increase rather than increase ventilation. When respiratory acidosis results from increased PCO_2, renal compensation usually occurs (Table 6-4).

Increased $PaCO_2$ may also be seen in patients who hypoventilate as a result of central nervous system or neuromuscular disorders. Whether CO_2 retention is the result of lung disease, central nervous system dysfunction, or neuromuscular disease, pH is usually maintained close to normal. The kidneys retain and produce bicarbonate (HCO_3^-) to match the increased $PaCO_2$. This response may completely compensate for a mildly elevated $PaCO_2$. However, it can seldom produce normal pH when the $PaCO_2$ is greater than 65 mm Hg. If the disorder causing the increased $PaCO_2$ is acute (e.g., foreign body aspiration), little or no renal compensation may be observed.

Hypoxemia is always present in patients who retain CO_2 while breathing air. As alveolar CO_2 increases, alveolar O_2 decreases. If the cause of hypercapnia is either obstructive or restrictive lung disease, hypoxemia may be severe because of $\dot{V}/\dot{Q}$ abnormalities. Because O_2

therapy is commonly used in these patients, changes in P_{CO_2} while breathing supplementary O_2 must be carefully monitored. Some patients with chronic hypoxemia have a decreased ventilatory response to CO_2. O_2 administered to these patients may reduce their hypoxic stimulus to ventilation. As a result, $PaCO_2$ may increase further. O_2 therapy is usually titrated to maintain $PaCO_2$ values less than 60 mm Hg without hypercapnia and acidosis.

Oxygen Tension

The PaO_2 of healthy young adults at sea level ranges from 85 to 100 mm Hg and decreases slightly with age. Breathing room air at sea level results in an inspired PO_2 of approximately 150 mm Hg:

$$P_IO_2 = F_{IO_2}(P_B - 47)$$
$$= 0.21(760 - 47)$$
$$= 0.21(713)$$
$$= 149.7$$

where:
F_{IO_2} = fractional concentration of inspired O_2
P_B = barometric pressure
47   = partial pressure of water vapor at 37° C

The partial pressure of O_2 in alveolar gas is usually close to 100 mm Hg and can be calculated using the alveolar air equation:

$$P_AO_2 = (F_{IO_2} \times [P_B - 47]) - PaCO_2 \left(F_{IO_2} + \frac{1 - F_{IO_2}}{R} \right)$$

where:
$PaCO_2$ = arterial CO_2 tension (presumed equal to alveolar CO_2 tension)
R   = respiratory exchange ratio (V_{CO_2}/V_{O_2})

Substituting 40 mm Hg for $PaCO_2$, and 0.8 for R:

$$P_AO_2 = (0.21 \times [760 - 47]) - 40 \left(0.21 + \frac{1 - 0.21}{0.8} \right)$$
$$= (0.21 \times 713) - 40(1.1975)$$
$$= 149.7 - 47.9$$
$$= 101.8$$

In healthy lungs with good gas exchange, arterial oxygen tension can approach the value of the alveolar PO_2. The difference between the alveolar and arterial oxygen tensions is described as the alveolar-arterial gradient, or A-a gradient. This gradient is usually less than 20 mm Hg in healthy individuals.

Hyperventilation may increase PaO_2 as high as 120 mm Hg in a patient with normal lung function (see the alveolar air equation in this section). Healthy patients breathing 100% O_2 may exhibit PaO_2 values higher than 600 mm Hg. The alveolar PO_2 (PaO_2) for a particular inspired O_2 fraction can be calculated as described above. Decreased PaO_2 can result from hypoventilation, diffusion defects, V/Q imbalances, and inadequate atmospheric O_2 (high altitude).

Table 6-1 lists changes that occur in PaO_2 because of body temperatures above and below normal (37° C). Changes in PO_2 and PCO_2 reflect solubility of the gas. Partial pressure of each gas is a measure of its activity. Hypothermia (low body temperature) is accompanied by decreased partial pressure. Hyperthermia (elevated body temperature) causes elevated gas tensions. All blood gas analyzers perform analyses at 37° C and allow temperature corrections to be made. Although blood gas tensions vary with temperature, the clinical significance of correcting measurements is unclear. Blood gas values should be reported at 37° C. Care must be taken to ensure that blood gas analyzers are maintained at 37° C. Measurements made at other temperatures can significantly alter results.

PO_2 is the pressure of O_2 dissolved in blood. The amount of Hb and whether it is capable of binding O_2 has a minimal effect on PO_2. Hypoxemia (decreased O_2 content of the blood) may occur even if PaO_2 is normal or elevated by breathing O_2. Hypoxemia commonly results from inadequate or abnormal Hb. Many automated blood gas analyzers calculate oxygen saturation (SaO_2). Saturation may be calculated from the PaO_2 and pH, assuming a normal oxygen-hemoglobin reaction occurs (Figure 6-1). Calculated SaO_2 may differ significantly from true saturation measured by a spectrophotometer (see Oxygen Saturation section).

A common example is the patient with elevated carboxyhemoglobin (COHb) resulting from smoking or smoke inhalation. The patient's PaO_2 may be normal while O_2 saturation is markedly decreased. Calculating saturation from PO_2 in this case overestimates the O_2 content of the blood. Measured SaO_2 is preferred to a calculated value.

In patients breathing air at sea level, the sum of PaO_2 and $PaCO_2$ is usually less than 150 mm Hg. If the sum is greater than 150 mm Hg, the patient was breathing supplementary O_2 or the blood gas values are erroneous. For patients breathing air, a quick estimate of alveolar PO_2 can be derived from the equation $150 - (PaCO_2/0.8)$.

Severity of impaired oxygenation is indicated by the PaO_2 at rest. PaO_2 is a good index of the lungs' ability to match pulmonary capillary blood flow with adequate ventilation. If ventilation matches perfusion, pulmonary capillary blood leaves the lungs with a PO_2 close to that of the alveoli. If ventilation is adequate, pulmonary capillary blood is almost completely saturated. If either of these conditions is not met (i.e., poor ventilation or V/Q mismatching), pulmonary capillary blood has reduced O_2 content. PaO_2 is reduced in proportion to the number of lung units contributing blood with low O_2 content. Lung units with good V/Q cannot compensate for their poorly functioning counterparts because pulmonary capillary blood leaving them is already almost fully oxygenated. O_2 binding to Hb is almost complete when the PaO_2 is greater than 60 mm Hg (90% saturation). As the PaO_2 decreases from 60 to 40 mm Hg, saturation decreases from 90% to 75%, with increasing symptoms of hypoxia (i.e., mental confusion, shortness of breath).

Delivery of O_2 to the tissues, however, depends on Hb concentration and cardiac output. Arterial oxygen content (CaO_2, ml/dl) is defined as follows:

$$CaO_2 = (1.34 \times Hb \times SaO_2) + (PaO_2 \times 0.0031)$$

where:
1.34 = O_2 binding capacity of Hb, ml/g
Hb = hemoglobin concentration, g/dl

Sao_2 = arterial oxygen saturation as a fraction
Pao_2 = arterial oxygen tension, mm Hg
0.0031 = solubility coefficient for O_2

Because most O_2 transported is bound to Hb, there must be an adequate supply (12 to 15 g/dl) of functional Hb. Adequate cardiac output (4 to 5 L/min) is necessary to deliver the oxygenated arterial blood to the tissues. Signs and symptoms of hypoxia may be present despite adequate Pao_2 because of severe anemia and/or reduced cardiac function.

The mixed venous oxygen tension ($P\bar{v}o_2$) in healthy patients at rest ranges from 37 to 43, with an average of 40 mm Hg (Figure 6-1). In healthy individuals, arterial oxygen content (Cao_2) averages 20 ml/dl. Mixed venous O_2 content ($C\bar{v}o_2$) averages 15 ml/dl. The resulting content difference, or $C(a-\bar{v})o_2$, is thus 5 ml/dl (or vol%). Although Pao_2 varies with the inspired O_2 fraction and matching of V/Q, $P\bar{v}o_2$ changes in response to alterations in cardiac output and O_2 consumption. If cardiac output increases while oxygen consumption (Vo_2) remains constant, the $C(a-\bar{v})o_2$ decreases. Conversely, if cardiac output decreases with no change in O_2 consumption, $C(a-\bar{v})o_2$ increases. Increased cardiac output sometimes occurs in response to pulmonary shunting. This allows mixed venous oxygen content to increase, reducing the deleterious effect of the shunt. Critically ill patients often have low $P\bar{v}o_2$ values

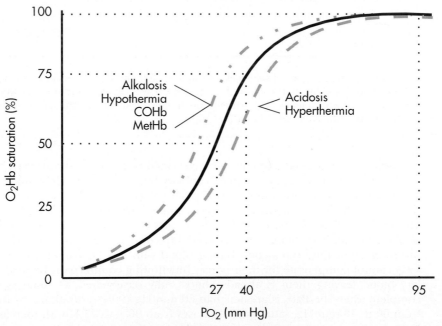

Figure 6-1 *Oxygen-hemoglobin dissociation curve.* The S-shaped curve represents the relationship between partial pressure of O_2 in blood *(x-axis)* and Hb saturation *(y-axis)*. The solid curve represents the reaction that occurs when Hb is normal, pH is 7.40, and temperature is 37° C. When Po_2 is 95 mm Hg, Hb is approximately 97% saturated; when Po_2 is 60 mm Hg, Hb is approximately 90% saturated; when Po_2 is 40 mm Hg (normal level for mixed venous blood), Hb is approximately 75% saturated. The P_{50} identifies the O_2 tension at which Hb is 50% saturated. For normal Hb, this is approximately 27 mm Hg. Conditions such as alkalosis, hypothermia, or elevated COHb or MetHb shift the dissociation curve to the left. This causes Hb to bind O_2 more tightly with less oxygen being unloaded as partial pressure decreases. Similarly, acidosis and hyperthermia shift the curve to the right, enhancing the delivery of O_2 as pressure decreases.

and increased $C(a-\bar{v})O_2$ as a result of poor cardiovascular performance. Alterations in $P\bar{v}O_2$ often occur even if PaO_2 is normal. $P\bar{v}O_2$ values less than 28 mm Hg in critically ill patients, accompanied by $C(a-\bar{v})O_2$ greater than 6 vol%, suggest marked cardiovascular decompensation.

Resting patients who have severe obstructive or restrictive diseases may have decreased PaO_2, occasionally as low as 40 mm Hg. Mild pulmonary disease may show little decrease in PaO_2 if hyperventilation is present. PaO_2 may be normal if the disease process affects ventilation and perfusion similarly. In patients with emphysema, destruction of alveolar septa may eliminate pulmonary capillaries as well, resulting in poor ventilation and equally poor blood flow. These patients may have severe airway obstruction but only a small decrease in PaO_2. Patients with chronic bronchitis or asthma, particularly during acute exacerbations, may have moderate or severe resting hypoxemia because of V/Q abnormalities.

During exercise in patients with obstructive disease, PaO_2 often decreases commensurate with the extent of the disease. PaO_2 during exercise is correlated with the patient's DL_{CO} and FEV_1, but wide variability exists. Patients with markedly decreased DL_{CO} (less than 50% to 60% of predicted) typically show low PaO_2 values at rest that decrease during exercise. The degree of arterial desaturation cannot be predicted from static pulmonary function measurements.

PaO_2 may be decreased for nonpulmonary reasons such as anatomic shunts (intracardiac) or hypoventilation because of neuromuscular disease. Tissue hypoxia can occur because of inadequate or nonfunctional Hb, or because of poor cardiac output. PaO_2 should be correlated with spirometry (FEV_1), DL_{CO}, ventilation ($\dot{V}_E$, tidal volume, dead space), and lung volumes (VC, RV, TLC) to distinguish pulmonary from nonpulmonary causes of inadequate oxygenation.

Oxygen Saturation

DESCRIPTION

Oxygen saturation is the ratio of oxygenated Hb (O_2Hb) to either total available Hb or functional Hb. Functional Hb is that portion of the total Hb that is capable of binding oxygen. This ratio of content to capacity is normally expressed as a percentage but is sometimes recorded as a simple fraction. The values may differ significantly depending on the method of calculation:

1. Oxyhemoglobin fraction of total Hb:

$$\frac{O_2Hb}{(O_2Hb + rHb + COHb + MetHb)}$$

2. Oxygen saturation of available Hb:

$$\frac{O_2Hb}{O_2Hb + rHb}$$

where:
rHb   = reduced hemoglobin concentration
COHb = carboxyhemoglobin concentration
MetHb = methemoglobin concentration

The first equation is used to measure O_2 saturation with a multiple-wavelength spectrophotometer (co-oximeter); the second equation is used to measure O_2 saturation with a pulse oximeter.

TECHNIQUE

O_2 saturation of Hb may be measured in several ways. In the first method, O_2 saturation is measured using a spectrophotometer (co-oximeter) (see Chapter 10). The total Hb, O_2Hb, COHb, and MetHb are usually reported.

In the second method, saturation is estimated noninvasively using a pulse oximeter (see Chapter 10). Pulse oximeters may use the ear, finger, or other capillary bed for attachment of the probe. Pulse oximeters typically use only two wavelengths of light.

A third method is used to measure mixed venous oxygen saturation. $S\bar{v}o_2$ may be measured by a reflective spectrophotometer in a pulmonary artery catheter (Swan-Ganz catheter). A special catheter that includes fiberoptic bundles is used to perform in vivo measurements.

Blood specimens for co-oximetry should be prepared as described for arterial blood gas specimens. Guidelines for quality control of blood gas analysis are included in Chapter 11.

Measurement of percent saturation allows calculation of the O_2 content of either arterial or mixed venous blood (Cao_2 and $C\bar{v}o_2$, respectively) (see Oxygen Tension section).

SIGNIFICANCE AND PATHOPHYSIOLOGY

See Blood Gases 6-3 for interpretive strategies. Sao_2 for a healthy young adult with a Pao_2 of 95 mm Hg is approximately 97%. The O_2Hb dissociation curve is relatively flat when the Pao_2 is above 60 mm Hg (i.e., Sao_2 is 90% or more). Saturation changes only slightly even when there is a marked change in Pao_2 at partial pressures above 60 mm Hg (Figure 6-1). Therefore, Pao_2 is a more sensitive indicator of oxygenation in lungs that do not have gross abnormalities. At Pao_2 values of approximately 150 mm Hg, Hb becomes completely saturated (Sao_2 is 100%). At Pao_2 values above 150 mm Hg, further increases in O_2 content are caused by increased dissolved oxygen. Alterations in $\dot{V}/\dot{Q}$ patterns in the lungs can be monitored by allowing the patient to breathe 100% O_2, and measuring the changes in dissolved oxygen. In practice, this is accomplished by using the clinical shunt equation (see Shunt Calculation section).

PF Tips

There are several key values to remember when assessing oxygen saturation. When Sao_2 is above 90%, Pao_2 is usually greater than 60 mm Hg. At a Pao_2 of 60, the saturation is 90% and O_2 therapy may be needed. At a Pao_2 of 55, the saturation is 85% and O_2 therapy is indicated. At a Pao_2 of 40, the saturation is approximately 75% (the same as mixed-venous blood).

When Pao_2 falls below 60 mm Hg, Sao_2 decreases rapidly. Small changes in Pao_2 result in large changes in saturation. As Sao_2 falls below 90%, O_2 content decreases rapidly. At saturations less than 85% (i.e., Pao_2 <55 mm Hg), symptoms of hypoxemia increase and supplementary O_2 may be indicated.

The ability of Hb to bind O_2 is measured by the P_{50}. P_{50} specifies the partial pressure at which Hb is 50% saturated (Figure 6-1). The P_{50} of normal adult Hb is approximately 26.7 mm Hg. P_{50} may be determined by tonometering (i.e., equilibrating) blood with several gases at low oxygen tensions. An Hb-O_2 dissociation curve is then constructed to estimate the partial pressure at which Hb is 50% saturated. A second method of estimating P_{50} compares measured Sao_2 (using a spectrophotometer) with the expected saturation. Calculated

BLOOD GASES 6-3 Interpretive Strategies—Oxygen Saturation

1 How was the estimate of saturation obtained? Co-oximeter? Calculated saturation? Pulse oximeter?
2 For co-oximetry or calculated saturation: was the specimen obtained anaerobically and handled properly?
3 Is Hb within normal limits? If low, oxygenation may be compromised; if elevated, look for clinical correlation.
4 Is O_2Hb > 90%? If so, oxygenation is probably adequate; if not, hypoxemia is likely.
5 Is O_2Hb < 85%? If so, supplementary oxygen may be indicated. Correlate with Pao_2 and clinical history.
6 Is COHb > 3%? If so, check for smoking history and/or environmental exposure.
7 Is MetHb > 1.5%? If so, check for environmental exposure to oxidizers.

saturations presume a P_{50} of 26 to 27 mm Hg, but it may differ significantly depending on the types of Hb and interfering substances present.

Healthy individuals have small amounts of Hb that cannot carry O_2. COHb is present in blood from metabolism and from environmental exposure to carbon monoxide (CO) gas. Normal COHb, expressed as a percentage, ranges from 0.5% to 2% of the total Hb. CO comes from smoking (cigarettes, cigars, and pipes), smoke inhalation, improperly vented furnaces, automobile emissions, and other sources of air pollution. In smokers, levels may increase from 3% to 15%, depending on recent smoking history. Smoke inhalation or CO poisoning from other sources also results in elevated COHb levels, sometimes as high as 50%. CO combines rapidly with Hb. Exposures of short duration can cause a high level of COHb if high concentrations of CO are present. Because O_2Hb saturation decreases as COHb increases, COHb levels greater than 15% almost always result in hypoxemia. High levels of COHb are rapidly fatal because of the profound hypoxemia that occurs.

COHb absorbs light at wavelengths similar to O_2Hb. When COHb is elevated, arterial blood appears bright red. Cyanosis, which appears when there is an increased concentration of reduced Hb, is absent. In addition, Pao_2 may be close to normal limits. Blood gas analysis that includes calculated saturation may give erroneously high O_2 saturations. For this reason, O_2Hb and COHb should be measured by co-oximetry whenever possible.

COHb interferes with O_2 transport in two ways. It binds competitively to Hb, and it shifts the O_2Hb curve to the left (Figure 6-1). Increased COHb causes reduced O_2Hb with a decrease in O_2 content. The left shift of the dissociation curve causes O_2 to be bound more tightly to Hb. The combination of these two effects can seriously reduce O_2 delivery to the tissues. COHb concentrations in blood begin to decrease once the source of CO has been removed. Removal of CO from the blood depends on the minute ventilation. Breathing air may require several hours to reduce even moderate levels to normal. Breathing 100% O_2 speeds the washout of CO. High concentrations of O_2 are indicated whenever dangerously high levels of COHb are encountered.

Methemoglobin (MetHb) forms when iron atoms of the Hb molecule are oxidized from Fe^{++} to Fe^{+++}. The normal MetHb level is less than 1.5% of the total Hb. High levels of MetHb can result from ingestion of, or exposure to, strong oxidizing agents. Like COHb, MetHb reduces O_2 carrying capacity of the blood by reducing the available Hb and shifting the O_2Hb dissociation curve to the left (Figure 6-1).

The saturation of mixed venous blood ($S\bar{v}o_2$) in healthy patients averages 75% at a $P\bar{v}o_2$ of 40 mm Hg. Healthy patients have a content difference, $C(a-\bar{v})o_2$, of 5 vol%. Arterial blood typically carries approximately 20 vol% O_2, and mixed venous blood carries 15 vol% O_2. Pulmonary diseases that cause arterial hypoxemia may reduce $S\bar{v}O_2$ if oxygen uptake and cardiac output remain constant. Cardiac output often increases to combat arterial hypoxemia caused by intrapulmonary shunting. Increased cardiac output increases O_2 delivery to the tissues. This results in a reduced extraction of O_2 from the blood. Mixed venous blood then returns to the lungs with normal or even increased O_2 saturation. When this blood is shunted, it has a higher O_2 content, thereby reducing the shunt effect. With or without arterial hypoxemia, $S\bar{v}O_2$ decreases if cardiac output is compromised.

$S\bar{v}O_2$ is useful in assessing cardiac function in the critical care setting and during exercise. Patients who have good cardiovascular reserves maintain a mixed venous saturation of 70% to 75%. Patients whose $S\bar{v}O_2$ values are in the 60% to 70% range have a limited ability to deliver more O_2 to the tissues. $S\bar{v}O_2$ values less than 60% usually indicate cardiovascular decompensation and tissue hypoxemia. The indwelling reflective spectrophotometer (see Chapter 10) allows continuous monitoring of this important parameter. $S\bar{v}O_2$ also decreases during exercise. Despite increased cardiac output, O_2 extraction by the exercising muscles reduces the content of blood returning to the lungs.

Estimation of SaO_2 by most pulse oximeters (SpO_2) is based on absorption of light at two wavelengths. When only two wavelengths are analyzed, only two species of Hb can be detected. Absorption in the red and near-infrared portions of the visible spectrum allows measurement of the oxyhemoglobin and reduced Hb, providing an estimate of the oxygen saturation of available Hb (see Pulse Oximetry section).

Pulse Oximetry

■ DESCRIPTION

SpO_2 estimates SaO_2 by analyzing absorption of light passing through a capillary bed. Pulse oximetry is noninvasive. SpO_2 is reported as percent saturation.

■ TECHNIQUE

Pulse oximeters (see Chapter 10) measure the light absorption of a mixture of two forms of Hb: O_2Hb and reduced Hb (rHb). The relative absorptions at 660 nm (red) and 940 nm of light (near infrared) can be used to calculate the combination of the two Hb forms. Absorption at two wavelengths provides an estimate of the saturation of available Hb (see Oxygen Saturation section). Most pulse oximeters use a stored calibration curve to estimate oxygen saturation.

Pulse oximetry may be used in any setting in which a noninvasive measure of oxygenation status is sufficient. This includes monitoring of O_2 therapy and ventilator management. Pulse oximetry is commonly used during diagnostic procedures such as bronchoscopy, sleep studies, or stress testing. It is also used for monitoring during patient transport or rehabilitation. Pulse oximetry may be used for continuous monitoring with inclusion of appropriate alarms to detect desaturation. Many pulse oximeter systems use memory (RAM) to record SpO_2 and heart rate for extended periods. This type of recorded monitoring allows pulse oximetry to be used for overnight studies of nocturnal desaturation. Alternatively, pulse oximetry can be used for discrete measurements or "spot checks."

Most pulse oximeters use a sensor that attaches to the finger (nail bed) or earlobe. The choice of attachment site should be dictated by the type of measurement being made. The ear site may be preferred in patients undergoing exercise testing or in whom arm movement

BLOOD GASES 6-4 Criteria for Acceptability—Pulse Oximetry

1 Documentation of adequate correlation with measured Sao_2 should be available. Spo_2 and Sao_2 should be within 2% from 85% to 100% saturation. Elevated COHb (>3%) or MetHb (>5%) may invalidate Spo_2.
2 Adequate perfusion of the sensor site should be documented by agreement between oximeter and patient's heart rate (ECG or palpation) and reproducible pulse waveforms (if available).
3 Known interfering substances or agents should be eliminated or accounted for.
4 Pulse oximeter readings should be stable long enough to answer the clinical question being investigated. Readings should be consistent with the patient's clinical history and presentation.

precludes use of the finger site. Both finger and earlobe sites presume pulsatile blood flow. Most oximeters adjust light output to compensate for tissue density or pigmentation. In some patients, impaired perfusion to one site determines which site is preferred. Low perfusion or poor vascularity can cause the oximeter to be unable to detect pulsatile blood flow. Rubbing or warming of the site often improves local blood flow and may be indicated to obtain reliable data. Some pulse oximeters can utilize reflective sensors that detect light reflected from bone underlying the tissue bed. These sensors are usually placed on the patient's forehead and may function when finger or ear sensors do not.

Some pulse oximeters display a representation of the pulse waveform derived from the absorption measurements (see Chapter 10). Such waveforms may be helpful in selecting an appropriate site or troubleshooting questionable Spo_2 values. Most pulse oximeters report heart rate (HR), which is also detected from pulsatile blood flow at the sensor site. Comparison of oximeter HR with palpated pulse or with an electrocardiograph (ECG) signal can assist with selection of an appropriate site. Inability to obtain a valid HR reading or acceptable pulse waveform suggests that Spo_2 values should be interpreted cautiously (Blood Gases 6-4).

A number of factors limit the validity of Spo_2 measurements (Table 6-5). To validate pulse oximetry readings, direct measurement of arterial saturation is required. Simultaneous measurement of Spo_2 and Sao_2 can be used initially to validate pulse oximetry. Pulse oximetry used during exercise testing has been shown to produce variable results. Co-oximetry may be necessary to validate pulse oximetry readings at peak exercise.

COHb absorbs light at wavelengths similar to oxyhemoglobin. The pulse oximeter senses COHb as O_2Hb and overestimates the O_2 saturation. MetHb increases absorption at both wavelengths used by pulse oximeters. This causes the ratio of the two Hb forms to approach 1, which is usually represented as a saturation of 85% (see Chapter 10). Other interfering substances may cause the pulse oximeter to underestimate saturation.

TABLE 6-5 Pulse Oximeter Limitations

Interfering Substances	Interfering Factors
Carboxyhemoglobin (COHb)	Motion artifact, shivering
Methemoglobin (MetHb)	Bright ambient lighting
Intravascular dyes (indocyanine green)	Hypotension, low perfusion (sensor site)
Nail polish or coverings (finger sensor)	Hypothermia
	Vasoconstrictor drugs
	Dark skin pigmentation

BLOOD GASES 6-5   Interpretive Strategies—Pulse Oximetry

1 Is the Spo_2 reading supported by blood oximetry? If not, interpret very cautiously.
2 Is there evidence of adequate perfusion at the sensor site? Consistent pulse waveform (if available)? Good correlation with palpated pulse or ECG heart rate? If not, consider alternate site or blood oximetry.
3 Is the patient a current smoker or smoke-inhalation victim? If so, blood oximetry is indicated.
4 Is the indicated Spo_2 >90%? If so, Hb saturation is probably adequate; correlate with clinical presentation.
5 Is indicated Spo_2 between 85% and 90%? If so, oxygen supplementation may be indicated; correlate with clinical presentation.
6 If indicated Spo_2 <85%, supplementary O_2 is indicated unless there is reason to suspect invalid Spo_2 data.
7 Does supplementary O_2 improve Spo_2 reading? If not, suspect shunt or invalid Spo_2 data.

■ SIGNIFICANCE AND PATHOPHYSIOLOGY

See Blood Gases 6-5 for interpretive strategies. Arterial oxygen saturation estimated by pulse oximetry should equal that measured by blood oximetry in healthy nonsmoking adults. Most pulse oximeters are capable of accuracy of ±2% of the actual saturation when Sao_2 is above 90%. For Sao_2 values of 85% to 90%, accuracy may be slightly less. For very low saturations (i.e., less than 80%), pulse oximeter accuracy is less of an issue because the clinical implications are the same.

Pulse oximetry is most useful when it has been shown to correlate with blood oximetry in a patient in a known circumstance. When this is the case, pulse oximetry can be used for noninvasive monitoring, either continuously or by taking discrete measurements. Uses include monitoring of O_2 therapy, ventilatory support, pulmonary or cardiac rehabilitation, bronchoscopy, surgical procedures, sleep studies, and cardiopulmonary exercise testing. In each of these applications, careful attention must be paid to minimizing known interfering agents or substances (Table 6-5).

Because of its limitations, pulse oximetry should be used cautiously when assessing oxygen need. This is particularly true when using pulse oximetry to detect exercise desaturation. Pulse oximetry may not accurately reflect Sao_2 during exertion. For this reason, Spo_2, even if demonstrated to correlate with Sao_2 at rest, may yield false-positive or false-negative results during exercise. Blood gas analysis with blood oximetry should be used to resolve discrepancies between the Spo_2 reading and the patient's clinical presentation.

Pulse oximetry may not be appropriate in all situations. To evaluate hyperoxemia (Pao_2 greater than 100 to 150 mm Hg) or acid-base status in a patient, blood gas analysis is required. Measurement of O_2 delivery, which depends on Hb concentration, cannot be adequately assessed by pulse oximetry alone.

Capnography

■ DESCRIPTION

Capnography includes continuous, noninvasive monitoring of expired CO_2 and analysis of the single-breath CO_2 waveform. Continuous monitoring of expired CO_2 allows trending of changes in alveolar and dead space ventilation. Analysis of a single breath of expired CO_2 measures the uniformity of both ventilation and pulmonary blood flow. End-tidal PCO_2 ($PetCO_2$) is reported in mm Hg.

TECHNIQUE

Continuous monitoring of expired CO_2 is performed by sampling gas from the proximal airway. This gas may be pumped to an infrared analyzer (see Chapter 10) or to a mass spectrometer. An alternative method inserts a "mainstream" sample window directly into the expired gas stream. The analyzer signal is then passed to either a recorder or a computer. CO_2 waveforms may be displayed either individually (Figure 6-2) or as a series of peaks to form a trend plot. $PetCO_2$ may be read from the peaks of the waveforms. It can also be obtained by a simple peak detector and displayed digitally. Continuous CO_2 monitoring is commonly used in patients with artificial airways in the critical care setting. $PaCO_2$ can be measured at intervals to establish a gradient with $PetCO_2$. Respiratory rate may be determined from the frequency of the CO_2 waveforms. The change in CO_2 concentration during a single expiration may be analyzed to detect ventilation-perfusion abnormalities (Figure 6-2).

Technical problems involved in capnography include the necessity of accurate calibration and management of the gas sampling system (Blood Gases 6-6). Calibration using known gases (preferably two gas concentrations) is required if the system will be used to monitor $PaCO_2$. Many systems use room air, containing minimal CO_2, and a 5% CO_2 mixture for calibration (see Chapter 11). Condensation of water in sample tubing, connectors, or the sample chamber can affect accuracy. Some infrared analyzers (see Chapter 10) may be

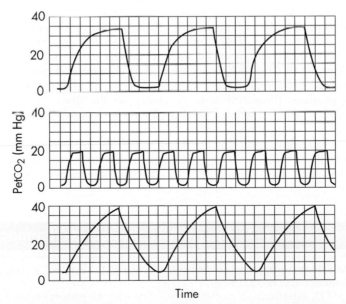

Figure 6-2 *Capnography tracings.* Plots of expired CO_2 versus time for three patients. In each example, expiration is marked by a rapid increase in carbon dioxide to a peak ($PetCO_2$) followed by a return to baseline during inspiration. *Top,* Normal respiratory pattern with $PetCO_2$ near 40 mm Hg and a relatively flat alveolar phase. *Middle,* Rapid respiratory rate and low $PetCO_2$ (20 mm Hg), which may be found in a patient who is hyperventilating; the expiratory waveform has a normal configuration. *Bottom,* Abnormal expired CO_2 waveform consistent with $\dot{V}/\dot{Q}$ abnormalities; no alveolar plateau is present, and the baseline does not return to zero.

BLOOD GASES 6-6   Criteria for Acceptability—Capnography

1 CO_2 analyzer should be calibrated on a frequency consistent with the types of measurements being made. Calibration with air and 5% CO_2 is suitable for most purposes.

2 Sample flow (except in mainstream analyzers) should be high enough to prevent damping of CO_2 waveforms. Sample flow should not be changed after calibration. The sample chamber and tubing should be free of secretions or condensation that may affect the accuracy of the results.

3 $Paco_2$ should be obtained to establish the gradient with $Petco_2$.

4 CO_2 waveforms (if displayed) should be consistent with the patient's clinical condition.

5 CO_2 waveforms (if displayed) should return to baseline during inspiration, indicating appropriate washout of dead space.

affected if flow changes after calibration. Saturation of a dessicator column, if used, can also lead to inaccurate readings. Long sample lines or low sample flows can cause damping of the CO_2 waveform, invalidating analysis of the shape of the expired gas curve.

■ SIGNIFICANCE AND PATHOPHYSIOLOGY

See Blood Gases 6-7 for interpretive strategies. In healthy patients, CO_2 rises to a plateau as alveolar gas is expired (Figure 6-2). If all lung units empty CO_2 evenly, the plateau appears flat. However, even healthy lungs have ventilation and blood flow imbalances. Healthy lung units empty CO_2 at varying rates. Alveolar CO_2 concentration increases slightly as the breath continues. $Petco_2$ theoretically should not exceed $Paco_2$. In healthy patients, the $Petco_2$ is usually close to the arterial value. When ventilation and perfusion become grossly mismatched (e.g., in severe obstruction), CO_2 concentration at the end of the alveolar plateau may exceed the $Paco_2$. $Paco_2$ reflects gas-exchange characteristics of the entire lung. Hence, $Petco_2$ may differ significantly if some lung units are poorly ventilated.

Continuous CO_2 analysis provides useful data for monitoring critically ill patients, particularly those requiring ventilatory support. $Petco_2$ measurements allow trending of changes in $Paco_2$ provided there is little or no change in the shape of the CO_2 waveform (indicating V/Q abnormalities). When a reference blood gas sample is obtained, $Petco_2$ can be used as a continuous, noninvasive monitor. Respiratory rate can be measured from the frequency of expired CO_2 waveforms. Marked changes (e.g., hyperpnea or apnea) can be detected quickly. Analysis of the individual CO_2 waveforms, along with $Paco_2$, may help identify abrupt changes in dead space. This can be useful in detecting pulmonary embolization or reduced cardiac output.

BLOOD GASES 6-7   Interpretive Strategies—Capnography

1 Was there an appropriate calibration of the CO_2 analyzer? If not, arterial–to–end-tidal CO_2 gradients may be inaccurate.

2 Are CO_2 waveforms (if available) consistent with the patient's clinical condition? Do waveforms show an obvious alveolar plateau?

3 Was $Paco_2$ measured? If so, what is the $Paco_2$-$Petco_2$ gradient? If greater than 5 mm Hg, consider marked ventilation-perfusion abnormalities.

4 Has $Petco_2$ changed (serial measurements)? Consider acute changes in dead space or cardiac output.

Problems related to ventilatory support devices can also be detected. Disconnection or leaks in breathing circuits can be quickly recognized by the loss of the CO_2 signal. Increased mechanical dead space (i.e., gas rebreathed in the ventilator circuit) can be identified by a baseline CO_2 concentration greater than zero. Irregularities in the CO_2 waveform often signal that the patient is "out of phase" with the ventilator.

The shape of the expired CO_2 curve is determined by ventilation-perfusion matching. Only lung units that are ventilated *and* perfused contribute CO_2 to expired gas. In patients without lung disease, the CO_2 waveform shows a flat initial segment of anatomic dead space gas containing little or no CO_2. This phase is followed by a rapid increase in CO_2 concentration, reflecting a mixture of dead space and alveolar gas. Finally, an "alveolar" plateau occurs in which gas composition changes only slightly. This slight change is caused by different emptying rates of various lung units. The absolute concentration of CO_2 at the alveolar plateau depends on factors such as minute ventilation and CO_2 production. Dead space–producing disease (e.g., pulmonary embolization or marked decrease in cardiac output) may show a profound decrease in expired CO_2 concentration. Patients who have pulmonary disease, especially obstruction, show poorly delineated phases of the CO_2 washout curve. The alveolar plateau may actually be a continuous slope throughout expiration, causing the measurement of $PetCO_2$ to be misleading.

Shunt Calculation

DESCRIPTION

A shunt is that portion of the cardiac output that passes from the right heart to the left heart without participating in gas exchange. When this occurs in the lungs, it is a pulmonary shunt. If it occurs in the heart (e.g., atrial or ventricular septal defects), it is referred to as an intracardiac shunt. The shunt calculation determines the ratio of shunted blood ($\dot{Q}s$) to total perfusion ($\dot{Q}t$). Shunt is reported as a percent of total cardiac output, or sometimes as a simple fraction.

TECHNIQUE

Two methods for measuring the shunt fraction are commonly used. The first uses O_2 content differences between arterial and mixed venous blood. This method is called the physiologic shunt equation:

1.

$$\frac{\dot{Q}s}{\dot{Q}t} = \frac{Cco_2 - Cao_2}{Cco_2 - C\bar{v}o_2}$$

where:
Cco_2 = O_2 content of end-capillary blood, estimated from saturation associated with calculated P_Ao_2
Cao_2 = arterial O_2 content, measured from an arterial sample
$C\bar{v}o_2$ = mixed venous O_2 content, measured from a sample obtained from a pulmonary artery catheter
The term in the denominator of this equation reflects potential arterialization of mixed venous blood. The term in the numerator reflects the actual arterialization.

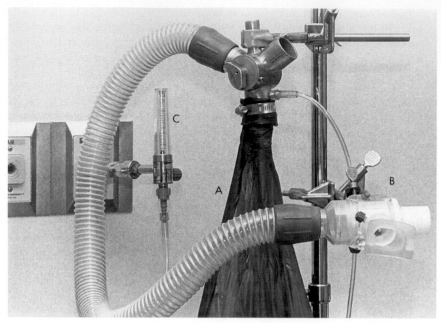

Figure 6-3 *Equipment used for clinical shunt measurement.* **A,** A large bag or balloon is used as a reservoir for 100% oxygen. **B,** A two-way nonrebreathing valve allows the patient to breathe gas from the balloon. **C,** An oxygen source allows the balloon to be refilled as necessary so the patient can breathe O_2 for at least 20 minutes. A blood gas syringe *(not shown)* is set up to obtain an arterial specimen at the end of the oxygen breathing. A pulse oximeter may be used to monitor the patient's saturation during the test. An oxygen analyzer (or appropriate blood gas analyzer) can be used to measure the actual FIO_2.

In the second method, the patient breathes 100% O_2 until the Hb is completely saturated (Figure 6-3). Twenty minutes of O_2 breathing is usually sufficient. Percent shunt is then calculated from differences in dissolved O_2. This method is called the clinical shunt equation:

2.

$$\frac{\dot{Q}s}{\dot{Q}t} = \frac{(P_{A}O_2 - PaO_2) \times 0.0031}{C(a - \bar{v})O_2 + [(P_{A}O_2 - PaO_2) \times 0.0031]}$$

where:
$P_{A}O_2$ = alveolar O_2 tension
PaO_2 = arterial O_2 tension
$C(a-\bar{v})O_2$ = arteriovenous O_2 content difference
0.0031   = solubility factor for O_2
When the patient is breathing 100% O_2, $P_{A}O_2$ can be estimated as follows:

$$P_{A}O_2 = P_B - PH_2O - \left(\frac{PaCO_2}{0.8}\right)$$

where:
P_B = barometric pressure
PH_2O = partial pressure of water vapor at body temperature (47 mm Hg)

Pa_{CO_2} = arterial CO_2 tension (as an estimate of alveolar P_{CO_2})
0.8   = normal respiratory exchange ratio

This calculation of alveolar P_{O_2} assumes that the inspired gas is 100% O_2. If the FIO_2 is measured and found to be less than 1, the standard alveolar air equation can be used (see Appendix E).

The clinical shunt calculation is accurate only when Hb is completely saturated. This normally requires a Pa_{O_2} greater than 150 mm Hg. A saturation of 100% is usually easily accomplished if O_2 is breathed long enough. If breathing 100% O_2 does not increase the Pa_{O_2} high enough to completely saturate Hb, the content difference method (physiologic method) should be used. With either method, shunt fraction may be multiplied by 100 and reported as a percentage (i.e., 0.20 ratio × 100 equals a 20% shunt).

Several technical considerations should be noted regarding shunt measurement (Blood Gases 6-8). Using O_2 content differences (equation 1) requires a pulmonary artery catheter to obtain mixed venous O_2 content. Using dissolved O_2 differences (equation 2) also relies on measured $C(a -\bar{v})O_2$. If placement of a pulmonary artery catheter is not practical, the clinical shunt equation may be used with an assumed a–v content difference (see Significance and Pathophysiology in this section).

The physiologic shunt equation may be used for patients on any known FIO_2. The clinical shunt measurement requires O_2 breathing for 20 minutes or longer. Prolonged O_2 breathing may be contraindicated in patients whose respiration is driven by hypoxemia. Breathing 100% O_2 washes nitrogen (N_2) out of the lungs. Washout of N_2 combined with O_2 uptake by perfusing blood flow can reduce the size of alveoli to their critical limit. In poorly ventilated lung units, this may cause alveolar collapse. The effect of this "nitrogen shunting" may be shunt values that are falsely high because some shunting was induced by the test itself.

■ SIGNIFICANCE AND PATHOPHYSIOLOGY

See Blood Gases 6-9 for interpretive strategies. In healthy individuals, approximately 5% of the cardiac output is shunted past the pulmonary system. An increased shunt fraction indicates that some lung units have little ventilation in relation to their blood flow. These patterns may be found in both obstructive and restrictive diseases. However, even in severe obstruction or restriction, blood flow to areas of poor ventilation may be reduced by the lesions themselves. In emphysema, destruction of the alveolar septa obliterates pulmonary capillaries.

BLOOD GASES 6-8   Criteria for Acceptability—Shunt Calculation

1 For physiologic shunt, patient must have simultaneous arterial and mixed venous blood specimens drawn over a 30-second interval.

2 For clinical shunt, patient should breathe 100% O_2 for at least 20 minutes, or until Hb is completely saturated (Pa_{O_2} >150 mm Hg). If Pa_{O_2} >150 mm Hg cannot be achieved, clinical shunt calculation may underestimate true shunt.

3 Ca_{O_2} and $C\bar{v}_{O_2}$ must be measured for physiologic shunt. Measured contents should be used for clinical shunt if available; otherwise estimated a-$\bar{v}$ content difference should be based on clinical status.

4 FIO_2 should be accurately determined; this is required to calculate capillary content for physiologic shunt. FIO_2 of 1.00 can be assumed for clinical shunt calculation, but measured value improves accuracy.

BLOOD GASES 6-9   Interpretive Strategies—Shunt Calculations

1 For physiologic shunt: Were arterial and mixed venous samples obtained correctly? Analyzed properly? F_{IO_2} accurately determined?

2 For clinical shunt: Did patient breathe O_2 long enough to maximally saturate Hb? Was estimated or measured content difference used?

3 Was calculated shunt ʺ5%? If so, no significant shunting is present.

4 Was calculated shunt >5% but <10%? If so, some shunting is likely. Consider technical causes (assumed content difference, assumed F_{IO_2}).

5 Was calculated shunt >10% but <30%? If so, significant shunting is present. Consider clinical correlation.

6 Was calculated shunt >30%? If so, severe shunting is present. Further testing is indicated to determine the site and physiologic basis for the shunt.

As the terminal airways lose their support, they also have reduced blood flow. In poorly ventilated lung units, vasoconstriction of pulmonary arterioles redirects blood flow away from the affected area. In these cases, there may be minimal shunting, even though severe ventilatory impairment exists.

Intrapulmonary shunting is common in acute disease patterns such as atelectasis or foreign body aspiration. Diseases such as pneumonia or adult respiratory distress syndrome (ARDS) often result in a shuntlike effect. This is caused by reduced ventilation in relation to blood flow in many lung units. Foreign body aspiration may cause shunting by blocking an airway and depriving all distal lung units of ventilation. Blood flow to the affected units cannot participate in gas exchange. The degree of shunting is directly related to the number of lung units with $\dot{V}/\dot{Q}$ ratios close to zero.

Intracardiac shunting occurs when defects in the atrial or ventricular septa allow mixed venous blood to pass from the right heart to the left heart without traversing the pulmonary capillaries. In the ventricles, shunting usually requires an elevated right-heart pressure to overcome the normal pressure difference between the systemic and pulmonary systems. Atrial septal defects, such as patent foramen ovale (PFO), allow blood to pass from the right atrium to the left atrium during systole.

Very large shunt values (greater than 30%) suggest that a significant volume of blood is moving from the right heart to the left heart without participating in gas exchange. Further testing may be required to determine whether the shunt is occurring in the lungs or in the heart. Echocardiography with contrast media or cardiac catheterization may be necessary to identify intracardiac shunts.

The accuracy of clinical shunt measurement (i.e., dissolved O_2 differences) depends on the accuracy of P_{O_2} determinations. In small shunts, Hb becomes 100% saturated. The difference between alveolar and arterial P_{O_2} values results simply from the amount of O_2 dissolved. The difference between the actual content of dissolved oxygen and the content that can potentially dissolve is the basis for the calculation. Measurements of P_{O_2} used for shunt calculations (200 to 600 mm Hg) are much higher than the normal physiologic range. Additional calibration and quality control of the P_{O_2} electrode may be necessary.

The calculated shunt fraction also depends on the O_2 content difference between arterial and mixed venous blood. $C(a-\bar{v})O_2$ is a component of the denominator in the clinical shunt equation. The a–$\bar{v}$ content difference is determined not only by the lungs but also by cardiac output and perfusion status of the tissues. Ideally, the value used in the equation should be measured rather than estimated. Arterial content can be determined easily from a sample taken from a peripheral artery. However, mixed venous content can only be measured accurately from a pulmonary artery sample. In patients with no pulmonary artery catheter in place, an estimated value must be used. $C(a\text{-}\bar{v})O_2$ values from 4.5 to 5.0 vol% are reasonable a–$\bar{v}$ content differences in patients who have good cardiac output and perfusion status. Values of 3.5 vol% are more realistic in patients who are critically ill.

In some instances, a–$\bar{v}$ content difference cannot be reliably estimated, or Hb cannot be maximally saturated by breathing 100% oxygen. In such cases, the alveolar-arterial oxygen gradient $P(A-a)O_2$ may be useful as an index for matching of ventilation to blood flow. In healthy patients breathing 100% O_2 at sea level, arterial PaO_2 should increase to approximately 600 mm Hg. $\dot{Q}s/\dot{Q}t$ does not directly provide absolute values for $\dot{Q}s$, but if the cardiac output $\dot{Q}t$ is known, $\dot{Q}s$ can be determined simply.

Measurement of the shunt fraction is sometimes performed in conjunction with the determination of the V_D/V_T ratio (see Chapter 4) to assess both types of gas exchange abnormalities together.

Summary

This chapter describes the measurement of pH, P_{CO_2}, P_{O_2}, and blood oximetry used as part of pulmonary function testing. Technical aspects of obtaining samples are discussed in detail because accurate interpretation makes numerous assumptions regarding proper specimen handling. Chapter 10 fully describes the design and function of blood gas electrodes and blood oximeters. Calibration and quality control issues as they apply to blood gas analyzers are discussed in Chapter 11.

Two noninvasive methods of assessing gas exchange are commonly used: pulse oximetry and capnography. Pulse oximetry offers a simple means of assessing oxyhemoglobin saturation. Attention to interfering factors and correlation with blood gases is necessary to make optimal use of pulse oximetry. Capnography is useful for monitoring changes in Pet_{CO_2}, particularly for patients in critical care settings.

Shunt measurements allow estimates of severe ventilation-perfusion imbalances in the lungs. Two methods are described: the clinical and physiologic equations. The advantages and disadvantages of each are also discussed.

CASE STUDIES

CASE 6-1

HISTORY

C.O. is a 57-year-old man referred to the pulmonary function laboratory for increasing shortness of breath. He admits having a chronic cough with production of thick white sputum, mainly upon awakening. C.O. reports that he quit smoking 3 months ago. He averaged approximately two packs of cigarettes per day for 30 years (60 pack-years) before quitting. C.O.'s referring physician performed pulse oximetry in an outpatient clinic and obtained readings of 90% to 91%. Complete pulmonary function studies with arterial blood gases were requested.

PULMONARY FUNCTION TESTS

Personal Data

Sex: Male
Age: 57 yr
Height: 66 in.
Weight: 197 lb

Spirometry

	Before Drug	Predicted	%	After Drug	%	%Chg
FVC (L)	3.97	4.10	97	4.04	99	2
FEV_1 (L)	2.31	2.99	77	2.50	84	8
$FEV_{1\%}$ (%)	58	73	—	62	—	7
$FEF_{25\%-75\%}$ (L/sec)	1.01	3.05	33	1.32	43	31
MVV (L)	83	116	72	92	79	11

Lung Volumes

	Before Drug	Predicted	%
VC (L)	3.97	4.10	97
IC (L)	2.66	2.76	96
ERV (L)	1.31	1.35	97
FRC (L)	3.65	3.42	107
RV (L)	2.34	2.07	113
TLC (L)	6.31	6.18	102
RV/TLC (%)	37	34	—

DL_{CO}

	Before Drug	Predicted	%
DL_{CO} (ml/min/mm Hg)	16.7	26.3	63
DL_{CO} (adj)	17.0	26.3	65
DL/V_A	5.09	4.38	86

Blood Gases

pH   7.37
Pco_2 (mm Hg)   44
Po_2 (mm Hg)   57
HCO_3^- (mEq/L)   26.4
BE (mEq/L)   −1.7
Hb (g/dl)   16.2
O_2Hb (%)   80.1
COHb (%)   5.9
MetHb (%)   0.2

TECHNOLOGIST'S COMMENTS

All spirometry maneuvers were performed acceptably. Lung volumes by helium (He) dilution were also performed acceptably. DL_{CO} was performed acceptably; DL_{CO} was corrected for an Hb of 16.2 and a COHb of 5.9.

QUESTIONS

1. What is the interpretation of:
   - Prebronchodilator and postbronchodilator spirometry?
   - Lung volumes?
   - DL_{CO}?
   - Blood gases?
2. What is the cause of the patient's symptoms?
3. What other treatment or tests might be indicated?

DISCUSSION

Interpretation

All spirometry, lung volumes, and diffusing capacity maneuvers were performed acceptably. Spirometry reveals moderate airway obstruction with minimal response to inhaled bronchodilators. Lung volumes by He dilution show a normal TLC, but with increased FRC, RV, and RV/TLC ratio. These changes are consistent with air trapping. DL_{CO} is moderately decreased even after correction for increased Hb and elevated COHb. Arterial blood gas results reveal normal acid-base status with a PCO_2 of 44. There is moderate to severe hypoxemia as indicated by a PO_2 of 57 and an oxyhemoglobin saturation of 80%. The hypoxemia is further aggravated by an increased COHb consistent with cigarette smoking or environmental exposure.

Impression: Moderate obstructive airways disease with no significant improvement after inhaled bronchodilator. There appears to be mild air trapping and a moderate loss of diffusing capacity. There is significant hypoxemia on room air, which is further increased by an elevation of COHb. Recommend further investigation of source of CO and clinical evaluation of O_2 supplementation.

Cause of Symptoms

This case demonstrates the importance of arterial blood gas analysis in the diagnosis of pulmonary disorders. The patient's complaint of increased shortness of breath was not explained by the borderline value of pulse oximetry (SpO_2). The referring physician correctly suspected a pulmonary problem resulting from the patient's previous smoking history.

The spirometric measurement shows moderate obstruction as evidenced by the FEV_1 of 58%. The response of FEV_1 to inhaled bronchodilator is less than 200 ml and represents only an 8% improvement over prebronchodilator values. Lung volumes are also consistent with an obstructive pattern showing a mild degree of air trapping.

Diffusing capacity is also reduced in a pattern consistent with mild to moderate airway obstruction. This abnormality persists even after the DL_{CO} is corrected for the elevated COHb. Correction for elevated CO in the blood increases the measured diffusing capacity. In this patient, the correction was offset by the elevated Hb level. When adjusted for the higher than normal Hb, his DL_{CO} decreased.

Of the variables measured, the arterial blood gas values are most abnormal. Although pH and PCO_2 are within normal limits, PO_2 is markedly decreased. As a result, oxygen saturation is low. Elevated CO further complicates oxygenation. This level is characteristic of individuals who currently smoke or who are chronically exposed to low levels of CO in their environment. The patient's spouse reported that he was still smoking 5 to 10 cigarettes per day.

Treatment and Other Tests

The patient was advised to refrain from smoking, which he did within a few days. Blood gas analysis 2 weeks later confirmed his smoking cessation (i.e., COHb was 1.7%). However, his P_{O_2} improved only slightly to 61 mm Hg (Sa_{O_2} was 87%). He was referred for evaluation of possible exercise desaturation. His arterial oxygenation was shown to actually increase with exercise, so O_2 supplementation was unnecessary. His lung function continued to improve over several months, presumably because of his smoking cessation.

CASE 6-2

HISTORY

Y.M. is a 31-year-old woman referred to the pulmonary function laboratory for a shunt study. Her chief complaint is shortness of breath with exertion as well as at other times. Her referring physician suspected a shunt and requested a shunt study. Y.M. was in no apparent distress on arrival at the laboratory. She never smoked and had no significant environmental exposure to respiratory irritants. Her mother died of a stroke at age 50, but there is no heart or lung disease in her immediate family.

SHUNT STUDY

Personal Data

Age:	31 yr
Height:	69 in
Weight:	200 lb
Race:	White

Blood Gases (Drawn After 20 Minutes of O_2 Breathing)

F_{IO_2}	1.00
P_B	752
pH	7.43
P_{CO_2}	38
P_{O_2}	557
HCO_3^-	24.1
BE	0.1
Hb	7.4
O_2Hb	99.6
COHb	0.3
MetHb	0.1

QUESTIONS

1. What is the patient's calculated shunt?
2. What is the interpretation of:
   a. Blood gases?
   b. Shunt?

3. What is the cause of the patient's symptoms?
4. What other treatment or tests might be indicated?

DISCUSSION

Calculations

The P_AO_2 is calculated as follows:

$$P_AO_2 = P_B - PH_2O \left(\frac{P_ACO_2}{0.8} \right)$$

$$= 752 - 47 - \left(\frac{38}{0.8} \right)$$

$$= 705 - 48$$

$$P_AO_2 = 657$$

Substituting this value in the clinical shunt equation and assuming an a–$\bar{v}$ content difference of 4.5:

$$\frac{\dot{Q}_S}{\dot{Q}_T} = \frac{(P_AO_2 - PaO_2) \times 0.0031}{C(a - \bar{v})O_2 + [(P_AO_2 - PaO_2) \times 0.0031]}$$

$$= \frac{(657 - 557) \times 0.0031}{4.5 + [(657 - 557) \times 0.0031]}$$

$$= \frac{0.31}{4.5 + (0.31)}$$

$$\frac{\dot{Q}_S}{\dot{Q}_T} - 0.06$$

Interpretation

The patient's blood gas results show a normal acid-base status. The PaO_2 reflects an appropriate increase after breathing 100% O_2 for 20 minutes. The Hb as measured by co-oximetry (7.4 mg/dl) is markedly decreased. The patient's shunt is 6% (0.06 as a fraction). This is very close to the normal range.

Impression: Normal arterial blood gas results and normal shunt with markedly reduced Hb. Recommend clinical correlation.

Cause of Symptoms

The patient's primary symptom of dyspnea does not appear to be caused by any significant shunting. In a shunt, blood passes from the right side of the heart to the left side without coming into contact with alveolar gas. The shunt may be in the heart or in the lungs themselves. Breathing high concentrations of oxygen will not relieve this problem. This patient increased her PaO_2 appropriately, which rules out a large shunt.

A more likely cause of the symptoms described is the patient's low Hb level. Severe anemia reduces the arterial oxygen content dramatically. Oxygen delivery to the tissues is reduced. Dyspnea can result during exertion or times of increased metabolic demand. The patient's arterial

dy state, however, is unnecessary if the primary objective of the evaluation is to deter-
e maximum values (oxygen uptake, heart rate, or ventilation). Short exercise inter-
lessen muscle fatigue that may occur with prolonged tests. Short-interval or ramp
ols may allow better delineation of gas exchange ($\dot{V}O_2$, $\dot{V}CO_2$) kinetics. Progressive
ultistage tests using intervals of 4 to 6 minutes may result in a steady state.

   Steady-state tests are designed to assess cardiopulmonary function under conditions of constant metabolic demand. Steady-state conditions are usually defined in terms of HR, oxygen
consumption ($\dot{V}O_2$), or ventilation ($\dot{V}_E$). If the HR remains unchanged for 1 minute at a given
workload, a steady state may be assumed. Steady-state tests are useful for assessing responses
to a known workload. Steady-state protocols may be used to evaluate the effectiveness of various therapies or pharmacologic agents on exercise ability. For example, an incremental test
may be performed initially to determine a patient's maximum tolerable workload. Then a
steady-state test may be used to evaluate specific variables at a submaximal level, such as 50%
and 75% of the highest $\dot{V}O_2$ achieved. The patient exercises for 5 to 8 minutes at a predetermined level to allow a steady state to develop. Measurements are performed during the last
1 or 2 minutes of the period. Successive steady-state determinations at higher power outputs
may be made continuously or spaced with short periods of light exercise or rest. A similar
protocol may be used for evaluation of exercise-induced bronchospasm (see Chapter 9).

The 6-minute walk test is a simple exercise test used to assess response to a medical or surgical
intervention. It is also used to assess functional capacity as well as morbidity and mortality. The
test is performed in an unobstructed hallway that is at least 100 feet in length. The objective of
the test is to have the patient cover as much ground as possible in 6 minutes. It is important to
use standardized phrases of encouragement during the test. Assessment of oxygen need should
be performed prior to the test and, when indicated, adequate flow rates of oxygen utilized.
Documentation should include the distance walked, the oxygen flow and delivery device if used,
the mode of oxygen transport (e.g., pulling an O_2 cart versus carrying a unit), and the ratings of
perceived exertion (RPE). Pulse oximetry is optional.

   The *6-minute walk test* is a simple test that does not require any sophisticated equipment.
It is typically performed to assess response to a medical or surgical intervention but has
also been used to assess functional capacity as well as to estimate morbidity and mortality.
A 100-foot (minimum) hallway that is free of obstructions is needed to perform the test.
Equipment needed includes:

- Countdown timer
- Mechanical lap counter
- A methodology to mark the endpoints of the course
- Chair
- Sphygmomanometer
- Rating of perceived exertion scale (Borg scale)
- Easy access to the emergency response team (e.g., telephone, nurse call light, etc.).

   An oxygen delivery device should be available, if appropriate. A pulse oximeter can be
used but is not required. The objective of the test is to have the patient walk as far as possible
in six minutes. The patient should be encouraged throughout the test, and it has been

TABLE 7-2   6-Minute Walk Log

Date	Distance (ft)	Inspired Gas	Mode of O_2 Transport	SpO_2 (End Exercise)	RPE (6-20)
5/18/2002	1,173	3.0 L/min NC	Patient carried unit	90	17
7/26/2002	1,266	3.0 L/min NC	Patient carried unit	94	18
8/15/2002	1,420	2.5 L/min	Patient carried unit	92	17

recommended that standard phrases be used to reduce test-to-test variability. Resting during the tests is permitted with encouragement to continue walking as soon as possible, while the timer continues to run. If pulse oximetry is measured, it should be done at the beginning and end of exercise, but not during exercise. Documentation should include the distance walked, the oxygen flow and delivery device if used, the mode of oxygen transport (e.g., pulling an O_2 cart has a different impact on work than carrying a unit), and the ratings of perceived exertion (RPE). See Table 7-2 for an example of a data record used to record 6-minute walk data from a patient.

Exercise Workload

Two methods of varying exercise workload are commonly used: the treadmill and the cycle ergometer (Figures 7-1 and 7-2). Each device has advantages and disadvantages (Table 7-3). Other methods sometimes used include arm ergometers, steps, and free running or walking (as previously described for the 6-minute walk test).

Workload on a treadmill is adjusted by changing the speed and/or slope of the walking surface. The speed of the treadmill may be calibrated either in miles per hour or in kilometers per hour. Treadmill slope is registered as "percent grade." Percent grade refers to the relationship between the length of the walking surface and the elevation of one end above level. A treadmill with a 6-foot surface and one end elevated 1 foot above level would have an elevation of $1/6 \times 100$, or approximately 17%. The primary advantage of a treadmill is that it elicits walking, jogging, or running, which are familiar forms of exercise. An additional advantage is that maximal levels of exercise can be easily attained, even in conditioned healthy patients. However, the actual work performed during treadmill walking is a function of the weight of the patient. Patients of different weights walking at the same speed and slope perform different workloads. Different walking patterns, or stride length, may also affect the actual amount of work being done. Patients who grip the handrails of the treadmill may use their arms to reduce the amount of work being performed. For these reasons, estimating $\dot{V}o_2$ from a patient's weight and the speed and slope of the treadmill may produce erroneous results. $\dot{V}o_{2max}$ has been shown to be measured slightly higher (approximately 7% to 10%) on a treadmill compared with a cycle ergometer.

The cycle ergometer allows workload to be varied by adjustment of the resistance to pedaling and by the pedaling frequency, usually specified in revolutions per minute (rpm). The flywheel of a mechanical ergometer turns against a belt or strap, both ends of which are connected to a weighted physical balance. The diameter of the wheel is known, and the resistance can be easily measured. When pedaling speed (usually 50 to 90 rpm) is determined, the amount of work performed can be accurately calculated. One of the chief advantages of the cycle ergometer is that the workload is independent of the weight of the patient. Unlike

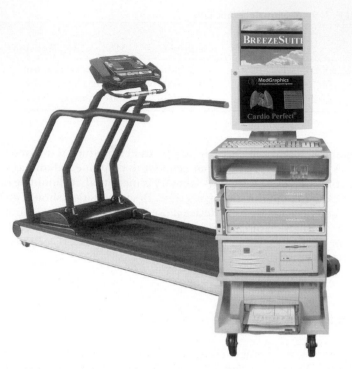

Figure 7-1 *Treadmill with computerized electrocardiogram (ECG) and controller.* The treadmill is controlled by a programmable interface so that different protocols (e.g., speeds and percent grade) can be selected. Manual control is also provided. Cardiac monitoring and exhaled gas analysis are integrated in a single computer system. The 12-lead ECG recordings or rhythm strips can be taken automatically at each exercise level. Most automated systems provide "freeze frame" technology that allows for close review during the test and storage of data for retrieval and analysis for significant arrhythmia and ST abnormalities after the test. The same system can be interfaced to a cycle ergometer (Figure 7-2). (Courtesy Medical Graphics Inc., St Paul, Minn.)

the treadmill, $\dot{V}O_2$ can be reasonably estimated if the pedaling speed and resistance are carefully measured. In addition, workload can be changed rapidly by adjusting the tension on the flywheel. Another advantage of ergometers is better stability of the patient for gas collection, blood sampling, and blood pressure monitoring. Electronically braked cycle ergometers (Figure 7-2) provide a smooth, rapid, and more reproducible means of changing exercise workload than mechanical ergometers. Electronically braked ergometers allow continuous adjustment of workload independent of pedaling speed. However, accuracy of the ergometer output may be dependent on a manufacturer's specified pedal cadence range (e.g., 40 to 100 rpm). This feature permits the exercise level to be ramped (i.e., the workload increases continuously rather than in increments). The ramp test allows the patient to advance from low to high workloads quickly and provides all the information normally sought during a progressive maximal exercise test. A ramp protocol typically requires electronic control (usually by a computer) for adjustment of the workload and rapid collection of physiologic data. Table 7-4 provides a systematic method of determining the desired workload increments using a cycle ergometer.

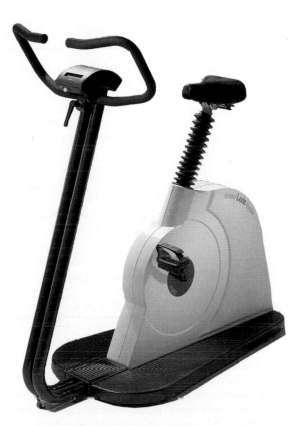

Figure 7-2 *Electronically braked cycle ergometer.* Typical cycle ergometer with continuous adjustable electronic braking. Workload (i.e., resistance) is usually managed by interfacing the ergometer to a computer. The computer allows selection of various cycle ergometer protocols. Changes in pedaling rate by the patient causes a change in resistance to maintain a constant workload. (Courtesy Medical Graphics Inc., St Paul, Minn.)

TABLE 7-3 Ergometers

	Advantages	Disadvantages
Treadmill	Natural form of exercise Easy to calibrate Higher $\dot{V}O_{2max}$	Risk of accidents Patient anxiety Motion artifact Difficult to obtain blood Difficult to quantify work
Cycle ergometer	Safer than treadmill Easy to monitor Easy to quantify work Easy to obtain blood	Difficult to calibrate Leg fatigue more of an issue Lower $\dot{V}O_{2max}$

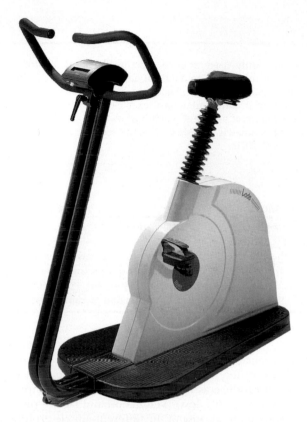

Figure 7-2 *Electronically braked cycle ergometer.* Typical cycle ergometer with continuous adjustable electronic braking. Workload (i.e., resistance) is usually managed by interfacing the ergometer to a computer. The computer allows selection of various cycle ergometer protocols. Changes in pedaling rate by the patient causes a change in resistance to maintain a constant workload. (Courtesy Medical Graphics Inc., St Paul, Minn.)

TABLE 7-3   Ergometers

	Advantages	Disadvantages
Treadmill	Natural form of exercise Easy to calibrate Higher $\dot{V}O_{2max}$	Risk of accidents Patient anxiety Motion artifact Difficult to obtain blood Difficult to quantify work
Cycle ergometer	Safer than treadmill Easy to monitor Easy to quantify work Easy to obtain blood	Difficult to calibrate Leg fatigue more of an issue Lower $\dot{V}O_{2max}$

TABLE 7-5 **Cardiopulmonary Exercise Variables**

Variables Measured	Uses
ECG, blood pressure, SpO_2	Limited to suspected or known coronary artery disease; pulse oximetry may be misleading if used without blood gases
All of the above plus ventilation Vo_2, Vco_2, and derived measurements	Noninvasive estimate of ventilatory threshold (AT), quantify workload; discriminate between cardiovascular and pulmonary limitation to work
All of the above plus arterial blood gases	Detailed assessment of gas exchange abnormalities; calculation of V_D/V_T; titration of O_2 in exercise desaturation; measurement of pH and lactate possible
All of the above plus mixed venous blood gases	Cardiac output by Fick method, noninvasive techniques, calculation of shunt, thermodilution cardiac output, pulmonary artery pressures, calculation of pulmonary and systemic vascular resistances

Measurement of ventilation, oxygen consumption, carbon dioxide production, and related variables permits a comprehensive evaluation of the cardiovascular system. Addition of these measurements to ECG, BP, and pulse oximetry makes it possible to grade the adequacy of cardiopulmonary function. In addition, analysis of exhaled gas allows the relative contributions of cardiovascular, pulmonary, or conditioning limitations to work to be determined. All of these variables can be measured noninvasively. When using pulse oximetry to assess gas exchange, the practitioner needs to be aware of the limitations of the device that may lead to a false positive result (e.g., motion artifact, peripheral vasoconstriction, etc.).

Adding blood gases to the exercise protocol enables detailed analysis of the pulmonary limitations to exercise. Placement of an arterial catheter is preferable to a single sample obtained at peak exercise. Multiple specimens permit comparison of blood gases at each workload. A single sample at peak exercise may be difficult to obtain and may not adequately describe the pattern of gas exchange abnormality. In some patients, measurement of cardiac output (CO) using either noninvasive or invasive techniques such as a pulmonary artery (Swan-Ganz) catheter may be indicated. Noninvasive CO determination depends on the availability of the technology and the underlying etiology of the patient (e.g., may not work well in patients with COPD). Invasive techniques require the placement of a catheter that allows measurement of mixed venous blood gases, cardiac output via the Fick method, and many other derived variables. Thermal dilution cardiac output is also available with most pulmonary artery catheters.

Cardiovascular Monitors During Exercise

Continuous monitoring of heart rate (HR) and ECG during exercise is essential to safe performance of the test. Intermittent or continuous monitoring of BP is equally important to ensure that exercise testing is safe. Recording of HR, ECG, and BP allows work limitations caused by cardiac or vascular disease to be identified and quantified. The level of fitness or conditioning can be gauged from the HR response in relation to the maximal work rate achieved during exercise.

> ### EXERCISE 7-1   Criteria for Acceptability—Cardiovascular Monitors During Exercise
>
> 1 Heart rate and rhythm (ECG) should be monitored continuously. At least one precordial lead is required; full 12-lead monitoring using modified limb leads is recommended.
> 2 A resting 12-lead ECG should be available for comparison with exercise tracings.
> 3 All exercise tracings should be free from artifact caused by motion or electrical interference.
> 4 ECG monitoring devices should allow manual or automated storage of arrhythmia events for later review.
> 5 "Raw" ECG tracings should be available for comparison with computer-averaged complexes.
> 6 Heart rates should be checked by visual inspection of the ECG tracing.
> 7 Systemic blood pressure (BP) should be monitored at appropriate intervals (i.e., at least once per exercise stage).
> 8 BP may be monitored using an appropriate-sized cuff or by automated noninvasive blood pressure (NIBP) monitor. A cuff/stethoscope should be available as backup for the NIBP.
> 9 If BP is monitored by an indwelling arterial catheter, the pressure transducer must be zeroed and calibrated appropriately. The catheter should be secured to minimize movement artifact.

■ HEART RATE AND ELECTROCARDIOGRAM

Heart rate and rhythm should be monitored continuously using one or more modified chest leads. Standard precordial chest lead configurations (V_1 to V_6) allow comparison with resting 12-lead tracings (Exercise 7-1). Twelve-lead monitoring during exercise is practical with electrocardiographs designed for exercise testing. These instruments incorporate filters (digital or analog) that eliminate movement artifact and provide ST-segment monitoring. Limb leads normally must be moved to the torso for ergometer or treadmill testing (modified leads). A resting ECG should be performed to record both the standard and modified leads. Single-lead monitoring allows only for gross arrhythmia detection and HR determination. It may not be adequate for testing patients with known or suspected cardiac disease.

Exercise tests are often performed to determine a patient's maximal exercise capacity. An end point that is commonly used is the patient's predicted maximal HR. Maximal HR is easily computed as 220 – age. A subject who is 40 years old would have a predicted maximal HR of 220 – 40, or 180 beats/min. If the subject achieves at least 85% of the predicted value (153 beats/min in this case), he or she is considered to have made a maximal effort. Because maximal HR varies among individuals, some patients may reach or exceed their predicted maximum. Many patients will reach a "symptom-limited" end point before reaching 85% of the predicted maximal HR. In these cases, the patient becomes exhausted, dyspneic, or has chest pain. The technologist should always record what symptoms caused the patient's inability to continue.

The ECG monitor should allow assessment of intervals and segments up to the patient's maximal heart rate (HR_{max}). Computerized arrhythmia recording or manual "freeze-frame" storage allows subsequent evaluation of conduction abnormalities while the testing protocol continues (Figure 7-3). Some digital ECG systems generate computerized

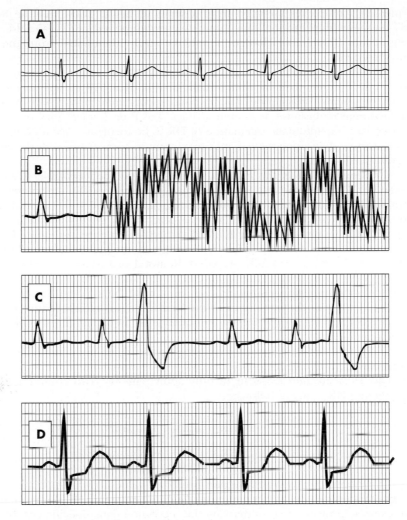

Figure 7-3 *Electrocardiographic (ECG) monitoring during exercise.* **A**, Standard rhythm lead showing normal sinus rhythm. Although testing can be done with 1 to 3 leads, 12-lead monitoring allows comparison with resting ECG tracings and better detection of ischemic changes. **B**, Motion artifact. The most common monitoring problem during exercise is poor ECG signals because of motion. These problems can be minimized by careful skin preparation and electrode application. Lead wires and cables should be supported so that movement and traction on electrodes is kept to a minimum. **C**, Premature ventricular contractions (PVCs). PVCs are a common occurrence during exercise in patients with underlying cardiac disease. Increased rate of PVCs, couplets (two in a row), or triplets (three in a row) may be indications for limiting the exercise test. **D**, ST-segment changes. Depression (and sometimes elevation) of the ST segment of the ECG is usually considered evidence of cardiac ischemia. Depression (or elevation) of the ST segment greater than 1 to 2 mm for 0.08 seconds or longer is consistent with significant ischemia. ST segments should be checked in multiple leads before, during, and after exercise.

"median" complexes averaged from a series of beats. These may be helpful in analyzing ST-segment depression. The "raw," or nondigitized, ECG should also be available. Significant ST-segment changes should be easily identifiable from the tracing up to the predicted HR_{max}.

Heart rate should be analyzed by visual inspection of the ECG, with manual measurement of the rate rather than by an automatic sensor. Most HR meters average RR intervals over multiple beats. Inaccurate HR measurements may occur with nodal or ventricular arrhythmias or because of motion artifact. Tall P or T waves may be falsely identified as R waves, causing automatic calculation of HR to be incorrect. Accurate measurement of HR is necessary to determine the patient's maximum in comparison with the age-related predicted value.

Motion artifact is the most common cause of unacceptable ECG recordings during exercise. Allowing the patient to practice pedaling on the ergometer or walking on the treadmill permits adequacy of the ECG signal to be checked. Carefully applied electrodes, proper skin preparation, and secured lead wires greatly minimize movement artifact (Exercise 7-1). Electrodes specifically designed for exercise testing are helpful. Most of these use extra adhesive to ensure electrical contact even when the patient begins perspiring. The skin sites should be carefully prepared. Removal of surface skin cells by gentle abrasion is recommended. Patients with excessive body hair may require shaving of the electrode site to ensure good electrical contact. Lead wires must be securely attached to the electrodes. Devices that limit the movement of the lead wires can greatly reduce motion artifact. Spare electrodes and lead wires should be available to avoid test interruption in the event of an electrode failure.

HR increases linearly with increasing workload, up to an age-related maximum. Several formulas are available for predicting HR_{max}. For most predicted HR_{max} values, a variability of ±10 to 15 beats/min exists in healthy adult patients. Two commonly used equations for predicting HR_{max} are as follows:

$$1.\ HR_{max} = 220 - Age\ (years)$$

$$2.\ HR_{max} = 210 - (0.65 \times Age\ [years])$$

Equation 1 yields slightly higher predicted values in young adults. Equation 2 produces higher values in older adults. Other methods of predicting HR_{max} vary depending on the type of exercise protocol used in deriving the regression data. Specific criteria for terminating an exercise test should include factors based on symptom limitation as well as HR and BP changes (see Safety section).

Heart rate increases almost linearly with increasing $\dot{V}O_2$. The increase in cardiac output (CO) depends on both HR and stroke volume (SV) according to the following equation:

$$CO = HR \times SV$$

Increases in stroke volume account for a smaller portion of the increase in CO, primarily at low and moderate workloads (Figure 7-4). While HR increases from 70 beats/min up to 200 beats/min in young healthy upright patients, SV increases from 80 ml to approximately 110 ml. At low workloads, increase in CO depends on the patient's ability to increase both HR and SV. At high workloads, further increases in CO result almost entirely from the increase in HR.

Deconditioned patients usually have a limited SV. High HR values occur with moderate workloads in deconditioned individuals because it is the primary mechanism for increasing CO.

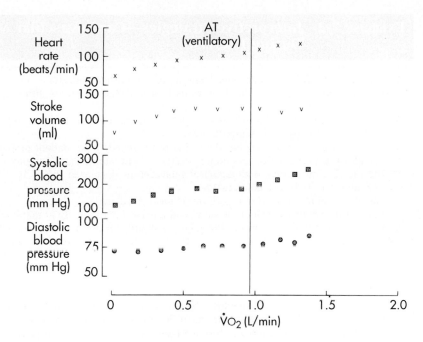

Figure 7-4 *Normal cardiovascular responses during exercise.* Four cardiovascular parameters are plotted against $\dot{V}O_2$ as a measure of work rate, as they might appear in a normal healthy adult. Heart rate (HR) increases linearly with work. Maximal HR is predicted by the age of the patient. Stroke volume (SV) increases initially at low to moderate workloads but then becomes relatively constant. Cardiac output (HR × SV) increases at low and moderate workloads because of increases in both HR and SV (*see text*). At higher levels of work, increases in HR are responsible for increasing cardiac output. Systolic blood pressure (BP) increases by approximately 100 mm Hg in a linear fashion, whereas diastolic BP increases only slightly.

Training (i.e., endurance or aerobic) typically improves SV. This allows the same cardiac output to be achieved at a lower HR. Training usually results in a lower resting HR as well as a higher tolerable maximum workload. Except in highly trained patients, maximal exercise in healthy individuals is limited by the inability to further increase the CO. Reductions in SV are usually related to the preload or afterload of the left ventricle. Increased HR response, in relation to the workload, implies that SV is compromised.

Reduced HR response may occur in patients who have ischemic heart disease or complete heart block (Exercise 7-2). Low HR is also common in patients who have been treated with drugs that block the effects of the sympathetic nervous system (β-blockers, calcium channel blockers). HR response may also be reduced if the autonomic nervous system is impaired or the heart is denervated, as occurs following cardiac transplantation (e.g. chronotopic insufficiency).

In patients who have heart disease (e.g., coronary artery disease, cardiomyopathy), increased HR is typically accompanied by ECG changes such as arrhythmias or ST-segment depression. Deconditioned patients without heart disease show a high HR at lower than maximal workloads but usually without ECG abnormalities. Horizontal or down-sloping ST-segment depression greater than 1 mm (from the resting baseline) for a duration of 0.08 seconds is usually considered evidence of ischemia. ST-segment depression at low workloads that increases with HR and continues into the postexercise period is usually indicative of

---

EXERCISE 7-2   Interpretive Strategies—Cardiovascular Monitors During Exercise

1. Is ECG recording acceptable? Free from motion and other artifact?
2. Is resting tracing consistent with previous 12-lead ECGs? If not, are differences caused by lead placement?
3. What is the rate and rhythm at rest? Is there evidence of heart block at rest? Is there evidence of ischemia (ST-segment changes) at rest?
4. Was maximal heart rate greater than 85% of predicted? If so, patient probably exerted maximal effort. If not, what factors limited exercise? Ventilation? Pain? Fatigue? Other?
5. Did the rhythm change with exercise? Increased or decreased PVCs? Was there evidence of ischemia (ST- or T-wave changes)?
6. Was BP normal at rest? If not, consider clinical correlation.
7. Did systolic BP increase appropriately? Did it exceed 250 mm Hg at maximal exercise?
8. Did diastolic BP remain constant or increase slightly? If not, consider clinical correlation.

---

multivessel coronary artery disease. ST-segment depression accompanied by exertional hypotension or marked increase in diastolic pressure is usually associated with significant coronary disease. The predictive value of ST-segment changes during exercise must be related to the patient's clinical history and risk factors for heart disease.

The most common arrhythmia that occurs during exercise testing is the premature ventricular contraction (PVC) (Figure 7-3). PVCs are associated with an increased incidence of myocardial ischemia and are considered dangerous because they may precede more serious, lethal arrhythmias. Exercise-induced PVCs occurring at a rate of more than 10 per minute are often found in ischemic heart disease. Increased PVCs during exercise may also be seen in mitral valve prolapse. Coupled PVCs (couplets) often precede ventricular tachycardia or ventricular fibrillation. Occurrence of couplets or frequent PVCs may be indications for terminating the exercise evaluation. Some patients with PVCs at rest or at low workloads may have these ectopic beats suppressed as exercise intensity increases. The most serious ventricular arrhythmias are sometimes seen in the immediate postexercise phase.

Shortness of breath (SOB) brought on by exertion is perhaps the most widespread indication for cardiopulmonary exercise evaluation. The combination of cardiovascular parameters (i.e., HR, SV) with data obtained from analysis of exhaled gas (i.e., $\dot{V}O_2$) permits assessment of dyspnea on exertion. Table 7-7 generalizes some of the basic relationships between cardiovascular and pulmonary exercise responses. These relationships help delineate whether exertional dyspnea is a result of cardiac or pulmonary disease, or whether the patient is simply deconditioned. In some instances, poor effort may mimic exertional dyspnea. Comparison of data from cardiovascular and exhaled gas variables can confirm inadequate patient effort.

BLOOD PRESSURE

Systemic BP may be monitored intermittently using the standard cuff method. Automated noninvasive cuff devices for monitoring BP are also available. Although these methods work well at rest and at low workloads, they may be difficult to implement during high levels of exercise. BP sounds may be difficult to detect because of treadmill noise or patient movement. It is important to monitor the pattern of BP response at low and moderate workloads to establish that both systolic and diastolic pressure respond as anticipated.

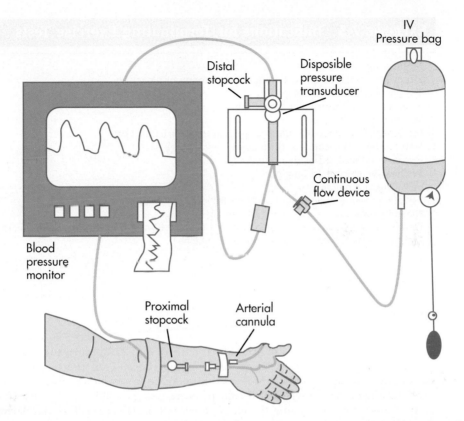

Figure 7-5 *Pressure transducer setup for continuous arterial monitoring.* A catheter is inserted into the radial or brachial artery. Pressure tubing connects the catheter to a continuous flow device that maintains a constant pressure (and a small flow of solution) against the arterial line to prevent backflow of blood into the system. The continuous flow device also allows flushing of the system. A pressure transducer assembly is connected in line with the tubing. Pressure changes in the system are transmitted via a thin membrane to the transducer. Blood samples may be drawn by inserting a heparinized syringe at a stopcock located near the indwelling catheter (blood pressure signal is temporarily lost during sampling). A similar assembly can be used for connection to a Swan-Ganz catheter for pulmonary artery monitoring during exercise.

Continuous monitoring of BP may be accomplished by connection of a pressure transducer to an indwelling arterial catheter (Figure 7-5). An indwelling line allows continuous display and recording of systolic, diastolic, and mean arterial pressures. In addition, the catheter provides ready access for arterial blood sampling. Arterial catheterization may be easily accomplished using either the radial or the brachial site. The catheter must be adequately secured to prevent loss of patency during vigorous exercise. Insertion of arterial catheters presents some risk of blood splashing or spills. Adequate protection for the individual inserting the catheter, as well as for those withdrawing specimens, is essential. See Chapter 11 for specific recommendations regarding arterial sampling via catheters.

Systolic BP increases in healthy patients during exercise from 120 mm Hg up to approximately 200 to 250 mm Hg (Figure 7-4). Diastolic pressure normally rises only slightly (10 to 15 mm Hg) or not at all. The mean arterial pressure rises from approximately 90 mm Hg to approximately 110 mm Hg, depending on the changes in systolic and diastolic pressures. Increased CO, particularly the SV, causes the increase in systolic pressure almost completely.

EXERCISE 7-3   Indications for Terminating Exercise Tests

Monitoring system failure
2-mm horizontal or down-sloping ST depression or elevation
T-wave inversion or Q waves
Sustained supraventricular tachycardia
Ventricular tachycardia
Increasing frequency of *multifocal* premature ventricular beats
Development of second- or third-degree heart block
Exercise-induced left or right *bundle branch block*
Progressive chest pain (angina)
Sweating and *pallor*
Systolic pressure greater than 250 mm Hg
Diastolic pressure greater than 120 mm Hg
Failure of systolic pressure to increase or a drop of 10 mm Hg with increasing workload
Lightheadedness, mental confusion, or headache
Cyanosis
Nausea or vomiting
Muscle cramping

Even though CO may increase fivefold, (e.g., from 5 to 25 L/min), the systolic pressure only increases twofold. Systolic pressure only doubles because of the tremendous decrease in peripheral vascular resistance. Most of this decrease in resistance results from vasodilatation in exercising muscles. Increased systolic pressure (>250 to 300 mm Hg) should be considered an indication for terminating the exercise evaluation (Exercise 7-3). Similarly, if the systolic pressure fails to rise with increasing workload, the CO is not increasing appropriately. The exercise test should be terminated and the patient's condition stabilized. Variations in BP during exercise are often caused by the patient's respiratory effort. Phasic changes with respiration are particularly common in patients who develop large transpulmonary pressures because of lung disease. Differences of as much as 30 mm Hg between inspiration and expiration may be seen during continuous monitoring of arterial pressure.

In maximal tests (i.e., the patient reaches HR_{max}), it may be impossible to obtain a reliable BP at peak exercise. Even with an arterial catheter, motion artifact may prevent recording of a usable tracing. Systolic pressure may transiently drop and diastolic pressure may drop to zero at the termination of exercise. To minimize the degree of hypotension resulting from abrupt cessation of heavy exercise, the patient should "cool down." This is accomplished easily by having the patient continue exercising at a low work rate until BP and HR have stabilized at or slightly above baseline levels.

◼ SAFETY

Safe and effective exercise testing for cardiopulmonary disorders requires careful pretest evaluation to identify contraindications to the test procedure (Exercise 7-4). A preliminary workup should include a complete history and physical examination by the referring physician or the physician performing the stress test. Preliminary laboratory tests should include a 12-lead ECG, chest x-ray study, baseline pulmonary function studies before and after bronchodilator therapy, and routine laboratory examinations such as complete blood count and serum electrolytes. Patients who take methylxanthine bronchodilators should have a recent

EXERCISE 7-4   Contraindications to Exercise Testing*

Recent (within 4 weeks) myocardial infarction
Unstable angina pectoris
Second- or third-degree heart block
Rapid ventricular/atrial arrhythmias
Orthopedic impairment
Severe *aortic stenosis*
Congestive heart failure
Uncontrolled hypertension
Limiting neurologic disorders
Dissecting/ventricular *aneurysms*
Severe pulmonary hypertension
Thrombophlebitis or intracardiac *thrombi*
Recent systemic or pulmonary embolus
Acute *pericarditis*
Pao_2 less than 40 mm Hg on room air
$Paco_2$ greater than 70 mm Hg
FEV_1 less than 30% of predicted

*These conditions represent *relative* contraindications to exercise testing; the risk to the patient must be evaluated on a case-by-case basis.

theophylline level measurement, particularly if the primary indication for exercise testing is ventilatory limitation.

The risks and benefits of the entire exercise procedure should be explained to the patient. Appropriate informed consent should be obtained. This includes an explanation of any alternate tests that might be done, and what the consequences of not performing the stress test might be. A physician experienced in exercise testing should supervise the test. Tests may be performed by qualified practitioners on patients younger than 40 years of age with no known risk factors provided a physician is immediately available. Criteria for terminating the exercise evaluation before the specified end point or symptom limitation occurs are listed in Exercise 7-4.

After termination of the exercise evaluation for whatever reason, the patient should be monitored until HR, BP, and ECG return to pretest levels. ECG monitoring should continue for at least 5 minutes (as recommended by the American College of Sports Medicine). Tracings should be made at frequent intervals immediately after exercise.

Personnel conducting exercise tests should be trained in handling cardiovascular emergencies and all aspects of cardiopulmonary resuscitation (ACLS). The laboratory should have available resuscitation equipment, including the following:

1. Standard intravenous (IV) medications (e.g., epinephrine, atropine, lidocaine, etc.)
2. Syringes, needles, IV infusion apparatus
3. Portable O_2 and suction equipment
4. Airway equipment, endotracheal tubes, and laryngoscope
5. DC defibrillator and appropriate monitor

All emergency equipment should be checked daily or immediately before any cardiopulmonary exercise evaluation. Equipment such as defibrillators, laryngoscopes, and suction apparatus should be routinely evaluated for proper function according to institutional policies.

Ventilation During Exercise

Collection and analysis of expired gas during cardiopulmonary exercise testing provides a noninvasive means of obtaining the following variables:

- Minute ventilation ($\dot{V}_E$)
- Tidal volume (V_T)
- Frequency of breathing; respiratory rate (f_b)
- Oxygen consumption; oxygen uptake ($\dot{V}o_2$)
- Carbon dioxide production ($\dot{V}co_2$)
- Respiratory exchange ratio (RER)
- Ventilatory equivalent for oxygen ($\dot{V}_E/\dot{V}o_2$)
- Ventilatory equivalent for CO_2 ($\dot{V}_E/\dot{V}co_2$)

■ EQUIPMENT SELECTION AND CALIBRATION

The two common methods of exhaled gas analysis use either a mixing chamber (Figure 7-6) or computerized breath-by-breath measurements (Figure 7-7). Pneumotachometers are used in both mixing chamber and breath-by-breath systems and should be calibrated using a

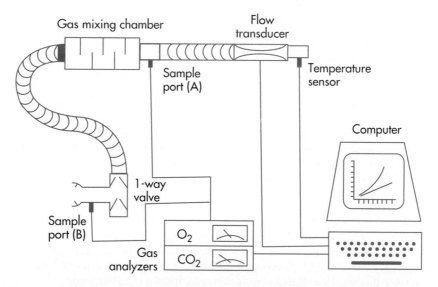

Figure 7-6 *Mixing chamber system for analysis of expired gas.* The patient inspires room air through a one-way valve and expires through large-bore tubing into a mixing chamber with a volume of approximately 5 L. Baffles in the chamber cause the gas to be thoroughly mixed so that it is representative of mixed expired gas. A small volume is extracted at *sample port A* and directed to the O_2 and CO_2 analyzers for determination of F_EO_2 and F_ECO_2. Expired gas then passes through a flow-sensing device (pneumotachometer) from which volume can be obtained by integration. A temperature probe at the flow transducer provides data for conversion of gas volume from ambient temperature to BTPS and STPD. Signals from the gas analyzers, flow transducer, and temperature sensor are recorded directly on an analog recorder or converted to digital signals for computer processing. Analysis of individual breaths of expired gas can be obtained by sampling at *port B*. This technique allows determination of respiratory rate and end-tidal CO_2 and O_2 concentrations. The mixing chamber system can be used for exercise protocols as well as for resting metabolic measurements.

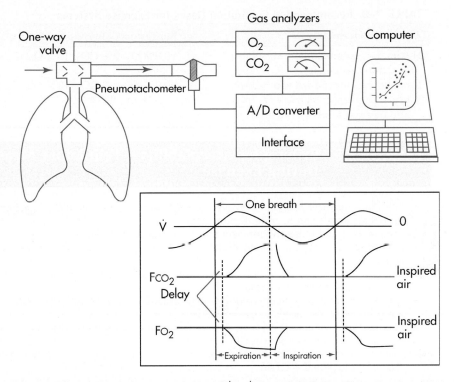

Figure 7-7 *Breath-by-breath system for determination of $\dot{V}O_2$, $\dot{V}CO_2$, and ventilation.* The patient inspires and expires through a pneumotachometer or similar flow-sensing device, which may or may not require the use of a unidirectional value. Gas is continuously sampled at the patient's mouth to determine fractional concentrations of O_2 and CO_2. The flow signal and signals from the gas analyzers are integrated to measure volume, F_EO_2, and F_ECO_2, and to calculate $\dot{V}_E$, $\dot{V}O_2$, $\dot{V}CO_2$, rate, and V_T. Computerization is required to perform calculations and corrections. Simultaneous recording of flow ($\dot{V}$) and fractional concentrations of O_2 and CO_2 are shown (*insert*). During expiration, FCO_2 increases and FO_2 decreases. Gas concentrations and flow are out of phase because of the time required to transport gas from the mouthpiece to the analyzers and the response time of the analyzers themselves. Storing appropriate phase-delay corrections (determined during calibration) in the computer can align signals. Ventilatory and gas-exchange parameters can be monitored and displayed on a breath-by-breath basis. For exercise tests or metabolic measurements, breath-by-breath data are averaged over a short interval (10 to 60 seconds) or specific number of breaths.

known volume (3-L syringe) or flow signal (Exercise 7-5). The flow sensor's accuracy should comply with the criteria set by the American Thoracic Society (ATS) for flow-measuring devices (e.g., ±3% or 50 ml, whichever is greater). Validation of a flow-measuring device can be performed by connecting it in series with a volume-based spirometer of known accuracy. Gas analyzers should also be calibrated and checked before each test procedure. Two-point calibration using gases that approximate the physiologic range to be tested provide the most appropriate means of ensuring accuracy. Three-point calibration is necessary to check the linearity of the analyzers. Table 7-6 lists some recommended gas concentrations for calibration of analyzers to be used for exercise tests.

If a gas collection valve (see Chapter 10) is used in the breathing circuit, it should have a low resistance (1 to 2 cm H_2O at 100 L/min) and a small dead space. In healthy adults, a valve dead space of 100 ml is acceptable. A valve with reduced dead space (25 to 50 ml) may be more appropriate for children or for patients who have dead space–producing disease or very

TABLE 7-6 Recommended Calibration Gases for Exercise Systems

Type of Exercise Test	Suggested Calibration Gases
Maximal or submaximal with subject breathing room air	20.9% O_2, 0% CO_2; 15% O_2, 5% CO_2
Maximal or submaximal with subject breathing supplementary O_2 (may also be used to check linearly)	20.9% O_2, 0% CO_2; 15% O_2, 5% CO_2; 26% O_2, 0% CO_2

EXERCISE 7-5   Criteria for Acceptability—Ventilatory Measurements During Exercise

1. Volume transducer calibration before exercise measurements should be performed according to ATS standards and kept for documentation.
2. Temperature and other environment factors should be recorded.
3. Breathing valve resistance and dead space should be appropriate for the patient tested if applicable.
4. Ventilatory variables should be measured over intervals appropriate for the type of exercise (incremental versus steady state).
5. Recent FEV_1 and MVV maneuvers should be available for interpretive purposes. The quality of the spirometry also needs to be considered.
6. Maximal flow-volume (F-V) loop should be measured before exercise, if exercise F-V or tidal volume loops are to be measured.
7. Inspiratory capacity (IC) should be accurately measured in order to plot exercise flows in relation to maximal F-V loop.

small tidal volumes. Some breath-by-breath systems can be programmed to reject small breaths (less than 100 ml). If this feature is used, the volume of rejected breaths should be matched to valve dead space. Breaths that do not clear valve dead space should be discarded. If valve dead space is too large for the patient, significant rebreathing may occur. In breath-by-breath exercise systems, this may show up as an expired CO_2 level that does not decrease to zero during inspiration. Many modern exercise systems have small flow sensors that do not require a valve system, so dead space and valve resistance become less critical.

If a mixing chamber is used, the patient should be allowed to breathe through the circuit with a nose clip in place long enough to wash out room air with expired gas. The exact washout volume, or time, depends on the volume of the mixing chamber. Breath-by-breath systems (Figure 7-7) normally require minimal washout because fractional gas concentrations are sampled directly at the mouthpiece. If supplemental O_2 is breathed, the inspiratory portion of the breathing circuit as well as the patient's lungs should be in equilibrium before gas sampling starts.

Depending on the protocol and equipment used, gas collection and analysis are performed over a specified interval during each exercise level. For steady-state protocols, gas collection is usually performed after 4 to 6 minutes at a constant workload. For incremental protocols, sampling may be performed during the last minute of each stage. In breath-by-breath systems, sampling is done continuously, with data being displayed for each breath. Breath-by-breath data may also be averaged over several breaths.

In gas collection or mixing chamber systems, raw data collected includes the following:

1. *Volume* expired, in liters
2. *Temperature* of gas at the measuring device (°C)

Patients who have lung disease may be limited by their ventilatory capacity during exercise. The maximal voluntary ventilation (MVV) is often used as an index of ventilatory capacity during exercise. Healthy patients typically use less than 70% of their MVV during maximal exertion. Patients with lung disease often have a reduced MVV and may reach or exceed 80% of their MVV during maximal exercise. In terms of absolute volumes, if the maximal ventilation during exercise is within 10 to 15 L/min of the patient's MVV, a ventilatory limitation to exercise is probably present. Some individuals may have flow limitation even though their ventilation is less than their MVV.

3. *Time* of collection, seconds or minutes
4. *Respiratory rate* during the collection interval
5. Fraction of mixed expired O_2 (Feo_2)
6. Fraction of mixed expired CO_2 ($Feco_2$)

These data can be recorded manually or by a multichannel recorder with appropriate analog signals. In most modern systems, the data are gathered into a computer by means of an analog-to-digital (A/D) converter (see Chapter 10). Computerized data reduction offers the advantage of immediate feedback for all measurements. Automated data collection also offers greater flexibility for using different exercise protocols (Table 7-1). Breath-by-breath gas analysis requires that signals from the flow sensor be integrated with the gas analyzer signals for Feo_2 and $Feco_2$. The phase delay between volume and gas concentration signals must be considered (Figure 7-7). This is done by measuring phase delay time (for each gas analyzer) during calibration. The phase delay is then stored, and subsequent measurements use this factor to align the volume and gas signals. Sampling flow or sample lines should not be altered after calibration because phase delay values may change. Water or particulate contamination of the gas analyzer sample line or damage to the sample line can also affect phase delay. Alterations of the phase delay can have a profound effect on the accuracy of the data (up to 30% error in the calculated $\dot{V}o_2$), especially at higher respiratory rates.

MINUTE VENTILATION

$\dot{V}_E$ is the volume of gas expired per minute by the exercising patient, expressed in liters, BTPS. For an exercise system in which gas is collected, $\dot{V}_E$ may be calculated as follows:

$$\dot{V}_E = \frac{\text{Volume expired} \times 60}{\text{Collection time (sec)}} \times \text{BTPS factor}$$

Sample calculations and BTPS factors are contained in Appendix F. Modern breath-by-breath systems measure the volume of each breath and continuously compute the minute ventilation.

Healthy adults at rest breathe 5 to 10 L/min. During exercise, this value may increase to more than 200 L/min in trained patients. It commonly exceeds 100 L/min in healthy adults (Figures 7-8 and 7-9). The increase in ventilation removes CO_2, the primary product of exercising muscles, as workload increases. Ventilation increases linearly with an increasing workload (i.e., $\dot{V}o_2$) at low and moderate levels of exercise. In healthy patients, this increase in ventilation during exercise follows the rise in $\dot{V}co_2$. As higher levels of work are achieved (greater than approximately 60% of $\dot{V}o_{2max}$), metabolic demand exceeds the capacity for energy production solely by aerobic pathways. To meet increasing energy demands, anaerobic

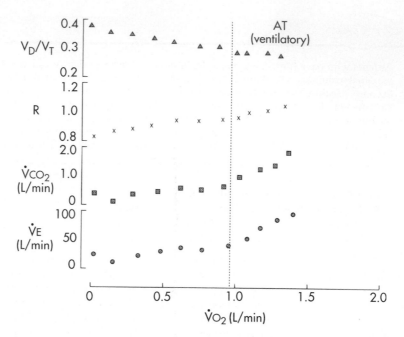

Figure 7-8 *Normal ventilation/gas exchange responses during exercise.* Four variables as they might appear in a healthy young adult are plotted against $\dot{V}O_2$. The *dotted vertical line* represents AT. $\dot{V}_E$ increases linearly with work rate at low and moderate workloads up to the AT, as does $\dot{V}CO_2$. At higher levels, $\dot{V}_E$ and $\dot{V}CO_2$ increase at a faster rate as HCO_3^- buffers lactic acid and as CO_2 is produced. The ratio of $\dot{V}CO_2$ to $\dot{V}O_2$ (RER) follows a similar pattern as RER approaches, and then exceeds 1. V_D/V_T initially decreases rapidly as V_T increases; it then continues to decrease but at a slower rate (*see text*).

glycolysis assumes an increasing role (Kreb's cycle). The main product of these reactions is lactate. As blood lactate rises, buffering occurs via the carbonic acid (H_2CO_3) pathway. The result is an increase in total $\dot{V}CO_2$. In healthy patients, ventilation increases further to remove CO_2 produced by the buffering of lactic acid.

   Relating the $\dot{V}_{E\ max}$ to resting ventilatory function provides an index of ventilatory limitations to exercise. MVV (see Chapter 2) can be related to the $\dot{V}_E$ achieved at the highest workload attained ($\dot{V}_{E\ max}$). Ventilatory capacity (sometimes called ventilatory ceiling) is defined by the measured MVV or the $FEV_1 \times 35$ (some clinicians prefer $FEV_1 \times 40$). The difference between $\dot{V}_{E\ max}$ and ventilatory capacity is often called *the ventilatory* (or *breathing*) *reserve* (Figure 7-10). Ventilatory reserve is calculated as follows:

$$\text{Ventilatory reserve} = \left[1 - \left(\frac{\dot{V}_{E max}}{MVV}\right)\right] \times 100$$

where:
$\dot{V}_{E\ max}$ = ventilation at highest exercise level reached, liters/minute
MVV   = maximal voluntary ventilation, liters/minute

   The ventilatory reserve is usually expressed as a percentage but can also be denoted as the actual difference. In healthy patients, the ventilatory reserve is typically 20% to 40%.

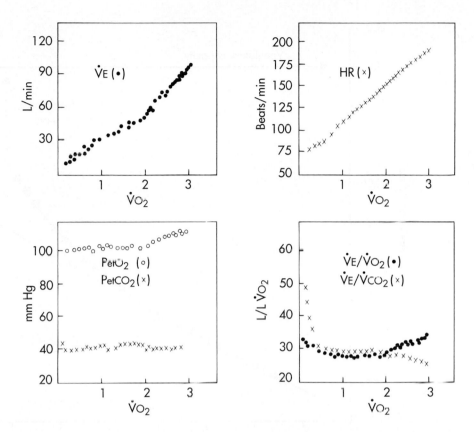

Figure 7-9 *Breath-by breath exercise data.* Four plots of data obtained using a breath-by-breath technique, as in Figure 7-7. Although data are recorded for each breath, the plots represent 30-second averages. All parameters are plotted against $\dot{V}O_2$ as the measure of work being performed. $\dot{V}_E$ increases linearly up to approximately 2 L/min $\dot{V}O_2$; HR increases linearly throughout the test. $PetO_2$ and $PetCO_2$ (end tidal partial pressures of O_2 and CO_2, respectively) remain relatively constant up to approximately 2 L/min $\dot{V}O_2$. At this point, end tidal O_2 begins to increase and end-tidal CO_2 begins to decrease. A similar pattern is seen on the plot of ventilatory equivalents for oxygen and carbon dioxide ($\dot{V}_E/\dot{V}O_2$ and $\dot{V}_E/\dot{V}CO_2$, respectively). A primary advantage of breath-by-breath analysis is that plots may be viewed in "real time," thus allowing modification of the testing protocol as required. Data in this example indicate the occurrence of ventilatory AT at approximately 2 L/min of $\dot{V}O_2$.

In patients with pulmonary disease, the reserve is less than 20% and/or the absolute difference between MVV and $\dot{V}_{E\ max}$ is less than 10 to 15 L. This latter relationship is important in individuals with a disease process that affects their ability to perform an MVV (i.e., those who have a low or abnormal MVV). In some cases, the abnormally low MVV can yield a $\dot{V}_{E\ max}$/MVV ratio that is in the normal range, but the actual difference is reduced (Table 7-7). A valid MVV maneuver is essential in order to compare exercise ventilation with MVV. Patients who have airway obstruction may actually achieve $\dot{V}_E$ during exercise that equals or exceeds their ventilatory capacity. In both scenarios, exercise is limited by their inability to further increase ventilation and they are therefore identified as being ventilatory limited.

At high levels of ventilation in healthy patients (greater than 120 L/min), increases in O_2 uptake gained by increased ventilation serve mainly to supply O_2 to the respiratory muscles.

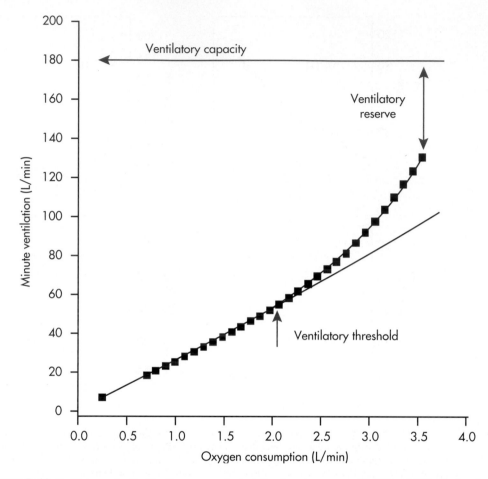

Figure 7-10 *Ventilatory capacity.* Ventilatory capacity is defined as the measured MVV or MVV calculated from $FEV_1 \times 35$ or 40. The difference between the $\dot{V}_{E\ max}$ (highest level of ventilation achieved during exercise) and the ventilatory capacity is termed the *ventilatory reserve* or *breathing reserve.*

The same phenomenon may occur at much lower levels of ventilation in patients with severe lung disease because of the increased work of breathing. Because of the ventilatory reserve in healthy patients, exercise is seldom limited by ventilation. Maximal exercise is normally limited by inability to further increase cardiac output, or inability to extract more O_2 at the tissue level in exercising muscles. Some highly trained athletes may achieve ventilatory limitation. Aerobic training can improve cardiovascular function so that ventilation, not cardiac output, limits maximal work.

■ TIDAL VOLUME AND RESPIRATORY RATE

V_T during exercise may be calculated by dividing $\dot{V}_E$ by f_b. Breath-by-breath systems record individual breaths and then report an average V_T over a short interval, or after a fixed number of breaths have been analyzed. Observation of the breathing kinetics or breathing strategy of a patient during exercise can be an important adjunct in interpretation of the exercise results.

TABLE 7-7   Exercise Variables and Dyspnea*

	Cardiac	Ventilatory	Deconditioned	Poor Effort
$\dot{V}O_{2max}$	Less than 80% of predicted	Less than 80% of predicted	Less than 80% of predicted	Less than 80% of predicted
$\dot{V}_{Emax}$	Less than 70% of MVV	Greater than 90% or MVV-$\dot{V}_{Emax}$ less than 15 L	Less than 70% of MVV	Variable
Anaerobic threshold	Achieved at low $\dot{V}O_2$	Usually not achieved	Achieved at low $\dot{V}O_2$	Not achieved
HR	Greater than 85% of predicted	Less than 85% of predicted	Greater than 85% of predicted	Less than 85% of predicted
ECG/signs of ischemia	ST changes, arrhythmias, chest pain	Usually normal	Normal	Normal
Sao_2	Greater than 90%	Often less than 90%, hypoxemia	Greater than 90%	Greater than 90%

*This table compares the usual findings for the exercise variables listed in subjects with dyspnea caused by cardiac disease, pulmonary disease, or deconditioning. Some subjects may have dyspnea because of a combination of causes. Poor effort during exercise may result from improper instruction, lack of understanding by the subject, or lack of motivation by the subject.

MVV, Maximal voluntary ventilation; *Sao₂*, arterial oxygen saturation.

The normal response to exercise is to increase the V_T at low and moderate workloads. Increased V_T accounts for most of the rise in ventilation at these workloads; only a small amount results from increased f_b. This pattern continues until the V_T approaches approximately 50% to 60% of vital capacity (VC). Further increases in total ventilation are accomplished by increasing f_b. These kinetic changes can be important in a patient complaining of SOB with normal lung function. A high-frequency, low-tidal volume breathing strategy will result in an increased V_D/V_T. More important, however, it may be the only physiologic reason for the patient's perceived SOB. Likewise, a patient using a large V_T and low f_b may also complain of SOB without a physiologic abnormality.

In healthy individuals, the increase in V_T is accomplished both by utilizing the inspiratory reserve volume (IRV) and by reducing the end-expiratory lung volume (EELV) (Figure 7-11, left panel). This allows efficient use of the respiratory muscles and chest wall pump. In patients with chronic airflow limitation, inability to increase ventilation may be related to dynamic compression of the airways and dynamic hyperinflation (i.e., increased lung volume) that can occur during exertion. These patients have large resting lung volumes (hyperinflation). During exercise, EELV tends to increase even more as the patient attempts to optimize expiratory flow to meet ventilatory demands. The dynamic shift in lung volume places the respiratory muscles at an even greater disadvantage. The sensation of dyspnea increases tremendously, and the patient is unable to continue exercise. The consequence for these patients is an increase in the work of breathing from both flow limitation and breathing at higher lung volumes (Figure 7-11, right panel). Patients who have airway obstruction may also be able to increase their $\dot{V}_E$ but cannot attain predicted values (Exercise 7-6). If VC is markedly reduced by the obstructive process, there may be little reserve to accommodate an increased V_T. Obstructed patients who have a normal VC but increased resistance to flow may increase

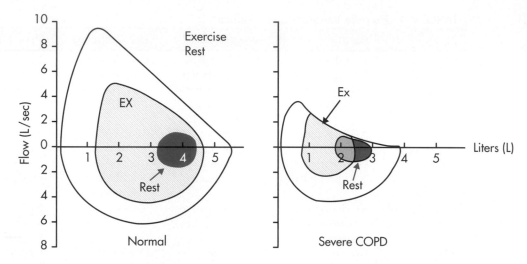

Figure 7-11 *Flow-volume loop kinetics.* Normal F-V loop kinetics are shown with recruitment of exercise tidal breathing from both the IRV and the ERV, and not touching the resting maximal F-V curve (MFVC) (*left*). Breathing kinetics of a patient with severe COPD are also shown (*right*). The patient has to move up in absolute lung volumes in order to recruit tidal volume. This, along with the fact that they are flow-limited throughout much of the tidal breath, increases the work of breathing.

their V_T at a low f_b during exercise in an effort to minimize the work of breathing. This pattern continues until the V_T reaches a plateau, as described previously. Then the f_b must be augmented to further increase $\dot{V}_E$. Because of flow limitation, particularly during the expiratory phase, increases in f_b must be accomplished by shortening the inspiratory portion of each breath. Reduction of the inspiratory time in relation to the total breath time (T_i/T_{tot}) requires the inspiratory muscles to generate increasingly greater flows. The increased load placed on the muscles of inspiration typically results in dyspnea.

EXERCISE 7-6   Interpretive Strategies—Ventilatory Measurements During Exercise

1 Were data collected over an interval appropriate to the type of exercise test?
2 Was resting ventilation within normal limits ($\approx$ 5 to 10 L/min)? If not, why?
3 Did minute ventilation increase appropriately with workload?
4 Was $\dot{V}_{Emax}$ less than 70% of MVV or $FEV_1 \times 35 - 40$? Was the absolute difference >10 to 15 L/min? If so, some ventilatory reserve is present. If not, ventilatory limitation to exercise is likely.
5 Were breathing kinetics appropriate? Did V_T increase to approximately 50% to 60% of VC? If not, why? Was increased respiratory rate primarily responsible for increased $\dot{V}_E$? If so, suspect a restrictive ventilatory pattern or inappropriate breathing kinetics.
6 Was there flow limitation evidenced by the tidal breathing superimposed on the maximal flow-volume curve? If so, to what extent?
7 Were changes in V_T consistent with an appropriate breathing strategy?
8 What reason did the patient offer for stopping exercise (if applicable)? Was this finding consistent with the pattern of ventilation observed?

Unlike the pattern in obstruction, in restrictive disease V_T may remain relatively fixed. Increases in $\dot{V}_E$ during exercise are accomplished primarily by rapid respiratory rates. It is usually more efficient for patients who have "stiff" lungs to move small tidal volumes at fast rates to increase ventilation. However, these tidal volumes may still comprise a relatively large portion of their vital capacity (60% to 70%). Flow-volume (F-V) loop profiles may be close to normal, whereas the work of distending the lung is increased in restrictive patterns. The mechanism of increasing ventilation primarily by increasing respiratory rate places a load on the respiratory muscles. In combination with hypoxemia, this increased load often results in extreme SOB.

■ FLOW-VOLUME LOOP ANALYSIS

Another method of determining the degree of ventilatory limitation is by monitoring F-V loop dynamics during exercise. Exercise tidal-volume loops may be plotted against the resting maximal F-V loop. This technique quantifies the amount of time the patient spends on the maximal flow-volume envelope and allows the clinician to identify the percent of flow limitation (Figure 7-12). This method may better define the increased work of breathing in individuals who do not reach a classic definition of ventilatory limitation, but have a substantial component of flow limitation during exercise. Monitoring the tidal flow-volume loop during exercise

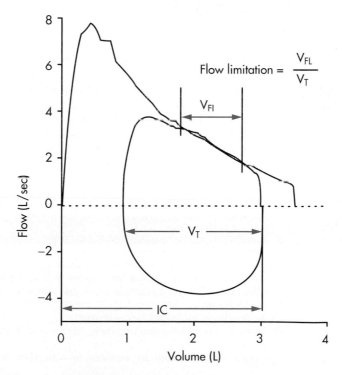

Figure 7-12 *Flow limitation during exercise.* Flow limitation can be quantified by plotting the exercise tidal breathing loop over the maximal F-V loop. The tidal loop is positioned by measuring the inspiratory capacity (IC) during exercise and positioning the end-expiratory level at an absolute lung volume equal to TLC − IC. Computer analysis can then quantify the percentage of time that the patient is breathing at or above maximal flow.

can also show dynamic changes in the flow pattern. These changes can alert the clinician to intrathoracic, extrathoracic, or fixed-airway abnormalities that are only demonstrated during exercise. This technique may also be useful in monitoring breathing kinetics during exercise. As discussed previously, the normal method of increasing tidal volume during exercise is to utilize both inspiratory and expiratory reserve volumes. Patients with obstructive lung disease have to "move up" in their lung volumes (Figure 7-11) in order to recruit tidal volume. In some cases, even individuals with normal lung function can use an inappropriate breathing strategy by moving up in their lung volumes to recruit tidal volume without evidence of flow limitation. Utilizing these inappropriate breathing strategies may cause a concomitant sensation of dyspnea. Some patients may breathe at very low lung volumes, which approach residual volume. Breathing at these low lung volumes can cause flow limitation secondary to the position of tidal breathing along the absolute lung volume scale. This breathing strategy can elicit wheezing and SOB that can mimic asthma, and has been coined a type of "pseudoasthma."

Oxygen Consumption, Carbon Dioxide Production, and Respiratory Exchange Ratio During Exercise

■ OXYGEN CONSUMPTION

$\dot{V}_{O_2}$ is the volume of O_2 taken up by the exercising (or resting) patient in liters, or milliliters/minute, STPD. Oxygen consumption is also commonly reported in milliliters/kilogram of body weight (ml/kg). $\dot{V}_{O_2}$ is the product of ventilation minute and the rate of extraction from the gas breathed (i.e., the difference between the F_IO_2 and the F_EO_2; see the following paragraph). Healthy patients at rest have a $\dot{V}_{O_2}$ of approximately 0.25 L/min (STPD), or approximately 3.5 ml O_2/min/kg (1 MET). During exercise, $\dot{V}_{O_2}$ may increase to over 4.0 L/min (STPD) in trained patients. $\dot{V}_{O_2}$ is the best single measure of external work being performed. Exercise limitation caused by ventilatory, gas exchange, or cardiovascular abnormalities may be quantified by relating exercise variables to $\dot{V}_{O_2}$. Figures 7-4 and 7-8

EXERCISE 7-7   Criterial for Acceptability—$\dot{V}_{O_2}$, $\dot{V}_{CO_2}$

1 There should be documentation of appropriate gas analyzer calibrations; 2-point calibration recommended for room air exercise, 3-point for exercise with supplemental oxygen.
2 Phase delay calibration (breath-by-breath systems) should be documented within manufacturer's specifications.
3 Volume transducer should be calibrated before testing.
4 Breathing valve (if used) should have appropriate resistance and dead space volume for patient tested.
5 There should be evidence of appropriate washout of collection device or mixing chamber (if used).
6 RER at rest should be within the physiologic range of 0.70 to 1.10; RER values greater than 1.0 may be present because of hyperventilation.
7 $\dot{V}_{O_2}$ and $\dot{V}_{CO_2}$ should be within normal limits with the patient at rest; each should increase with increasing workloads.

provide examples of ventilatory and cardiovascular variables related to $\dot{V}O_2$ in healthy patients. The causes of work limitation may be defined by comparing these patterns in the exercising patient. Exercise limitation may be a result of pulmonary disease, cardiovascular disease, muscular abnormalities, deconditioning, poor effort, or a combination of these factors.

To calculate $\dot{V}O_2$ and $\dot{V}CO_2$, the fractional concentrations of O_2 and CO_2 in expired gas must be analyzed (Exercise 7-7). Exhaled gas is sampled from a mixing chamber (Figure 7-6) or a breath-by-breath system (Figure 7-7). In systems that accumulate gas (e.g., mixing chamber), a pump is used to draw the sample through the O_2 and CO_2 analyzers. Water vapor is removed from the mixed expired sample by passing the gas through a drying tube (usually containing calcium chloride). In breath-by-breath systems, fractional gas concentrations are sampled at the mouth using rapid gas analyzers. Most systems use sample tubing that is permeable to water vapor, so that the effects of humidity can be accomodated (see Chapter 10). Gas concentration signals from the analyzers are integrated with the expiratory flow signal to measure the volumes of O_2 and CO_2 exchanged for each breath (Figure 7-7).

$\dot{V}O_2$ is calculated from an accumulated gas volume using the following equation:

$$\dot{V}O_2 = \left(\left[\frac{1 - F_EO_2 - F_ECO_2}{1 - F_IO_2} \times F_IO_2 \right] - F_EO_2 \right) \times \dot{V}_E(STPD)$$

where:

F_EO_2 = fraction of O_2 in the expired sample
F_ECO_2 = fraction of CO_2 in the expired sample
F_IO_2 = fraction of O_2 in inspired gas (room air − 0.2093)

The term

$$\left(\frac{1 - F_EO_2 - F_ECO_2}{1 - F_IO_2} \right)$$

is a factor to correct for the small differences between inspired and expired volumes when only expired volumes are measured. Ventilation is corrected to STPD as follows:

$$\dot{V}_E(STPD) = \dot{V}_E(BTPS) \times \left(\frac{P_B - 47}{760} \right) \times 0.881$$

O_2 consumption at the highest level of work attainable by normal patients is termed the $\dot{V}O_{2max}$. $\dot{V}O_{2max}$ is characterized by a plateau of the oxygen uptake despite increasing external workloads. $\dot{V}O_{2max}$ is useful for comparing exercise capacity between patients. $\dot{V}O_{2max}$ may also be used to compare a patient with his or her age-related predicted value of $\dot{V}O_{2max}$. Equations for deriving predicted $\dot{V}O_{2max}$ are included in Appendix B.

One measure of impairment is the percentage of expected $\dot{V}O_{2max}$ attained by the exercising patient. Height, gender, age, and fitness level all affect the "normal" maximal oxygen consumption. Because of these factors, most reference equations show a large variability (±20%). Patients who have a of 20% to 40% reduction in their $\dot{V}O_{2max}$ have mild to moderate impairment. Those who have $\dot{V}O_{2max}$ values less than 50% of their predicted values have severe exercise impairment. Some studies have attempted to estimate $\dot{V}O_2$ based on the height and weight of the patient and the speed and slope of a treadmill. O_2 consumption estimated from treadmill walking is sufficiently variable so that its use is limited. Power output from a calibrated cycle ergometer may be used to estimate $\dot{V}O_2$ more accurately than from treadmill exercise. Workload estimated from cycle ergometry is not influenced by weight or stride. Actual $\dot{V}_{O_2}$ may differ significantly from the estimated value even using an ergometer. Cycle ergometry usually produces slightly lower maximal $\dot{V}_{O_2}$ values than treadmill walking in healthy patients (see Exercise Protocols section).

■ CARBON DIOXIDE PRODUCTION

$\dot{V}_{CO_2}$ is a direct reflection of metabolism. It is expressed in liters or milliliters per minute, STPD. $\dot{V}_{CO_2}$ may be calculated using the following equation:

$$\dot{V}_{CO_2} = (F_E CO_2 - 0.0003) \times \dot{V}_E (STPD)$$

where:

$F_E CO_2$ = fraction of CO_2 in expired gas
0.0003 = fraction of CO_2 in room air (may vary)
$\dot{V}_E(STPD)$ = calculated as in the equation for $\dot{V}_{O_2}$

Pulmonary ventilation, consisting of alveolar ventilation ($\dot{V}_A$) and dead space ventilation ($\dot{V}_D$), may be related in terms of the $\dot{V}_{CO_2}$. The fraction of alveolar carbon dioxide ($F_A CO_2$) is directly proportional to $\dot{V}_{CO_2}$ and inversely proportional to $\dot{V}_A$. The concentration of CO_2 in the lung is determined by CO_2 production and the rate of removal from the lung by ventilation. This relationship may be expressed as follows:

$$F_A CO_2 = \frac{\dot{V}_{CO_2}}{\dot{V}_A}$$

$\dot{V}_{CO_2}$ in a healthy patient at rest is approximately 0.20 L/min (STPD). It may increase to more than 4 L/min (STPD) during maximal exercise in trained individuals. The adequacy of $\dot{V}_A$ in response to the increase in $\dot{V}_{CO_2}$ is indicated by how well Pa_{CO_2} is maintained near normal levels. Alveolar ventilation keeps Pa_{CO_2} in equilibrium with alveolar gas at low and moderate workloads. At high workloads, $\dot{V}_A$ increases dramatically to reduce Pa_{CO_2} when buffering of lactic acid takes place. At maximal workloads, even high levels of ventilation cannot keep pace with CO_2 produced metabolically and from lactate buffering. As a result, acidosis develops.

■ RESPIRATORY EXCHANGE RATIO

The respiratory exchange ratio (RER) is defined as the ratio of $\dot{V}_{CO_2}$ to $\dot{V}_{O_2}$ at the mouth. RER is calculated by dividing $\dot{V}_{CO_2}$ by $\dot{V}_{O_2}$; it is expressed as a fraction. In some circumstances, RER at rest is assumed to be equal to 0.8. For exercise evaluation or metabolic studies, however, the actual value is calculated. RER normally varies between 0.70 and 1.00 in resting patients, depending on the nutritional substrate being metabolized (see Chapter 9). RER reflects the respiratory quotient (RQ) at the cellular level only when the patient is in a true steady state. RER may differ significantly from RQ, depending on the patient's ventilation.

RER typically increases from a resting level of between 0.75 and 0.85 as work increases. When anaerobic metabolism (see next paragraph) begins to produce CO_2 from the buffering of lactate, $\dot{V}_{CO_2}$ approaches $\dot{V}_{O_2}$. As exercise continues, $\dot{V}_{CO_2}$ exceeds $\dot{V}_{O_2}$ and the RER becomes greater than 1. RER is commonly elevated at rest because many patients hyperventilate during exhaled gas analysis before exercise begins (Exercise 7-7). In steady-state exercise tests (i.e., 4 to 6 minutes at a constant workload), RER may equal RQ, and it then reflects the ratio of

$\dot{V}co_2/\dot{V}o_2$ at the cellular level. Under steady-state conditions, $\dot{V}co_2$ reflects the CO_2 produced metabolically at the cellular level.

The respiratory exchange ratio (RER) is a good indicator of maximal effort during a cardiopulmonary exercise test. Patients who exert maximal effort are usually able to exceed their anaerobic threshold (AT). During exercise, the RER increases; at the highest workloads, it exceeds 1.00. An RER value greater than 1.15 is usually consistent with a maximal effort. Patients with pulmonary disease are often limited by ventilation and may not reach an RER greater than 1.

ANAEROBIC OR VENTILATORY THRESHOLD

Measurement of and analysis of exhaled gases during exercise allows a noninvasive estimate of the *anaerobic threshold (AT)*. This threshold is also termed the *ventilatory threshold* when it is denoted by a change in ventilation and CO_2 production. The AT occurs when the energy demands of the exercising muscles exceed the body's ability to produce energy by aerobic metabolism. The workload at which AT occurs is considered an index of fitness in healthy patients. The AT is also used to assess cardiac performance in patients with heart disease.

Historically, anaerobic metabolism was detected by noting an increase in the blood lactate level of an exercising patient. Analysis of $\dot{V}_E$ and $\dot{V}co_2$ in relation to workload ($\dot{V}o_2$) can be used to detect the onset of anaerobic metabolism without drawing blood. This threshold is commonly referred to as the ventilatory threshold.

At low and moderate workloads, $\dot{V}_E$ increases linearly with increases in $\dot{V}co_2$. When the body's energy demands exceed the capacity of aerobic pathways, further increases in energy are produced anaerobically. The primary product of anaerobic metabolism is lactate. The increased lactic acid (from lactate) is buffered by HCO_3^-, resulting in an increase in CO_2 in the blood. $\dot{V}co_2$ measured from exhaled gas increases because CO_2 is being produced by both the exercising muscles and the buffering of lactate. To maintain the pH near normal, $\dot{V}_E$ increases to match the increased $\dot{V}co_2$. This pattern of increasing ventilation and CO_2 production can be detected when these parameters are plotted against $\dot{V}o_2$ (Figure 7-8). Determination of the ventilatory AT may be accomplished by visual inspection of an appropriate plot. Statistical analysis can also be used to determine the inflection point as displayed by the graph in Figure 7-13. Several different algorithms may be used to identify the ventilatory AT. One of the most common techniques uses regression analysis to determine the "breakpoint" at which $\dot{V}_E$ and $\dot{V}co_2$ change abruptly (V-slope method).

Noninvasive AT determination may be useful in assessing cardiovascular or pulmonary diseases (Exercise 7-8). In healthy patients, AT occurs at 60% to 70% of the $\dot{V}o_{2max}$. Patients who have cardiac disease often reach their AT at a lower workload ($\dot{V}o_2$). Early onset of anaerobic metabolism occurs when the demands of exercising muscles exceed the capacity of the heart to supply O_2. Occurrence of the anaerobic threshold at less than 40% of the $\dot{V}o_{2max}$ is considered abnormally low. Patients who have a ventilatory limitation to exercise (i.e., pulmonary disease) may be unable to exercise at a high enough workload to reach their anaerobic threshold. In these patients, O_2 delivery is limited by the lungs, rather than by cardiac output or extraction by the exercising muscle.

Aerobic training improves cardiac performance, specifically the stroke volume (SV). Training allows more O_2 to be delivered to the tissues, resulting in a delay in the AT until higher workloads are reached. Measurement of the AT is often used to select a training level

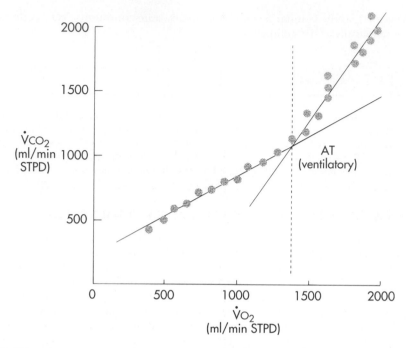

Figure 7-13 *V-slope determination of ventilatory AT.* By plotting $\dot{V}CO_2$ against $\dot{V}O_2$, an infection point can typically be identified, indicating an abrupt increase in CO_2 production. A more precise method fits two regression lines to the data gathered. One line is a best-fit line through the low and moderate workload portion of the data; the second is fit through the high workload points. These lines are recalculated repeatedly until the best statistical "fit" is obtained. The point at which the two lines intersect represents the onset of lactate production (anaerobic threshold).

EXERCISE 7-8   Interpretive Strategies—$\dot{V}O_2$, $\dot{V}CO_2$

1 Were the data obtained acceptably? Were all calibrations appropriate? Gas analyzers? Volume transducer? Phase delay?

2 Were appropriate reference values selected? Age? Sex? Height? Weight?

3 Was $\dot{V}O_{2max}$ (ml/kg) achieved? If so, there is no aerobic impairment.

4 Was $\dot{V}O_{2max}$ (ml/kg) less than 80% of predicted? If so, some aerobic impairment is present. Was $\dot{V}O_{2max}$ (ml/kg) less than 60% of predicted? If so, there is moderate to severe exercise limitation.

5 Was ventilatory AT reached? If so, at what % $\dot{V}O_{2max}$? If less than 50% to 60%, early onset of anaerobic metabolism is likely. Consider clinical correlation.

6 What factors contributed to the reduced $\dot{V}O_{2max}$?
   Cardiac (arrhythmias, ischemic changes)?
   Vascular (BP response)?
   Pulmonary (ventilation, hypoxemia, V_D/V_T)?
   Other (poor effort, deconditioning, pain, orthopedic problems)?

7 What reason did the patient cite for stopping exercise (incremental tests)? Is it consistent with physiologic patterns observed?

(e.g., exercise prescription). Maximum training effects seem to occur when the patient exercises at a workload slightly below the AT. In sedentary patients, deconditioning may occur. Deconditioning is characterized by reduced SV and poor O_2 extraction by the muscles from lack of use. Deconditioning may be present when the AT occurs at a lower than expected workload and there is no evidence of cardiovascular disease.

The AT may also be determined by inspecting graphs of the ventilatory equivalents for O_2 and CO_2 (see the next section) plotted against workload ($\dot{V}O_2$). When $\dot{V}_E/\dot{V}O_2$ increases without an increase in $\dot{V}_E/\dot{V}O_2$, the AT has been reached. A similar pattern can be seen when the end-tidal O_2 and CO_2 gas tensions are plotted (Figure 7-9).

Sample calculations of $\dot{V}_E$, $\dot{V}O_2$, $\dot{V}CO_2$, and RER, as used with one of the gas collection methods, are included in Appendix F.

VENTILATORY EQUIVALENT FOR OXYGEN

Minute ventilation during exercise may be related to the work being performed (expressed as $\dot{V}O_2$). This ratio is termed the *ventilatory equivalent for O_2*, or $\dot{V}_E/\dot{V}O_2$. It is calculated by dividing $\dot{V}_E$ (BTPS) by $\dot{V}O_2$ (STPD) and expressing the ratio in liters of ventilation/liters of O_2 consumed per minute. The $\dot{V}_E/\dot{V}O_2$ is a measure of the efficiency of the ventilatory pump at various workloads.

During resting data collection in healthy patients, the ratio is in the range of 30 to 40 L/L depending on the degree of ventilation, including anticipatory hyperventilation. As the patient begins to exercise, this ratio decreases to about 25 ± 4 (Figure 7-14). This initial kinetic change is assumed to be related to an improvement in $\dot{V}/\dot{Q}$ matching with increased cardiac output during exercise. At low and moderate workloads, ventilation increases linearly with increasing $\dot{V}O_2$ and $\dot{V}CO_2$. The absolute level of ventilation depends on the response to CO_2, the adequacy of $\dot{V}_A$, and the V_D/V_T ratio. At workloads above 60% to 75% of the $\dot{V}O_{2max}$, $\dot{V}_E$ is more closely related to $\dot{V}CO_2$. As ventilation increases to match the $\dot{V}CO_2$ above the AT, the ventilatory equivalent for O_2 also increases.

Ventilation helps determine how much O_2 can be transported per minute. Therefore, it is often useful to evaluate the level of total ventilation required for a particular workload to assess the role of the lungs in exercise limitations. In some pulmonary disease patterns, the $\dot{V}_E/\dot{V}O_2$ may be close to normal at rest but increases with exercise out of proportion to increases in either $\dot{V}O_2$ or $\dot{V}CO_2$. This usually occurs in individuals who have $\dot{V}/\dot{Q}$ abnormalities that worsen as cardiac output increases during exercise. Some patients who have pulmonary disease may have an elevated $\dot{V}_E/\dot{V}O_2$ at rest (i.e., greater than 40 L/L $\dot{V}O_2$) that decreases during exercise but does not return to the normal range. Many patients hyperventilate during the resting phase at the beginning of an exercise evaluation. The result is an increased $\dot{V}_E/\dot{V}O_2$ that usually returns to the normal range during exercise. This pretest hyperventilation is usually denoted by an RER of greater than 1 that returns to a normal level when the patient begins to exercise.

VENTILATORY EQUIVALENT FOR CARBON DIOXIDE

The ventilatory equivalent for CO_2 ($\dot{V}_E/\dot{V}CO_2$) is calculated in a manner similar to that used for the $\dot{V}_E/\dot{V}O_2$. Minute ventilation (BTPS) is divided by CO_2 production (STPD). The $\dot{V}_E/\dot{V}CO_2$ mimics the initial $\dot{V}_E/\dot{V}O_2$ kinetic change, decreasing to a normal range of 25 to 35 L/L $\dot{V}CO_2$. $\dot{V}_E$ tends to match $\dot{V}CO_2$ from low up to high workloads. Hence the $\dot{V}_E/\dot{V}CO_2$ remains constant in healthy patients until the highest workloads are reached. The $\dot{V}_E/\dot{V}CO_2$ may be useful for estimating the maximum tolerable workload in patients who have moderate or severe ventilatory limitations. The ventilatory equivalents for O_2 and CO_2, measured using a breath-by-breath technique, may be useful in identifying the onset of the AT. Anaerobic metabolism is usually

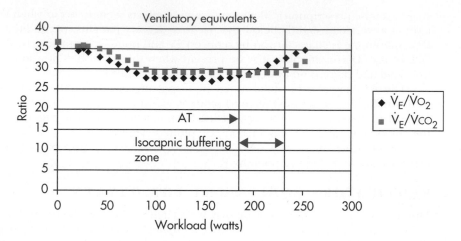

Figure 7–14 *Determination of ventilatory AT using ventilatory equivalents data.* The ventilatory threshold is defined as the point where the $\dot{V}_E/\dot{V}O_2$ begins to increase while the $\dot{V}_E/\dot{V}CO_2$ remains constant or begins to decrease. The period from the onset of AT until $\dot{V}_E/\dot{V}CO_2$ increases is the *isocapnic buffering zone.* Minute ventilation is appropriate for $\dot{V}CO_2$, which now exceeds $\dot{V}O_2$ because of acid buffering created by anaerobic metabolism ($H^+ + HCO_3^- \leftrightarrow H_2CO_3 \leftrightarrow H_2O + CO_2$).

accompanied by a steady increase in the $\dot{V}_E/\dot{V}O_2$ while the $\dot{V}_E/\dot{V}CO_2$ remains constant, or decreases slightly. The period in which $\dot{V}_E/\dot{V}O_2$ is increasing yet $\dot{V}_E/\dot{V}O_2$ is constant is called the *isocapnic buffering zone* (Figure 7-14). This zone indicates the onset of metabolic acidosis, where $\dot{V}_E$ is no longer proportional to $\dot{V}O_2$ but is appropriate for $\dot{V}CO_2$. Occurrence of this pattern coincides with the buffering of the lactate ($H^+ + HCO_3^- \leftrightarrow H_2CO_3 \leftrightarrow CO_2 + H_2O$). Eventually, the buffering system cannot keep pace with the metabolic acidemia, and the $\dot{V}_E/\dot{V}CO_2$ increases as attempts to maintain pH. This same pattern may also be seen on a breath-by-breath display of $PetO_2$ and $PetCO_2$ (Figure 7-9). A markedly elevated $\dot{V}_E/\dot{V}CO_2$ (>50) may also be observed in pulmonary hypertensive disease.

■ OXYGEN PULSE

The efficiency of the circulatory pump may be related to the workload (i.e., $\dot{V}O_2$) during exercise by the O_2 pulse. O_2 pulse is defined as the volume of O_2 consumed per heartbeat and is derived from the Fick Equation:

$$Cardiac\ output = \frac{\dot{V}O_2}{CaO_2 - C\bar{v}O_2}$$

$$HR \times SV = \frac{\dot{V}O_2}{CaO_2 - C\bar{v}O_2}$$

$$\frac{\dot{V}O_2}{HR}(O_2\ pulse) = SV \times (CaO_2 - C\bar{v}O_2)$$

O_2 pulse is sometimes called the "poor man's" estimate of stroke volume because of the relatively small change in the $CaO_2-C\bar{v}O_2$ difference with exercise. The ratio is expressed as milliliters of O_2 per heartbeat. In healthy patients, O_2 pulse varies between 2.5 and 4.0 ml O_2/beats at rest. It increases to 10 to 15 ml O_2/beats during strenuous exercise.

In patients with cardiac disease, the O_2 pulse may be normal or even low at rest but does not increase to expected levels during exercise. This pattern is consistent with an inappropriately high HR for a particular level of work. Cardiac output normally increases linearly with increasing exercise (Figure 7-4). A low O_2 pulse is consistent with an inability to increase the SV because of the relationship noted above. O_2 pulse may even decrease in patients with poor left ventricular function. The pattern of low O_2 pulse with increasing work rate may be seen in patients with coronary artery disease or valvular insufficiency, but it is most pronounced in cardiomyopathy. Tachycardia or tachyarrythmias tend to lower the O_2 pulse because of the abnormally elevated heart rate. Conversely, β-blocking agents, which tend to reduce HR, may elevate the O_2 pulse.

O_2 pulse is often used as an index of fitness. At similar power outputs, a fit patient will have a higher O_2 pulse than one who is deconditioned. Fitness is generally accompanied by a lower HR, both at rest and at maximal workloads. Lower HR occurs because conditioning exercises (e.g., aerobic training) tend to increase SV. As a result, the heart beats less frequently but produces the same CO. Trained patients can thus achieve higher work rates before reaching their limiting cardiac frequency (i.e., attain a higher O_2 pulse).

Exercise Blood Gases

■ ARTERIAL CATHETERIZATION

Although invasive, blood gas sampling during exercise testing is often indicated in patients with primary pulmonary disorders. An indwelling arterial catheter permits analysis of blood gas tensions (PaO_2, $PaCO_2$), saturation (SaO_2), O_2 content (CaO_2), pH, and lactate levels at various workloads. Table 7-8 lists some of the indications for arterial catheterization for exercise testing.

Arterial catheterization, at either the radial or the brachial site, has been demonstrated to be relatively safe. The modified Allen's test is performed to ascertain adequate collateral circulation (see Chapter 6). The site is cleaned with povidone-iodine or similar disinfectant. Local anesthetic (1% to 2% Xylocaine [lidocaine]) is injected subcutaneously. An appropriate-size catheter is inserted percutaneously. The catheter needs to be secured in order to prevent being dislodged during the exercise study. The catheter is then connected to a high-pressure flush system to maintain patency. Care must be taken when drawing blood samples from the catheter not to contaminate the specimen with flush solution (Exercise 7-9). If flush solution mixes with the specimen, dilution occurs and can affect pH, PCO_2, PO_2, and hemoglobin (Hb) values.

TABLE 7-8 Indications for Arterial Catheterization with Exercise Testing

Moderate or severe pulmonary disease
Clinical suspicion of a gas exchange abnormality
Low diffusion capacity for carbon monoxide (less than 50% predicted)
Low or borderline PaO_2 at rest (55 to 60 mm Hg)
Multiple blood specimens required (blood gases, lactate)
Titration of supplemental O_2

EXERCISE 7-9   Criteria for Acceptability—Exercise Blood Gases

1 Blood gases should be drawn from either a radial or a brachial catheter. Care should be taken that specimens are not contaminated with flush solution.

2 Exercise blood gas specimens should be handled like any other sample for blood gas analysis, according to the National Committee for Clinical Laboratory Standards (NCCLS) publication C46-A, *Blood Gas and pH Analysis and Related Measurements.*

3 Specimens from multiple exercise levels should be labeled to indicate the exercise workload and related conditions.

4 Blood obtained by a single arterial puncture at peak exercise should be obtained within 15 seconds of the observed maximal workload.

5 If pulse oximetry is used to evaluate exercise desaturation, it should be validated by correlation with co-oximetry, preferably at rest and peak exercise.

6 If pulse oximetry is used to titrate supplemental O_2 administration and SpO_2 does not increase, an arterial blood specimen may be required.

The catheter may also be connected to a suitable pressure transducer (Figure 7-5) for continuous monitoring of systemic BP. The BP transducer should be balanced ("zeroed") at the level of the left ventricle during exercise. See Chapter 11 for precautions concerning insertion of arterial catheters.

ARTERIAL PUNCTURE

An alternate technique is to obtain a specimen by a simple arterial puncture at peak exercise. Use of a cycle ergometer for testing allows better stabilization of the radial or brachial artery sites. The site should be identified and the modified Allen's test performed before beginning exercise. The sample should be obtained within 15 seconds of peak exercise. Blood gas tensions, particularly PaO_2, may change rapidly as blood recirculates. A serious disadvantage of the single puncture is that if the specimen cannot be obtained within 15 seconds, the procedure must be repeated. If any of the conditions listed in Table 7-8 are present, arterial catheterization should be considered.

PULSE OXIMETRY

Oxygen saturation during exercise may be monitored using a pulse oximeter (SpO_2) using the ear, finger, or forehead sites (see Chapter 10). Wherever the pulse oximeter is attached, the probe should be adequately secured. Motion artifact is a common problem, particularly with treadmill exercise.

An advantage of pulse oximetry is that it provides continuous measurements of saturation, compared with discrete measurements of arterial sampling. Continuous measurements can be very helpful in evaluating patients who have pulmonary disease. These patients often display rapid changes in PaO_2 and SaO_2 during exercise. A decrease of 4% to 5% in SaO_2 is indicative of exercise desaturation, even if some other factor (e.g., ventilation, arrhythmia) limits exercise.

Pulse oximetry may overestimate the true saturation if a significant concentration of COHb is present (Exercise 7-9). A low total Hb level (i.e., anemia) sometimes contributes to exercise limitation. This condition may not be detected by pulse oximetry alone. Inadequate perfusion at the site of the probe (e.g., ear or finger) may also cause erroneous readings during exercise testing. Motion artifact, light scattering within the tissue at the probe site, and dark skin pigmentation may all cause discrepancies between SpO_2 and actual SaO_2 (see Chapter 6). A single arterial sample, preferably at peak exercise, may be used to correlate the SpO_2 reading with true saturation if the specimen is analyzed with a multiwavelength blood oximeter (see Chapter 10). If adequate correlation between SaO_2 and SpO_2 during exercise is established, further blood sampling may be unnecessary.

■ Pao_2 DURING EXERCISE

In healthy patients, PaO_2 remains relatively constant even at high workloads (Exercise 7-10). Alveolar PO_2 increases at maximal exercise from the increased ventilation accompanying the increase in $\dot{V}CO_2$. The alveolar-arterial (A-a) gradient (normally approximately 10 mm Hg) widens as a result of the increase in alveolar oxygen tension. The A-a gradient also increases somewhat because of a lower mixed venous O_2 content during exercise. The A-a gradient may increase to 20 to 30 mm Hg in healthy patients during heavy exercise because of these mechanisms.

A decrease in PaO_2 with increasing exercise can result from increased right-to-left shunting. Similarly, inequality of $\dot{V}_A$ in relation to pulmonary capillary perfusion may result in reduced PaO_2. Diffusion limitation at the alveolocapillary interface can also affect PaO_2. Because exercise reduces the mixed venous oxygen tension ($P\bar{v}O_2$), a shunt or $\dot{V}/\dot{Q}$ inequality may result in a decrease in the PaO_2 or widening of the A-a gradient. This change in PaO_2 may occur without an absolute change in the magnitude of the shunt. Mixed venous blood with a lowered O_2 content (from extraction by the exercising muscles) passes through abnormal lung units and then mixes with normally arterialized blood.

In some patients who have decreased PaO_2 and increased $P(A-a)O_2$ at rest, oxygenation may improve with exercise. Increased cardiac output or redistribution of ventilation during exercise may actually cause an increase in PaO_2. Some improvement of PaO_2 may occur as a result of an increased PaO_2 caused by a reduction of $PaCO_2$ at moderate to high work rates.

EXERCISE 7-10   Interpretive Strategies—Exercise Blood Gases

1. Were blood gas samples obtained acceptably? No dilution or contamination with flush solution or air?
2. Were blood gas samples obtained at each exercise level or just at peak exercise? If drawn by arterial puncture at peak exercise only, were they obtained within 15 seconds?
3. Did PaO_2 decrease with increasing workloads? Did the A-a gradient increase to greater than 30 mm Hg? If so, exercise desaturation is likely.
4. Did PaO_2 decrease to less than 55 mm Hg or SaO_2 decrease to less than 85%? If so, supplemental O_2 is indicated. Retesting on O_2 may be indicated.
5. Did $PaCO_2$ remain constant or decrease slightly with increasing workloads? If not, respiratory acidosis may be contributing to work limitation.
6. Did pH decrease to the range of 7.20 to 7.35 (or lower) at the highest workload? If so, metabolic acidosis is present; the patient made a good effort. If not, did ventilation limit work below the anaerobic threshold?
7. Was V_D/V_T normal at rest? Did it decrease with increasing workloads? If not, suspect pulmonary hypertension, pulmonary vascular disease, or inappropriate breathing strategy.
8. Are blood gas test results consistent with observed changes in ventilatory and cardiovascular variables during exercise?

Improved $\dot{V}/\dot{Q}$ relationships resulting directly from the changes in ventilation or cardiac output may also improve Pao_2. Because Pao_2 may either increase or decrease during exercise, measuring Pao_2 during exercise may be particularly valuable in patients with pulmonary disorders.

When Pao_2 decreases to less than 55 mm Hg or Sao_2 decreases to less than 85%, the exercise evaluation should be terminated. Patients with hypoxemia at rest or who desaturate at very low work rates should be tested with supplemental O_2 (e.g., a nasal cannula) to determine an appropriate exercise O_2 prescription. Different flows of supplemental O_2 may be required at rest and for various levels of exertion. Correlation of Pao_2 while breathing supplemental O_2 at different exercise workloads allows precise titration of therapy to the patient's needs. Measurement of $\dot{V}o_2$ while the patient breathes supplemental O_2 presents special problems. A closed system in which the patient breathes from a reservoir containing blended gas is usually required.

Reported in some elite athletes at very high levels of work (e.g., 400 to 500 watts or 9 mph/18% grade) is a widening of the A-a gradient with Pao_2 values falling into the range of 50 to 60 mm Hg. This phenomenon is thought to be related to the time constants of blood in the lung with very high cardiac outputs and high oxygen extraction at the cellular level.

▌ $Paco_2$ DURING EXERCISE

In healthy patients, $Paco_2$ remains relatively constant at low and moderate work rates (Exercise 7-10). $\dot{V}_A$ increases to match the increase in $\dot{V}co_2$. End-tidal CO_2 increases at submaximal workloads, indicating that less ventilation is "wasted" (V_D/V_T decreases). At workloads in excess of 50% to 60% of the $\dot{V}o_{2max}$, metabolic acidosis from anaerobic metabolism stimulates an increase in $\dot{V}_E$. This occurs in response to the augmented $\dot{V}co_2$ from the buffering of lactic acid as noted previously. Ventilation thus increases in excess of that required to keep $Paco_2$ constant. A progressive decrease in $Paco_2$ results, causing respiratory compensation for the acidosis associated with anaerobic metabolism (Figures 7-8 and 7-9). $Petco_2$ decreases along with $Paco_2$ at high work rates.

PF Tips

The V_D/V_T ratio is often measured during cardiopulmonary exercise testing. This ratio is usually about 0.3 at rest and should decrease with exercise in healthy subjects. V_D/V_T can be estimated noninvasively with a breath-by-breath metabolic measurement system. These systems use the end-tidal pco_2 ($Petco_2$) along with mixed expired CO_2 to calculate the ratio. In patients with pulmonary disease, $Petco_2$ may not accurately reflect the arterial pco_2 ($Paco_2$). For such patients, arterial blood gases drawn during exercise may be required to accurately assess the V_D/V_T ratio.

Some individuals who have airway obstruction can increase $\dot{V}_A$ to maintain a normal $Paco_2$ at low workloads. At higher workloads, however, they may be unable to reduce $Paco_2$ to compensate for the metabolic acidosis. In many patients with airway obstruction, maximal exercise is limited by lack of ventilatory reserve. These individuals typically do not reach the AT. Ventilatory limitation prevents them from attaining a workload high enough to induce anaerobic metabolism. In patients with severe airflow obstruction, $\dot{V}_A$ may be unable to match any increment in $\dot{V}co_2$, resulting in hypercapnia and respiratory acidosis. Increased work of breathing and reduced sensitivity to CO_2, combined with the increased $\dot{V}co_2$ of exercise, allow $Paco_2$ to increase.

ACID-BASE STATUS DURING EXERCISE

The pH, like $Paco_2$, is regulated by the $\dot{V}_A$ at low work rates. $\dot{V}_A$ increases in proportion to $\dot{V}co_2$ up to the ventilatory AT. At work rates above AT, proportional increases in ventilation maintain the pH at near-normal levels. Most of the buffering of lactic acid is provided by HCO_3^- and a decrease in $Paco_2$. At the highest work rates (above 80% of the $\dot{V}o_{2max}$), pH decreases despite hyperventilation because compensation for lactic acidosis becomes incomplete. In the presence of airway obstruction, ventilatory limitations may prevent compensation above the anaerobic threshold, with the development of significant respiratory acidosis. However, patients who have moderate or severe obstruction generally cannot exercise up to a level that elicits anaerobic metabolism. Increased $Paco_2$ (respiratory acidosis) may be the primary cause of acidosis in these patients.

EXERCISE VARIABLES CALCULATED FROM BLOOD GASES

Arterial blood gases drawn during exercise allow several other parameters of gas exchange to be determined (Exercise 7-10). These include physiologic dead space, alveolar ventilation, and the V_D/V_T ratio.

Calculation of V_D, $\dot{V}_A$, and V_D/V_T requires measurement of $Paco_2$. V_D may be calculated using the following equation:

$$V_D = \left(V_T \times \left[1 - \frac{F_Eco_2 \times (P_B - 47)}{Paco_2} \right] \right) - V_{Dsys}$$

where:

V_T = tidal volume, liters (BTPS)
F_Eco_2 = fraction of expired CO_2
$P_B - 47$ = dry barometric pressure
$Paco_2$ = arterial CO_2 tension
V_{Dsys} = dead space of one-way breathing valve, liters

When V_D has been determined, $\dot{V}_A$ can be calculated using the following equation:

$$\dot{V}_A = \dot{V}_E - (f_b \times V_D)$$

where:

$\dot{V}_E$ = minute ventilation (BTPS)
f_b = respiratory rate (breaths/minute)
V_D = respiratory dead space (BTPS)

V_D/V_T ratio may be calculated as the quotient of the V_D (as just determined) and the V_T, averaged from the $\dot{V}_E$ divided by f_b. Alternately, V_D/V_T may be derived simply from the difference between arterial and mixed expired CO_2 at each exercise level:

$$V_D / V_T = \frac{(Paco_2 - P_{\bar{E}}co_2)}{Paco_2}$$

where:

$P_{\bar{E}}co_2$ = partial pressure of CO_2 in expired gas

Most breath-by-breath systems calculate V_D/V_T noninvasively by substituting end-tidal CO_2 for $Paco_2$. This method assumes that $Petco_2$ and $Paco_2$ are equal. This may not be the case at higher workloads and in patients who have pulmonary disease.

V_D, comprised of anatomic and alveolar dead space, is the part of $\dot{V}_E$ that does not participate in gas exchange. V_D/V_T expresses the relationship between "wasted" and tidal ventilation for the average breath. The healthy adult at rest has a $\dot{V}_A$ of 4 to 7 L/min (BTPS) and a V_D/V_T ratio of approximately 0.20 to 0.35. The absolute volume of dead space increases during exercise in conjunction with increased $\dot{V}_E$. Because of increases in V_T and increased perfusion of well-ventilated lung units (e.g., at the apices), the V_D/V_T ratio decreases. This pattern is expected in healthy patients (Figure 7-8). V_D/V_T increases with age, but the kinetic change with exercise remains the same. V_D/V_T may decrease in mild or moderate pulmonary disease states as well. In severe airway obstruction or in pulmonary vascular disease, V_D/V_T remains fixed or may even increase. An increase in V_D/V_T with exertion indicates ventilation increasing in excess of perfusion. This pattern is often associated with pulmonary hypertension. The vascular "space" is fixed in pulmonary hypertension; additional lung units cannot be recruited to handle the increased CO during exercise. V_D/V_T may also be elevated in individuals who use inappropriate breathing strategies. Small tidal volumes and high respiratory rates to recruit $\dot{V}_E$ in an otherwise normal patient can yield falsely high ratios. Coaching a patient to increase tidal volume and utilize a more normal breathing pattern can alleviate a falsely elevated V_D/V_T ratio.

$\dot{V}_A$ during exercise in healthy patients increases more than $\dot{V}_E$ as V_D/V_T decreases. In patients whose V_D/V_T ratio remains fixed or increases, adequacy of $\dot{V}_A$ must be assessed in terms of $Paco_2$ and not simply by the magnitude of $\dot{V}_E$.

Cardiac Output During Exercise

There are several methods for calculating cardiac output (CO) during exercise. Noninvasive methods include CO_2 rebreathing, soluble gas, and Doppler (ultrasound) techniques. Invasive methods measure CO by the direct Fick method or by thermal dilution. The invasive methods require placement of a pulmonary artery catheter (Swan-Ganz) (Exercise 7-11).

EXERCISE 7-11   Criteria for Acceptability—Cardiac Output During Exercise

1 If a noninvasive technique (e.g., soluble gas, CO_2 rebreathing) was used, were the laboratory's quality standards for the test satisfied?
2 For the Fick cardiac output method, the pulmonary artery catheter must be properly placed. The distal port should be located in a pulmonary arteriole and must not be in the "wedge" position. For thermodilution, the catheter must also be properly placed; the proximal (injection) port must be in the right atrium with the thermistor in a pulmonary arteriole.
3 For Fick measurements, arterial and mixed venous blood should be drawn simultaneously over 15 to 30 seconds (or longer). Care should be taken to avoid dilution with flush solution; dilution can markedly alter content calculations and hence cardiac output.
4 Oxygen consumption should be measured over the same interval as blood sampling for the Fick method.
5 Thermodilution measurements should be performed according to the manufacture's recommendations, particularly in regard to temperature of injectate and rate of injection.
6 Two or more acceptable measurements should be averaged if possible; multiple measurements may not be practical during exercise.

Noninvasive Cardiac Output Techniques

The CO_2 rebreathing technique (also termed the *indirect Fick method*) utilizes the Fick equation for carbon dioxide:

$$\dot{Q}_T = \frac{\dot{V}CO_2}{C\bar{v}CO_2 - CaCO_2}$$

where:

$\dot{Q}_T$ = cardiac output (CO), L/min
$\dot{V}CO_2$ = CO_2 production calculated from exhaled gases
$CaCO_2$ = arterial CO_2 content, calculated from $PaCO_2$
$C\bar{v}CO_2$ = mixed venous CO_2 content, calculated from alveolar PCO_2 after rebreathing to allow equilibrium of alveolar gas with mixed venous blood

The acetylene technique, also known as the soluble gas technique, can be performed using either closed-circuit or open-circuit methods. This method depends on the rate of uptake of a soluble gas (e.g., acetylene) that has a very low diffusion coefficient. The rate of uptake is directly proportional to the pulmonary blood flow. As long as there is no intracardiac or pulmonary shunt, pulmonary blood flow equals cardiac output. Both of these breathing techniques correlate well with invasive techniques in normal patients but have limited use in patients with maldistribution of ventilation.

Instrumentation using Doppler technology to estimate CO works on the principle of measuring flow with an ultrasound signal directed at the arch of the aorta. A measurement of the diameter of the aorta is also made using echocardiography. These two measurements allow for the determination of cardiac output (i.e., flow × cross-sectional area = total output). This method works well at rest and at low levels of exercise using a cycle ergometer, but motion artifact and increasing tidal volumes limit its usefulness at higher workloads.

Direct Fick Method

The direct Fick method is based on measurement of O_2 consumption and arterial-venous content difference for O_2:

$$\dot{Q}_T = \frac{\dot{V}O_2}{C(a-\bar{v})O_2} \times 100$$

where:

$\dot{Q}_T$ = cardiac output (CO), L/min
$\dot{V}O_2$ = oxygen consumption, L/min (STPD)
$C(a-\bar{v})O_2$ = arterial-mixed venous O_2 content difference, ml/dl
100 = factor to correct $C(a-\bar{v})O_2$ to liters (content differences are normally reported in vol% or milliliters/deciliter)

$\dot{V}O_2$ is measured using one of the methods described previously. $C(a-\bar{v})O_2$ is obtained by measuring or calculating oxygen content in both arterial and mixed venous blood (see Chapter 6). Arterial and mixed venous blood specimens should be drawn simultaneously during the last 15 to 30 seconds of each exercise level. Oxygen consumption averaged over the same interval should be used for the calculation.

Thermodilution Method

Most pulmonary artery (Swan-Ganz) catheters include circuitry for measurement of CO by thermodilution. A sensitive thermistor is placed near the tip of the catheter. A chilled saline solution (usually 10° to 20° C) is injected through a catheter port that is located in the right atrium. The thermistor senses the change in temperature as the solution is pumped through the right ventricle and into the pulmonary artery. The computer then integrates the change in temperature and the time required for the change to occur, and CO is calculated.

The thermodilution method is commonly used in critical care settings. It can also be used during exercise testing. Multiple measurements (2 to 4) should be made at each exercise level and the results averaged. Some automated systems allow other cardiopulmonary variables (e.g., ejection fraction) to be calculated as well.

▆ CARDIAC OUTPUT DURING EXERCISE

Cardiac output in healthy adults is approximately 4 to 6 L/min at rest. During exercise, it may increase to 25 to 35 L/min (Exercise 7-12). CO is the product of HR and SV:

$$\dot{Q}_T = HR \times SV$$

where:
$\dot{Q}_T$ = cardiac output (CO), liters or milliliters
HR = heart rate, beats/minute
SV = stroke volume, liters or milliliters

In healthy upright adults, SV is approximately 70 to 100 ml at rest. SV may be slightly higher if the patient is supine or semirecumbent because of increased venous return from the lower extremities. SV increases to 100 to 140 ml with low or moderate exercise. HR increases almost linearly with increasing work rate as described earlier, so at low workloads an increase in CO is caused by a combination of HR and SV. At moderate and high workloads, further increases in CO result mainly from increased HR. Derivation of SV (dividing $\dot{Q}_T$ by HR) is useful for quantifying poor cardiac performance in patients with coronary artery disease, cardiomyopathy, or other diseases that affect myocardial contractility.

Patients who are able to reach their predicted $\dot{V}o_{2max}$ and their predicted HR_{max} typically have normal CO and SV. A patient who has a reduced $\dot{V}o_{2max}$ but achieves maximal predicted HR often has low CO because of low SV. Limited CO with increasing workload is often accompanied by early onset of anaerobic metabolism (anaerobic or ventilatory threshold). Reduced CO may be seen in both atrial and ventricular arrhythmias, valvular insufficiency, and cardiomyopathies.

EXERCISE 7-12   Interpretive Strategies—Cardiac Output During Exercise

1 Were cardiac output measurements acceptable by laboratory standards? If a pulmonary artery catheter was used, were the measurements reproducible within 10% (as applicable)? If not, interpret cautiously.
2 Did cardiac output increase appropriately with increasing workloads? If not, consider cardiomyopathy, myocardial hypokinesis, valvular insufficiency, and other outflow tract abnormalities.
3 Was stroke volume normal at rest? Did it increase at low and medium workloads?
4 Was there evidence of ischemic changes or arrhythmias (on ECG) that might explain reduced cardiac output?
5 Was cardiac output compromised by increased systemic or pulmonary vascular resistance?
6 If cardiac output was not available, did the O_2 pulse (surrogate for SV) increase appropriately with exercise?

In fit patients, SV is increased both at rest and during exercise. Endurance (aerobic) training normally results in increased SV. Other benefits of aerobic training include reductions in systolic BP and ventilation. Fit patients typically have a lower resting HR than their sedentary counterparts. Because HR (i.e., cardiac output) is the factor that limits exercise in most individuals, fit patients reach a higher $\dot{V}o_{2max}$. Depending on the frequency, intensity, and duration of training, fit individuals are able to maintain a higher level or work for longer periods because of improved CO.

SYMPTOMS SCALES

The measurement of RPE (or Borg scale) and other symptom scales can be essential for connecting subjective symptoms and the physiologic responses to exercise. Rating scales, when they are discordant, can assist the physician in counseling the patient. There are two versions of the RPE scale, often referred as the Borg and Modified-Borg scales (Table 7-9). These scales are usually printed on a card or poster that the patient can see and/or point to during exercise testing. The scales should be reviewed with the patient before exercise begins. This is particularly important if exhaled gas is being collected because the patient may have a mouthpiece in place. The patient should be able to indicate his or her level of exertion even without vocalizing. General symptom scales can be adapted to any chief complaint the patient may be vocalizing by simply using a 0-to-4 scale and grading intensity from "nothing at all" to "severe." A patient complaining of lightheadedness or chest tightness can then alert the testing staff to his or her level of discomfort during the test using hand signals.

QUALITY OF TEST

Quality assurance and quality control of instrumentation is discussed in detail in Chapter 11. However, the complexity of cardiopulmonary exercise testing warrants consideration of a quality system approach to testing. The National Committee for Clinical Laboratory

TABLE 7-9 Ratings of Perceived Exertion (Borg) Scales

Perceived Exertion Scale		Modified Perceived Exertion Scale	
6		0	Nothing at all
7	Very, very light	0.5	Very, very slight (just noticeable)
8		1	Very slight
9	Very light	2	Slight
10		3	Moderate
11	Fairly light	4	Somewhat moderate
12		5	Severe
13	Somewhat hard	6	
14		7	Very severe
15	Hard	8	
16		9	Very, very severe (almost maximal)
17	Very hard	10	Maximal
18			
19	Very, very hard		
20			

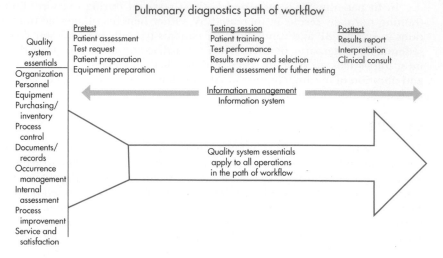

Figure 7-15 *Pulmonary diagnostics path of workflow.*

Standards (NCCLS) has published *A Quality System Model for Health Care.* This document champions the approach that a quality model has to address the continuum of patient care, and incorporates the concept of a path of workflow process (Figure 7-15). This concept integrates pretest, test, posttest, and information management with all processes that can affect any section across the path of workflow. Pretest processes include patient assessment, test request, patient preparation, and equipment preparation. Patient assessment, as it relates to cardiopulmonary exercise testing, might include laboratory results, current medications affecting exercise performance (e.g., β-blockers, digitalis, etc.), or orthopedic issues that may affect ergometer selection. Each quality system essential is applied to all operations in the path of workflow, which in turn allows for complete quality analysis of all processes.

■ INTERPRETATION STRATEGIES

In order to interpret a study appropriately, the clinician first needs to assess the degree of effort and determine whether the test is a maximal study (Table 7-10). Once the test has been qualified as maximal or submaximal, an algorithmic approach to data review and interpretation is essential (see Interpretive Strategies—boxed material, this chapter).

The following scheme can assist in a stepwise approach to data analysis:

- Determine maximal study
- Cardiovascular response (Exercises 7-2 and 7-11)
  - ECG, BP, CO, O_2, pulse, and symptoms
- Ventilatory response (Exercise 7-6)
  - Ventilatory reserve, breathing kinetics
- Gas exchange (Exercise 7-10)
  - A-a gradient, V_D/V_T, $Paco_2$

- Metabolic and oxygen uptake (Exercise 7-8)
  - Anaerobic/ventilatory threshold, lactate, $\dot{V}O_{2max}$, $\dot{V}O_2/kg$
- Impression

TABLE 7-10 Determining Maximal Effort

***	Heart rate	>85% to 90% of predicted
***	End exercise	50% to 80% $\dot{V}_E$ of MVV or $FEV_1 \times 40$; MVV $- \dot{V}_{Emax} \leq 15$ L
**	SaO_2	<80%
*	Metabolic work	RER >1.10 or lactate >7
*	Clinical investigator	Opinion of effort or early termination criteria met

* = Weight of variable.
Once a single criterion is met, test is graded a maximal effort.

Summary

This chapter examines the measurement of cardiopulmonary variables during exercise. Various protocols for assessing exercise responses are described, including treadmill and cycle ergometry methods, as well as the 6-minute walk. Monitoring of the cardiovascular system with a special concern for patient safety is discussed. Techniques for measuring ventilation, oxygen consumption, carbon dioxide production, and the associated variables during exercise are delineated. The measurement of breathing kinetics and flow volume analysis during exercise are described. Special emphasis is given to criteria for acceptability and interpretive strategies for the various measurements described. Assessment of blood gases and cardiac output is also discussed. Case studies and self-assessment questions on the topic of cardiopulmonary exercise testing are included.

CASE STUDIES

CASE 7-1

HISTORY

The patient is a 54-year-old man complaining of dyspnea on exertion. Several months ago, he had an initial episode of SOB, which has worsened during the past 2 months. He has a 15 to 20 pack-year smoking history. He works as a foreman for a utility company and does not have any related environmental exposures. His laboratory results were all normal. His echocardiogram, chest x-ray, and CT scan of the chest were also normal. His spirometry results are as follows:

PULMONARY FUNCTION TESTS

Personal Data

Sex: Male
Age: 54 yr
Height: 69.3 in (176 cm)
Weight: 195 lb (88.4 kg; BMI 28.6)

Spirometry

	Predicted		Control	
	Normal	Range	Found	%Pred
VC	4.73	>3.89	5.12	108
FVC	4.73	>3.89	5.03	106
FEV$_1$	3.74	>3.06	4.19	112
FEV$_1$/FVC	79.1	>69.9	83.3	
FEF$_{25\%-75\%}$	3.4	>1.9	4.0	119
FEF$_{max}$	8.7	>5.2	9.0	104
MVV	148	>115	141	95

TECHNOLOGIST'S COMMENTS

Spirometry testing was performed meeting criteria for acceptability and reproducibility.

QUESTIONS

1. What is the interpretation of the spirometry results?

TABLE 7-11 Exercise Test—Case 7-1

		Rest	AT	Max	Pred Max	%Pred Max
Exercise						
Workload	watts		160	180		
Time	min:sec	4:40	8:56	10:50		
$\dot{V}O_2$	L/min	0.167	1.938	2.108	2.424	87
$\dot{V}O_2$/kg	ml/kg	1.9	21.9	23.9		
R		0.80	1.07	1.13		
Cardiac function						
Heart rate	beats/min	78	139	156	175	89
Blood pressure (direct)	mm Hg	145/90	235/110	235/110		
Oxygen pulse	ml/beat	2.1	13.9	13.5		
Ventilation						
Minute ventilation	L/min	6.7	56.0	69.3	141.0	49
Respiratory rate	per min	14	20	23		
Tidal volume	ml, BTPS	498	2803	2975		
Tidal volume/FVC	%	10	56	59		
Vent equiv for O_2	$\dot{V}_E$/VO$_2$	40.5	29.2	32.8		
Blood gases						
Arterial pH		7.42		7.37		
Arterial PCO_2	mm Hg	38		39		
Arterial PO_2	mm Hg	82		98		
Arterial O_2 sat	%	98		96		
Arterial bicarbonate	mEq/L	24.0		22.0		
(A-a) gradient O_2	mm Hg	16.3		11.1		
P(ET-a) CO_2	mm Hg	−1.9		6.3		
V_D/V_T	%	55		2.4		
Arterial lactate	mM/L	0.7		4.9		

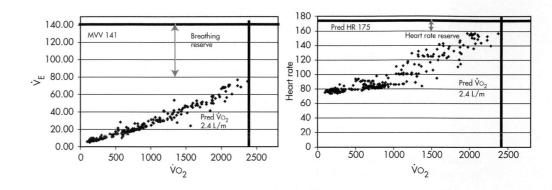

Spirom [content obscured]

Diffusin [content obscured]

TECHI [content obscured]

Spirome [content obscured]

QUEST [content obscured]

1. Wha [content obscured]

2. What is the interpretation of:

- Cardiovascular response?
- Ventilation during exercise?
- Gas exchange during exercise?
- Oxygen consumption and ventilatory threshold during exercise?
- Impression?

3. Discussion of the patient's exercise response.
4. What treatment might be recommended based on these findings?

DISCUSSION

Interpretation (Pulmonary Function)

Normal spirometry.

Interpretation (Exercise)

The patient exercised on a cycle ergometer to a maximum workload of 180 watts using a 20-watt incremental protocol. He terminated the test complaining of SOB and leg fatigue. This appears to be a near-maximal study based on heart rate criterion.

Cardiovascular Response: Heart increased from 78 to 156 beats/min. Electrocardiogram showed normal sinus rhythm at rest with rare PVCs with exercise. There is no evidence of ischemic changes. Blood pressure shows exercise-induced hypertension.

Ventilatory Response: There was a normal ventilatory reserve with normal breathing kinetics. Tidal volume increased to 59% of FVC.

Gas Exchange: Arterial blood gases were normal at rest and at exercise. The V_D/V_T ratio decreased appropriately with exercise. Maximal oxygen consumption and ventilatory threshold were within normal limits.

Impression: Normal study with the exception of exercised-induced hypertension.

Discussion of Patient's Exercise Response

The testing staff selected an incremental protocol of 20 watts/min, based on what appeared to be a normal patient with a predicted $\dot{V}O_{2max}$ of 2.424 L (increment based on $\dot{V}O_2 = 2400 - 300/100 = 21$). The test was determined to be a near-maximal study based on a heart rate response of 89% of predicted, a large ventilatory reserve, and a lactate level of 4.9 mM/L.

C
His bl
this te
increa
V
resulti
tidal v
G
being
ing fr
remai
increa
O

Treati

The p
prescri

CAS

HIST

A 69-y
dyspne
curren
primar
is norn

PULM

Persor

Sex:
Age:
Height
Weight

Lung

TLC
VC
RV
RV/T
FRC

*Outsi
†Bronc

CASE 7-3

HISTORY

The patient is a 53-year-old office worker who was referred for evaluation of SOB. She has a 44 pack-year history of smoking and continued to smoke up to the time of her test. She has a morning cough that produces 50 to 100 ml/day of thick white sputum. Her chest x-ray shows increased vascular markings and mild hyperinflation. She was taking no medications at the time of this test. No familial history of lung disease or cancer was found, and she had no unusual environmental exposure.

PULMONARY FUNCTION TESTS

Personal Data

Sex: Female
Age: 53 yr
Height: 65 in
Weight: 131 lb

Spirometry

	Predicted	Control	%Pred	Postdilator	%Change
FVC	3.35	3.24	97	3.34	100
FEV_1 (L)	2.53	1.49	59	1.56	62
$FEV_{1\%}$ (%)	75	46	—	47	—
$FEF_{25\%-75\%}$ (L/sec)	2.86	0.79	27	1.19	42
$\dot{V}_{max50}$ (L/sec)	4.24	1.99	47	2.25	53
$\dot{V}_{max50}$ (L/sec)	1.86	0.68	37	0.99	53
MVV (L/min)	97.9	52	53	55	56
Raw (cm H_2O/L/sec)	0.6-2.4	2.22		2.1	—
SGaw (L/sec/cm H_2O/L)	0.14-0.58	0.12		0.13	—

Lung Volumes (by Plethysmograph)

	Predicted	Control	%Pred
VC (L)	3.35	3.27	98
IC (L)	2.31	1.80	78
ERV (L)	1.04	0.99	95
FRC (L)	2.88	3.54	123
RV (L)	1.84	2.55	136
TLC (L)	5.20	5.82	112
RV/TLC (%)	35	44	—

Diffusing Capacity (Single-Breath)

	Predicted	Control	%Pred
DL_{CO} (ml CO/min/mm Hg)	20	8.8	44
DL_{CO} (adj)	20	10.3	51
$\dot{V}_A$ (L)	—	5.67	—
DL/V_A	3.85	1.55	—

Blood Gases (F$_{IO_2}$ 0.21)

pH	7.38
Pa$_{CO_2}$ (mm Hg)	43
Pa$_{O_2}$ (mm Hg)	59
Sa$_{O_2}$ (%)	85.1
Hb (g/dl)	11.7
coHb (%)	5.7

TECHNOLOGIST'S COMMENTS

All spirometric efforts were acceptable, both before and after bronchodilator administration. Lung volume and DL$_{CO}$ testing were performed acceptably. DL$_{CO}$ was corrected for an Hb of 11.7 and COHb of 5.7.

Three days later, a treadmill test was performed with an arterial catheter in place. The test was repeated with oxygen supplementation. Gas with an F$_{IO_2}$ of 0.28 was prepared in a meteorologic balloon for the portion of the exercise test using O$_2$ (Table 7-12).

QUESTIONS

1. What is the interpretation of:

   ■ Prebronchodilator and postbronchodilator spirometry?
   ■ Lung volumes and diffusing capacity?
   ■ Room air blood gases at rest?

TABLE 7-13 Exercise Test—Case 7-3

Exercise	Air		Oxygen		
Workload					
mph	0	1.5	0	1.5	2
Grade (%)	0	0	0	0	4
Time (min)	10	3	10	3	3
Ventilation					
f (breaths/min)	16	28	13	20	31
$\dot{V}_E$ (L/BTPS)	10.20	23.40	6.23	16.59	27.81
$\dot{V}_A$ (L/BTPS)	6.02	14.74	3.74	10.45	17.80
VT (L/BTPS)	0.638	0.836	0.479	0.830	0.897
V$_D$ (L/BTPS)	0.262	0.309	0.190	0.307	0.323
V$_D$/V$_T$	0.41	0.37	0.40	0.37	0.36
Gas exchange					
$\dot{V}_{O_2}$ (L/STPD)	0.310	0.835	0.279	0.649	0.986
$\dot{V}_{CO_2}$ (L/STPD)	0.303	0.743	0.251	0.617	0.976
RER	0.98	0.89	0.90	0.95	0.99
$\dot{V}_E/\dot{V}_{O_2}$ (L/L)	32.90	28.00	22.33	25.50	28.20
$\dot{V}_{O_2}$/HR (ml/beat)	3.44	7.59	3.29	6.18	8.57
Pulse oximeter					
Sp$_{O_2}$ (%)	92	87	97	93	93

Table continued on next page.

TABLE 7-13 Exercise Test—Case 7-3—Cont'd

Blood gases	Air		Oxygen		
pH	7.45	7.39	7.39	7.38	7.36
$Paco_2$ (mm Hg)	34	39	44	45	46
Pao_2 (mm Hg)	61	47	84	71	66
Sao_2 (%)	87.4	77.3	91.4	88.9	87.0
COHb (%)	5.1	4.7	4.8	4.7	4.6
$P(A-a)o_2$ (mm Hg)	51	56	64	78	84
Hemodynamics					
HR (beats/min)	90	110	92	105	115
Systolic BP (mm Hg)	130	145	134	145	150
Diastolic BP (mm Hg)	85	88	90	90	90

2. What is the interpretation of:

   ■ Ventilation during exercise?
   ■ Gas exchange during exercise?
   ■ Blood gas levels during exercise?

3. What is the cause of the patient's exercise limitation?
4. What treatment might be recommended based on these findings?

DISCUSSION

Interpretation (Pulmonary Function Tests)

All spirometry, lung volume, diffusing capacity, and blood gas measurements were acceptable.

Spirometry results show an obstructive process with a well-preserved FVC. There is only a 5% improvement in the FEV_1 after bronchodilator administration. Lung volumes by plethysmography show increased FRC and RV consistent with air trapping. TLC is close to normal, so there is little hyperinflation. DL_{CO}sb is decreased, even after correction for Hb and COHb. Arterial blood gases on air show hypoxemia that is complicated by an elevated COHb.

Impression: Moderately severe obstructive disease with no significant response to bronchodilators. Air trapping is present, and DL_{CO} is severely decreased. Exercise evaluation for oxygen desaturation is recommended.

Interpretation (Cardiopulmonary Exercise Test)

The exercise test was performed in two parts; the first part of the test was stopped because the patient's Pao_2 decreased to 46 mm Hg with an Sao_2 of 77.3%. The second phase, using oxygen, was terminated because of SOB. The patient tolerated very low workloads even with supplemental O_2.

Ventilation was slightly elevated at rest but increased normally. When given O_2, the patient's ventilation was slightly lower both at rest and at similar workloads. The V_D/V_T ratio was mildly elevated but decreased with exercise, on both air and oxygen. The patient's minute ventilation was only 51% of her observed MVV after bronchodilator administration, indicating some ventilatory reserve.

The patient achieved a peak $\dot{V}o_2$ of only 0.986 L/min on oxygen, which is 53% of her age-related predicted value of 1.858 L/min. This is consistent with moderately severe exercise impairment. The ventilatory equivalent for O_2 is within normal limits, and the O_2 pulse increased normally, although not to maximal values.

Blood gas analysis during exercise shows borderline hypoxemia at rest resulting from PaO_2 of 61 mm Hg in combination with elevated COHb. PaO_2 decreased to 47 mm Hg with only slight exertion. On 28% oxygen, the PaO_2 improved to 84 mm Hg at rest but decreased as workload increased. $PaCO_2$ increased slightly during oxygen breathing, possibly because of respiratory depression. COHb was elevated, likely resulting from the patient's continued smoking. Pulse oximetry (SpO_2) during exercise shows readings higher than the actual saturation, presumably because of the elevated COHb.

The HR and BP responses were appropriate for the workloads achieved while breathing both air and oxygen. The low maximal HR suggests an exercise limitation other than cardiovascular pathology or deconditioning. The ECG was unremarkable.

Impression: Moderately severe exercise impairment primarily caused by desaturation during exercise. Some ventilatory limitation is probably present as well. Desaturation is aggravated by an elevated COHb.

Cause of the Patient's Exercise Limitation

This patient characterizes an individual with obstructive lung disease in whom derangement of blood gases limits exercise more than impaired ventilation does. Her ventilation and gas exchange are close to normal at rest and at 1.5 mph, 0% grade. PaO_2 is low, however, and decreases abruptly with just a small increase in workload. The decrease is severe enough that desaturation may occur with daily activities or during sleep. The elevated COHb further impairs O_2 delivery. Although a pulse oximeter was used during the exercise test, its readings were falsely high because of the elevated COHb. Even if pulse oximeter readings are corrected for COHb, a discrepancy often exists between SpO_2 and SaO_2 during exercise. This error in pulse oximeter readings may result from changes in blood flow at the sensor site or motion artifact during exercise. Desaturation might be expected because of her low DL_{CO}. There is some evidence that DL_{CO} values less than 50% of predicted values are accompanied by exercise desaturation.

To evaluate the effect of oxygen therapy, a controlled trial of walking while breathing supplemental O_2 was performed. The patient breathed from a balloon containing gas blended to have an FIO_2 of approximately 0.28. The most notable change was the increase in resting PaO_2 from 61 to 84 mm Hg. However, the pattern of desaturation persisted. Her O_2 tension decreased dramatically, just as when she breathed room air. Because her PaO_2 was elevated by the supplemental O_2, it remained above 55 mm Hg. This is the level at which serious symptoms of hypoxemia begin to occur. Supplemental O_2 also may be responsible for the decrease in ventilation exhibited by the patient at rest and during exercise. The mild increase in $PaCO_2$ may be evidence of increased sensitivity to hypoxemia. When she breathes O_2, her respiratory drive decreases slightly, allowing CO_2 to increase. Abnormal $\dot{V}/\dot{Q}$ is the most likely explanation of desaturation observed in the patient. The bronchitic component of her obstructive disease results in shunting and venous admixture.

While breathing oxygen, she did not desaturate to a level at which hypoxemia might be considered as a cause of the exercise limitation. She also did not increase ventilation to her maximal level. This may suggest that deconditioning was responsible for the low maximal workload achieved. However, her HR and BP did not increase as typical in significant deconditioning. Other possible causes for the low workload achieved while breathing oxygen may be inadequate patient effort, development of bronchospasm, or greatly increased work of breathing.

Treatment

The patient began a formal effort to stop smoking and eventually quit. She was also referred for pulmonary rehabilitation, which included bronchial hygiene, breathing retraining, and exercise with supplemental O_2. She began using nasal oxygen at 1 to 2 L/min for exertion. A follow-up evaluation was recommended 3 to 6 months after smoking cessation.

CASE 7-4

HISTORY

The patient is a 62-year-old woman complaining of dyspnea on exertion. Her past medical history includes severe subglottic stenosis, which has been managed with several rigid dilatations over the past 2 years. She had a surgically corrected endarterectomy and a significant family history of coronary artery disease. Her current medications include metaprolol (Toprol), levothyroxine (Synthroid), and amlodipine (Norvasc). On physical examination, her lungs were clear to auscultation and she was in no apparent distress. Chest x-ray showed some narrowing of the subglottic trachea with no significant change since 1 year ago.

PULMONARY FUNCTION TESTS

Personal Data

Sex: Female
Age: 62 yr
Height: 62.5 in (158.8 cm)
Weight: 179 lb (81.3 kg; BMI 32.3)

Lung Volumes

	Predicted		Control		Postdilator*	
	Normal	Range	Found	%Pred	Found	%Change
TLC (Pleth)	4.82	>3.72	4.06	84		
VC	2.96	>2.22	2.28	77	2.42	+6
RV	1.86	<2.41	1.79	96		
RV/TLC	38.5	<50.5	44.0	114		
FRC			2.2			

*Bronchodilator was albuterol.

Spirometry

	Predicted		Control		Postdilator†	
	Normal	Range	Found	%Pred	Found	%Change
FVC	2.96	>2.22	*2.07	70	*2.20	+6
FEV_1	2.40	>1.85	*1.70	71	*1.78	+5
FEV_1/FVC	81.2	>70.0	82.3		80.9	
$FEF_{25\%-75\%}$	2.3	>1.0	1.5	67	1.5	
FEF_{max}	5.5	>2.9	3.1	55	3.6	+17
FIF_{max}					1.5	
$FEF_{50\%}/FIF_{50\%}$					1.5	

*Outside normal range.
†Bronchodilator was albuterol.

Airway Function

	Predicted		Control	
	Normal	**Range**	**Found**	**%Pred**
SRaw	4.7	>7.9	5.5	117

Diffusing Capacity

	Predicted		Control	
	Normal	**Range**	**Found**	**%Pred**
$DL_{CO}sb$	20.9	>14.4	14.4	69
V_A	1.64	>3.72	*3.58	77

*Outside normal range.

Oximetry

	Predicted		Rest	Exercise (step 3 min)
	Normal	**Range**		
O_2 sat	96	≥93	95	97
Pulse			66	104

TECHNOLOGIST'S COMMENTS

Spirometry testing was performed meeting criteria for acceptability and reproducibility.

QUESTIONS

1. What is the interpretation of:
   - Prebronchodilator and postbronchodilator spirometry?
   - Lung volumes and diffusing capacity?

TABLE 7-14 Exercise Test—Case 7-4

		Rest	Maximum	Pred Max	% Pred Max
Exercise					
Workload	watts		60		
Time	min:sec		7:00		
Oxygen saturation	%	99	98		
$\dot{V}O_2$	L/min	0.191	0.801	1.674	48
$\dot{V}O_2$/kg	ml/kg	2.3	9.9		
R		0.68	1.05		

Table continued on next page.

TABLE 7-14 Exercise Test—Case 7-4—Cont'd

		Rest	Maximum	Pred Max	% Pred Max
Cardiac function					
Heart rate	beats/min	67	110	170	65
Blood pressure (cuff)	mm Hg	122/60	148/72		
Oxygen pulse	ml/beat	2.9	7.3		
Ventilation					
Minute ventilation	L/min	6.2	29.2	68.0	43
Respiratory rate	per min	12	20		
Tidal volume	ml, BTPS	528	1564		
Tidal volume/FVC	%	26	76		
Vent equiv for O_2	$\dot{V}_E/\dot{V}O_2$	34.7	36.7		

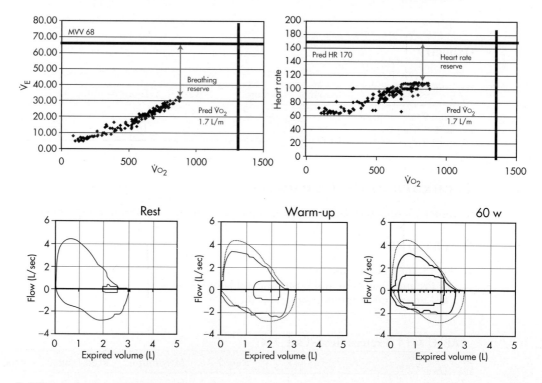

2. What is the interpretation of:
   - Cardiovascular response?
   - Ventilation during exercise?
   - Gas exchange during exercise?
   - Oxygen consumption and ventilatory threshold during exercise?
   - Impression?

3. Discussion of patient's exercise response.

4. What treatment might be recommended based on these findings?

DISCUSSION

Interpretation (Pulmonary Function)

Spirometry results show a nonspecific reduction in vital capacity and FEV_1 with a normal FEV_1/FVC ratio. Lung volumes were within normal limits. There was no response to bronchodilator. The DL_{CO} was at the lower limit of normal. A cardiopulmonary exercise test was ordered with F-V loop analysis to determine whether there was flow limitation that would require repeat dilation of the trachea, versus deconditioning or decreased exercise tolerance.

Interpretation (Exercise)

The patient exercised on a cycle ergometer to a maximal workload of 60 watts using a 10-watt protocol. The patient terminated the test complaining of SOB. This appears to be a submaximal study.

Cardiovascular Response: The heart rate increased to 110 beats/min, which was 65% of predicted. The ECG was a normal sinus rhythm at rest. During exercise, there were no arrhythmias and/or evidence of ischemic changes. The reduced heart rate response may also be secondary to the beta-blocker the patient was taking. Blood pressure and the O_2 pulse increased appropriately with exercise.

Ventilatory Response: There was an adequate ventilatory reserve; breathing kinetics were appropriate with increasing tidal volumes to 76% of the forced vital capacity. It should be noted that the tidal volume to FVC ratio is somewhat elevated at 76%, but this can be seen in individuals with reduced lung volumes.

Gas Exchange: Pulse oximetry was 99% at rest and 98% at end exercise, suggesting normal oxygen saturation.

Oxygen consumption in this submaximal study was 48% of predicted, and the ventilatory threshold could not be determined.

F-V loops were performed at rest, during warm-up, and at maximal workload. There was no evidence of either inspiratory or expiratory flow limitation, when compared with either the resting maximum F-V loop or the partial loops performed during exercise.

Impression: Submaximal study with reduced exercise tolerance and no evidence of flow limitation.

Discussion of Exercise Response

A 10-watt incremental protocol was selected based on a predicted $\dot{V}O_{2max}$ of 1.674 L ((1600 − 300)/ 100 = 13) and because of the patient's stated reduced exercise tolerance.

In evaluating whether a study represents maximal effort, five categories are examined. These are cardiovascular response, ventilatory response, oxygen saturation, metabolic parameters, and clinical observation (Table 7-10). Her heart rate was 65% of predicted; $\dot{V}_{Emax}$ reached 43% of her calculated MVV. SpO_2 was 98%, and her metabolic work showed an RER of 1.05. Clinical observation revealed poor effort. These factors all suggest a submaximal study. Based on these findings, the study can still be interpreted accordingly.

Cardiovascular Response: Heart rate response was reduced, either related to the poor effort or secondary to a beta blockade effect.

Ventilatory Response: There was adequate ventilatory reserve based on both a normal ratio ($\dot{V}_{Emax}/MVV$) and an absolute difference of 39 L. Tidal volume increased appropriately with exercise; however, it did comprise a significant portion of the forced vital capacity. This is often seen in individuals with restrictive patterns and/or reduced lung volumes.

Gas-exchange analysis was limited to oxygen saturation, which was normal.

Oxygen consumption was 48% of predicted in this submaximal study, and the ventilatory threshold could not be determined. This is not surprising in a submaximal test.

Flow-Volume Loops: F-V loops showed no evidence of flow limitation. The resting graph is a plot of the maximal F-V loop versus her tidal breathing. The warm-up and 60-watt graphs demonstrate her tidal breathing plotted against both her resting maximal F-V loop (dotted line) and partial loops performed during exercise.

Treatment

The purpose of this test was to discover whether the patient needed another surgical dilation for subglottic stenosis. Visual inspection via bronchoscopy showed the area to be the same diameter as measured earlier. Despite this, she had an increase in dyspnea on exertion. The surgical procedure was deferred based on the results of the F-V loop analysis during exercise. The patient was enrolled in a pulmonary rehabilitation program to improve her exercise tolerance.

■ SELF-ASSESSMENT QUESTIONS

Entry-level

1. *Which of the following equipment is required to perform a 6-minute walk test?*
   I. Countdown timer
   II. Lap counter
   III. Pulse oximeter
   IV. Sphygmomanometer
   a. I and II
   b. I, II, and III
   c. I, II, and IV
   d. II, III, and IV

2. *In an adult patient with a resting BP of 130/90, which of the following responses would be an indication to stop an exercise test?*
   a. Systolic increase to 180, diastolic increase to 95
   b. Systolic increase to 255, diastolic increase to 130
   c. Systolic increase to 160, diastolic increase to 100
   d. Systolic remains at 130, diastolic decrease to 85

3. *What cycle ergometer protocol should the technologist select based on the information provided?*

Pred HR: 175	Pred $\dot{V}o_2$:	2.40 L/min
Height: 69 in	Weight:	190 lb
FVC: 4.65 L	FEV_1:	3.74 L

   a. 10 watts/min
   b. 15 watts/min
   c. 20 watts/min
   d. 25 watts/min

4. *Which of the following is an indication for terminating a cardiopulmonary exercise test?*

   a. SoB (Borg = 4)
   b. 2-mm downsloping ST-segment depression
   c. 5 premature ventricular contractions/min
   d. Failure of pulse oximeter sensor

5. *The following graph plots $\dot{V}_E$ and $\dot{V}co_2$ against $\dot{V}o_2$:*

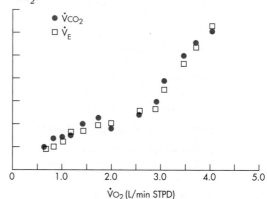

   At approximately what $\dot{V}o_2$ does the ventilatory threshold occur?
   a. 1.0 L/min
   b. 2.0 L/min
   c. 3.0 L/min
   d. 4.0 L/min

6. *The "phase delay" between flow at the mouth and analysis of O_2 and CO_2 is necessary for calibration of a:*
   a. Mixing chamber–type exercise system
   b. Rebreathing cardiac output system
   c. Standard Fick cardiac output determination
   d. Breath-by-breath exhaled gas analysis system

Advanced

7. Which results from a maximal exercise test would be consistent for a patient who has severe COPD?

   I. $\dot{V}_E$/MVV   90%
   II. V_T/FVC   48%
   III. V_D/V_T 12%
   IV. A-a gradient 45

   a. I and IV
   b. I and II
   c. II, III, and IV
   d. I, II, and IV

8. A 61-year-old woman with dyspnea on exertion has the following results from a cardiopulmonary exercise test.

	Rest	Maximal Exercise	Pred
HR	88	154	170
$\dot{V}_{O_2}$ (ml/kg)	4	17	23
$\dot{V}_E$ (L)	9.0	44.0	90.0
V_T (ml)	575	685	
RR (per min)	12	64	
V_D/V_T (%)	45	50	

These findings are most consistent with:

a. Ventilatory limitation
b. Pulmonary hypertension
c. Inappropriate breathing strategy
d. Pulmonary fibrosis

9. Tidal breathing loops at different stages of exercise are plotted against the resting maximal F-V curve. Which of the following best describes the data?

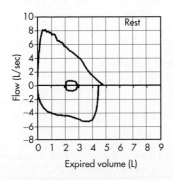
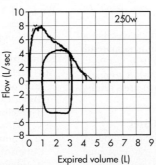
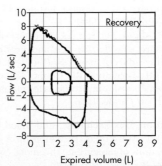

a. Inappropriate breathing strategy
b. Dynamic hyperinflation
c. No significant flow limitation
d. Fixed obstruction

10. A patient has the following results of a cardiopulmonary exercise test (values in parentheses are percentages of predicted):

$\dot{V}_{O_2 max}$	L/min (STPD)	3.44	(97%)
HR_{max}	b/min	171	(95%)
$\dot{V}_{Emax}$	L/min (BTPS)	60	(47%)

Which of the following best describes these results?

a. Mild aerobic impairment, consistent with deconditioning
b. Poor patient effort indicated by low maximal ventilation
c. Moderate exercise impairment with ventilatory limitation
d. Normal exercise response

11. A patient performs a symptom-limited maximal exercise test on a cycle ergometer using a ramp protocol of 20 watts/min. The ventilatory threshold is measured at 39% of the patient's peak $\dot{V}_{O_2}$. These findings are consistent with which of the following?

a. Inappropriate ergometer protocol
b. Poor patient effort
c. Early onset of anaerobic metabolism
d. Normal cardiovascular response

12. *A patient has the following results of an exercise test:*

	Maximal Exercise	Predicted
HR (beats/min)	119	159
ST change (mm)	0.5	<1
$\dot{V}O_2$ (ml/min/kg)	10.2	22
$\dot{V}_E$ (L/min)	37	42
PaO_2 (mm Hg)	53	>85

Which of the following clinical conditions is most consistent with these findings?

a. COPD
b. Poor patient effort
c. Exercise induced bronchospasm
d. Coronary artery disease

SELECTED BIBLIOGRAPHY

General References

ACSM: *Resource manual for guidelines for exercise testing and prescription,* ed 4, American College of Sports Medicine, Jeffrey L. Roitman (Ed), Philadelphia, 2001, Lippincott Williams & Wilkins.

American College of Sports Medicine: *Guidelines for exercise testing and exercise prescription,* ed 6, Philadelphia, 2000, Lippincott Williams & Wilkins.

Hansen JE: Exercise instruments, schemes, and protocols for evaluating the dyspneic patient, *Am Rev Respir Dis* 129(suppl):S25, 1984.

Hansen JE, Sue DY, Wasserman K: Predicted values for clinical exercise testing, *Am Rev Respir Dis* 129(suppl): S49, 1984.

Jones NL: *Clinical exercise testing,* ed 4, Philadelphia, 1997, WB Saunders.

Wasserman K, Hansen J, Sue D, et al: *Principles of exercise testing and interpretation,* ed 3, Philadelphia, 1999, Lippincott, Williams & Wilkins.

Weber KT, Janicki JS: *Cardiopulmonary exercise testing: physiologic principles and clinical applications,* Philadelphia, 1986, WB Saunders.

Cardiovascular Monitoring During Exercise

Bruce RA: Value and limitations of the electrocardiogram in progressive exercise testing, *Am Rev Respir Dis* 129(suppl):S28, 1984.

Daida H, Allison TG, Squires TW, et al: Peak exercise blood pressure stratified by age and gender in apparently healthy subjects, *Mayo Clin Proc* 71:445, 1996.

Pollack ML, Bohannon RL, Cooper KH, et al: A comparative analysis of four protocols for maximal stress testing, *Am Heart J* 92:39, 1976.

Ventilation, Gas Exchange, and Blood Gases

Beaver WL, Wasserman K, Whipp BJ: A new method for detection of anaerobic threshold by gas exchange, *J Appl Physiol* 60:2020, 1986.

Blackie SP, Fairbarn MS, McElvaney NG, et al: Normal values and ranges for ventilation and breathing pattern at maximal exercise, *Chest* 100:136-142, 1991.

Blackie SP, Fairbarn MS, McElvaney GN, et al: Prediction of maximal oxygen uptake and power during cycle ergometry in subjects older than 55 years of age, *Am Rev Respir Dis* 139:1424-1429, 1989.

Eschenbacher WL, Mannina A: An algorithm for the interpretation of cardiopulmonary exercise tests, *Chest* 97:263-267, 1990.

Escourrou PJL, Delaperche MF, Visseaux A: Reliability of pulse oximetry during exercise in pulmonary patients, *Chest* 97:635-638, 1990.

Johnson BD, Beck KC, Zeballos RJ, et al: Advances in pulmonary laboratory testing, *Chest* 116:1377-1387, 1999.

Johnson BD, Weisman IM, Zeballos RJ, et al: Emerging concepts in the evaluation of ventilatory limitation during exercise—the exercise tidal flow-volume loop, *Chest* 116:488-503, 1999.

Jones NL: Normal values for pulmonary gas exchange during exercise, *Am Rev Respir Dis* 129(suppl):S44, 1984.

Proctor DN, Beck KC: Delay time adjustments to minimize errors in breath-by-breath measurement of Vo2 during exercise, *Appl Physiol* 81:2495-2499, 1996.

Whipp BJ, Ward SA, Wasserman K: Ventilatory responses to exercise and their control in man, *Am Rev Respir Dis* 129(suppl):S17, 1984.

Standards and Guidelines

ACC/AHA 2002 guideline update for exercise testing: a report of the American College of Cardiology/ American Heart Association Task Force on Practice Guidelines, *Circulation* 106:1883-1892, 2002.

ACC/AHA 2002 guideline update for exercise testing: a report of the American College of Cardiology/ American Heart Association Task Force on Practice Guidelines, *J Am Coll Cardiol* 40:1531-1540, 2002.

American Association for Respiratory Care: Clinical practice guideline: exercise testing for evaluation of hypoxemia and/or desaturation, *Respir Care* 46:514-522, 2001.

American Thoracic Society statement: cardiopulmonary exercise testing, *Am J Respir Crit Care Med* 167:211-277, 2003.

American Thoracic Society statement: guidelines for the six-minute walk test, *Am J Respir Crit Care Med* 166:111-117, 2002.

ATS/ACCP statement on cardiopulmonary exercise testing, *Am J Respir Crit Care Med* 167:211-277, 2003.

Fletcher GF, Froelicher VF, Hartley LH, et al: Exercise standards: a statement for health professionals from the American Heart Association, *Circulation* 82:2286-2322, 1990.

NCCLS: A quality system model for health care, approved guideline, HS01-A, Wayne, Penn, 2002.

NCCLS: Blood gas and pH analysis and related measurements, approved guideline, C46-A Wayne, Penn, 2001.

NCCLS: Procedures for the collection of arterial blood specimens, approved standard, H11-A3, Wayne Penn, 1999.

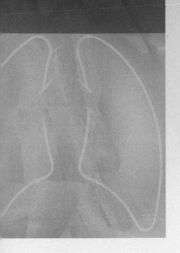

CHAPTER 8

PEDIATRIC PULMONARY FUNCTION TESTING

Deborah White

OBJECTIVES

After studying this chapter and reviewing its tables and case studies, you should be able to do the following:

Entry-level and Advanced

1. State how American Thoracic Society (ATS) guidelines relate to pulmonary function testing in children, and resultant interpretative strategies.
2. Suggest techniques for approaching young children and modifications to testing protocols for standard pulmonary function tests.
3. Relate specific pediatric disease states to anticipated changes in standard pulmonary function measurements.
4. State the physiologic and testing effects that sedation may produce in infants.
5. State differences in procedures and techniques between pulmonary function testing in infants as compared with older children.

nfant and pediatric pulmonary function testing is one of the most dynamic and challenging aspects of pulmonary physiology. Although technologic improvements have affected all areas of pulmonary function testing, the implications for infant and pediatric testing are especially evident. Improved accuracy and precision of flow sensors, combined with user-friendly computer software, make respiratory system measurements reproducible and readily available for physician offices as well as for sophisticated research-oriented laboratories. Infants, of course, are unable to follow specific instructions. Respiratory measurements in this age group are limited to techniques that are independent of effort, or that involve mechanical manipulation of the infant's chest. The specialized equipment and techniques needed for these measurements are discussed in this chapter. Children 3 years and older present a different array of challenges for the pulmonary function technologist. The primary limiting factor for the young child is the "effort and cooperation" component. This chapter focuses on practical tips, techniques, and guidelines for obtaining pulmonary function data that are reliable and relevant in assessing pediatric respiratory ailments.

Spirometry

The basics of spirometry apply to both pediatrics and adults (see Chapter 2). The same principles for testing and equipment are used. The indications for testing are similar, although disease processes in pediatrics often differ. The anatomy and physiology of the respiratory system changes significantly from the young child to the older adolescent. As for adults, the goals of spirometry are:

1. To identify the presence of an obstructive or restrictive defect
2. To quantify the degree of the abnormality
3. To test for a response to a bronchodilator

Spirometry in pediatrics has several pitfalls and special challenges, however. These can be addressed by posing several questions and giving specific examples.

■ AT WHAT AGE CAN A CHILD PERFORM SPIROMETRY?

This question is commonly asked, but it cannot be answered until spirometry is attempted. Children as young as 3 years of age have the potential of performing the maneuver, but with limitations. On average, by age 5, most children can perform spirometry with adequate technique and reproducibility. There are, of course, many exceptions. Spirometry is an effort-dependent test that requires cooperation and attention from the child. Equally important is the experience and patience of a well-trained pulmonary function technologist. Children who are mentally delayed or not capable of following directions may not perform adequate spirometry at any age, regardless of the coach or technologist. Patients who are not feeling well or having chest pain, for example, may follow instructions, but not perform maximally.

■ WHAT CAN BE DONE TO ENSURE MAXIMAL EFFORT ON THE PART OF THE CHILD?

First, gain the child's confidence and do not rush into testing. Children are very fearful that the testing will hurt. When possible, reassure the child by carrying on a conversation that is directed toward the child. See Figure 8-1 for a list of suggestions that will "break the ice" and get things going in a positive direction. Try to demonstrate the test and reassure the child that it is easy. Prepare the child for testing. When possible, the child should be standing and the technologist at eye level with the child. The use of nose clips is recommended, but depends on the age and cooperation of the child. The anatomy of the nasopharyngeal

For spirometry, different "catch phrases" can help the child more clearly understand instructions. Examples are:
- ■ "Take a big breath in until you feel like a balloon ready to burst!"
- ■ "Punch that air out like a dump truck is rolling over your belly!"
- ■ "Keep blowing until the air comes out of your toes!"

Be creative and think like a kid!

TIPS for SUCCESS with SPIROMETRY

1. Greet the child, introduce yourself, and engage in conversation
   * Compliment the child on a pretty dress or cool T-shirt
   * Ask about vacations, school, sports activities, etc.
   * Ask if the child would like to play a 'blowing game' on the computer

2. Demonstrate the test
   * Blow on a tissue, pinwheel, or similar toy
   * Reassure the child how easy the test is

3. Encourage the child to stand straight and hold the flow sensor upright
   * Use nose clips if possible, but compromise if necessary
   * Get at the same eye level of the child

4. Be expressive with body language
   * Change the intonation of your voice and be enthusiastic
   * Use your hands to emphasize action

5. Use words the child can understand and keep directions simple
   * "Breathe in, breathe out"
   * "Take little baby breaths"
   * "Take a giant breath in until you feel ready to burst"
   * "Blast the air out. Keep blowing until it comes out of your toes"

6. Think like a kid!
   * "Race" with the child to see who can blow longer
   * Pretend it's the child's birthday and he or she has to blow out the same number of candles as his or her age
   * Show the child the "mountains" he or she has blown and explain how the mountains can be made taller and wider

7. Be prepared to try different techniques (open vs. closed) and offer rest periods

8. Offer praise and prizes
   * High fives
   * "Best Blower of the Day" awards
   * Small toys or stickers
   * Smiley faces or A+ on PFT reports

9. *Be patient*, and know when to quit. Repeated efforts can be frustrating and counterproductive for the next visit

---

Figure 8-1 *Tips for success with spirometry in pediatric patients.*

structures in younger children is such that the use of nose clips may not be necessary. If the child is willing to wear nose clips, encourage him or her to do so.

Many pulmonary function systems offer two mouthpiece techniques for performing spirometry: "closed" and "open" techniques. Each offers advantages and disadvantages. Attempt the technique with which laboratory personnel are most comfortable and consistent. For the closed technique, have the child stand with nose clips in place and the mouthpiece situated securely. Ask the patient to breathe tidally for several breaths. This offers the opportunity to observe the child and ensure that the seal around the mouthpiece is tight. It also gives the child a feeling of security that he or she will get plenty of air through the mouthpiece. The child should be reassured during tidal breathing that he or she is doing very well.

If the spirometer permits real-time visualization of flow, the child may even see himself "drawing pictures" with his or her breathing. It is essential to gain the child's confidence and offer praise whenever possible. It is very important to talk the child through the maneuver. Use simple words and phrases. For example, "Breathe in; breathe out," "Take easy, little, baby breaths," or "One more little breath. Now take a giant breath in." The technologist should be vocal and use hands and arms to demonstrate. The intonation of the voice should mimic the action, for example "easy, gentle breaths" in a soft voice versus "big, fast and long breath" in a louder tone. Sometimes having the child "race" with another technologist, both blowing tissues into the air, may be helpful. Other simple toys, such as pinwheels, may offer incentive.

If the child is having particular difficulty, changing the technique may lead to success. For example, use a different mouthpiece or try the open technique. The child may have a sensitive gag reflex, or for unclear reasons, become anxious with tidal breathing. With the open technique, the child should first be instructed to hold the mouthpiece close to his or her face, perhaps supported on the cheek. Next, open the mouth wide, take in the deepest breath possible, place the mouthpiece in the mouth, and immediately blow. The disadvantage of this technique is that air may be lost as the child tries to get the mouthpiece into his or her mouth and form a seal. It is often helpful to graduate the child from the open to the closed technique once he or she becomes more comfortable performing spirometry.

■ WHY IS EFFORT SO IMPORTANT?

As mentioned previously, the biggest challenge with children is ensuring a maximal breath in prior to the forced expiration. The concept is simple: The more air in, the more air out. The technologist should strive to get the child to breathe in as deeply as possible and observe the child's chest excursion. Movement of the shoulders upward without chest excursion is common and can fool the technologist into believing it is a maximal inspiratory capacity. This may also be a pitfall when comparing pre- and postbronchodilator spirometry. Figure 8-2 is from a 6-year-old patient performing spirometry for the first time. The prebronchodilator spirometry (8-2, A) appears to be normal and may be entirely reproducible. Following bronchodilator (8-2, B), both FVC and FEV_1 improve significantly. However, the increase in FVC and FEV_1 is symmetrical with little change in the FEV_1/FVC ratio. Although a bronchodilator response cannot be ruled out, learning effect is also a strong possibility for this change. Contrast this with Figure 8-3, A and B. In this example, both FVC and FEV_1 increase; however, the increase in FEV_1 is proportionately higher, which also increases the FEV_1/FVC ratio. Although learning may have some effect in this example, it is evident that mild intrathoracic airflow obstruction is completely reversed. Once a child has learned the technique and is capable of performing spirometry, the results are remarkably reproducible. With practice, it is unusual to have a child who cannot reproduce his or her FVC and FEV_1 within 5%.

Once a maximal inspiration is accomplished, most young children do not have difficulty blowing out forcefully. As for adult spirometry, the technologist should minimize hesitation prior to the forced maneuver that may create a "time zero" or back-extrapolated volume error. Do not encourage a breath hold. Delayed exhalation can result in a poor peak flow measurement and falsely raise the FEV_1. Figure 8-4 shows an example of this. Figure 8-4, A is an acceptable FVC maneuver. Note how the delayed exhalation in Figure 8-4, B can skew the curve to the right and falsely elevate timed parameters. Young children have a desire to please and, unless they are feeling poorly, will usually respond to the direction of "blast the air out." Obtaining a maximal peak flow can actually be more difficult in an adolescent. Teenage children often can be reluctant to perform maximally unless strongly encouraged to do so. This may be due to chest pain, embarrassment, or fear that something is wrong with them. Occasionally, this poor effort may be related to typical teenage angst or attention-seeking

Spirometry		Pred	Pre-RX (A)		Post-RX (B)		%Chg
			Best	%Pred	Best	%Pred	
FVC	Liters	1.50	1.34	89	1.61	108	21
FEV$_1$	Liters	1.34	1.21	90	1.50	112	24
FEV$_1$/FVC	%	90	90		93		
FEF$_{25\%-75\%}$	L/sec		1.27		2.02		59
PEF	L/sec	3.33	2.62	79	3.03	91	15

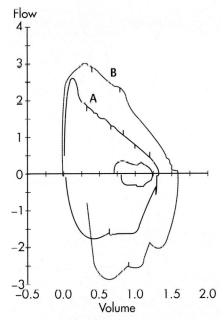

Figure 8-2 *First-time spirometry in a 6-year-old patient.* **A**, Prebronchodilator. **B**, Postbronchodilator.

motivation. A sensitive and perceptive technologist can often combine the right amount of compassion with the necessary verbal encouragement to obtain optimal results. Variability, due to effort alone, may be especially important if the patient is performing serial measurements, as in a methacholine challenge. A change in treatment regimen or admission to the hospital is often based on spirometric changes; therefore reproducibility is critical.

HOW LONG SHOULD A CHILD EXHALE DURING AN FVC MANEUVER?

ATS criteria recommend an expiration of at least 6 seconds and until a flow plateau is reached. Young children may not be able to meet these criteria. Their lung volume is significantly smaller, and the lungs may completely empty in only 2 or 3 seconds. When a child feels empty, the natural instinct is take a breath back in. With instruction and practice, the child can

Spirometry		Pred	Pre-RX (A)		Post-RX (B)		%Chg
			Best	%Pred	Best	%Pred	
FVC	Liters	2.09	2.04	98	2.17	104	6
FEV$_1$	Liters	1.80	1.61	89	1.91	106	19
FEV$_1$/FVC	%	86	79		88		
FEF$_{25\%-75\%}$	L/sec	2.05	1.40	69	2.25	110	60
PEF	L/sec	3.33	3.92	95	4.78	115	22

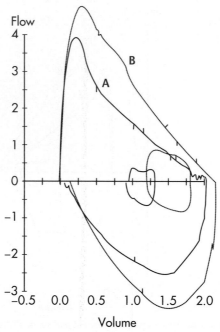

Figure 8-3 *Spirometry in an 8-year-old patient.* **A,** Prebronchodilator spirometry in a child showing mild intrathoracic airflow obstruction. **B,** Postbronchodilator response.

learn to continue the expiration; however, this may not be possible on the first visit to the lab. This does not invalidate the FVC maneuvers, but requires that the child be evaluated carefully. Figure 8-5, *A* represents three prebronchodilator flow-volume (F-V) loops superimposed over each other. Although this 5-year-old child does not meet ATS end-of-test criteria, the FEV$_1$ and shape of the F-V loop are remarkably reproducible. Postbronchodilator (Figure 8-5, *B*) ATS criteria are not met, but F-V loops are significantly improved and reproducible. The 6-second expiration and zero flow rules may not be appropriate for pediatric testing, suggesting the need for specific pediatric criteria. Optional end-of-test criteria have been proposed, but not universally accepted. Children who are severely obstructed, like their adult counterparts, may have the ability to exhale for an extended time. Figure 8-6 shows the F-V loop and volume-time tracing of a 10-year-old girl with cystic fibrosis. This child is able to sustain expiration for 15 seconds. However, the additional volume measured in this prolonged expiration is small and may exhaust the child performing the test. She approaches a flow plateau at

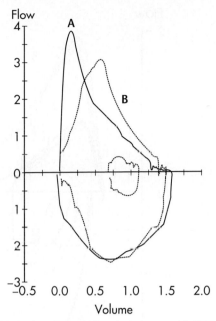

Figure 8-4 *Spirometry in a child showing effects of effort.* **A,** An acceptable FVC effort. **B,** Poor effort/ technique, resulting in delayed exhalation (see text).

approximately 7 to 8 seconds, and the maneuver can be terminated at this point. Although end-of-test criteria are not met, the spirometry is still valid for interpretation. Many decisions regarding acceptability of pulmonary function test results require good judgment from the technologist and careful interpretation from the physician.

Children may not successfully meet all ATS recommendations for spirometry; however, this does *not* necessarily invalidate the FVC maneuver. Careful interpretation of incomplete maneuvers is very important.

IS THE $FEF_{25\%-75\%}$ A RELIABLE PARAMETER IN CHILDREN?

Historically, $FEF_{25\%-75\%}$ has been used to evaluate flow from the "small airways." More precisely, the $FEF_{25\%-75\%}$ should be considered a measurement of flow at lower lung volumes, not merely flow from medium-sized and smaller airways. As in adults, the variability of the $FEF_{25\%-75\%}$ is greater than that of the FVC and FEV_1. Because children may be even less reproducible at baseline, the reliability of this measurement in pediatric testing may be questionable. In addition, if the child does not fully exhale to RV, $FEF_{25\%-75\%}$ may be artificially elevated due to reduced vital capacity. If it is reported, the $FEF_{25\%-75\%}$ in a pediatric subject should

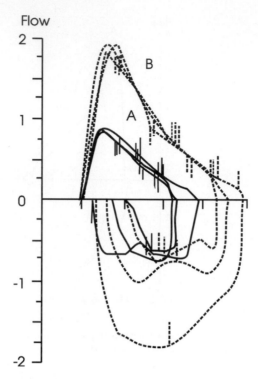

Figure 8-5 *Reproducibility of efforts in a 5-year-old patient.* **A,** Prebronchodilator spirometry that is reproducible, although the usual end-of-test criteria are not met (see text). **B,** Postbronchodilator spirometry in the same patient, again demonstrating reproducible efforts (see text).

be interpreted with caution. A substantially greater change postbronchodilator is needed before a change can be considered significant. Figure 8-7 considers a young child who performs very reproducibly, but whose vital capacity is almost completely exhaled in one second, and is at the lower limits of normal. Observe the shape of the F-V curve pre- and postbronchodilator. This patient has a less than significant change in FEV_1 following bronchodilator, but a large change in $FEF_{25\%-75\%}$. If the $FEV_{0.5}$ had been reported, it would certainly have indicated a significant change consistent with the change in $FEF_{25\%-75\%}$. An $FEF_{25\%-75\%}$ that improves by more than 35% to 45% after bronchodilator suggests reversal of obstruction from peripheral airways. As noted above, $FEF_{25\%-75\%}$ can be reduced for several reasons that are not always related to small airway disease. The F-V loop in Figure 8-8 is an example of a child with a severe fixed airflow obstruction from an endobronchial lesion in a mainstem bronchus. The $FEF_{25\%-75\%}$ of this patient is extremely low but is due to an obstruction in a large central airway.

ARE ANY OTHER PARAMETERS OF FORCED FLOW HELPFUL IN PEDIATRICS?

Spirometry yields a variety of expiratory and inspiratory flows, including $FEF_{25\%}$, $FEF_{50\%}$, $FEF_{75\%}$, $FEF_{85\%}$, $FIF_{50\%}$, and the $FEF_{50\%}/FIF_{50\%}$ ratio. Each of these parameters relates to flow at a particular lung volume and may have some benefit for particular instances. These flows, like the $FEF_{25\%-75\%}$, are less reproducible than the FEV_1 and FVC, and do not have any

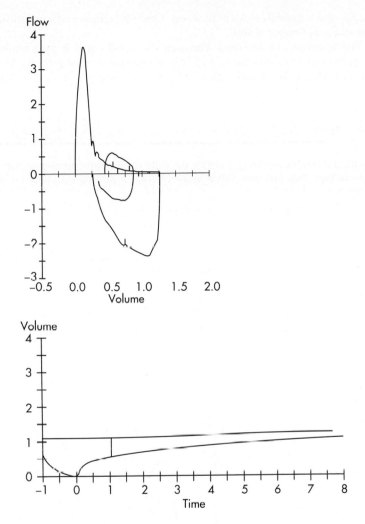

Figure 8–6 *F-V loop and volume-time tracing of a 10-year-old girl with cystic fibrosis* (see text). Note prolonged exhalation and severe airflow obstruction.

reference values. The $FEF_{50\%}/FIF_{50\%}$ ratio may be helpful in identifying intrathoracic versus extrathoracic airflow obstruction (see Chapter 2). Unlike the expiratory limb of the F-V loop, the inspiratory limb has not been well characterized in pediatric subjects. There are several reasons for this; however, the most important are energy expenditure and effort dependence. Expiration from TLC is far more reproducible due to the elastic recoil of the lung. The $FEF_{50\%}$ occurs in the portion of the expiratory limb that is considered effort independent. The inspiratory limb, conversely, is effort dependent and energy dependent for the entire maneuver. Therefore, optimal patient effort is vital for analyzing the inspiratory loop. A great deal of important information can be obtained from an appropriately performed maneuver. Too often, the inspiratory limb is ignored. When teaching children how to perform spirometry, certainly the emphasis is on expiration. Once it is mastered, attention should be paid to the inspiratory maneuver as well.

The aperture, or opening, through the vocal cords is approximately the same at both 50% of expiratory vital capacity and 50% of inspiratory vital capacity. Hence, the $FEF_{50\%}/FIF_{50\%}$ ratio should not be greater than 1.0. A ratio greater than 1.0 suggests an extrathoracic

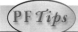

Assuming maximal effort is given by the child for the entire maneuver, the inspiratory limb of the flow-volume loop can give valuable information regarding extrathoracic obstruction in pediatric patients.

Spirometry		Pred	Pre-RX Best	%Pred	Post-RX Best	%Pred	%Chg
FVC	Liters	1.45	1.19	82	1.20	83	1
FEV_1	Liters	1.30	1.11	85	1.20	92	8
FEV_1/FVC	%	89	93		100		
$FEF_{25\%-75\%}$	L/sec		1.07		2.05		92
PEF	L/sec	3.59	2.66	74	3.11	87	17
FET 100%	Sec		7.06		5.05		−28

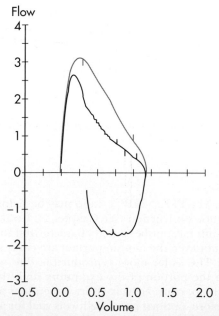

Figure 8-7 *Prebronchodilator and postbronchodilator spirometry in a child showing minimal improvement in FEV1.* Note the large improvement in $FEF_{25\%-75\%}$ consistent with a marked improvement in airflow (see text).

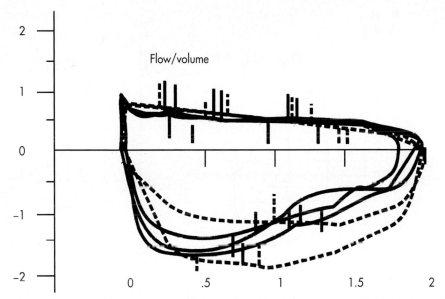

Figure 8-8 *F-V loop in a child with a severe fixed airflow obstruction from an endobronchial lesion in a mainstem bronchus* (see text).

obstruction; however, this relationship has not been closely studied or reported in pediatric patients. Conversely, an $FEF_{50\%}/FIF_{50\%}$ ratio of less than 1.0 may be normal or may represent significant intrathoracic obstruction. In addition, a ratio close to normal is possible if significant obstruction is seen on both inspiration and expiration (fixed obstruction), yielding a ratio of 1.0. This underlies the importance of correlating the F-V loop with the child's clinical picture and symptoms. Figure 8-9, *A* to *E* shows examples of F-V loops with differing $FEF_{50\%}/FIF_{50\%}$ ratios and the shape of the loops represented by them. Although $FEF_{50\%}/FIF_{50\%}$ may not always discriminate between intrathoracic versus extrathoracic airflow obstruction, the importance of extrathoracic obstruction should not be underestimated. Laryngeal webs, subglottic stenosis, tracheal malacia, and other lesions of the laryngeal-tracheal airway are important causes of upper airway obstruction in the pediatric population. In addition, the vocal cords represent a major "choke point" to airflow. The cords may have a structural abnormality, such as nodules or granulomas, or may become edematous, as in croup. The recurrent laryngeal nerve may be damaged, resulting in inappropriate movement or paralyzed cords. These conditions are generally easy to diagnose with direct visualization of the vocal cords. Vocal cord dysfunction (VCD) may also be responsible for poor abduction (opening) of the vocal cords during inspiration. VCD has become increasingly recognized as a reason for shortness of breath and sternal chest pain, often mimicking asthma. Adolescents who are competitive athletes or exceptionally goal-oriented and children who suffer from stress-related disorders are at highest risk. Unfortunately, vocal cord dysfunction is highly variable and may only be detectable when the patient is stressed in a manner that provokes the condition. In very severe forms, "clipping" of the inspiratory loop with a completely normal expiratory loop is the classic presentation (Figure 8-9, *E*). The child may or may not sound very stridorous during inspiration. The patient may try to speak while inspiring in short, gasping sentences. More common is a completely normal-appearing child with normal expiratory

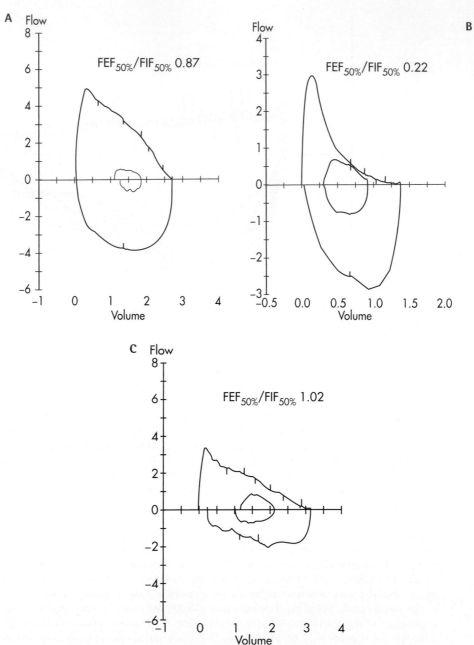

Figure 8-9 *F-V loops and FEF$_{50\%}$/FIF$_{50\%}$ ratios in various types of airflow obstruction.* **A,** Normal. **B,** Intrathoracic airflow obstruction. **C,** Fixed airflow obstruction.

Figure continued on next page.

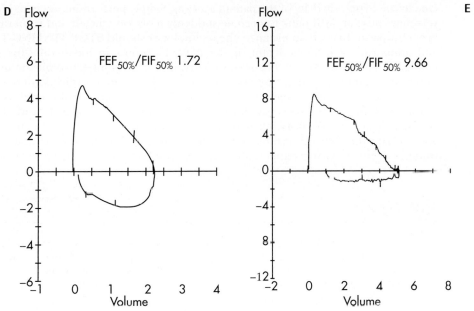

Figure 8-9—Cont'd D, Extrathoracic airflow obstruction. **E,** Extrathoracic airflow obstruction with severe clipping of the inspiratory flow pattern (see text).

loops, but highly variable inspiratory loops. Some inspiratory loops may be normal ($FEF_{50\%}/FIF_{50\%}$ <1.0); however, often many are abnormal with an $FEF_{50\%}/FIF_{50\%}$ >1.0. If the patient is challenged with exercise, cold air, or methacholine, the expiratory loops remain normal while the clipping of the inspiratory loop may become more apparent. VCD is an example of a disorder in which the variability in the patient's inspiratory loop is the hallmark of the dysfunction. This variability is associated with involuntary adduction (closing) of the vocal cords. Direct visualization of the vocal cords via a laryngoscopy (during an episode) will conclusively make the diagnosis. However, laryngoscopy may not be practical or available, and a series of well-performed F-V loops are very helpful in making this presumptive diagnosis. It should be emphasized that vocal cord dysfunction, in less-than-severe cases, is primarily a diagnosis of exclusion, and absence of inspiratory clipping on F-V loops does not rule out the diagnosis.

HOW ELSE CAN SPIROMETRY BE BENEFICIAL IN THE PEDIATRIC POPULATION?

ATS recommendations emphasize the importance of reproducibility for the FVC, FEV_1, and peak expiratory flow rate (PEFR). In some instances, patients cannot reproduce these parameters, and effort is not the reason. Figure 8-10 shows an example of such an instance. If only a single (best) F-V loop (Trial 1) were reported to the physician, the interpretation would state that this patient has mild intrathoracic airflow obstruction. However, the next three successive maneuvers that this 17-year-old asthmatic performed are also provided (Figure 8-10, Trials 2, 3, and 4). These successive trials reveal progressively significant drops in FEV_1 and FEV_1/FVC, which are not reproducible with Trial 1. This pattern is an extremely important clue to the hyperreactivity of the patient's airway. Simply performing repeated forced maneuvers may cause an asthmatic to become suddenly more obstructed and vulnerable to further bronchospasm. In such an instance, the technologist should STOP TESTING THE PATIENT and administer a bronchodilator. If the patient's report included only his best prebronchodilator and postbronchodilator spirometry, it would completely omit the most important information and may prevent necessary changes in his asthma medication regimen. An interesting but opposite phenomenon may be seen in the spirometry of a mild asthmatic. Deep inspirations may cause progressive bronchodilation with improving FEV_1 and FEV_1/FVC. This is a beneficial compensatory mechanism and is likely similar to the asthmatic athlete who is able to "run through" his asthma with bronchodilation during exercise. After exercise, tidal volumes decrease, airway temperature changes, and bronchoconstriction may be provoked.

Variability (or lack of reproducibility) in spirometric efforts may be important for identifying diseases such as asthma and vocal cord dysfunction. Reporting or displaying all flow-volume loops can assist in the data interpretation. The technologist performing the test should look for characteristic patterns of variability and include the most appropriate data in the final report.

Unusual F-V curve shapes may be very helpful in providing clues to the location of fixed or variable obstruction. However, increased variability is inherent in testing children, and may be effort- or technique-related. Conclusions based on abnormally shaped curves should be made with great care. One scenario common in pediatrics is tracheal and/or bronchial malacia. Malacia refers to one or more airways that is soft and pliable due to lack of supportive connective or cartilaginous tissue. Depending on the location (intrathoracic, extrathoracic, or both), these airways may collapse during inspiration or be compressed during exhalation.

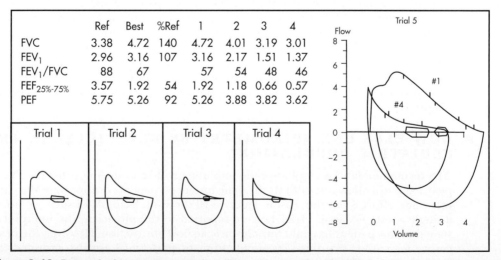

Figure 8-10 *Repeated spirometry maneuvers in a 17-year-old asthmatic patient.* Trials 2, 3, and 4 reveal progressively significant drops in FEV_1 and FEV_1/FVC that are not reproducible with Trial 1 (see text).

Some bizarre-shaped F-V curves may result. Figure 8-11 shows a 12-year-old boy who underwent double-lung transplantation. Following transplantation, he developed malacia at one of the anastomotic sites (mainstem bronchus). Curve A represents a forced exhalation that is normal in shape. Immediately following this, the patient tried to blow harder, resulting in curve B. Obtaining reproducible and acceptable F-V loops in the face of malaciac airways can be challenging. A similar phenomenon can be seen primarily in infants with malacia of the upper trachea. This condition can produce significant stridor and clipping of inspiratory loops. F-V loops that are abnormal in one phase of the breathing cycle are referred to as variable intrathoracic or variable extrathoracic obstructions (see Chapter 2). If the obstruction appears on both inspiration and expiration, it is termed a fixed obstruction and is more likely a structural abnormality. Figure 8-12 is the F-V loop of a 13-year-old child who developed tracheal stenosis following prolonged intubation. The square-wave nature of the loop with flow limitation evident even from the peak flow measurement is characteristic of fixed obstruction.

■ CHALLENGE OR PROVOCATION SPIROMETRY

As with adults, children can be exposed to a variety of inhaled, ingested, or topically applied substances to challenge the airways. The purpose of any challenge study is to identify and/or stage the level of airway hyperreactivity (see Chapter 9). Examples of conditions that cause

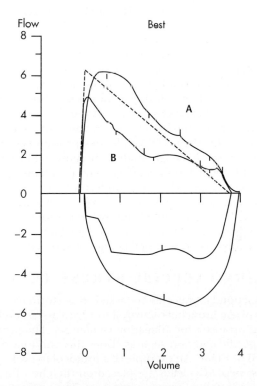

Figure 8-11 *F-V loops from a 12-year-old boy after double-lung transplantation.* Following transplantation, the patient developed malacia at one of the anastomotic sites *(mainstem bronchus).* **A,** F-V loop shows a forced exhalation that is normal in shape. **B,** F-V loop immediately following, in which the patient tried to blow harder (see text). The predicted F-V curve is also shown *(dotted line).*

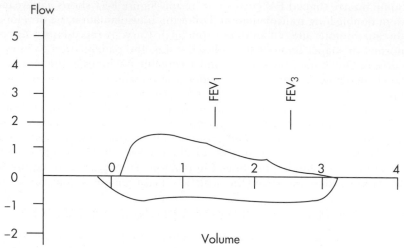

Figure 8–12 *Flow-volume loop of a 13-year-old child who developed tracheal stenosis following a prolonged intubation* (see text).

bronchoconstriction in children are asthma, gastroesophageal reflux, and anaphylactic reactions. Airway hyperreactivity may range from a very mild condition that produces only intermittent cough to sudden death from status asthmaticus or life-threatening anaphylaxis. Therefore, it can be very important to identify if a child is reactive to a substance, or to stage the level of reactivity. Examples of provocative agents include methacholine, histamine, adenosine, cold air, hyperventilation, aspirin, latex, and others. The mechanism of the bronchoconstriction may differ with the agent administered; however, serial spirometry at specified time intervals and close observation of the child is required. Specific protocols for each type of challenge should be established by the pulmonary laboratory and approved by the medical director. The 1999 ATS Guidelines provide specific recommendations for methacholine and exercise challenge studies. Because children can become fatigued or easily distracted with prolonged testing, abbreviated protocols have been published. It is also possible to perform challenges on young children who cannot perform spirometry. This requires very close monitoring of breath sounds, oxygen saturation, respiratory rate, and symptoms. Challenges in pediatric patients are not recommended in any facility unfamiliar or inexperienced with children. Immediate physician availability and a fully stocked emergency cart are also essential. Patient safety and well-being are always the number-one priority.

■ PULMONARY EXERCISE STRESS TESTING

Pulmonary function laboratories are asked to perform exercise stress tests for two main reasons: (1) to provoke bronchoreactivity and (2) to assess level of fitness. Protocols for exercise are as varied as protocols for inhalation challenges. The protocol used is often geared toward answering a specific question such as "Does this child have exercise-induced bronchospasm or asthma (EIB or EIA)?" An example of a protocol to evoke EIB includes preexercise spirometry as the first step. ECG leads are placed on the chest for heart rate assessment, and pulse oximetry is used to follow oxygen saturation. The patient performs a "free run" on a treadmill, with nose clips in place, but without a mouthpiece. Jogging on a treadmill is the most "asthmagenic" exercise because it mimics natural exercise and uses many muscle groups. This protocol also permits the technologist to watch and listen to the child without a mouthpiece in place. Evaluation of hyperventilation and/or stridorous respirations can be made. Vocal cord dysfunction (VCD) is very common in children during exercise. Several of the symptoms manifested (i.e., intense shortness of breath and sternal chest pain) are also symptoms of asthma. The speed and elevation of the treadmill are increased every minute to increase the patient's heart rate to a sustained 180 beats/min or higher for approximately 3 to 4 minutes. The entire exercise study should take no more than 8 to 9 minutes and should end abruptly without a cool-down period. Postexercise spirometry is performed every 3 to 5 minutes until 20 minutes after exercise. Laboratories differ as to the parameter and percent decrease needed to signify EIB. A decrease in the FEV_1 of at least 15% to 20% associated with a decreased FEV_1/FVC is considered diagnostic of EIB. Maximal bronchoconstriction most often occurs 6 to 12 minutes after exercise. Cough, desaturation, and worsening shortness of breath usually accompany changes in pulmonary function. A decrease in flow immediately after exercise with a quick return to normal is suspect and may be effort-related. Children who exhibit vocal cord dysfunction tend to recover very quickly after the stress of exercise, although abnormal inspiratory flows may persist.

Protocols for exercise stress tests may vary according to the patient being studied and the indication for testing.

The indication for a maximal cardiopulmonary exercise test is to evaluate how well the respiratory and cardiovascular systems work together. The clinical question asked is often whether the child has normal exercise tolerance. If not, is the child limited by the lungs (ventilatory limitation), the heart (cardiovascular limitation), or both? Maximal tests are performed with a full 12-lead EKG, pulse oximetry, and a mouthpiece in place to measure ventilation, oxygen consumption, and carbon dioxide production (See Chapter 7 for a detailed discussion of indications, protocols, analysis, etc.). Use of an ergometer versus a treadmill may be a laboratory preference. Maximal oxygen consumption is usually slightly higher on a treadmill. The advantage of an ergometer, however, is that the child is relatively still, using legs only. This decreases movement of head and leaks around the mouthpiece. Pulse oximetry is often problematic during exercise. In general, there are fewer artifacts with less body motion. The disadvantages of cycle ergometry in children are (1) modifying the equipment to fit the child, (2) keeping the child cycling consistently, and (3) obtaining true maximal oxygen consumption. Children may simply stop cycling when they feel fatigued. Unless a plateau in oxygen consumption ($\dot{V}o_2$) can be identified, the highest level reached is termed *peak oxygen consumption.*

Lung Volumes

Lung volume measurements in the pediatric population are extremely valuable, and often reveal information not obtained from spirometry only. Not all children need lung volume determination. It is preferable that the child be comfortable performing spirometry before attempting lung volumes, but many children adapt easily to a new test situation. The choice of techniques for measuring lung volume is similar to that with adults. Lung volume determination via gas dilution techniques often underestimates lung volumes in patients with obstructive airway disease. This problem becomes even more relevant in the pediatric population because the size of the airway is smaller and easier to obstruct. Helium dilution and/or nitrogen washout may not be as well tolerated as body plethysmography. Problems with keeping a mouth seal and breathing a dry gas for several minutes make these techniques less desirable. Conversely, a child who performs even less than optimal spirometry may "jump" into the body box and pant appropriately. Many commercial body plethysmographs require minimal effort in determining thoracic gas volume (V_{TG}). Vigorous panting is no longer required to obtain V_{TG}. With most systems, limited panting or only tidal breathing is necessary. Some commercial systems permit the technologist to alter the timing of the panting to minimize patient discomfort. Technical advances in body plethysmography, the ease and versatility of making measurements, and the accuracy of the measurement make this technique the preferred choice for lung volumes in pediatric patients. A detailed description of the functioning of a body plethysmograph is included in Chapter 3.

Versatility and accuracy of commercially available body plethysmographs make this method of lung volume determination the preferred technique, even in young patients.

WHAT IS THE FIRST STEP?

The first step in performing plethysmography in the pediatric population is getting the child into the body box. This is usually not a major obstacle. In many cases, the child has been to the pulmonary function laboratory on previous occasions and is familiar with the environment and personnel. The child often asks, "What's that?" This becomes an opportunity to appeal to the child's imagination. A body box, in a child's eye, can be a spaceship or Cinderella's coach. Sometimes the child only sits in the body box on the first or second visit, but ultimately this is a valuable experience. It may be possible to have the parent also sit in the body box and perform some testing until the child feels comfortable alone. The instructions should be kept simple and be demonstrated to the child. In many instances, the child will perform adequately without the need to modify instructions. Too many instructions can lead to confusion. A fitted mouthpiece and nose clips are required for testing in the body box. Some technologists suggest supporting the cheeks during the test. It may be preferable not to hold the cheeks. This may cause the child to raise his or her shoulders and not breathe at a true resting level. The child should sit up straight with hands relaxed in the lap. The instructions can be modified if the child pouches his cheeks, producing open loops rather than closed loops during panting. Although newer body boxes vent to the atmosphere, the door should be opened periodically to let the child rest and converse with the technologist or parent. Children requiring oxygen should also be given a break between trials to replace their cannula or mask until their oxygenation is back to baseline.

WHAT PLETHYSMOGRAPHIC PARAMETERS ARE MOST IMPORTANT?

The tests performed and parameters examined depend on the reason for performing the study, and on the ability of the child. In very young children, obtaining a stable resting level and reproducible FRC may be all that can be accomplished. Once spirometry is mastered, the child can quickly learn to perform a full IC and VC in the body box. A skilled technologist and user-friendly software allow data to be manipulated or edited to provide TLC, FRC, RV, and RV/TLC. It is important that the technologist understand when and how to average data versus deleting data, and when to accept the "best test" data. This is especially true with pediatric patients who may not reproduce the entire maneuver with each trial.

Although spirometry is the first test performed in many patients, spirometry alone may not accurately predict lung volumes in children. Figure 8-13, *A* to *C* shows case presentations of obstructive and restrictive lung disease, as well as a mixed presentation. The case in Figure 8-13, *A* is a 15-year-old boy with advanced cystic fibrosis. Severe obstruction is evident in the spirometry data. Both FEV_1 and FEV_1/FVC are reduced consistent with an obstructive disorder. Lung volume measurements confirm the severity of obstruction and air trapping. Although the TLC is within normal limits, FRC, RV, and RV/TLC are significantly elevated. Compare these findings with the spirometry and lung volumes in Figure 8-13, *B.* This case is a 13-year-old girl with scoliosis. Her pulmonary function results represent a restrictive defect. FVC and FEV_1 are reduced in a symmetrical pattern; however, the ratio is normal. Restrictive disorders often present with a normal or elevated FEV_1/FVC. The lung volume measurements are also consistent with a pure restrictive defect, showing reduced volumes (TLC, FRC, RV, ERV) and a normal RV/TLC.

Many pediatric and adult diseases do not present as a purely obstructive or restrictive process, but as a combination of obstruction and restriction. The case in Figure 8-13, *C* is a 21-year-old woman recovering from histiocytosis (eosinophilic granuloma). Some elements of her pulmonary function study point to an obstructive component, whereas others are consistent with restriction. Her spirometry reveals a severely reduced FVC, FEV_1, and reduced FEV_1/FVC, all indicative of airflow obstruction. Her lung volumes reveal a reduced TLC, however, consistent with restrictive lung disease. The combination of an obstructive pattern on spirometry and a reduced total lung capacity is usually associated with air trapping, or elevated RV/TLC. This pattern is the hallmark of a mixed obstructive and restrictive disorder.

A

Spirometry		Pred	Pre-Rx Best	%Pred
FVC	Liters	3.42	1.11	32
FEV$_1$	Liters	3.01	0.62	21
FEV$_1$/FVC	%	88%	56%	
FEF$_{25\%-75\%}$	L/sec	3.42	0.21	6
PEF	L/sec	5.99	2.07	35
FET100%	Sec		9.2	
Lung volumes				
VC	Liters	3.42	1.11	33
TLC	Liters	4.45	4.83	109
FRC PL	Liters	2.19	3.88	177
RV	Liters	1.01	3.72	368
RV/TLC	%	24%	77%	
IC	Liters		0.95	
ERV	Liters		0.14	

Figure 8-13 *Pulmonary function studies in obstruction, restriction, and mixed disease.* **A,** Data from a 15-year-old boy with advanced cystic fibrosis.

Figure continued on next page.

B *Spirometry*

		Pred	Pre-Rx Best	%Pred
FVC	Liters	3.98	2.47	62
FEV$_1$	Liters	3.82	2.16	57
FEV$_1$/FVC	%	86%	87%	
FEF$_{25\%-75\%}$	L/sec	4.21	2.74	65
PEF	L/sec	6.71	5.45	81
FET100%	Sec			

Lung volumes

		Pred	Best	%Pred
VC	Liters	3.98	2.62	66
TLC	Liters	5.21	3.31	64
FRC PL	Liters	2.47	1.66	67
RV	Liters	1.08	0.69	64
RV/TLC	%	21%	21%	
IC	Liters		1.65	
ERV	Liters		0.97	

C *Spirometry*

		Pred	Pre-Rx Best	%Pred	Post-Rx Best	%Pred	%Chg
FVC	Liters	3.89	1.81	47	1.91	49	6
FEV$_1$	Liters	3.15	1.14	36	1.16	37	2
FEV$_1$/FVC	%	81%	63%		61%		
FEF$_{25\%-75\%}$	L/sec	3.7	0.61	16	0.58	16	−5
PEF	L/sec	7.22	3.33	46	3.39	47	2
FET100%	Sec		7.32		8.11		

Lung volumes

		Pred	Best	%Pred
VC	Liters	3.89	1.87	48
TLC	Liters	5.01	3.63	72
FRC PL	Liters	2.96	2.52	85
RV	Liters	1.41	1.76	125
RV/TLC	%	27%	48%	
IC	Liters		1.11	
ERV	Liters		0.66	

Diffusion capacity

		Pred	Best	%Pred
DL$_{CO}$	ml/mm Hg/min	27.1	4.1	15
D$_L$ Adj	ml/mm Hg/min	27.1	4.2	16
DL$_{CO}$/V$_A$	ml/mm Hg/min	6.41	1.4	22
V$_A$	ml/mm Hg/min		2.84	

Figure 8-13—Cont'd **B,** Data from a 13-year-old girl with scoliosis. **C,** Data from a 21-year-old woman recovering from histiocytosis (See text for complete descriptions of each case).

Are lung volumes necessary? The cases in Figure 8-13, *A* and *B* are straightforward presentations in which spirometry alone is very representative of the child's disease process. The lung volumes merely confirm the degree of airflow obstruction (Figure 8-13, *A*) and lung restriction (Figure 8-13, *B*). Mixed obstructive and restrictive disorders (Figure 8-13, *C*) definitely require lung volume determination to better define the child's lung mechanics. In addition, a seemingly restrictive pattern in spirometry may be observed in the pediatric population. Subsequent lung volumes may identify a completely normal TLC, with an elevated RV/TLC. What appears to be a restrictive process on spirometry is, indeed, an obstructive disorder once lung volumes are examined. This pattern may be seen quite often in the pediatric population because of the relatively smaller size of intrathoracic airways. Airflow obstruction in these small peripheral airways may occur early in the course of respiratory disorders, leading to significant air trapping in the pediatric lung.

■ DOES MEASUREMENT OF AIRWAY RESISTANCE PLAY A ROLE?

Depending on the equipment and software being used, measurement of airway resistance during plethysmography may be an option. Airway resistance (Raw) is measured while having the patient pant prior to closing a shutter or valve to obtain the thoracic gas volume (V_{TG}). Patients, including children, have a tendency to pant at an elevated lung volume. In other words, they do not return to the resting expiratory level with every pant, and progressively increase their chest volume. If V_{TG} is measured at the very end of the maneuver, it will be artificially elevated. Although this is not the patient's true FRC, the application software makes a correction and reports separate values for V_{TG} and FRC. Raw should always be reported and interpreted at the lung volume at which it was measured (i.e., using V_{TG} to calculate specific airway resistance and specific conductance). Except in trained patients, Raw tends to be less reproducible than other pulmonary function parameters. Measurement of Raw complicates and prolongs the test, and may not be necessary for routine testing. However, Raw can be significantly increased in patients with central airway intrathoracic obstruction, as well as in extrathoracic obstruction. Many laboratories find measurement of Raw, specific airway resistance (SRaw), and specific conductance (SGaw) very helpful during methacholine challenges. Because the variability of these measurements is greater, a greater change is required to meet clinical significance. Whereas a decrease of 20% in FEV_1 is considered a positive response to methacholine, a corresponding increase of 35% to 40% in Raw is required. The measurement of Raw may be a more sensitive test and may identify changes in airflow earlier in the challenge.

Diffusion Capacity

The DL_{CO} in the pediatric population can be a very important indicator of gas transport difficulties at the alveolar level. This may be due to problems with perfusion of the pulmonary capillary bed, bleeding within the lung, or thickening of the alveolocapillary membrane. Several serious pediatric disorders fall into these categories, and the DL_{CO} may provide an answer to a very specific question. Examples of pediatric pulmonary diseases that may produce a reduced DL_{CO} include pulmonary fibrosis (primary disease or secondary to radiation treatment or chemotherapy), immunologic disorders (scleroderma, systemic lupus erythematosis), bronchiolitis obliterans, pulmonary edema, and hematologic disorders. An abnormally high DL_{CO} may be seen in acute hemorrhagenous bleeds, as in pulmonary vasculitis. The single-breath DL_{CO} (DL_{CO}sb) is the most common method utilized for assessing diffusion capacity. The problems already discussed in performing pulmonary function studies in the pediatric patient are compounded for this particular test. However, the guidelines and recommendations offered by the ATS for DL_{CO} testing in adults are also applicable to pediatrics (see Chapter 5). The single-breath maneuver is difficult for very small children to perform, and often requires several sessions of practice. Even older children may have difficulty accomplishing the important components of the DL_{CO} maneuver. These components include emptying to RV prior to a deep inspiration, obtaining an IVC of at least 90% of FVC, a relaxed 10-second breath hold, and a smooth, complete exhalation. In addition, other technical considerations may alter results, such as inappropriate mechanical or anatomic dead space corrections. Depending on the system used, if end-tidal gas is collected in a sample bag, the bag should be an appropriate size for pediatric patients. Similarly, if a demand value is used for inspiration of test gas, the triggering mechanism should be sensitive enough to be opened easily by a child. Some commercial systems also provide an option for a slow exhalation against a resistor in place of the breath hold. The advantage of this technique is that a breath hold is not necessary; however, a target flow for exhaled gas must be maintained. Unfortunately, children who cannot perform a breath hold are generally not able to perform this technique well.

Other confounders that alter the measurement of DL_{CO} are abnormal levels of hemoglobin and the presence of carboxyhemoglobin (COHb). Children who require repeated DL_{CO} measurements may have conditions that cause anemia (e.g., chemotherapy, sickle cell disease, transplantations). Correction of DL_{CO} for hemoglobin is essential (see Chapter 5). It should not be assumed that pediatric patients do not smoke. Older teenagers should be asked if they smoke and told honestly that smoking may affect the results of the test. If the patient has been smoking prior to testing, a COHb level can be obtained to correct for carbon monoxide already present in the circulating blood.

As with adults, diffusion capacity is dependent on the size of the lungs. An estimation of lung size known as the V_A (alveolar volume) is also made during the single-breath maneuver. In addition to carbon monoxide, the test gas also contains an inert gas such as helium, methane, or neon that is used to estimate V_A by a dilution method. As with all gas dilution techniques, V_A will be increasingly underestimated as airflow obstruction worsens. The case in Figure 8-13, C includes the DL_{CO}. This young woman has a severely reduced raw DL_{CO}, corrected DL_{CO}, and DL/V_A. This is consistent with the diffusion block and fibrotic interstitial space associated with severe histiocytosis. V_A is also significantly less than TLC, supporting further the obstructive defect in her lung.

WHAT OTHER PULMONARY FUNCTION PARAMETERS ARE MEASURED AND CLINICALLY FOLLOWED IN PEDIATRICS?

Maximal Respiratory Pressures

Measurement of muscle strength can be a very important parameter in the pediatric population. Children suffer from a variety of congenital and acquired neuromuscular disorders and thoracic deformities that reduce the strength of the diaphragm and intercostal muscles. Examples of neuromuscular diseases include, but are not limited to, muscular dystrophies, spinal muscle atrophy, meningomyeloceles, Guillian-Barré syndrome, myasthenia gravis, trauma-related paralysis, and steroid-induced myopathies. Thoracic deformities include scoliosis, kyphoscoliosis, pectus excavatum or carinatum, and undefined congenital syndrome abnormalities. Measuring maximal inspiratory pressure (MIP) and maximal expiratory pressure (MEP) may help (1) identify the degree of weakness and (2) follow the progression of the specific disorder. See Chapter 2 for a discussion of the technique for performing MIP and

MEP. This test can be very scary for children. The patient and parent should be gently warned that the measurement of the MIP might be uncomfortable and cause the child to cry. For this reason, this test should be performed after all other measurements are made. In children, it may be necessary to attach a mask and one-way valve to the pressure manometer and apply the mask snugly to the child's face. It may also be necessary to hold the mask in place until the child becomes "air hungry" and feels a need to gasp for air. It is understandable why this test is so unpopular with children. A similar measurement of spontaneous inspiratory strength may be made while a child is being mechanically ventilated, and this parameter is often referred to as the negative inspiratory force (NIF). While the measurement of inspiratory strength may ultimately be involuntary, the expiratory strength measurement (MEP) is completely effort dependent. The child cannot be forced to push as hard as possible unless he or she chooses to do so. For this reason, MEP results should be viewed cautiously. Although predicted values are available for MIP and MEP, a single measurement in time may be difficult to interpret. Rather, trending serial measurements often provides information that is more useful once the child is accustomed to the test.

Maximal Voluntary Ventilation

In a cooperative and inspired child, the maximal voluntary ventilation (MVV) can be a very useful measure of muscle strength, as well as maximal ventilation (see Chapter 2). If the child has significant muscle weakness, he or she may not be able to sustain maximal ventilation for the required 12 seconds. In this case, comparing the MVV for 6 seconds with that of 12 seconds may explain the disparity. The MVV may also be used prior to a maximal exercise test to identify the maximal level of ventilation of which the child is capable. Ventilatory limitation during exercise can be identified by comparing the minute ventilation at maximal oxygen consumption to the MVV obtained prior to exercise.

Arterial Blood Gases

An arterial blood gas is sometimes considered the most important measurement of pulmonary function. Regardless of what spirometry, lung volumes, or DL_{CO} reveal, PaO_2 and $PaCO_2$ ultimately signify how well the lungs are performing. Arterial blood gases in children are, for obvious reasons, not popular. Pediatricians tend not to order blood gas analysis as frequently as physicians who treat adults because of the trauma of drawing arterial blood. Pulse oximetry can often be substituted for a blood gas for oxygen saturation, and a capillary blood gas obtained for PCO_2. There are definite indications, however, for obtaining arterial blood gases. Examples are (1) impending ventilatory failure, (2) prior problem with anesthesia or sedation, and (3) impending thoracic surgery in a child unable to perform routine pulmonary function tests. Children tolerate arterial punctures much better with reassurance and local anesthesia at the puncture site. The use of topical Emla cream or subcutaneous lidocaine (1%) is extremely helpful.

Infant and Toddler Pulmonary Function Testing

The challenge for diagnostic testing in infants and toddlers is their lack of comprehension of instruction. Even obtaining a value as simple as an oximetry reading may not be so simple in a crying young child or a wiggling baby. Toddlers may be capable of understanding simple instructions but can be very fearful of the hospital environment, unfamiliar faces, or strange-looking equipment. Expecting full cooperation and maximal effort is unrealistic.

Alternate methods of assessing pulmonary function have been developed. The ability to obtain forced flows and lung volume measurements remains the cornerstone of pulmonary function testing, even in the youngest patient. Modifications of technique and specialized equipment are necessary, however. Newer, less invasive methods of measuring airway resistance and airway inflammation continue to be investigated and are promising techniques for the near future.

■ HOW CAN INFANTS PERFORM PULMONARY FUNCTION TESTING?

Newborn babies and older infants are not capable of following directions needed to perform conscious pulmonary function tests. Placing a mask on an infant is usually not tolerated, and results in a screaming baby. Even an infant who permits a mask over his nose and mouth invariably changes his breathing pattern (i.e., volume and frequency of breathing). Only premature babies and very young newborns will tolerate a mask while sleeping. In these specific and rare instances, it may be possible to assess passive tidal breathing mechanics. More sophisticated pulmonary function tests that measure lung volumes and forced flows require the infant to be in a quiet sleep, fully relaxed, and spontaneously breathing. To accomplish this state of sleep and cooperation, the infant must be sedated.

■ WHAT TYPE OF SEDATION IS APPROPRIATE?

Sedation of infants and toddlers is a common practice in pediatric hospitals because many procedures require a calm, motionless child. Procedures and protocols for sedation of children that follow the Joint Commission on Accreditation of Healthcare Organizations (JCAHO) guidelines are usually established by the hospital anesthesia department (see Appendix D). It is essential that established procedures be closely observed for the protection of the child, the pulmonary laboratory, and the hospital. The sedating agent chosen, the personnel needed, and the required recovery time all depend on the extent of testing needed and patient history. A very straightforward test in an uncomplicated infant can be safely performed by laboratory personnel with the use of a conscious sedating agent, such as chloral hydrate. At the other end of the spectrum may be an infant with an unstable airway, severe pulmonary compromise, or other organ complications. This scenario warrants an anesthesiologist and sedation nurse in addition to the technologist performing the study. Chloral hydrate is probably the safest and easiest sedating medication to administer, although several other agents are available with the current armamentarium of drugs. The advantages of chloral hydrate are that it is usually administered orally, does not necessarily require a nurse or physician, and is a conscious sedating agent. This implies that the child can be roused from sleep with stimulation. The major disadvantage is that a large dose of a very unpleasant medicine must be swallowed. Vomiting, crying, and upset stomachs are not unusual side effects. Nevertheless, chloral hydrate works very well in the majority of cases. IV narcotics, such as pentobarbital or secobarbital, need to administered and monitored by a sedation nurse. The advantage of IV medications is that intravenous access is available if needed, and the medication can be titrated to the child's need. Additional options include ketamine and propofol. Both of these require a physician, and possibly an anesthesiologist, to administer. The rapid onset of action and quick recovery make these attractive sedating agents, but also require close monitoring for apnea. Regardless of the agent chosen, safety is the primary concern. The child must be closely monitored throughout the entire procedure, including recovery, and written documentation of the sedation procedure placed in the patient's record. A fully stocked crash cart should be close at hand, and a resuscitation bag and mask on the patient's bed. Loss of a patent airway is always possible with any sedating agent. It is also extremely important to remember that sleep induced with sedation is *not* natural sleep. Changes in respiratory pattern, depth of respiration, and breathing rate should be noted. Interpretation of infant pulmonary function tests should also be made with the level of sedation in mind.

Sedated sleep in infants is *never* natural sleep, and respiratory measurements made during sedated sleep may be influenced by the altered sleep state.

WHAT PURPOSE IS SERVED BY PERFORMING INFANT PULMONARY FUNCTION TESTS?

Infant pulmonary function tests provide important data regarding growth of the lungs, identification of airflow obstruction, progression of a disease state, and response to therapeutic interventions. Infant pulmonary function tests require a significant time commitment, and competent and patient technologists. Sedation carries some risk, and testing should not be viewed as routine. Commercially available equipment typically uses the most technically advanced flow sensors and analyzers and may be very expensive for a pulmonary laboratory to purchase. Prior to pursuing this type of testing, the laboratory should thoroughly evaluate its expectations, goals, and resources available to perform quality testing.

Lung Volumes

As with measurement of lung volumes in adults, the lung volume compartments in the infant can be measured by several techniques, including gas dilution and whole-body plethysmography. Until recently, body plethysmography in infants was performed almost exclusively by infant pulmonary research laboratories. Only a few manufacturers produce commercially available body boxes for infants (Figure 8-14). Whole-body plethysmography in an infant presents a unique set of challenges. The theory and technical aspects of measuring V_{TG}, previously discussed in Chapter 3, are essentially the same for adults and infants, but with several additional caveats. The infant is placed in a supine position with nose and mouth surrounded by a tight-fitting mask with a small dead space volume. Rapid-moving valves may make airway occlusions at end-inspiration or end-expiration for determination of V_{TG} and Raw. The infant does not pant. However, tidal breaths may be quite shallow; therefore the pressure transducers and flow sensors must be critically precise and accurate. In addition, the infant body box is relatively small, and temperature changes can drastically alter these measurements. Therefore, the temperature in the box must be controlled, and the air vented. Signal-to-noise ratios are particularly critical in an infant plethysmograph. Although the child is motionless, safety features must permit rapid access to the box and the baby. The breathing apparatus should be easily removable in case the child is in distress or vomits. The advantage of plethysmography in infants is that it accurately measures V_{TG}, and hence, FRC may be determined. Since the infant is not capable of performing a voluntary maximal inspiration or expiration, residual volume and TLC cannot be obtained in the traditional manner. However, if the infant pulmonary function system is capable of performing raised volumes and forced thoracic compressions, then a full set of fractional lung volumes can be estimated. A forced squeeze from TLC provides a volume very close to a vital capacity measurement and can be used to calculate ERV, RV, TLC, FRC/TLC, and RV/TLC.

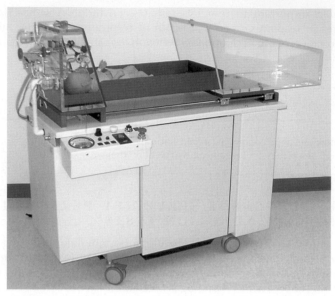

Figure 8–14 *Infant pulmonary lab (IPL).* Whole-body infant plethysmograph directly measures V_{TG} (FRC at resting level). The IPL also has the capability of obtaining passive mechanics and forced flows (partial and raised volume), and provides close estimation of fractional lung volumes (TLC, RV, RV/TLC, FRC/TLC). *(Courtesy Collins Medical [Ferraris CardioRespiratory], Toledo, Ohio.)*

Optional methods of determining lung volumes are available. These include gas equilibration techniques such as helium dilution and nitrogen washout. Although technically easier to perform, gas equilibration techniques have several disadvantages. Leaks in the systems may falsely elevate FRC. Children with intrathoracic airflow obstruction may have poor ventilation distal to obstructed airways causing an incomplete washout or equilibration, and have falsely low FRC values. Considering that infants have significantly smaller airways than older children or adults, only mild inflammation or obstruction with secretions can alter ventilation in a sedated child. Infants also have an incredible ability to adjust their FRC depending on their clinical status. Children may respond to hypoxia by dynamically elevating their FRC to create a PEEP-like effect (dynamic FRC). Grunting is a clinical sign that an infant may be hypoxic. In this situation, sedation and supplemental oxygen tend to relax a child. It is possible to see consecutive FRC measurements decrease as the child falls into a deeper sedation and static lung volume decreases to a resting FRC. Nevertheless, measurement of FRC is a very important parameter in infant pulmonary function testing. The normal FRC range is between 15 and 25 ml/kg of weight, and 2 to 3 ml/cm of length. It serves as a reference lung volume when analyzing flows or compliance. When a parameter is referenced to a lung volume such as FRC, it is termed *specific* (e.g., specific flow at FRC, specific compliance, or specific resistance).

Passive Tidal Mechanics

Many studies have examined the passive tidal loops of infants and have attempted to differentiate normal tidal loops from loops associated with airflow obstruction. Several parameters have been suggested to examine intrathoracic airflow obstructions during tidal breathing, such as t_{pef}/t_e (ratio of time to reach tidal peak flow to total expiratory time). Passive loops are highly variable. They are especially subject to changes in upper airway tone, as may be seen with sedation, or with laryngeal or diaphragmatic "braking." As mentioned previously, infants can adduct their vocal cords (grunt) during exhalation to create a physiologic PEEP. Likewise, they have the ability to modulate their diaphragms and intercostal muscles in an attempt to dynamically elevate their FRC and improve oxygenation. Therefore, the shape of tidal loops, and the parameters used to describe the shape may change from minute to minute. As with standard pulmonary function testing, passive tidal loops are not maximal maneuvers. Therefore, identification of flow limitation with forced flows is the desired measurement.

Passive Compliance, Resistance, and Time Constants

The chest wall of the infant is extremely compliant, unlike that of an adult. It does not contribute significantly to the compliance of the total respiratory system. Measuring pulmonary mechanics in the infant takes advantage of this very important difference. Noninvasive measures of respiratory system compliance, therefore, directly reflect the child's lung compliance. In simplest terms, compliance is defined as change in volume divided by change in pressure (see Chapter 2). In a quiet, relaxed baby (usually sedated), these parameters can be measured quite easily. The method is referred to as *the passive occlusion technique*. Rapid occlusion of the airway may occur once (single occlusion) at the end of a tidal breath, or with multiple occlusions at different lung volumes. Young infants will hold their breath when their airway is occluded. This phenomenon is known as the Hering-Breuer reflex and is present in children until approximately 1 year of age. During this occlusion and breath hold, alveolar pressure equalizes and can be measured by a pressure transducer at the airway opening (mouth). Once the occlusion valve opens, the child can passively exhale, and the exhaled volume is measured by a flow sensor. The two components of lung compliance, change in alveolar pressure and change in volume, are obtained. Airway resistance (Raw) can be easily calculated from the same maneuver. Raw is defined as change in driving pressure divided by flow. With the maneuver described, the driving pressure is the peak airway (alveolar) pressure developed during the occlusion, and the flow is the peak flow. Figure 8-15, *A* shows an infant's passive tidal exhalation after an airway occlusion. The slope of the curve is linear as the baby exhales to a relaxed FRC. Children with airflow obstruction do not empty their lungs at a constant rate. The expiration may be forced with paradoxical movement of the diaphragm and belly. The accuracy of compliance and airway resistance measurements made under these conditions is poor. The exhaled curve will appear very "scooped out" or curvilinear, and may end abruptly with the child at an elevated FRC. Figure 8-15, *B* shows a lung with multiple time constants, meaning that the lungs do not empty homogeneously or uniformly. The term *time constant* is defined as compliance × resistance and can be easily calculated from the parameters above. Since compliance and airway resistance are both dependent on the lung volume at which they are measured, it is important to correct these measured parameters by the infant's FRC.

PF Tips

Diameter of the airway is an important determinant of flow. Inflammation and/or secretions in the airways of a young child can cause significant intrathoracic obstruction and profound clinical symptoms.

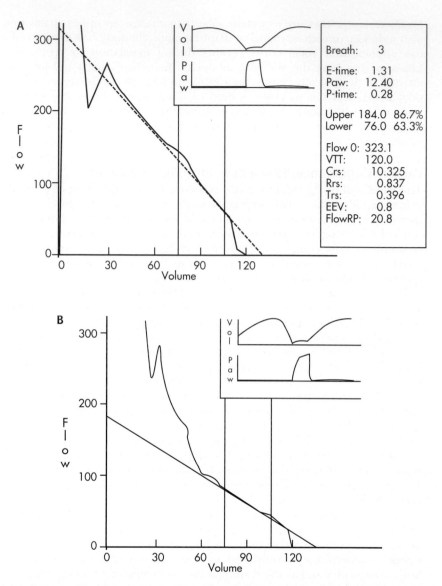

Figure 8-15 *Passive exhalation mechanics in infants.* **A,** An infant's passive tidal exhalation after an airway occlusion. The slope of the curve is linear, and the infant exhales to a relaxed FRC. **B,** Passive tidal exhalation showing a lung with multiple time constants, meaning that the lung does not empty homogeneously (see text).

Dividing the raw compliance or airway resistance measurement by the FRC yields specific compliance and specific airway resistance.

Compliance in infants can also be determined by other methods, including insertion of an esophageal catheter or by weighted spirometry. Although inserting an esophageal catheter into an infant is usually not difficult, it is invasive, and the exact placement of the catheter may affect measurements. In addition, distortion of pleural pressure in children with airflow obstruction causes associated artifactual changes, yielding inaccurate compliance values. Under ideal circumstances, when accurate pleural pressures are measured, total respiratory system compliance can be subdivided into the chest wall and lung compliance components.

Intubated and ventilated children represent an additional challenge when assessing pulmonary mechanics. Several of the parameters discussed can also be obtained in babies on ventilators; however, several technical and mechanical problems must be considered. The endotracheal tube represents a resistor, and can limit flow and alter pressure readings at the airway opening. Endotracheal tubes in infants are generally uncuffed, and leaks around the tubes are common. Secretions in the endotracheal tube and water condensation in the tubing easily clog pneumotachometers. Ventilators offer a variety of operational modes, such as pressure or volume control, IMV or SIMV, and pressure support. Depending on the mode chosen, auxiliary flow through the ventilator circuit will result in inaccurate flow measurements at the child's airway. Children on ventilators are often sedated, and passive mechanics are dependent on the sleep state. For all the reasons stated, pulmonary mechanics on ventilated children should only be done by experienced technologists who are familiar with the child and the ventilator. In addition, measurements made under artificial conditions (ventilator, PEEP, etc.) do not necessary reflect the infant's own lung mechanics when not ventilated.

Partial Expiratory Flow–Volume (PEFV) Curves

Flow is related to the volume of air in the chest during the forced exhalation. Stated simply, the larger the volume, the faster the flow. The advantage and reason for spirometry's reproducibility is that it is performed from TLC with every maneuver. With reasonable effort, exhaled flows and volumes are quite reproducible. However, if the patient does not inhale to TLC, significant variability in flows and volumes will be observed. This is a very common problem in young children ages 3 to 6 years. If inspiratory capacity is altered, traditional spirometric measurements (FVC, FEV1, PEFR) are not reproducible. Forced flows in very young children are not without merit. However, it is necessary to relate these flows to a lung volume that the child can reproduce. This can be accomplished if the child is able to breathe quietly and relaxed for several breaths. Most important, if he or she returns to a stable resting level with each exhalation, then this relaxed resting level represents the child's FRC. It is not necessary to measure FRC; rather, it represents a reference point (static lung volume) to which flow can then be related. After several tidal breaths, the child is asked to take a slightly deeper breath in and blow out as hard and long as possible. It does not matter how deep the breath is, but the forced exhalation has to extend beyond the FRC point from the previous tidal breaths. Once the FRC point is identified, the flow corresponding to that point is then recorded. Because FRC is approximately 40% of TLC, flows at this relatively low lung volume correspond to flows such as $FEF_{25\%-75\%}$, $FEF_{50\%}$, and $FEF_{75\%}$ seen in standard spirometry. These flow rates are only as reproducible as the resting level FRC. If the child's tidal loops are highly variable, a stable FRC cannot be identified. The corresponding flow at FRC will not be reproducible in such instances. An additional confounding factor is the lack of predicted values for partial forced flows in the toddler age range. The technique may be of value in a cooperative child when assessing response to bronchodilator therapy or performing a methacholine challenge.

The technique of performing partial forced F-V curves is used much more commonly in the sedated infant. The principle is similar to that described previously, but the child's chest is mechanically squeezed (or "hugged") by an inflatable jacket that surrounds the chest.

The technique is referred to as rapid thoracoabdominal compression (RTC). The flows that are generated are maximal flows from within tidal range (partial forced flows). They are measured by a flow sensor (usually a pneumotachometer) attached to a mask placed on the infant's face. The lung volume that can be identified and referenced is the FRC; therefore, the flow is referred to as flow at FRC or $\dot{V}_{max}$ FRC. Figure 8-16, A shows the point identified as FRC on the volume axis of an F-V curve. As with the partial forced flows, this point can be easily identified. The flow at that point represents the $\dot{V}_{max}$ FRC. It is important that several tidal loops are observed prior to the hugging maneuver to ensure that the infant returns with each breath to a stable resting level, or FRC. The RTCs are done at progressively higher pressures until maximal flow at FRC from the child is attained. The pressures are generated from a large air reservoir connected to the hugging bag. The pressure within the hugging bag usually does not exceed 100 cm H_2O. A significantly lower pressure is transmitted across the chest wall to the lung tissue. With progressively higher hugging pressures, flow at FRC increases until flow limitation is reached. At this point, higher hugging pressures do not yield higher flows, and flow at FRC may in fact decrease. Reaching flow limitation while doing these maneuvers is a very important concept, and is somewhat controversial. Because infants grow (length and weight) at such different rates and because males differ from females, the question of whether flow limitation is achieved with partial forced flows often arises. This question is especially difficult in infants with normal lung function. The problem is complicated when trying to identify normal flows for any particular child. Several infant research centers have published a collaborative study combining data from normal infants, but technique-related differences still exist. It is recommended that PFT labs performing infant studies test a group of infants without respiratory difficulties to confirm that the normal values obtained concur with published reference normals. Although this type of comparison is desirable, some hospital internal review boards may not permit sedation of infants for collection of normative data. Another method of standardizing flow is to compare maximal flow at FRC with the actual FRC measured. This parameter is known as the specific flow at FRC ($S\dot{V}_{max}$FRC or $\dot{V}_{max}$FRC/FRC). As discussed, FRC serves as static measured reference volume. Because flow increases with higher volumes, a fixed relationship or constant value, independent of age or height, can be determined for flow at that volume. This constant value is termed *specific flow*, and normal specific flow should equal or exceed 1.20.

PF Tips

Infant growth and development is highly variable. Since pulmonary function parameters, such as flow rates, compliance, and resistance, are directly related to lung volume, a method to standardize these parameters is recommended. The infant's measured FRC may be used to "volume correct" each parameter (e.g., specific flow at FRC).

Figure 8-16, A shows the flow curve of a child with a $\dot{V}_{max}$FRC of 440 ml/sec and an $S\dot{V}_{max}$FRC of 1.63. The specific flow at FRC was obtained by dividing the child's $\dot{V}_{max}$FRC of 440 ml/sec by the previously measured FRC of 270 ml.

Forced Flows from Raised Lung Volume

Success in standardization of spirometry has been dependent on the patient inspiring to total lung capacity (TLC) prior to performing a maximal expiration. This is the key to

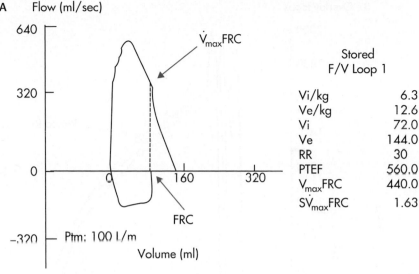

Figure 8-16 *Rapid thoracoabdominal compression (RTC) in infants.* **A,** Flow-volume curve (RTC) of a child with a $\dot{V}_{max}$ FRC of 440 ml/sec and an $S\dot{V}_{max}$ FRC of 1.63. The specific flow at FRC was obtained by dividing the child's $\dot{V}_{max}$ FRC of 440 ml/sec by the previously measured FRC of 270 ml.

Figure continued on next page

standardization in infants as well. Techniques have been developed to raise the volume of the infant's lungs prior to forced exhalation. This may be accomplished by stacking inspirations or by a method known as the raised volume technique. For this maneuver, a bias flow of air is provided to the child during inspiration. The exhalation port is simultaneously occluded, raising the intrathoracic pressure and volume in the child's lungs. A pressure of −30 cm H_2O is required to inflate the infant's lung to near TLC. Once inflated, the child is then permitted to passively exhale. After several cycles of inflation and deflation, the child's Pco_2 decreases, relaxing the child further. The final inflation is then followed by a forced compression from the inflatable jacket. The maneuver is repeated at increasingly higher jacket pressure until expired volume and flows at mid-lung volumes maximize. The advantage of this method compared with partial forced flows is that the expired volume is nearly an FVC measurement. The traditional FEV_1 is not measured because the infant reaches residual volume before 1 second of exhalation occurs. However, the volume expired in 0.5 sec or 0.75 sec can be calculated, and is analogous to the FEV_1 in standard spirometry. Figure 8-16, *B* shows several F-V curves obtained after rapid thoracic compressions (from raised lung volume) superimposed. Progressively higher squeeze pressures do not yield higher flows or volumes, indicating that flow limitation has been met. In addition, a partial F-V curve (from a lower lung volume) is superimposed in the diagram.

Forced Deflation Technique
As with the RTC technique, forced deflations also produce maximal expiratory F-V curves (MEFV). The method, however, is exactly opposite to the positive pressure generated during the RTC method. Instead, a negative pressure is applied to the airway opening and the lungs are deflated quickly. This technique is usually reserved for intubated infants in a critical care setting and performed by technologists and physicians familiar with its possible complications.

B Overlay loops

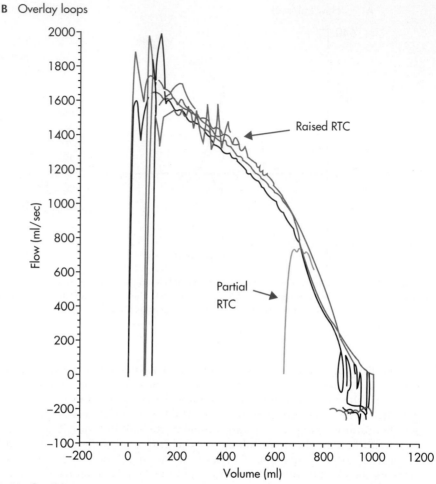

Figure 8–16—Cont'd B, Raised lung volume RTC. F-V curves obtained after rapid thoracic compressions (from raised lung volume) are superimposed. Progressively higher squeeze pressures do not yield higher flows or volumes, indicating that flow limitation has been met. In addition, a partial F-V curve (from a lower lung volume) is superimposed in the diagram (see text).

The size of the endotracheal tube may limit flow. The child must be maximally sedated and paralyzed, and therefore must be ventilated between maneuvers. Prior to the deflation, the lungs of the infant are manually inflated to TLC using approximately +30 to +40 cm H_2O. This inflation is performed four times with a 2- to 3-second breath hold at TLC. The airway is then switched into a source of negative pressure (approximately −30 to −40 cm H_2O). Air is evacuated for a maximum of 3 seconds or until expiratory flow ceases (i.e., residual volume is reached). As the lungs empty, an F-V curve is produced, and flows at lower lung volumes are analyzed. The lungs are then reinflated with 100% O_2, and the procedure is repeated until flow limitation is obtained.

Standards for Testing

For several specific pulmonary function tests, regardless of age, maximal effort and cooperation are needed to optimize results. It has often been assumed that small children are incapable of performing adequate pulmonary function tests. Laboratories that specialize in working with pediatric patients have proven this untrue. However, not every small child can or will perform up to desired expectations. Criteria and standards for many pulmonary function tests have been established by the ATS (see Chapter 2), but these guidelines are intended for the adult population. Well-defined standards for pediatrics are not widely available. The goal for any patient performing pulmonary function studies, regardless of age, should be to meet or exceed ATS criteria. However, age-appropriate criteria are needed for the pediatric population. Interpretation of pulmonary function tests should note if ATS criteria have not been reached. The physician's interpretation should state whether age and/or effort-related limitations are evident, and these should be taken into consideration.

■ VARIABILITY IN REFERENCE SETS AND PREDICTED VALUES FOR PEDIATRICS

Until recently, a limiting factor for interpretation of pediatric pulmonary function tests was the lack of consistent predicted values. Caution is warranted regarding the choice of an appropriate reference set. Reference sets are often named for an author or primary investigator; examples are the Dickman and Knudson reference sets. However, reference sets may contain regression equations from one author only, or several researchers (or studies) may contribute to a single reference set. An example is the Polgar and Promadhat reference set, which is actually a compilation of regression equations from several different population studies and authors. When choosing a reference set for a population of children, consideration must be given to selecting the set that most closely represents the population being tested. Several questions should be considered carefully:

- How many normal patients were studied, and how was it determined that these patients were free of respiratory disease?
- What are the demographics of the population represented (i.e., age range, sex, race, etc.)?
- What equipment and techniques were used to collect the data?

The number of patients studied is critically important to the value of the reference set. Many common pediatric reference sets developed between the 1960s and the 1980s (e.g., Polgar, Knudson, Hsu, Zapletal) were based on relatively small numbers (several hundred children). Each child was tested only once, and therefore the sample is cross-sectional. Repeat studies were not performed on the same children as they aged and grew. By 2000, population studies on many thousands of children had been completed. In addition, these studies were *longitudinal* by design. Longitudinal means that repeated measurements were made on the same children as they grew. The power of the regression equations generated from these population studies is far greater than those of preceding decades. Examples of pediatric reference sets now available based on very large numbers of children are those of Wang-Dockery and the NHANES III (National Health and Nutrition Evaluation Survey III) study. One difficulty is that these reference sets are for spirometry only. It is relatively easy to bring a portable spirometer into a school and test a group of children quickly. Repeat studies can be performed at intervals to gather longitudinal data. It is not easy to bring a large number of children into a pulmonary function laboratory and perform tests such as lung volumes, DL_{CO}, etc. Predicted values for these pulmonary function tests are still lacking. A further problem arises when trying to combine "older" predicted values for lung volumes and DL_{CO} with newer, updated spirometric reference sets. Many commercial pulmonary function systems permit the user to "mix and match" regression equations and build their own reference set. Caution must be exercised when doing this. It is important that the laboratory personnel know if their reference set is a standard (unaltered) set, or if it is compiled from available reference sets. It is also advisable that the reference sets be identified on the final pulmonary function reports. Consulting physicians who are not associated with the laboratory performing the studies may be interested in knowing the source of the predicted values.

Biologic variability for physiologic measurements, including pulmonary function, is critically dependent on the populations' sex, age, race, and body dimensions. Several reference sets only considered white subjects. Race correction for African Americans were applied as a constant correction factor (see Appendix B). In addition, the ages for children tested were often in the range of 8 to 18 years. There is tremendous growth during these years, but at different rates, depending on sex and pubertal changes. Attempting to apply a simple regression for each parameter tested (FVC, FEV_1, etc.) based on one independent variable (usually height) may be misleading. Although distribution of pulmonary function values may follow the normal Gaussian (bell-shaped) curve (see Appendix B), there is increasing disparity at both ends of the age range. Further error is introduced if these regression equations are extrapolated to ages younger than actually tested (e.g., down to 6 years of age). Newer reference sets for spirometry now examine races separately and have even developed regression equations for each age child (Wang and Dockery).

PF Tips

In pediatric patients, lung growth is closely correlated with age, height, and sex. Trending of pulmonary function measurements must be done on a percent-predicted basis. Actual values will continue to increase through the somatic growth stage.

Measurement technique can also significantly alter physiologic data; lung volumes measured via gas dilution versus those measured by body plethysmography are one example. In pediatrics, even simple differences in performing tests may affect results. Examples include the use of nose clips versus no nose clips, or standing versus sitting while performing testing. Consistency is the key, although there may be no absolutes in the correct methodology for a particular test. The technologist should be aware of the methods employed in his or her laboratory as compared with those of the reference sets utilized.

WHAT IS IN THE FUTURE?

One of the most difficult challenges is assessing lung function of a very young child (2 to 4 years) because he or she cannot perform standard measurements of pulmonary function. Sedation may not be an alternative, or the size and/or compliance of the child's chest may not be conducive to thoracoabdominal compressions. Physical examination, auscultation, and other indirect indices, such as pulse oximetry, are often very misleading in this age group. Presence or absence of wheezing is not necessarily correlated with oxygen status or the clinical presentation of the child. There is a tremendous need for a noninvasive measurement of airflow limitation that is sensitive enough to use for clinical decisions. Several alternative methods of assessing pulmonary function in very young children and infants are currently in clinical trials. These techniques are not as simple as techniques that measure volume and flow, and they require sophisticated equipment. Respiratory impulse oscillometry and measurement of exhaled nitric oxide are two promising techniques.

■ RESPIRATORY IMPULSE OSCILLOMETRY (ROS, IOS)

This procedure is also referred to as the forced oscillation technique (FOT). A miniature loudspeaker is placed proximal to the device's flow sensor and produces forced oscillations with a range of frequencies into the airway. They are sensed as popping pulsations as the child breathes tidally. The pressure oscillations generated by the soundwaves are of two types: (1) those in phase with airflow, termed *airway resistance* (Rrs), and (2) those out of phase with airflow, termed *reactance* (Xrs). The reactance component is quite complex and relates to delays of pressure change due to elastic components of the respiratory system, as well as inertia. The interaction of airway resistance and reactance constitutes respiratory impedance. The advantage of this procedure is that it is very easy for a child to accomplish. Even a 2-year-old toddler can be taught to breathe on a mouthpiece for approximately 1 minute to obtain a stable reading of 15 to 20 seconds. The disadvantage is that reference standards are not yet available for the pediatric population, and the clinical significance of these parameters is still unclear. Patients, including children, may be able to serve as their own controls, and perform this procedure serially at every clinic visit. The procedure is far less time-consuming, strenuous, and effort-dependent than spirometry. The sensitivity of this test may be greater than that of the FEV_1, especially with methacholine challenges, although its variability is somewhat greater.

■ EXHALED NITRIC OXIDE (eNO)

Nitric oxide (NO) is a normally occurring substance found in reproducible levels in exhaled air. This gas can be measured in single or multiple breaths by a number of techniques. Levels of nitric oxide have been shown to significantly increase from tissues that are inflamed. The measurement of exhaled nitric oxide has therefore been proposed as an index of airway inflammation, such as occurs in asthma. The ease of measurement makes it an attractive diagnostic clinical tool for use with young children. As with IOS, protocols for testing have not yet been standardized, nor reference values in pediatrics determined.

Summary

This chapter describes techniques for performing pulmonary function tests in pediatric patients. Spirometry, lung volumes, DL_{CO}, blood gases, pulmonary mechanics, and challenge tests are all discussed with attention to how these measurements differ in the pediatric population. For each category of tests, relevant questions are posed to relate pediatric testing to adult testing. Special emphasis is given to how the pulmonary function technologist should approach testing in young children and adolescents. Measurement of airflow and lung volumes in infants is also described,

c. Obstruction on spirometry with increased RV/TLV in the body box

d. Restriction on spirometry with normal lung volumes

5. *A 7-year-old child is capable of several "pants" during plethysmography and takes a maximal inspiratory capacity; however, expiration is incomplete. Which of the following parameters would be increased?*

a. TLC
b. FRC
c. VC
d. RV

6. *Which of the following statement is TRUE regarding DL_{CO} in the pediatric population?*

a. DL_{CO} is an inappropriate test for children because they cannot perform it correctly.

b. DL_{CO} may be decreased for several reasons, but it is never increased.

c. Smoking history is irrelevant in teenagers because they do not develop increased carbon monoxide levels as adults do.

d. Although sometimes difficult to perform in children, DL_{CO} can give valuable insight into abnormalities in gas transfer at the alveolar level.

7. *In infants, measurement of raised lung volume forced flows has an advantage over partial forced flows because:*

a. Infants do not require sedation to perform raised forced flows, but do require sedation to perform partial forced flows.

b. Partial forced flows require intubation, whereas forced flows from raised lung volume do not.

c. The volume of the forced expiration approximates a vital capacity measurement similar to standard spirometry.

d. FRC measurements and calculation of specific flow at FRC are unnecessary.

8. *During infant pulmonary function tests, a baby who has been very stable starts to stir and flicker her eyelids. Concurrently, the measurements being made are significantly changed. Which of the following is the most likely cause?*

a. There has been a change in sleep state.

b. The equipment has lost its calibration and needs to be recalibrated.

c. The baby is having a serious adverse reaction to the sedating agent and the sedation should be reversed.

d. A hypoxic episode has occurred.

9. *Chloral hydrate is often used for sedation of infants during pulmonary function testing because:*

a. It is administered intravenously and easily titrated to the patient's need.

b. It is rapid acting, usually within 2 to 3 minutes.

c. It can be quickly reversed when testing is complete.

d. It is safe, relatively easy to administer, and does not require a full "sedation team."

10. *Which factors are important to consider when choosing a pediatric reference set?*

   I. The number of normal children tested
   II. The distributions of age, sex, and race of the population
   III. Consistency of technique in performing testing
   IV. Standardization of equipment

   a. I and III
   b. II and IV
   c. I, III, and IV
   d. I, II, III, and IV

SELECTED BIBLIOGRAPHY

General References

Hyatt RE: Forced Expiration. In *Handbook of physiology: the respiratory system*, Bethesda, Md, 1986, American Physiological Society.

Mueller GA, Eigen H: Pulmonary function testing in pediatric practise, *Pediatr Rev* 15:403-411, 1994.

Pfaff JK, Morgan WJ: Pulmonary function in infants and children, *Pediatr Clin North Am* 41(2):401-423, 1994.

Polgar G, Promadhat V: *Pulmonary function testing in children: techniques and standards*, Philadelphia, 1971, WB Saunders.

Stocks J, Sly PD, Tepper RS, et al: *Infant respiratory function testing*, New York, 1996, Wiley-Liss.

Zapletal A, Samanck M, Paul T: Lung function in children and adolescents—methods, reference values. In *Progress in respiration research*, New York, 1987, Karger.

Spirometry

Brugman SM, Howell JH, Rosenburg DM, et al: The spectrum of pediatric vocal cord dysfunction, *Am J Respir Crit Care Med* 149:A353, 1994.

Crenesse D, Berlioz M, Bourrier T, et al: Spirometry in children aged 3 to 5 years: reliability of forced expiratory maneuvers, *Pediatr Pulmonol* 32:56-61, 2001.

Desmond KJ, Allen PD, Demizio DL, et al: Redefining end of test (EOT) criteria for pulmonary testing in children, *Am J Respir Crit Care Med* 156:542-545, 1997.

Elshami AA, Tino G: Coexistent asthma and functional upper airway obstruction, *Chest* 110:1358-1361, 1996.

Krowka MJ, Enright PL, Rodarte JR, et al: Effect of effort on measurement of forced expiratory volume in one second, *Am Rev Respir Dis* 136:829-833, 1987.

Landwehr LP, Wood RP, Blager FB, et al: Vocal cord dysfunction mimicking exercise-induced bronchospasm in adolescents, *Pediatr* 98:971-974, 1996.

Lebowitz MD, Sherrill DL: The assessment and interpretation of spirometry during the transition from childhood to adulthood, *Pediatr Pulmonol* 19:143-149, 1995.

McFadden ER Jr, Zawadski DK: Vocal cord dysfunction masquerading as exercise-induced asthma: a physiologic cause for "choking" during athletic activities, *Am J Respir Crit Care Med* 153:942-947, 1996.

Miller RD, Hyatt RE: Evaluation of obstructing lesions of the trachea and larynx by flow-volume loops, *Am Rev Respir Dis* 108:475-482, 1975.

Wanger JS, Ikle DN, Cherniack RM: The effect of inspiratory maneuvers on expiratory flow rates in health and asthma: influences of lung elastic recoil, *Am J Respir Crit Care Med* 153:1302-1308, 1996.

Predicted Values and Reference Equations

Cook CD, Hamann JH: Relation of lung volumes to height in healthy persons between the ages of 5 and 38 years, *J Pediatr* 59:710-715, 1961.

Hankinson JL, Odencrantz JR, Fedan KB: Spirometric reference values from a sample of the general U.S. population, *Am J Respir Crit Care Med* 159:179-187, 1999.

Hsu KHK, Jenkins DE, Hsi BP, et al: Ventilatory functions of normal children and young adults—Mexican-American, white, and black—I. Spirometry, *J Pediatr* 95:14-23, 1979.

Knudson RJ, Lebowitz MD, Holberg CJ, et al: Changes in the normal maximal expiratory flow-volume curve with growth and aging, *Am Rev Respir Dis* 127:725, 1983.

Pattishall EN: Pulmonary function testing references values and interpretations in pediatric training programs, *Pediatr* 85:768-773, 1990.

Pattishall EN, Helms RW, Strope GL: Noncomparability of cross-sectional and longitudinal estimates of lung growth in children, *Pediatr Pulmonol* 7:22-28, 1989.

Wang X, Dockery DW, Wypij D, et al: Pulmonary function between 6 and 18 years of age, *Pediatr Pulmonol* 15:75-88, 1993.

Inhalational Challenges

Cockcroft DW, Killian DN, Mellon JJA, et al: Bronchial reactivity to inhaled histamine: a method and clinical survey, *Clin Allergy* 7:235-243, 1977.

Eggleston PA: A comparison of the asthmatic response to methacholine and exercise, *J Allergy Clin Immunol* 63:104-110, 1979.

Hargreave FE, Ryan A, Thomson NC, et al: Bronchial responsiveness to histamine or methacholine in asthma measurement and clinical significance, *J Allergy Clin Immunol* 68:345-347, 1981.

Irvin CG: Bronchial challenge testing, *Respir Clin North Am* 1:265-285, 1995.

Seiner JC, Staudenmayer H, Koepke JW, et al: Vocal cord dysfunction: the importance of psychologic factors and provocation challenge testing, *J Allergy Clin Immunol* 79:726-733, 1987.

Provocational and Maximal Exercise Stress Testing

Cooper DM: Rethinking exercise testing in children: a challenge, *Am J Respir Crit Care Med* 152:1154-1157, 1995.

Godfrey S: Exercise-induced asthma—clinical, physiological, and therapeutic implications, *J Allergy Clin Immunol* 56:1-17, 1975.

James FW, et al: Responses of normal children and young adults to controlled bicycle exercise, *Circulation* 61:902-912, 1980.

McFadden ER Jr: Exercise-induced asthma—assessment of current etiologic concepts, *Chest* 91:151S-157S, 1987.

Nixon PA, Orenstein DM: Exercise testing in children, *Pediatr Pulmonol* 5:107-122, 1988.

Strauss RH, McFadden ER Jr, Ingram RH Jr, et al: Enhancement of exercise-induced asthma by cold air, *N Engl J Med* 297:743-747, 1977.

Weisman IM, Zeballos RJ: Clinical exercise testing, *Clin Chest Med* 22:679-701, 2002.

Pulmonary Function Testing in Infants and Very Young Children

Castile R, Filbrun D, Flucke R, et al: Adult-type pulmonary function tests in infants without respiratory disease, *Pediatr Pulmonol* 30:215-227, 2000.

Clarke JR, Aston H, Silverman M: Evaluation of a tidal expiratory flow index in healthy and diseased infants, *Pediatr Pulmonol* 17:285-290, 1994.

Hanrahan JP, Brown RW, Carey VJ, et al: Passive respiratory mechanics in healthy infants, *Am J Respir Crit Care Med* 154:670-680, 1996.

Hanrahan JP, Tager IB, Castile RG, et al: Pulmonary function measures in healthy infants: variability and size correction, *Am Rev Resp Dis* 141:1127, 1990.

Hoo AF, Dezateux C, Hanrahan JP, et al: Sex-specific prediction equations for $\dot{V}_{max}$ FRC in infancy, *Am J Respir Crit Care Med* 165:1084-1092, 2002.

Jones M, Castile R, Davis S, et al: Forced expiratory flows and volumes in infants—normative data and lung growth, *Am J Respir Crit Care Med* 161:353-359, 2000.

Jones MH, Davis SD, Grant D, et al: Forced expiratory maneuvers in very young children: assessment of flow limitation, *Am J Respir Crit Care Med* 159:791-795, 1999.

LeSouef PN, England SJ, Bryan AC: Passive respiratory mechanics in newborns and children, *Am Rev Respir Dis* 129:552-556, 1984.

Lodrup KC, Mowinckel P, Carlsen KH: Lung function measurements in awake compared to sleeping newborn infants, *Pediatr Pulmonol* 12: 99-104, 1992.

McCoy KS, Castile RG, Allen ED, et al: Functional residual capacity (FRC) measurements by plethysmography and helium dilution in normal infants, *Pediatr Pulmonol* 19:282-290, 1995.

Morgan WJ, Geller DE, Tepper RS, et al: Partial expiratory flow-volume curves in infants and young children, *Pediatr Pulmonol* 5:232-243, 1988.

Neto GS, Gerhardt T, Silberberg A, et al: Nonlinear pressure/volume relationship and measurements of lung mechanics in infants, *Pediatr Pulmonol* 12:146-152, 1992.

Panitch HB, Kekklian EN, Motley RA, et al: Effect of altering smooth muscle tone on maximal expiratory flows in patients with tracheomalacia, *Pediatr Pulmonol* 9:170-176, 1990.

Taussig LM, Landau LI, Godfrey S, et al: Determinants of forced expiratory flows in newborn infants, *J Appl Physiol* 53:1220-1227, 1982.

Tepper RS, Asdell S: Comparison of helium dilution and nitrogen washout measurements of functional residual capacity in infants and very young children, *Pediatr Pulmonol* 13:250-254, 1992.

Tepper RS, Reister T: Forced expiratory flows and lung volumes in normal infants, *Pediatr Pulmonol* 15:357-361, 1993.

Turner DJ, Stick SM, LeSouef KL, et al: A new technique to generate and assess forced expiration from raised lung volume in infants, *Am J Respir Crit Care Med* 51:1441-1450, 1995.

Sivan Y, Deakers TW, Newth CJL: An automated bedside method for measuring functional residual capacity by N_2 washout in mechanically ventilated children, *Pediatr Res* 28:446-451, 1990.

Sly PD, Brown KA, Bates JHT, et al: Non-invasive determination of respiratory mechanics during mechanical ventilation of neonates: a review of current and future techniques, *Pediatr Pulmonol* 4:39-47, 1988.

Stocks J: Assessment of lung function in infants, *Perfusion* 8:71-80, 1993.

Oscillometry and Nitric Oxide

Bisgaard H, Klug B: Lung function measurement in awake young children, *Eur Respir J* 8:2067-2075, 1995.

Buchvald F, Bisgaard H: FeNO measured at fixed exhalation flow rate during controlled tidal breathing in children from the age of 2 years, *Am J Respir Crit Care Med* 163:699-704, 2001.

Ducharme FM, Davis GM: Respiratory resistance in the emergency department—a reproducible and responsive measure of asthma severity, *Chest* 113:1566-1572, 1998.

Standards and Guidelines

American Association for Respiratory Care: Clinical practice guideline: infant/toddler pulmonary function tests, *Respir Care* 40:761-768, 1995.

American Association for Respiratory Care: Clinical practice guideline: methacholine challenge testing 2001 revision and update, *Respir Care* 46:523-530, 2001.

American Thoracic Society: Guidelines for methacholine and exercise challenge testing—1999, *Am J Respir Crit Care Med* 161:309-329, 2000.

American Thoracic Society: Lung function testing: selection of reference values and interpretative strategies, *Am Rev Respir Dis* 144:1202-1218, 1991.

American Thoracic Society/European Respiratory Society: Respiratory function measurements in infants: measurement conditions, *Am J Respir Crit Care Med* 151:2058-2064, 1995.

American Thoracic Society/European Respiratory Society: Respiratory mechanics in infants: physiologic evaluation in health and disease, *Am Rev Respir Dis* 147:474-496, 1993.

American Thoracic Society/European Respiratory Society Workshop Summary: The raised volume rapid thoracoabdominal compression technique, *Am J Respir Care Med* 161:1760-1762, 2000.

Official Statement of the American Thoracic Society: Recommendations for standardized procedures for the online and offline measurement of exhaled lower respiratory nitric oxide and nasal nitric oxide in adults and children—1999, *Am J Respir Crit Care Med* 160(6):2104-2117, 1999.

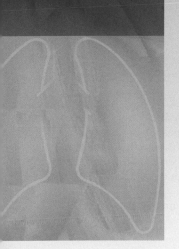

CHAPTER 9

SPECIALIZED TEST REGIMENS

After studying this chapter, you should be able to do the following:

Entry-level

1. Describe two methods of performing bronchial challenge tests
2. Identify a positive response to a methacholine challenge test
3. List two indications for preoperative pulmonary function testing

Advanced

1. Interpret a test for exercise-induced asthma
2. Suggest appropriate tests to evaluate disability in either chronic obstructive pulmonary disease (COPD) or pulmonary fibrosis
3. Judge the acceptability of metabolic measurements

Diagnosis of specific pulmonary disorders requires that appropriate tests be performed. Specialized test regimens, such as those described in this chapter, often consist of standard tests performed under special conditions. For example, forced expiratory volume (FEV_1) may be analyzed after inhalation challenge, hyperventilation, or exercise to quantify airway reactivity. The clinical question asked regarding a patient might be whether he or she qualifies for disability or if it is safe to undergo surgery. Spirometry, lung volumes, diffusing capacity (DL_{CO}), or blood gas analysis may be required to answer these questions.

Metabolic measurements are widely used to assess caloric needs and nutritional support in a variety of patients. The methods used are similar to those used in gas exchange measurements during exercise. Specialized calculations allow very precise description of the nutritional status of the patient.

Bronchial Challenge Testing

Bronchial challenge testing is used to identify and characterize airway hyperresponsiveness. Challenge tests are performed in patients with symptoms of bronchospasm who have normal pulmonary function studies or uncertain results of bronchodilator studies. Bronchial challenge can also be used to assess changes in hyperreactivity of the airways or to quantify its severity. Bronchial challenge tests are sometimes used to screen individuals who may be at risk from environmental or occupational exposure to toxins.

Several commonly used provocative agents can be used to assess airway hyperreactivity. These include the following:

- Methacholine challenge
- Histamine challenge
- Eucapnic voluntary hyperventilation (using either cold or room-temperature gas)
- Exercise

Each of these agents may trigger bronchospasm, but in slightly different ways. Methacholine is a chemical that increases parasympathetic tone in bronchial smooth muscle. Histamine triggers a similar response producing bronchoconstriction. Hyperventilation, either at rest or during exercise, results in heat and water loss from the airway. This provokes bronchospasm in susceptible patients. With each of these agents, pulmonary function variables are assessed before and after exposure to the challenge. FEV_1 is the variable most commonly used. Other flow measurements, as well as airway resistance (Raw) and specific conductance (SGaw), may also be evaluated before and after challenge. Additional parameters that have been used to assess response to bronchial challenge include breath sounds, transcutaneous Po_2 ($tcPo_2$, see Chapter 10), and forced oscillation measurements of resistance.

■ METHACHOLINE CHALLENGE

Bronchial challenge by inhalation of methacholine is performed by having the patient inhale increasing doses of the drug. Spirometry, and sometimes SGaw, is measured after each dose. Most clinicians consider the test positive when inhalation of methacholine precipitates a 20% decrease in FEV_1. The methacholine concentration at which this 20% decrease occurs is called the *provocative concentration* or $PC_{20\%}$. In the doses usually employed (Table 9-1), normal patients do not display decreases greater than 20% in FEV_1. Therefore, the methacholine challenge test is highly specific for airway hyperreactivity. Many patients who have asthma experience a 20% reduction in FEV_1 with doses of 8 mg/ml or less. However, bronchial hyperresponsiveness may also be seen in other pulmonary disorders such as COPD, cystic fibrosis, and bronchitis.

Patients to be tested should be asymptomatic, with no coughing or obvious wheezing. Their baseline FEV_1 should be normal or at least greater than 70% of their expected value. For patients with known obstruction or restriction, FEV_1 should be close to their highest previously observed value. Obvious airway obstruction (i.e., $FEV_{1\%}$ less than predicted, SGaw less than 0.09 L/sec/cm H_2O/L) is a relative contraindication. If the patient has an FEV_1 less than 1.0 to 1.5 L, there is a risk that a large drop in FEV_1 following methacholine challenge might leave the individual with compromised lung function. Bronchial challenge may be indicated in obstructed patients if the clinical question is related to the degree of responsiveness.

If the patient has been taking bronchodilators, they should be withheld according to the schedule listed in Table 9-2. Other medications or substances can affect the validity of the challenge as well.

TABLE 9-1 Methacholine Dosing Schedules

4 × Increase*	2 × Increase†
0.0625 mg/ml	0.031 mg/ml
0.250 mg/ml	0.0625 mg/ml
1.0 mg/ml	0.125 mg/ml
4.0 mg/ml	0.25 mg/ml
16.0 mg/ml	1.0 mg/ml
	2.0 mg/ml
	4.0 mg/ml
	8.0 mg/ml
	16.0 mg/ml

*As used for the 5-breath dosimeter protocol.
†As used for the 2-minute tidal breathing protocol.

TABLE 9-2 Withholding Medications Before Bronchial Challenge

Short-acting β-adrenergic agents (inhaled)	8 hours
Long-acting β-adrenergic agents (inhaled)	48 hours
Standard β-adrenergic agents (oral)	12 hours
Long-acting β-adrenergic agents (oral)	24 hours
Anticholinergic agents (ipratropium)	24 hours
Standard theophylline preparations	12-24 hours
Sustained-action theophylline preparations	48 hours
Cromolyn sodium	8 hours
Nedocromil	48 hours
Antihistamines	72-96 hours
Corticosteroids (inhaled or oral)	Patients challenged while taking a stable dosage*
Leukotriene modifiers	24 hours
Caffeine-containing drinks (cola, coffee)	6 hours
β-blocking agents	May increase the response

*Corticosteroids may decrease bronchial hyperreactivity.

Baseline spirometry is performed to establish that the patient's FEV_1 is greater than 60% to 70% of predicted or the previously observed best value. Patients who demonstrate obstruction based on reduced $FEV_{1\%}$ or other flows do not require challenge testing to document airway hyperreactivity. However, obstructed patients may be tested to establish the degree of hyperreactivity. Patients who have a restrictive process (i.e., reduced FEV_1, forced vital capacity [FVC], and total lung capacity [TLC]) may also be tested for hyperreactive airways. If the patient is unable to perform acceptable baseline spirometry (i.e., acceptable and reproducible FEV_1 measurements), any change following inhalation challenge may be difficult to interpret. In these situations, another parameter (such as SGaw) that is less dependent on patient effort may be preferable as an end point.

Two methods of delivering methacholine to the airway have been recommended by the American Thoracic Society (ATS): the *5-breath dosimeter method* and the *2-minute tidal breathing method*. Several other methods and variations on each are also used. A dosimeter can provide a true "quantitative" challenge test by delivering a consistent volume of drug. The dosimeter (or nebulizer) is activated during inspiration, either automatically (by a flow sensor) or manually (by the technologist). A driving pressure of approximately 20 psi is used for most dosimeters. An activation time of 0.5 to 0.6 seconds allows a fixed volume of aerosol to be generated for each breath. By limiting the period of aerosol production, the last part of the inhalation carries the aerosol into the lung. The tidal breathing method is somewhat simpler because only a nebulizer is used.

A small-volume, gas-powered nebulizer is used to generate the methacholine aerosol (Figure 9-1). The nebulizer should generate an aerosol with a particle size in the range of 1.0 to 3.6 μm (mass median aerodynamic diameter). This particle range promotes deposition in the medium and small airways. For the tidal breathing method, the nebulizer output should be 0.13 ml/min; for use with a dosimeter (5-breath method) the output should be 0.009 ml for each 0.6-second actuation of the dosimeter. Because the output of each nebulizer varies by manufacturer and can change over time, it should be measured. This can be done by weighing the nebulizer on an accurate scale before and after a sham administration of drug. The output should be measured using the protocol to be used for testing. For the 5-breath dosimeter method, more breaths may be needed to measure the small output. The delivered dose of methacholine is standardized by using a fixed number of breaths (5), or breathing for a fixed length of time (2 minutes).

PF Tips

Despite different techniques for administering methacholine, patients who truly have asthma usually display a 20% decrease in FEV_1. The lower the dose of methacholine, the more sensitive, or hyperresponsive, the patient's airways are. Detecting a 20% decrease in FEV_1 requires that acceptable and reproducible baseline spirometry is obtained.

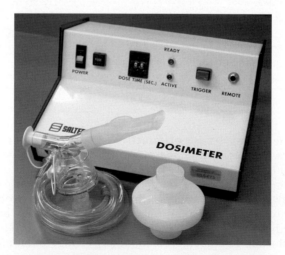

Figure 9-1 *Nebulizer and dosimeter.* A DeVilbiss 646 nebulizer capable of delivering a prescribed volume of aerosol with 1- to 3-micron particles is shown. A dosimeter that controls the flow of gas to the nebulizer is also shown. The dosimeter provides a timer so that nebulization occurs for 0.6 seconds during inhalation. A manual trigger is used; some dosimeters sense the patient's inspiratory effort and trigger flow automatically. Also shown is a bacterial filter that may be attached to the expiratory port of the nebulizer to reduce the volume of aerosol in the room.

5-Breath Dosimeter Method

Methacholine is prepared in 5 concentrations so that each dose is 4 times larger than the previous dose (Table 9-3). Methacholine may be stored under refrigeration, but should be brought to room temperature before administration. Baseline spirometry is performed.

The patient begins by inhaling 5 breaths of nebulized diluent, usually normal saline. The diluent step is optional but provides a means of checking that the patient understands the procedure and that the system is working properly. If the diluent step is performed, the FEV_1 following diluent becomes the "control" and the target FEV_1 for a positive test is 80% of this value. If the diluent step is omitted, the target FEV_1 is 80% of the baseline spirometry value. The breaths should be slow and deep, and the patient should wear a nose clip. The patient should inspire from FRC to TLC. The dosimeter should be triggered as inspiration begins; this may be done manually or automatically. The nebulizer should be activated for 0.6 seconds. Inspiration should last about 5 seconds, with a 5-second breath hold at TLC to maximize aerosol deposition. Inhalations are repeated for 5 breaths, lasting 2 minutes or less.

Spirometry is repeated at approximately 30 and 90 seconds following the last inhalation. A timer or stopwatch is useful for staging the maneuvers. The FVC maneuver should be acceptable and may be repeated if necessary. The number of attempts should be limited to three or four efforts, so that two acceptable maneuvers are obtained within 5 minutes. If Raw and SGaw are also measured, the patient should be seated in the plethysmograph and the door closed as soon as spirometry has been completed. With practice and careful timing, spirometry and resistance measurements can be completed within about 5 minutes after each dose of methacholine.

TABLE 0 3   Preparation of Methacholine for Two Common Dosing Schedules*

Methacholine	Diluent (0.9% NaCl)	Dilution
Doubling dosage, as used in the 2-minute tidal breathing protocol		
100 mg (dry powder)	6.25 ml	16.0 mg/ml
3 ml of 16.0 mg/ml	3 ml	8.0 mg/ml
3 ml of 8.0 mg/ml	3 ml	4.0 mg/ml
3 ml of 4.0 mg/ml	3 ml	2.0 mg/ml
3 ml of 2.0 mg/ml	3 ml	1.0 mg/ml
3 ml of 1.0 mg/ml	3 ml	0.5 mg/ml
3 ml of 0.5 mg/ml	3 ml	0.25 mg/ml
3 ml of 0.25 mg/ml	3 ml	0.125 mg/ml
3 ml of 0.125 mg/ml	3 ml	0.0625 mg/ml
3 ml of 0.625 mg/ml	3 ml	0.031 mg/ml
Quadrupling dosage, as used in the 5-breath dosimeter protocol		
100 mg (dry powder)	6.25 ml	16.0 mg/ml
3 ml of 16.0 mg/ml	9 ml	4.0 mg/ml
3 ml of 4.0 mg/ml	9 ml	1.0 mg/ml
3 ml of 1.0 mg/ml	9 ml	0.25 mg/ml
3 ml of 0.25 mg/ml	9 ml	0.0625 mg/ml

*For each schedule, 6.25 ml of saline is added to dry powdered methacholine. Subsequent dilutions then use 3 or 9 ml of saline added to 3 ml of the previous dilution.

The largest FEV_1 after each dose should be reported. If airway resistance measurements are also made, the average of two acceptable panting maneuvers should be reported. If FEV_1 decreases less than 20%, or specific conductance (SGaw) decreases less than 35%, the next highest dose is administered. If FEV_1 decreases more than 20%, or SGaw decreases 35%, the test is complete. Signs and symptoms related to asthma should be recorded. A β-adrenergic bronchodilator should be administered, and spirometry repeated after a 10-minute delay.

2-Minute Tidal Breathing Method

In this method, normal relaxed breathing is used as the patient inhales the aerosol. Methacholine is prepared in ten doses of doubling concentrations (Table 9-3). If the methacholine has been refrigerated, it should be allowed to come to room temperature for 30 minutes. A nebulizer capable of delivering 0.13 ml/min (±10%) driven by compressed air should be used. An accurate flow meter allows adjustment to the flow necessary to deliver the desired volume.

The patient should hold the nebulizer upright and breathe quietly through the mouthpiece with nose clip in place. A facemask may be used in place of a mouthpiece, but the nose clip should not be omitted. A filter may be placed on the expiratory limb of the nebulizer circuit to limit the amount of methacholine released in aerosol form in the testing area. A timer or stopwatch should be used to ensure the breathing interval is exactly 2 minutes long.

As in the dosimeter method, spirometry is repeated at 30 and 90 seconds after the end of the 2-minute tidal breathing interval. If a diluent step is included, the target FEV_1 (for a positive response) is 80% of the largest value obtained after the diluent. If the diluent step is omitted, the target FEV_1 is 80% of the baseline value. Patients with highly reactive airways may have a positive response (i.e., a 20% decrease in FEV_1) to the diluent. The FVC maneuvers should be completed within about 3 minutes; if Raw or SGaw is to be measured, the measurement should be performed as quickly as possible following spirometry. If FEV_1 decreases less than 20%, the next highest dose should be administered. If FEV_1 decreases by 20% or more, or if SGaw decreases by 35%, the challenge is complete. A β-adrenergic bronchodilator should be administered to reverse the bronchospasm, and spirometry repeated after 10 minutes.

These two dosing protocols use different methacholine concentrations. The 2-minute tidal breathing method uses a doubling dosage, whereas the 5-breath dosimeter method quadruples the concentration. Each of these dilutions may be prepared from a 16 mg/ml stock solution. The stock solution is prepared by dissolving the powdered drug in a saline diluent. A preservative (0.4% phenol) may be added to the solution but is not required. Methacholine concentrations greater than 0.125 mg/ml are stable after mixing and usually may be kept for 3 months if refrigerated at 4° C. The smallest dose (0.025 mg/ml) is the least stable and may need to be prepared immediately before testing. Methacholine solutions should be prepared by a pharmacist or similarly trained individual using sterile technique. Vials of methacholine should be carefully marked with labels that clearly identify the concentration.

Spirometry or plethysmographic measurements are the most commonly used end points for bronchial challenge tests. For each parameter, the percent of decrease is calculated as follows:

$$\% \text{ Decrease} = \frac{x - y}{x} \times 100$$

where:
x = control FEV_1 (baseline, or after diluent)
y = current FEV_1 after methacholine inhalation

A 20% or greater decrease in the FEV_1 is considered a positive test. The decrease should be sustained. Additional spirometry efforts may be necessary to distinguish an actual decrease from variability in the maneuvers. The same equation may be used to calculate changes in airway resistance or specific conductance. A decrease of 35% to 45% in SGaw is consistent with bronchial hyperresponsiveness. In patients suspected of having vocal cord dysfunction (VCD), complete flow-volume (F-V) loops may be helpful. VCD is sometimes mistaken for asthma in patients referred for bronchial challenge testing. Limitation of inspiratory flow (with little or no change in FEV_1) is usually observed in VCD.

Several methods of quantifying the results of the challenge are commonly used. The concentration of methacholine that results in a 20% decrease (PC_{20}) can be calculated from the last and second-to-last doses administered:

$$PC_{20} = \text{antilog}\left[\log C_1 + \frac{(\log C_2 - \log C_1)(20 - R_1)}{R_2 - R_1}\right]$$

where:
C_1 = second-to-last methacholine concentration
C_2 = final methacholine concentration (causing 20% or greater decrease)
R_1 = percent decrease in FEV_1 after C_1
R_2 = percent decrease in FEV_1 after C_2

PC_{20} calculated this way provides a single index of bronchial responsiveness. PC_{20} may also be identified directly from a graph in which change in FEV_1 is plotted against the log concentration of methacholine (Figure 9-2). Provocative concentrations for other variables,

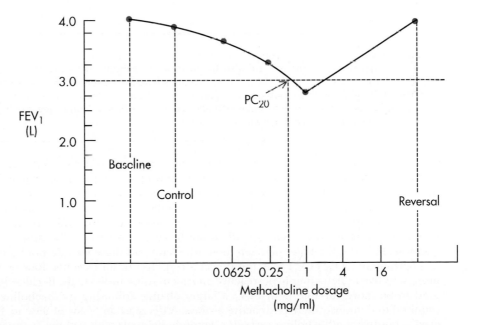

Figure 9-2 *Methacholine challenge test.* Results of data gathered during a bronchial challenge test are shown. The dosage of the challenge agent (methacholine in this case) is plotted on a logarithmic scale on the *x*-axis. FEV_1 (or other variable) is plotted on the *y*-axis. The first point represents a baseline FEV_1 of 4 L. The control (FEV_1 after inhalation of the diluent) is plotted next. FEV_1 after each dose of methacholine is plotted until a 20% decrease occurs. FEV_1 decreased by more than 20% with a dose of 1 mg/ml. A vertical line drawn from the point at which the dose response curve crosses the 20% line defines the PC_{20}. The patient is then given an inhaled bronchodilator to reverse the effect of the provocative agent, and the response is plotted.

such as SGaw, can be calculated similarly by substituting the appropriate percentage for 20 in the above equation and substituting the percent decrease for that variable for R_1 and R_2. Note that this calculation requires that at least two concentrations of methacholine have been given. If FEV_1 decreases 20% after the diluent or the first dose of methacholine, PC_{20} should be reported as less than the lowest concentration administered. If FEV_1 does not decrease by at least 20% after the highest dose, PC_{20} should be reported as "greater than 16 mg/ml."

See Test Regimens 9-2 for interpretive strategies. Airway responsiveness to methacholine can be described using the PC_{20}. Most patients referred for bronchial challenge testing have a history or symptoms suggestive of asthma, but not a definite diagnosis. For these patients, if FEV_1 decreases less than 20% at the highest dose (PC_{20} >16 mg/ml), bronchial responsiveness is probably normal and asthma is unlikely. For patients whose FEV_1 decreases 20% or more at low doses of methacholine (PC_{20} <1.0 mg/ml), the diagnosis of asthma is highly likely. For patients with PC_{20} values from 1 to 16 mg/ml, the diagnosis of asthma must be considered based on the pretest probability of asthma, the history of symptoms, and other possible causes for bronchial hyperreactivity. In practice, patients who have a PC_{20} greater than 8 to 16 mg/ml usually do not have asthma. Patients who have a negative methacholine challenge (PC_{20} >8 to 16 mg/ml) may have asthma that has been suppressed by antiinflammatory medications or occupational asthma that is triggered by a specific agent. Conversely, some individuals who have PC_{20} values less than 8 mg/ml may not have asthma. Patients with allergic rhinitis and smokers with COPD often have bronchial hyperreactivity, but not asthma.

PF Tips

Some patients whose FEV_1 drops 20% or more at low doses of methacholine may not have asthma. Hyperreactive airways are also found in some patients with COPD who smoke or in patients who have allergic rhinitis. A negative methacholine challenge (i.e., a decrease in FEV_1 <20% at the highest dose) may occur in patients who have asthma that has been suppressed by anti-inflammatory medications. Some asthmatics may have their asthma triggered by exposure to a specific agent such as cold dry air.

A number of physiologic factors affect the sensitivity and specificity of methacholine challenge testing. Methacholine causes constriction of bronchial smooth muscle. In healthy individuals, taking a deep breath before performing the FVC maneuver may cause bronchodilatation for several minutes. In patients who have mild asthma, a similar response is sometimes observed. In patients who have severe asthma, the bronchodilating effect of a deep inspiration is reduced; a deep breath may actually cause bronchoconstriction. Because of this differing response, FEV_1 discriminates between those who have and those who do not have asthma.

Spirometry (i.e., FEV_1) may not detect a response in all patients. Raw or SGaw may be more sensitive in detecting hyperreactive airways in some individuals. Because Raw and SGaw tend to be more variable than FEV_1, a larger change following methacholine challenge is required to demonstrate hyperreactive airways. A decrease in SGaw of 35% to 45% is considered a positive methacholine response. Some individuals with asthma symptoms may have primarily large airway changes in response to methacholine. These changes may manifest themselves as a decrease in SGaw or blunting of the inspiratory limb of the F-V loop. Although PEF is useful for monitoring asthma, it is less reproducible and more effort-dependent than FEV_1 for detecting changes following bronchial challenge.

Technical factors can also make methacholine challenge tests difficult or impossible to interpret (Test Regimens 9-1). Changes in FEV_1 following bronchial challenge are usually not

TEST REGIMENS 9-1   Criteria for Acceptability—Bronchial Challenge Tests

1 The patient should withhold all bronchodilators before the test. The patient should also be free of upper or lower respiratory infection and not ingest any caffeinated beverages before the test.

2 Spirometric and/or plethysmographic efforts must meet standard criteria for acceptability and reproducibility. For adults, two FEV_1 measurements should be within 200 ml or 5% (depending on the criteria used by the laboratory) before the challenge. SGaw measurements should be within 10% before the challenge level. During the challenge, acceptable efforts should be obtained; reproducibility is desirable but may not be attained.

3 For methacholine and histamine challenges, a nebulizer that produces aerosol particles in the 1.0 to 3.6 μm range should be used. Nebulizer output, inspiratory flow, lung volume, and breath-hold time should be consistent for all levels (doses) of challenge.

4 For exercise challenge, the patient should attain at least 80% to 90% of the predicted maximal heart rate (or $\dot{V}o_{2max}$, if measured). This level should be maintained for 4 to 6 minutes. Measurements of $\dot{V}_E$ is recommended.

5 For hyperventilation challenges (cold or room air), the target ventilation level should be maintained for the specified interval (dependent on protocol used). For EVH, a target ventilation of $30 \times FEV_1$ for 6 minutes is recommended. For all challenge protocols, clinical signs and symptoms (e.g., presence or absence of coughing, wheezing) should be documented.

diagnostic in patients who cannot perform acceptable and reproducible baseline spirometry. Variable efforts by the patient may produce a false-positive test result (apparent reduction in FEV_1 but not asthma). FEV_1 values obtained at 30 and 90 seconds after each dose of methacholine should be similar. The maneuvers should meet criteria for an acceptable effort (see Chapter 2). However, because the primary end point is the FEV_1, it may not be necessary for the patient to exhale for 6 seconds. Using a shortened exhalation requires that the patient inspires fully to TLC, and this may be difficult to determine unless a full FVC effort is performed. The usual reproducibility criteria (FEV_1 efforts within 200 ml) may not be met because of the effects of methacholine. Additional maneuvers may be needed at 30 and 90 seconds to verify that a real decrease has occurred. The FEV_1 reported for each dose of methacholine should be the largest value obtained at that level.

The type of nebulizer and dosimeter affects the amount of agonist reaching the airways. Factors that should be controlled as much as possible include type of nebulizer, nebulizer output, particle size, inhaled volumes, breath-hold times, and inspiratory flow. Nebulizer driving pressure and/or flow should be consistent throughout the test. If a single nebulizer is used, it should be thoroughly emptied between doses. If multiple nebulizers are used (one for each dose), each should be checked for similar output. Although the dosimeter and tidal breathing techniques deliver different volumes of methacholine, the sensitivity and specificity of the test is similar for both methods in adults as well as children. The spirometer used should meet the minimal standards set by the ATS (see Chapter 11). It should provide spirometric tracings or F-V loops for later evaluation.

Methacholine challenge testing is a safe procedure. The main risk to the patient is that severe bronchospasm may occur, so a physician experienced in treating acute bronchospasm should be immediately available. The technologist administering the bronchial challenge test should be thoroughly familiar with the procedure, and with the signs and symptoms of bronchospasm. The technologist must know when to stop the test and how to administer bronchodilators to reverse acute bronchospasm. Medications for reversal of the bronchospasm (i.e., epinephrine, atropine) and for resuscitation should be immediately available in the event of an adverse reaction. Because of the risks involved, some laboratories require written consent from the patient. The test should be administered in a well-ventilated room to protect other patients and the technologist from exposure. The addition of a filter to the exhalation port of the nebulizer may help reduce the volume of aerosolized methacholine in the room. Technologists with known sensitivity to methacholine should not perform this procedure unless appropriate methods are used to avoid exposure to the drug.

HISTAMINE CHALLENGE

Aerosolized histamine extract (histamine phosphate) may be used for inhalation challenge in a manner similar to methacholine challenge. Histamine produces bronchoconstriction by an uncertain pathway. Antihistamines or H1-receptor antagonists can block the response to histamine. Histamine-induced bronchospasm is also partially blocked by most classes of bronchodilators. Histamine differs from methacholine in its side effects, half-life, and cumulative effects. Flushing and headache are two common side effects of histamine inhalation. The peak action of histamine occurs within 30 seconds to 2 minutes, which is similar to that observed in methacholine. Recovery of baseline function is significantly shorter for histamine than for methacholine. The action of histamine, unlike that of methacholine, is thought to be less cumulative.

Patient preparation for histamine challenge is similar to that used for methacholine (Table 9-2). Antihistamines and H_1-receptor antagonists should be withheld for 48 hours before testing.

Table 9-4 lists one dosing protocol for histamine challenge. These increments approximately double the concentration of drug at each level. The same criteria as those used for baseline spirometry in methacholine challenge are observed. Diluent may be administered first to determine a control value for FEV_1.

If FEV_1 does not decrease by more than 10%, then 5 breaths of the first dilution are administered. Spirometric measurements are performed immediately, then repeated at 3 minutes. A response is considered positive if FEV_1 decreases by 20% or more below the control at 3 minutes. If there is a negative response (FEV_1 decreases <20%), the next dose is given and measurements are repeated.

The results of histamine challenge are reported in a manner similar to that described for methacholine. The histamine concentration that produces a 20% decrease in FEV_1 is termed the PC_{20}. Response may also be reported by graphing the percentage of change in FEV_1 against the concentration (or its logarithm) of the drug. This type of plot is commonly called a dose-response graph. It permits interpolation of the precise concentration of drug that elicits the 20% decrease (Figure 9-2).

Histamine, like methacholine, is relatively safe if testing follows the procedures described. Baseline and control values should always be established (Test Regimens 9-2).

TABLE 9-4 Histamine Dosing Schedule

0.03 mg/ml
0.06 mg/ml
0.12 mg/ml
0.25 mg/ml
1.00 mg/ml
2.50 mg/ml
5.00 mg/ml
10.00 mg/ml

TEST REGIMENS 9-2   Interpretive Strategies—Bronchial Challenge Tests

1 Was the challenge agent administered appropriately?
  For methacholine or histamine, were the doses of agonist appropriate?
  Were nebulizer output, inspiratory flow, etc., consistent for each dose?
  For exercise, did the patient maintain an appropriate workload for 6 to 8 minutes?
  For hyperventilation, did the patient maintain the target level of ventilation?
2 Were there any pretest factors that might influence results? Failure to withhold bronchodilators? Respiratory infection? If so, interpret cautiously or not at all.
3 Were spirometric efforts acceptable and reproducible before and after challenge? If not, interpret very cautiously or not at all.
4 For methacholine or histamine challenge, was there a 20% decrease in FEV_1 after inhaling diluent? If so, test is positive. Was there a 20% decrease in FEV_1 after inhalation of the agonist? If so, test is positive. Was there a 35% decrease in SGaw (if measured)? If so, test is positive.
5 For exercise or hyperventilation challenge, was there a 15% decrease in FEV_1 after challenge? If so, test is positive.
6 Were there signs or symptoms of airway hyperreactivity (coughing, wheezing, shortness of breath)? If so, test suggests bronchial hyperresponsiveness.
7 Were the results borderline? If so, consider repeat testing in the future.
8 Were symptoms present despite little or no change in FEV_1? Consider additional measurements such as SGaw, or related conditions such as vocal cord dysfunction.

Bronchial challenge should always begin with a low concentration of drug. The range of concentrations used should be appropriate for the patient tested. For adult patients in whom airway hyperreactivity is the suspected diagnosis, the dosing schedules previously described are recommended. Patients who have a positive response to histamine challenge recover more quickly than if tested with methacholine. Histamine challenge can be repeated within 2 hours after the patient has returned to baseline level of function.

■ EUCAPNIC VOLUNTARY HYPERVENTILATION

Airway hyperreactivity may also be assessed by having the patient breathe at a high level of ventilation. Heat or water loss from the upper airways has been demonstrated to provoke bronchospasm in susceptible individuals. These physiologic changes are most pronounced when the patient inhales cold, dry gas, but they can also be demonstrated with gas at room temperature. To prevent respiratory alkalosis (i.e., true hyperventilation), carbon dioxide (CO_2) is mixed with inspired air. This gas mixture allows high levels of ventilation with little change in pH.

Patients to be tested using EVH should withhold bronchodilators as suggested in Table 9-2. Baseline spirometry is performed to ascertain that airway obstruction is not present. In ventilation challenges, the baseline is the control value with which subsequent measurements will be compared.

If cold air is to be used, the mixture is passed through a heat exchanger or over a cooling coil. These devices lower the temperature and remove water vapor from the gas. Gas temperatures are reduced to a subfreezing level in the range $-10°$ to $-20°$ C. The relative humidity is usually very near 0%.

The patient breathes the gas at an elevated level of ventilation. In one method, the patient breathes at a fraction of his or her maximal voluntary ventilation (MVV) (e.g., 30% to 70% of the MVV). CO_2 is added to the gas to maintain a stable $Petco_2$. This is accomplished either by titrating CO_2 into the mixture or by using a gas composed of 5% CO_2, 21% O_2, and balance N_2. The patient maintains the specified level of ventilation for 4 to 6 minutes. Spirometry or SGaw is then measured at fixed intervals after the hyperventilation (e.g., 1, 5, and 10 minutes). A second method has the patient breathe at increasing levels of ventilation up to the MVV (e.g., 7.5, 15, 30, 60 L/min and MVV). Again CO_2 is added to the inspired gas to maintain isocapnia (i.e., $Paco_2$ of approximately 40 mm Hg).

Eucapnic voluntary hyperventilation (EVH) with room-temperature gas also provides a ready stimulus for bronchospasm. In this technique, the patient breathes a mixture of 5% CO_2, 21% O_2, and balance N_2 at room temperature. The gas is used to fill a "target" bag or balloon of approximately 5 L (Figure 9-3). The patient breathes from the bag via a nonrebreathing valve (see Chapter 10) and large-bore tubing. The patient wears a nose clip. A high-output flow meter is used to fill the target bag. The flow meter is adjusted to deliver gas at approximately 30 times the patient's FEV_1. The patient breathes from the bag and tries to match ventilation to keep the bag partly deflated. The high level of ventilation is continued for 6 minutes. Spirometry is performed immediately after hyperventilation and then at 5-minute intervals (i.e., at 5, 10, 15, and 20 minutes).

For both the cold-air and room-temperature protocols, if no decrease in FEV_1 occurs within 20 minutes after hyperventilation, the test may be considered negative. The percentage decrease is calculated just as for methacholine challenge testing, described previously. A decrease of 15% is consistent with some degree of airway hyperreactivity (Test Regimens 9-2). EVH in normal patients usually results in bronchodilatation. Therefore, a 15% decrease

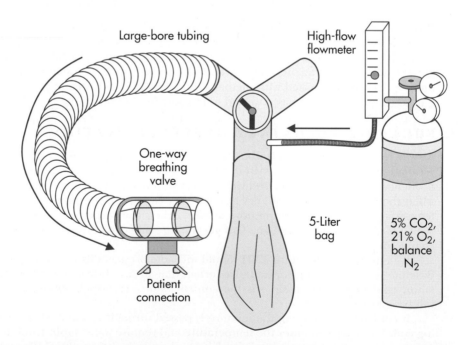

Figure 9-3 *Breathing circuit for EVH.* A gas containing 5% CO_2, 21% O_2, and balance N_2 is directed through a precision high-flow flowmeter to a reservoir bag. Flow is adjusted to a target ventilation level, such as 30 times the patient's FEV_1. The patient then breathes from the bag via a one-way valve with large-bore tubing. The patient is coached to increase ventilation to keep the bag partially deflated. The test is continued for a predetermined interval, usually 6 minutes.

is abnormal and highly specific for increased bronchial responsiveness. Some asthmatic patients may experience significant decreases in FEV_1 (20% to 60%). Bronchospasm should be reversed with inhaled bronchodilators, and the reversal documented with spirometry. The technologist performing the procedure should be prepared to manage severe bronchospasm if it occurs.

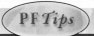

PF *Tips*

EVH testing may be a good substitute for exercise-induced asthma testing. High levels of eucapnic ventilation produce heat and water loss from the upper airway similar to that which occurs with exercise. By setting a target ventilation that represents a significant fraction of the patient's maximal value (i.e., $FEV_1 \times 30$), airway hyperreactivity can be demonstrated. High levels of ventilation are not always achieved during exercise, especially if patients are limited by their maximal heart rate or by deconditioning.

Raw and SGaw can be measured easily when hyperventilation tests are used. Because the airway challenge is applied once, the patient can remain in the body plethysmograph for measurements at defined intervals. Cold-air testing requires specialized equipment to refrigerate and dry inspired gas. Testing with cold air is slightly more sensitive and specific than testing with room-temperature gas. Both techniques correlate well with the results of methacholine challenge tests, although they are slightly less specific. If multiple levels of ventilation are evaluated, a dose-response curve can be constructed. However, the single challenge is less complicated and can be used to evaluate patients with suspected asthma, particularly exercise-induced asthma.

■ EXERCISE CHALLENGE

Exercise-induced asthma (EIA) is typified by bronchospasm during or immediately after vigorous exercise. EIA is related to heat and water loss from the upper airway that accompanies increased ventilation during exercise. Evaluation of exercise-induced bronchospasm (EIB) may be helpful in the following instances:

1. In patients who have shortness of breath on exertion but exhibit normal resting pulmonary function
2. In symptomatic patients in whom other bronchial provocation tests (such as methacholine challenge) produce negative or ambiguous results
3. In patients with known EIA in whom therapy is being evaluated
4. In screening patients where some risk to asthmatics might be involved (e.g., athletics, military service, etc.)

Patients referred for exercise challenge should be evaluated by means of an appropriate history and physical examination. The evaluation should include a resting electrocardiogram (ECG) to ascertain potential contraindications to exercise testing (see Chapter 7). Bronchodilators should be withheld as for methacholine challenge testing (Table 9-2). Before exercise, the patient's FEV_1 should not be less than 65% of the predicted value. Patients with overt obstruction do not require an exercise challenge to demonstrate airway hyperreactivity. Patients should refrain from vigorous exercise for 4 hours before the test because there is a refractory period after exercise. Patients referred for EIB testing should be free from respiratory infections for 3 to 6 weeks before testing.

Either a treadmill or a cycle ergometer may be used, depending on the type of physiologic measurements being made. Exercise should be vigorous enough to elicit work rates of 80% to 90% of the patient's predicted heart rate (HR) for 6 to 8 minutes. The patient's response to an increasing workload should be monitored via continuous ECG and blood pressure (BP). A pulse oximeter should be used to determine whether oxygen desaturation occurs with exercise. Because pulse oximetry is not always accurate during exercise, an arterial line may be indicated if there is a high probability that exercise desaturation will occur. Measurement of variables such as minute ventilation $\dot{V}_E$ and tidal volume (V_T) may be helpful in assessing the ventilatory load imposed by the exercise. Measurement of F-V curves during exercise may be a useful adjunct in assessing the ventilatory response to increasing workloads (see Chapter 7). A spirometer that meets ATS requirements (see Chapter 10) is necessary. Resuscitation equipment, as described in Chapter 7, should be available.

Because EIB is related to heat and water loss from the upper airway, environmental conditions should be controlled. Room temperature should be less than 25° C with relative humidity of 50% or less. The patient should wear nose clips, even if exhaled gas is not collected, to reduce gas conditioning by nasal airflow. The patient may also be allowed to breathe dry gas from a compressed air source using a setup similar to that described for EVH (without added CO_2). Ambient temperature, relative humidity, and barometric pressure (P_B) should be recorded.

Low-intensity exercise for 1 to 2 minutes allows evaluation of ventilatory and cardiovascular responses to work. As soon as a normal cardiovascular response is observed, workload should be increased until the patient attains 85% of predicted maximal HR or predicted maximal oxygen consumption $\dot{V}_{O_2}$. Alternately, the minute ventilation ($\dot{V}_E$) may be used as a target for exercise intensity if exhaled gas is collected. Ventilation should reach 40% to 60% of the patient's predicted MVV. The treadmill or cycle ergometer can be adjusted to increase or decrease the workload to maintain the correct intensity for the desired length of time.

In most instances, a short period of moderately heavy work is all that is required to trigger exercise-induced bronchospasm. The goal is to have the patient exercise at high intensity for 4 to 6 minutes, with a total exercise duration of 6 to 8 minutes. Bronchospasm usually occurs immediately after the exercise, not during it, unless the test is extended over a longer interval (Test Regimens 9-2). Repeated testing should be delayed for 4 hours because of a "refractory period" during which the severity of the bronchoconstriction lessens. This response is presumably caused by the release of catecholamines during exercise. An extended warm-up period before the actual exercise may also protect the airways and lessen subsequent bronchoconstriction.

Baseline spirometry values are established before testing. The patient should be able to perform acceptable and reproducible FEV_1 measurements. Inability to perform acceptable spirometry will make interpretation of postexercise changes very difficult. As for hyperventilation challenge, the baseline value is also the control. After exercise, spirometry is performed at 1 to 2 minutes, then every 5 minutes as the selected variable (usually FEV_1 or SGaw) decreases to a minimum. For spirometry, the highest value of acceptable measurements is recorded; FEV_1 should be reproducible. The preferred method of reporting response to exercise is:

$$\% \, \text{Decrease} = \frac{x - y}{x} \times 100$$

where:
x = baseline value (FEV_1 or SGaw)
y = lowest postexercise value

Testing is continued until the parameter returns to baseline. Maximal decreases are typically seen in the first 5 to 10 minutes after cessation of exercise. A decrease in FEV_1 of 10% to 15% is consistent with increased airway reactivity. Spontaneous recovery occurs within 20 to 40 minutes.

Severe bronchospasm may occur, and the technologist performing the test should be prepared to manage it. If the bronchospasm is severe, it should be reversed using an inhaled bronchodilator. FEV_1 should return to within 10% of the pretest baseline value. Administration of a bronchodilator may also be useful in assessing borderline decreases in FEV_1 (<10%) following exercise challenge. Patients who show a minimal decrease after exercise may improve dramatically with an inhaled bronchodilator, suggesting increased airway responsiveness.

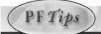

PF Tips

The normal response to exercise is for the FEV_1 (and specific conductance) to increase slightly. Patients who have exercise-induced bronchospasm usually have a decrease in flows (FEV_1). When an increase is expected, a decrease of 10% to 15% is consistent with airway hyperreactivity. Some patients have a much greater decrease in response to even moderate exercise, so the pulmonary function technologist should be prepared to reverse severe bronchospasm.

Patients who have VCD or other upper airway abnormalities are often referred for EIA tests. F-V curves (including inspiratory flows) should be performed if the history or physical examination suggests these disorders. Measurement of F-V loops during exercise may also help to define the pattern of ventilatory limitation.

One potential problem with using exercise to elicit EIB is that the level of exercise chosen may not mimic real-world triggers. Sedentary patients may not attain a level of ventilation high enough to trigger EIB when exercising at 85% of their maximal HR. Patients who are very fit (elite athletes, etc.) may require very high workloads to reach 85% of their predicted HR. Measurement of $\dot{V}_E$ during exercise may be needed to determine the level of ventilation attained. Patients whose asthma is triggered by cold, dry air may not show a maximal response if tested under standard laboratory conditions. Exercise-induced bronchospasm may be evaluated using one of the hyperventilation techniques described previously. These techniques eliminate the need for more complicated exercise testing. EVH (using a target ventilation level) may be more sensitive in detecting airway hyperreactivity than exercise testing.

Preoperative Pulmonary Function Testing

Preoperative pulmonary function testing is one of several means available to clinicians to evaluate surgical candidates at risk for developing respiratory complications. Preoperative testing, in conjunction with history and physical examination, ECG, and chest x-ray examination, may be indicated for any of the following reasons:

1. To estimate postoperative lung function in candidates for pneumonectomy or lobectomy
2. To plan perioperative care (preoperative preparation, type and duration of anesthetic during surgery, postoperative care) to minimize complications
3. To enhance the estimate of risk involved in the surgical procedure (i.e., morbidity and mortality) derived from history and physical examination

The need for preoperative pulmonary function testing is controversial. Some studies show increased odds of postoperative complications related to low FEV_1, hypoxemia, low DL_{CO}, hypercarbia, or low $\dot{V}O_2$. Other studies show little relationship between pulmonary function and postoperative risk, especially for general surgical and cardiovascular operations. Many investigations, both prospective and retrospective, have identified that the risk of postoperative pulmonary complications is highest in thoracic procedures, followed by upper and lower abdominal procedures. Postoperative pulmonary complications may occur in as many as 25% to 50% of major surgical procedures. Patients who have pulmonary disease are at higher risk in proportion to the degree of their pulmonary impairment. Specific tests, such as spirometry or DL_{CO}, seem to be most useful in candidates for lung resection or esophagectomy.

Preoperative pulmonary function testing may be indicated in patients who have the following:

1. A smoking history
2. Symptoms of pulmonary disease (e.g., cough, sputum production, shortness of breath)
3. Abnormal physical examination findings, particularly of the chest (e.g., abnormal breath sounds, ventilatory pattern, respiratory rate)
4. Abnormal chest radiographs

Preoperative testing may also be indicated in the following:

1. Patients who are obese (more than 30% above ideal body weight)
2. Patients who are advanced in age, usually more than 70 years of age
3. Patients who have current or recent respiratory infections or a history of respiratory infections
4. Patients who are markedly debilitated or malnourished

The value of pulmonary function studies to predict perioperative complications is controversial. Some studies have shown that FEV_1, DL_{CO}, PaO_2, and $PaCO_2$ are useful in assessing preoperative risk. Other studies have shown no clear indicators of postoperative complications. PFTs seem to be most useful in patients undergoing lung resection or esophagectomy. FEV_1 and DL_{CO} have been used to predict postoperative lung function in lung resection.

In these patients, the primary purpose of pulmonary function testing is to reveal preexisting pulmonary impairment. VC may decrease more than 50% from the preoperative value in thoracic or upper abdominal procedures. This places individuals with compromised function at risk of developing atelectasis and pneumonia. Postoperative decreases in FRC and increases in closing volume (CV) may lead to ventilation-perfusion ($\dot{V}/\dot{Q}$) abnormalities and hypoxemia. Abnormal ventilatory function related to the central control of respiration or to the ventilatory muscles may also play a role in postoperative complications.

Certain tests of pulmonary function appear to be better predictors of postoperative complications. These tests should be used both for risk evaluation and to assist in planning the perioperative care of the individual.

1. *Spirometry.* FVC, FEV_1, $FEF_{25\%-75\%}$, MVV. Obstructive disease can be easily identified with simple spirometry. A significant percentage of patients who may develop postoperative problems can be detected with minimal screening. Patients who have reduced FVC, with

or without airways obstruction, typically have an impaired ability to cough effectively when VC decreases further during the immediate postoperative period. The FEV_1 is also used to predict postoperative pulmonary function in lung resection or pneumonectomy.

2. *Bronchodilator studies.* Operative candidates with airway obstruction should also be tested with bronchodilators. Postbronchodilator values for FVC, FEV_1, $FEF_{25\%-75\%}$, and MVV may be used in estimating surgical risk. There may be significantly less risk if the patient's airway obstruction is reversible. Bronchodilator studies are similarly helpful in planning perioperative care. Bronchodilator therapy may improve the patient's bronchial hygiene both before and after surgery.

3. *Blood gas analysis.* Arterial blood gas analysis is helpful in assessing patients with documented lung disease to determine the response to pulmonary changes that occur postoperatively. PaO_2 is not a good predictor of postoperative problems. Individuals with hypoxemia at rest usually also have abnormal spirometry results, and hence are at risk. PaO_2 may improve postoperatively in patients undergoing thoracotomy for lung resection if the resected portion contributed to $\dot{V}/\dot{Q}$ abnormalities. $PaCO_2$ appears to be the most useful blood gas indicator of surgical risk. $PaCO_2$ above 45 mm Hg in combination with airway obstruction and pulmonary symptoms (wheezing, cough, etc.) presents an increased risk of postoperative morbidity and mortality.

4. *Exercise testing.* Exercise studies can accurately predict patients at risk. Individuals who cannot tolerate moderate workloads often have airway obstruction or similar ventilatory limitations. Patients who can attain an oxygen uptake ($\dot{V}O_2$) greater than 20 ml/min/kg typically have a low incidence of cardiopulmonary complications. Those unable to attain a $\dot{V}O_2$ of 15 ml/min/kg almost always have complications.

5. DL_{CO}. A few studies have indicated that a low percent predicted postoperative diffusing capacity is an independent indicator of increased morbidity and mortality in patients undergoing lung resection.

In addition to routine pulmonary function studies, several other tests are used in predicting postoperative lung function in candidates for pneumonectomy or lobectomy. These procedures are normally used in addition to spirometry and blood gas analysis.

1. *Perfusion and $\dot{V}/\dot{Q}$ scans.* Lung scans are particularly useful in estimating the remaining lung function in patients who are likely to require removal of all or part of a lung. Split-function scans are performed. These allow partitioning of lungs into right and left halves, or into multiple lung regions. Although ventilation-perfusion scans give the best estimate of overall function, simple perfusion scans yield similar information. Lung scan data, in the form of regional function percentages, are used in combination with simple spirometric indices to calculate the patient's postoperative capacity. An example follows:

$$\text{Postoperative } FEV_1 = \text{Preoperative } FEV_1 \times \%\text{Perfusion to unaffected regions}$$

Patients whose postoperative FEV_1 is less than 800 ml are typically not considered surgical candidates. Resection of any lung parenchyma resulting in an FEV_1 less than 800 ml would leave the patient more severely impaired. One exception to this general guideline occurs in patients referred for lung volume reduction surgery (LVRS). These candidates are usually end-stage COPD patients, often with FEV_1 values less than 800 ml and significant air trapping. Removal of poorly ventilated lung tissue often results in an improvement in spirometry, with significant increases in both FVC and FEV_1.

2. *Pulmonary artery occlusion pressure.* In some candidates for pneumonectomy, the development of postoperative pulmonary hypertension may be a limiting factor. To estimate the effect of redirecting the entire right ventricular output to the remaining lung,

TABLE 9-5 Preoperative Pulmonary Function

Test	Increased Postoperative Risk	High Postoperative Risk	Candidate for Pneumonectomy*
FVC	Less than 50% of predicted	Less than 1.5 L	
FEV_1	Less than 2.0 L or 50% of predicted	Less than 1.0 L	Greater than 2.0 L
$FEF_{25\%-75\%}$	Less than 50% of predicted		
MVV		Less than 50 L/min or 50% of predicted	Greater than 50 L/min or 50% of predicted
$Paco_2$		Greater than 45 mm Hg	
$\dot{V}o_{2max}$	15-20 ml/min/kg	Less than 15 ml/min/kg	
Predicted postoperative FEV_1			Greater than 0.8 L/min
Pulmonary artery occlusion			Less than 35 mm Hg

*Values in this column determine whether the patient is to be considered a candidate for lung resection (see text).

a catheter is inserted into the pulmonary artery of the affected lung and blood flow occluded by means of a balloon. The resulting pressure increase in the remaining lung is then measured. A pressure increasing to less than 35 mm Hg is usually considered consistent with acceptable postoperative pressures. The effect of redirected blood flow on oxygenation may also be a consideration. This can also be examined during occlusion to estimate postoperative Pao_2.

Tests that predict the effects of resection on the remaining lung are normally done in series, with spirometry done first, followed by split-function lung scans (if spirometry results are acceptable), and then pulmonary artery occlusion pressure (if cor pulmonale is a concern). Table 9-5 summarizes general value ranges used for preoperative pulmonary function testing.

Pulmonary Function Testing for Disability

Pulmonary function tests are one of several means of determining a patient's inability to perform certain tasks. Respiratory impairment and disability, however, are not synonymous. Respiratory impairment relates to the failure of one or more of the functions of the lungs, as measured by pulmonary function studies. Disability is the inability to perform tasks required for employment and includes medically determinable physical or mental impairment. The impairment must be expected to either result in death or last for at least 12 months. Impairment in children must be comparable to that which would disable an adult.

Pulmonary function tests used to determine impairment leading to disability should characterize the type, extent, and cause of impairment. Pulmonary function testing may not completely describe all factors involved in the disabling impairment. Other factors involved may be age, educational background, and patient motivation. The energy requirements of the task in question also affect the level of disability.

Determination of the level of impairment caused by pulmonary disease usually includes history and physical examination, chest x-ray examination, other appropriate imaging techniques, and pulmonary function tests.

Pulmonary function tests are often used in assessing disability from lung disease. Because tests such as FVC and FEV_1 are effort-dependent, it is important that all tests meet established criteria for acceptability and reproducibility. Low values for FVC and FEV_1 may be due to lung disease or poor effort. Careful attention to test acceptability and reproducibility can help distinguish pathophysiology from poor effort.

Physical examination does not allow measurement of disabling symptoms but is useful in grading shortness of breath. Shortness of breath is the most prominent feature of respiratory impairment. Shortness of breath, like pain, is subjective. Tachypnea, cyanosis, and abnormal respiratory patterns are not indicative of the extent of impairment but may be helpful in interpreting pulmonary function studies.

Chest x-ray studies do not correlate well with shortness of breath or pulmonary function studies, except in advanced cases of pneumoconioses (i.e., "dust" diseases). Absence of usual findings in the pneumoconioses may be helpful in excluding occupational exposure to toxins as part of the impairment.

Pulmonary function studies should be objective and reproducible and, most important, specific to the disorder being investigated. Impairments caused by chronic respiratory disorders usually produce irreversible loss of function because of ventilatory impairment, gas exchange abnormalities, or a combination of both.

◼ FORCED VITAL CAPACITY AND FORCED EXPIRATORY VOLUME

Spirometry is the most useful index for the assessment of impairment caused by airway obstruction. The test should not be performed unless the patient is stable. The reported FVC and FEV_1 should be the largest values obtained from at least three acceptable maneuvers. The two largest FVC values and FEV_1 values should be reproducible within 5% or 0.1 L, whichever is greater. Spirometric efforts before and after bronchodilators should meet these reproducibility criteria. Computation of the FEV_1 should be done using back-extrapolated volumes (see Chapter 2). The spirogram is acceptable if the back-extrapolated volume is less than 5% of the FVC, or 0.1 L, whichever is greater. Each maneuver should be continued for 6 seconds or until there is no detectable change in volume for the last 2 seconds of the maneuver. It is unacceptable to report FEV_1 when only an F-V curve is recorded. It is *required* to provide a volume-time tracing from which FEV_1 can be measured. Spirometry should be repeated 10 minutes after bronchodilator if the prebronchodilator FEV_1 is less than 70% of predicted. All lung volumes and flows must be reported at body temperature, pressure, and saturation (BTPS). Standing height, without shoes, should be used for comparison of measured values with limits for disability (Table 9-6). In case of marked spinal deformity, arm-span measurement should be used (see Chapter 1).

TABLE 9-6 FEV₁ and FVC Values for Disability Determinations

Height Without Shoes (in)	FEV₁ Equal to or Less Than (L/BTPS)	FVC Equal to or Less Than (L/BTPS)
60 or less	1.05	1.25
61 to 63	1.15	1.35
64 to 65	1.25	1.45
66 to 67	1.35	1.55
68 to 69	1.45	1.65
70 to 71	1.55	1.75
72 to more	1.65	1.85

Adapted from Disability Evaluation under Social Security, US Department of Health and Human Services, Publication No 64-055, 1999.

Volume calibration of the spirometer should agree to within 1% of a 3-L syringe. If spirometer accuracy is less than 99% but within 3% of the calibration syringe, a calibration correction factor should be used (see Chapter 11). If a flow-sensing spirometer is used, linearity should be documented by performing calibration at three different flows (3 L/6 sec, 3 L/3 sec, and 3 L/1 sec). The volume-time tracing should have the time sensitivity marked on the horizontal axis and the volume sensitivity marked on the vertical axis. The paper speed should be at least 20 mm/sec and the volume excursion at least 10 mm/L. The manufacturer and model of the spirometer should be stated in the report (Test Regimens 9-3).

TEST REGIMENS 9-3   Criteria for Acceptability—Disability Testing

1 Spirometer must show a 3-L calibration that is within 1% or corrected within 3%. Flow-based spirometers should be calibrated at three different flows to demonstrate linearity. The manufacturer and model of spirometer should be stated.
2 All FVC maneuvers should be recorded before and after bronchodilator challenge. Time scale must be at least 20 mm/sec, volume scale at least 10 mm/L. FEV₁ may *not* be calculated from a flow-volume tracing.
3 There must be at least three acceptable FVC maneuvers before bronchodilator; the two largest values (FVC, FEV₁) should be within 5% or 0.1 L, whichever is greater.
4 The spirogram must show peak flow early in expiration with a smooth, gradually decreasing flow. The maneuver is acceptable if the effort continues for 6 seconds or if there is a plateau with no change in volume for 2 seconds. The FEV₁ should be measured using back-extrapolation; the back-extrapolated volume should be less than 5% of FVC or 0.1 L, whichever is greater.
5 Postbronchodilator studies should be performed if FEV₁ is less than 70% of predicted. Postbronchodilator testing should be done 10 minutes after administration of the drug. The name of the drug should be included.
6 DL_{CO} testing (if performed) should meet all current American Thoracic Society recommendations. DL_{CO} uncorrected for Hb is reported.
7 Exercise testing (if performed) should be for 6 to 8 minutes at a workload of approximately 5 METS. Blood gas samples should be obtained at rest and during exercise.
8 Statements regarding the patient's ability to understand directions, as well as effort and cooperation, should be included with all tests.

DIFFUSING CAPACITY

The DL_{CO} is useful in determining impairment in restrictive disorders such as pulmonary fibrosis. The single-breath method should be used. The standard criteria for acceptability for the DL_{CO} maneuver should be applied (see Chapter 5). The reported value should be uncorrected for hemoglobin (Hb), but abnormal Hb or carboxyhemoglobin (COHb) values should be reported. If the DL_{CO} is greater than 40% of predicted but less than 60%, resting blood gas analysis is indicated.

ARTERIAL BLOOD GAS ANALYSIS

Although blood gas results are objective, they are largely nonspecific in determining impairment. The A-aO_2 gradient may not be reliable because it can be affected by hyperventilation (Table 9-7). Blood gas analysis may be required in diffuse pulmonary fibrosis and should include PaO_2 and $PaCO_2$. Blood gases (and A-a gradient) may also be assessed during exercise. The requirement for supplemental oxygen (O_2) may also be quantified by exercise blood gas analysis. Pulse oximetry or capillary blood gas analysis is not an acceptable substitute for arterial blood gas analysis.

EXERCISE TESTING

Patients considered for exercise evaluation should first have resting blood gas evaluation, either sitting or standing. A steady-state exercise test (see Chapter 7) is then performed, preferably using a treadmill. The patient should exercise for 4 to 6 minutes at an O_2 consumption rate of approximately 17.5 ml/min/kg (approximately 5 METS) breathing room air. An equivalent workload should be used for cycle ergometry (e.g., 75 W for a 175-lb patient). Blood gas samples should be drawn at this workload to determine whether significant hypoxemia is present (see Table 9-7). If the patient does not desaturate at this level, a higher workload can be used to determine exercise capacity. If the patient cannot achieve a workload of 5 METS, a lower workload can be selected to determine exercise capacity. Blood gas samples obtained after completion of exercise are unacceptable.

TABLE 9-7 Arterial Oxygen Tension for Disability Determinations

PCO_2 (mm Hg)	Less Than 3000 ft Above Sea Level	3000 to 6000 ft Above Sea Level	More Than 6000 ft Above Sea Level
	PO_2 (mm Hg)	PO_2 (mm Hg)	PO_2 (mm Hg)
30 or below	≤65	≤60	≤55
31	≤64	≤59	≤54
32	≤63	≤58	≤53
33	≤62	≤57	≤52
34	≤61	≤56	≤51
35	≤60	≤55	≤50
36	≤59	≤54	≤49
37	≤58	≤53	≤48
38	≤57	≤52	≤47
39	≤56	≤51	≤46
40 or above	≤55	≤50	≤45

Adapted from *Disability evaluation under Social Security*, US Department of Health and Human Services, Publication No 64-055, 1999.

TEST REGIMENS 9-4   Interpretive Strategies—Disability Testing

1 Were spirometry, diffusing capacity, blood gases, and exercise tests performed acceptably? If not, interpret very cautiously or not at all.

2 Was FEV_1 less than the predicted limit for the patient's height? If so, disabling obstruction is very likely.

3 Was FVC less than the predicted limit for the patient's height? If so, disabling restrictive disease is likely.

4 Was the $D_{L_{CO}}$ (if measured) less than 10.5 ml/min/mm Hg or less than 40% of predicted? If so, the patient has a marked gas-exchange abnormality.

5 Was the patient's Pa_{O_2}, measured while clinically stable on two occasions at least 3 weeks apart but within 6 months, equal to or less than published limits (adjusted for Pa_{CO_2} and altitude)? If so disabling hypoxemia is present.

6 Was Pa_{O_2} equal to or less than published limits during steady-state exercise (less than or equivalent to 5 METS) breathing air? If so, disabling hypoxemia is present.

7 Are lung function measurements consistent with history, physical examination, chest x-ray study, and other imaging techniques?

ECG should be monitored continuously throughout the exercise evaluation, and blood gases drawn during the final 2 minutes of the test. It may be helpful to measure $\dot{V}_{O_2}$, $\dot{V}_{CO_2}$, and $\dot{V}_E$. The altitude of the test site and barometric pressure should be included in the report to assist with interpretation of blood gas values.

In reporting impairment for the purpose of determining disability, the remaining functional capacity is as important in determining the patient's ability to perform a certain task as the percentage of lost function. Some statement of the patient's ability to understand and cooperate during pulmonary function measurements should accompany the tabular and graphic data.

Limits for determining disability based on respiratory impairment have been set for the United States by the Social Security Administration. Criteria are set according to the disease category (Test Regimens 9-4). COPD is evaluated by comparing FEV_1 with the values in Table 9-6. Restrictive ventilatory disorders are evaluated by comparing FVC with the values in Table 9-6. Impaired gas exchange is evaluated by comparing Pa_{O_2} with the values in Table 9-7. Disability caused by asthma is also evaluated using FEV_1. Episodes of asthma (requiring emergency treatment or hospitalization) occurring at least every 2 months or at least 6 times per year may also be evidence of disability.

Metabolic Measurements: Indirect Calorimetry

■ DESCRIPTION

Measurements of $\dot{V}_{O_2}$, $\dot{V}_{CO_2}$, and the respiratory exchange ratio (RER, $\dot{V}_{O_2}/\dot{V}_{CO_2}$) may be used to determine resting energy expenditure (REE). REE is usually expressed in kilocalories/day (kcal/day). These measurements allow nutritional assessment and management. In combination with measurements of urinary nitrogen (UN), indirect calorimetry allows calories to be partitioned among various substrates (e.g., fat, carbohydrate, protein).

■ TECHNIQUE

Indirect calorimetry may be performed using either an open-circuit or closed-circuit system to measure O_2 consumption, CO_2 production, and RER.

Open-Circuit Calorimetry

Exchange of O_2 and CO_2 may be measured by recording and the fractional differences of O_2 and CO_2 between inspired and expired gas. These measurements are accomplished using either a mixing chamber, dilution system, or breath-by-breath system similar to those used for expired gas analysis during exercise (see Chapter 7). $\dot{V}O_2$ and $\dot{V}CO_2$ are measured as described for exercise testing using mixing chamber and breath-by-breath systems. $\dot{V}_E$, V_T, and f_B (respiratory rate) may be measured simultaneously. In systems that use the dilution principle, a constant flow of gas is mixed with expired air. The dilution of CO_2 is then used to calculate ventilation. Connection to the patient may be made by a standard directional breathing valve with mouthpiece and nose clips. A ventilated hood or canopy (Figure 9-4) may also be used.

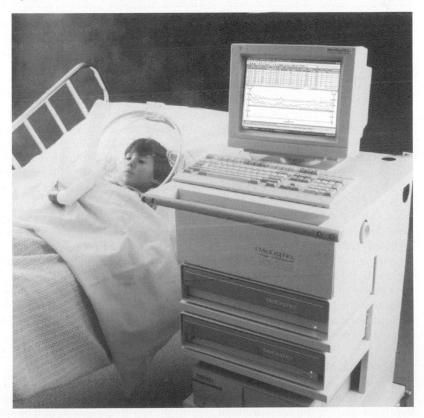

Figure 9-4 *Canopy for metabolic measurements (indirect calorimetry).* REE may be measured from changes in gas flow and fractional concentrations of expired air drawn from a hood or canopy. A continuous or "bias" flow of gas is drawn through the canopy. Changes (increases or decreases) in the bias flow are measured to determine ventilation. Fractional gas concentrations are determined from the gas drawn from the hood. The canopy offers the advantage of not requiring direct connection to the patient's airway, which may affect ventilation and the measurement of REE. For patients requiring mechanical support of ventilation, the measuring apparatus samples gas from the ventilator circuit. *(Courtesy Medical Graphics Corporation, St. Paul, Minn.)*

Almost all metabolic measurement systems provide for connection to a mechanical ventilator circuit.

A hood or canopy allows long-term measurements without direct connection to the patient's airway. The hood is ventilated by drawing a flow of gas through it that exceeds the patient's peak inspiratory demand (40 L/min is usually adequate). Ventilation can be calculated by measuring the change in flow into and out of the hood during breathing ("bias" flow).

Estimation of caloric needs for a 24-hour period from a metabolic study requires that the measurements be made with the patient in a steady state. The short interval during which measurements are made (usually 10 to 20 minutes) should be free of interruptions that may alter the patient's metabolic rate. These include ventilator changes or suctioning. Nutritional support (if given) should be continuous, and the patient should be resting.

Connection to a ventilator requires a means of measuring exhaled volume along with fractional concentrations of both inspired and expired gas. Breath-by-breath metabolic measurement systems usually sample gas at the patient-ventilator connection.

Closed-Circuit Calorimetry

The simplest type of closed-circuit calorimeter is one that measures $\dot{V}O_2$ volumetrically. The patient rebreathes from a closed system that contains a spirometer filled with oxygen. CO_2 is scrubbed from the circuit using a chemical absorber. A recorder is used to measure the decrease in spirometer volume, equal to the rate of O_2 uptake ($\dot{V}O_2$). A similar approach uses a closed spirometer system to measure the volume of oxygen added as the patient rebreathes and consumes oxygen. $\dot{V}O_2$ is equal to the volume of O_2 that must be added per minute to maintain a constant volume. CO_2 production cannot be measured using a closed-circuit system unless a CO_2 analyzer is added to the device. $\dot{V}_E$, V_T, and respiratory rate may all be determined from volume excursions of the spirometer. Closed-circuit systems may be used with spontaneously breathing patients by means of a simple breathing valve and mouthpiece. Use of a closed-circuit calorimeter with a mechanical ventilator requires that the spirometer system be connected between the patient and ventilator. The ventilator then "ventilates" the spirometer, which in turn ventilates the patient. This technique usually requires a bellows-type spirometer in a fixed container so that the positive pressure generated by the ventilator can compress the bellows. The volume delivered by the ventilator (V_I) must be increased to compensate for the volume of gas compressed in the closed-circuit spirometer during positive pressure breaths.

Performing Metabolic Measurements

The primary purpose of indirect calorimetry is to estimate REE over an extended period, usually 24 hours. To extrapolate the values obtained during the sampling period, the patient's condition during the measurement is critical (Test Regimens 9-5). The following guidelines help ensure that measurements are made under steady-state conditions:

1. The patient should be recumbent or supine for 20 to 30 minutes before beginning measurements and should stay quiet during the test. Ideally, the patient should be awake and aware during testing. The testing apparatus should not cause discomfort or exertion for the patient. Breathing valves, mouthpieces, and nose clips may alter the patient's breathing pattern.

2. The patient should fast for 2 to 4 hours before the test starts. If the patient is receiving either enteral or parenteral feedings, the feedings should be continuous rather than in bolus form. Information about the type and amount of nutritional support in the previous 24 hours may be helpful in interpreting test results.

3. The patient should be in a neutral thermal environment. Special corrections may be required for patients who are febrile or hypothermic. The patient's temperature at the time of the test should be recorded along with a temperature history of the previous 24 hours. Temperature changes of 1° C can result in a 13% change in REE.

4. Drugs or substances that alter metabolism should be avoided. Substances such as caffeine and nicotine are particularly common stimulants. Theophylline-based drugs may also increase metabolic rate.

5. Data collection should continue long enough to establish a stable baseline and verify steady-state conditions (Figure 9-5) Ten to fifteen minutes of stable readings for $\dot{V}O_2$ and $\dot{V}CO_2$ are recommended. Common indicators of steady-state conditions are the parameters assessed as part of the metabolic study. $\dot{V}O_2$ should not vary more than 10% from the mean value measured during the test. $\dot{V}CO_2$ should be within 6% of the mean

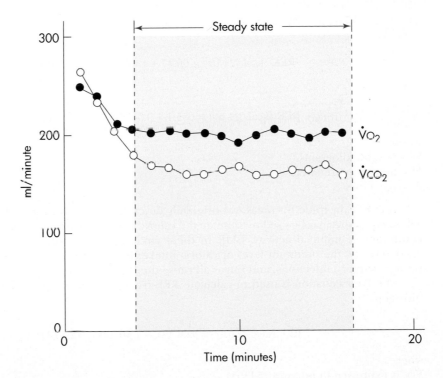

Figure 9-5 *Indirect calorimetry.* Typical tracing of continuous measurement of $\dot{V}O_2$ and $\dot{V}CO_2$ as performed during open-circuit indirect calorimetry. The patient's expired gas is analyzed to determine O_2 consumption, CO_2 production, and RQ during a resting state. Measurements are observed until a metabolic steady state can be determined (usually 10 to 15 minutes). During the steady-state interval, values representing REE are measured. Daily caloric requirements are estimated from these measurements. If a 24-hour urinary urea nitrogen (UUN) sample is obtained, the percentages of energy derived from fats, carbohydrates, and proteins can be calculated (see text).

during the same interval. RER (RQ) values should be within the normal physiologic range (0.67 to 1.30). If the patient does not achieve steady-state conditions, a longer test interval may be required to average representative periods of metabolic activity.

6. Patients on ventilators should be in a stable condition. No ventilator adjustments should be made 1 to 2 hours before the test period. Modifications in minute ventilation or FIO_2 settings can cause gross changes in the patterns of gas exchange, particularly in patients with pulmonary disease. The ventilator must have a stable delivered oxygen concentration; FIO_2 settings greater than 0.60 may result in erroneous $\dot{V}O_2$ measurements. Appropriate valves may need to be used for ventilator modes that involve continuous gas flow.

7. The calorimeter or metabolic cart should be calibrated at least daily, preferably before each test. Gas analyzers should be calibrated using gas concentrations appropriate for the clinical situation. Sample lines and gas-conditioning devices (absorbers) should be checked before each test. If calibration or testing produces questionable values, the device should be checked against a known standard. Burning ethanol or other material with a fixed RQ can be used. A large-volume syringe can be used to simulate a patient with $\dot{V}O_2$ and $\dot{V}CO_2$ values near zero.

Metabolic Calculations

The Harris-Benedict equations are used to estimate REE:
   Men:

$$REE \text{ (kcal/24 hr)} = 66.47 + 13.75W + 5H - 6.76A$$

   Women:

$$REE \text{ (kcal/24 hr)} = 655.1 + 9.56W + 1.85H - 4.68A$$

where:
W = weight, kilograms
H = height, centimeters
A = age, years

The REE by these formulas was originally described as the basal metabolic rate (BMR). These equations may be used to estimate the caloric expenditure in normal individuals under conditions of minimal activity. BMR in these circumstances is related to lean body mass. To determine the optimum level of caloric intake, BMR must be adjusted upward because trauma, surgery, infections, and burns all cause the REE to increase.

The Weir equation is used to calculate REE from respiratory gas exchange and urinary nitrogen:

$$REE \text{ (kcal/24 hr)} = 5.68\,\dot{V}O_2 + 1.59\,\dot{V}CO_2 - 2.17\,UN$$

where:
$\dot{V}O_2$ is expressed in ml/min (STPD)
$\dot{V}CO_2$ is expressed in ml/min (STPD)
UN = urinary nitrogen (g/24 hr)

If UN is unknown, REE may be calculated:

$$REE \text{ (kcal/24 hr)} = 5.46\,\dot{V}O_2 + 1.75\,\dot{V}CO_2$$

Indirect calorimetry by the open-circuit method provides measures of both O_2 consumption and CO_2 production. As previously mentioned, RER is the ratio $\dot{V}_{CO_2}/\dot{V}_{O_2}$. Under steady-state conditions, RER approximates the mean respiratory quotient (RQ) at the cell level. RQ normally varies from 0.71 to 1.00, depending on the substrates being metabolized. Carbohydrate oxidation produces an RQ near 1.0, fat oxidation produces an RQ near 0.71, and protein oxidation produces an RQ of 0.82. RQ attributable to carbohydrates and fats may be determined by subtracting $\dot{V}_{O_2}$ and $\dot{V}_{CO_2}$ derived from protein. This form of the RQ is termed the nonprotein RQ or RQnp and is calculated as follows:

$$RQnp = \frac{1.44\,\dot{V}_{CO_2} - 4.754\,UN}{1.44\,\dot{V}_{O_2} - 5.923\,UN}$$

where:
$\dot{V}_{CO_2}$ is expressed in ml/min
$\dot{V}_{O_2}$ is expressed in ml/min
UN = urinary nitrogen (g/24 hr)
1.44 – factor to convert ml/min to L/24 hr

Because CO_2 production varies with O_2 uptake, deviations of the RQ from the average value of 0.85 result in differences of less than 5% in the calculation of REE if only $\dot{V}_{O_2}$ and RQ are used. Indirect calorimetry by the closed-circuit (volumetric) method takes advantage of this small difference by assuming a fixed RQ (usually 0.85) and measuring only $\dot{V}_{O_2}$. UN is obtained from a 24-hour urine collection. Because protein metabolism accounts for only a small portion of total calories per day (approximately 12%), omission of the UN in the Weir equation changes the calculated REE by only 2%.

The Consolazio equations can be used to determine energy expenditure from gas exchange ($\dot{V}_{O_2}$, $\dot{V}_{CO_2}$), UN, and the caloric equivalents of carbohydrates, fats, and proteins:

$$CHO = 5.926\,\dot{V}_{CO_2} - 4.189\,\dot{V}_{O_2} - 2.539\,UN$$
$$FAT = 2.432\,\dot{V}_{O_2} - 2.432\,\dot{V}_{CO_2} - 1.943\,UN$$
$$PRO = 6.250\,UN$$

where:
CHO = Carbohydrates oxidized in grams/24 hours
FAT = Fat oxidized in grams/24 hours
PRO = Protein oxidized in grams/24 hours

From the grams of each substrate used, the kilocalories derived from that source can be computed:

$$\text{carbohydrates (in kcal)} = 4.18\ \text{carbohydrates (in g)}$$
$$\text{fat (in kcal)} = 9.46\ \text{fat (in g)}$$
$$\text{protein (in kcal)} = 4.32\ \text{protein (in g)}$$
$$\text{total (in Kcal)} = \text{carbohydrate} + \text{fat} + \text{protein}$$

The percentage of calories from each substrate may also be calculated by dividing the kilocalories derived from that substrate by the total kilocalories. Because the Consolazio equations are intended for analysis of normal substrate partitioning, RQ values outside of the range of 0.71 to 1.00 will result in negative values for either carbohydrates or lipids (fat). These negative values are erroneous if RER does not equal RQ (i.e., the patient is not in a metabolic steady state).

TEST REGIMENS 9-5   Criteria for Acceptability—Indirect Calorimetry

1 Appropriate calibration of gas analyzers and volume transducers should be documented daily, preferably before each test.
2 RQ should be within the normal physiologic range of 0.67 to 1.30.
3 Measured $\dot{V}o_2$ values should vary by no more than ±10% around the mean; $\dot{V}co_2$ values should vary by less than ±6% of the mean.
4 Data should be collected for a minimum of 10 to 15 minutes with minimal variability.
5 RQ values should be consistent with the patient's current nutritional intake.
6 Documentation should include the patient's medications, nutritional support, body temperature at time of test, and ventilatory support setting (if applicable).
7 The patient should be resting; no bolus feedings or pharmacologic stimulants or depressants. There should be no physical therapy, airway care, or major ventilator changes immediately before assessment.
8 If a 24-hour urinary urea nitrogen (UUN) is collected for substrate use, it should be concurrent with the metabolic study.

■ SIGNIFICANCE AND PATHOPHYSIOLOGY

See Test Regimens 9-6 for interpretive strategies. Indirect calorimetry assesses nutritional status in patients whose daily energy needs are altered by disease, injury, or therapeutic interventions. REE accounts for approximately two thirds of the daily energy requirements in healthy patients. The Harris-Benedict equations, or similar predictive equations, are commonly used to estimate REE. Various factors can be used to adjust estimated REE to account for additional caloric needs imposed by the patient's clinical status. This approach works well in many patients. However, metabolic requirements of critically ill patients vary widely. Indirect calorimetry is indicated for patients who do not respond favorably to traditional methods of nutritional assessment and support. Indirect calorimetry can be used to detect undernourishment, overnourishment, or use of inappropriate substrates (Table 9-8).

TEST REGIMENS 9-6   Interpretive Strategies—Indirect Calorimetry

1 Were metabolic data collected acceptably? Did $\dot{V}o_2$ values vary by less than 10%? Did $\dot{V}co_2$ values vary by less than 6%? If not, interpret cautiously. Was RQ between 0.67 and 1.30? If not, interpret very cautiously or not at all.
2 Was measured REE less than predicted (Harris-Benedict equation)? If so, consider technical error or hypometabolic state.
3 Was RQ less than 0.70? If so, consider ketosis or starvation.
4 Was RQ greater than 1.00? If so, consider lipogenesis or nonsteady state (hyperventilation).
5 Is the measured REE significantly greater than the patient's intake in the previous 24 hours? If so, the patient is probably being underfed or may be febrile.
6 Is the measured REE significantly less than the patient's intake in the previous 24 hours? If so, the patient is probably being overfed.
7 Is the nonprotein RQ near 1.00? If so, the main substrate being used is carbohydrate. Is the nonprotein RQ near 0.70? If so, the main substrate is fat.
8 Are metabolic measurements consistent with the patient's clinical status? Is nutritional support (if provided) appropriate for metabolic needs?

TABLE 9-8 Indications for Indirect Calorimetry*

Head trauma or paralysis
COPD
Multiple trauma
Acute pancreatitis
Patients in whom height or weight is indeterminate
Poor response to enteral or parenteral support
Patients receiving total parenteral nutrition at home
Transplant patients
Morbidly obese patients
Patients with demonstrated hypermetabolism or hypometabolism
Patients on prolonged mechanical ventilation who are unable to eat

*Risk and/or stress factors known to interfere with calculation of energy expenditure.

Undernourishment or starvation can occur during illness. It may be detected by caloric expenditure in excess of caloric intake (negative energy balance). Both fat stores and protein from muscle breakdown may contribute to metabolism during periods of undernourishment. Indirect calorimetry is often used along with measurement of body weight, triceps skinfold measurements, and other approximations of energy reserves. These measurements allow planning of nutritional therapy to replenish diminished reserves.

Overnourishment occurs when any substrate is supplied in excess of the energy requirements. Overfeeding is most deleterious when the patient's nutritional status is already adequate. Excess lipid or carbohydrate calories are stored as fat, which may place stress on one or more organ systems.

Patients with pulmonary disease present a special dilemma. Excessive carbohydrate intake results in increased CO_2 production because the RQ of carbohydrates is 1. For patients in respiratory failure, excess CO_2 production increases the ventilatory load on the respiratory system. Adjustments in substrate use can be made after the nonprotein RQ is determined by indirect calorimetry. Lipids (i.e., fats) are typically substituted for glucose so that the RQ can be reduced while the caloric intake is maintained. Patients in respiratory failure may also experience atrophy of ventilatory muscles. Substrate analysis can be used to assess N_2 balance related to the breakdown of muscle protein. Substrate analysis permits measurement of nutritional requirements necessary to maintain N_2 balance.

Technical considerations involved in indirect calorimetry include the accuracy of gas analysis and measurement of expired volume during the test. The most common problem during metabolic measurements is attainment of a true steady state. Only if the measurements are made under steady-state conditions is the metabolic rate representative of caloric expenditure over 24 hours. Hyperventilation resulting from connection to a mask or mouthpiece, or from ventilator manipulation, occurs frequently. Head hoods or continuous-flow canopies can eliminate much of the stimulation associated with connection to the metabolic measurement system (Figure 9-4) but cannot be used for patients on mechanical ventilators. An RER greater than 1 should always be evaluated in relation to $\dot{V}_E$ and end-tidal CO_2. Abnormally high and low end-tidal CO_2 values may indicate hyperventilation. RER values in excess of 1 that cannot be explained as hyperventilation may be caused by storage of excess calories as fat (lipogenesis). RER values between 0.67 and 0.70 may occur in ketosis caused by extreme fasting or diabetic ketoacidosis. However, more commonly, low RER values (less than 0.67) signal improper calibration of the CO_2 or O_2 analyzers. Inaccurate calibration or improper performance of gas analyzers can result in RER values outside of the usual metabolic range of 0.70 to 1.

Special problems may be encountered in performing metabolic measurements on patients requiring mechanical ventilatory support. A common difficulty relates to measurements of O_2 consumption in patients receiving supplemental O_2. Measurement of $\dot{V}O_2$ by respiratory gas exchange requires analysis of the difference between inspired and expired O_2 along with $\dot{V}_E$. In patients breathing room air, inspired FIO_2 is constant. Many oxygen-blending systems, such as those used on ventilators, may not provide a constant fraction of inspired O_2. Large differences in calculated $\dot{V}O_2$ may result from small fluctuations in FIO_2, even if F_EO_2 remains relatively constant. Small differences in inspired and expired volumes (resulting from the RER) are corrected by adjusting the inspired fraction of oxygen according to the following equation:

$$\frac{(1 - F_EO_2 - F_ECO_2)}{1 - FIO_2} \times FIO_2$$

The correction of inspired FIO_2 for gas balance in the lung (i.e., the Haldane transformation) limits the accuracy of the open-circuit method of determining $\dot{V}O_2$. As FIO_2 increases, the value in the denominator of the equation becomes smaller. Even with very accurate gas analyzers, measurement of differences between FIO_2 and F_EO_2 (when FIO_2 is above 0.60) is variable. Indirect calorimetry by the volumetric method (i.e., a closed system) avoids this problem by measuring the actual volume of O_2 removed during rebreathing. Allowing the patient to breathe from a reservoir bag containing an elevated FIO_2 can usually accommodate measurement of $\dot{V}O_2$ and $\dot{V}CO_2$ in spontaneously breathing patients who require supplemental O_2.

Other considerations involved in metabolic measurements of ventilated patients include the effects of positive pressure on gas analysis and on volume determination. Analysis of O_2 and CO_2 in the ventilator circuit must take into account the effect of positive pressure breaths on the gas analyzers. Depending on the sampling method used, positive pressure swings during each breath may generate falsely high partial pressure readings. Closed-circuit calorimetry places a volumetric device in the breathing circuit between the ventilator and the patient. The volume delivered by the ventilator must be increased to accommodate the higher compressible gas volume in the circuit, approximately 1 ml/cm H_2O for each liter of added volume.

Summary

This chapter discusses the application of pulmonary function tests for specific purposes. Each special regimen uses tests that have been discussed previously. Spirometry is used for bronchial challenge tests, preoperative testing, and tests designed to evaluate disability. Other tests (e.g., lung volumes, blood gases) are used because they answer specific clinical questions. Metabolic studies that use techniques associated with exhaled gas analysis are an additional tool used to manage critically ill patients.

Bronchial challenge tests can be done using several different agents, all of which test the airway responsiveness in slightly different ways. Methacholine challenge is the most commonly used and best-standardized test of airway hyperreactivity. Histamine and antigenic agents are also used. Exercise testing can be specifically used to evaluate exercise-induced bronchospasm. Hyperventilation tests, with cold or room-temperature air, mimic the ventilatory load that occurs with exercise.

Preoperative and disability testing use spirometry, lung volumes, diffusing capacity, blood gases, and exercise testing. Each test examines a specific aspect of either preoperative risk or respiratory impairment that prevents work.

Metabolic measurements, specifically indirect calorimetry, provide a means of assessing nutritional status and support. Indirect calorimetry has been shown to be more accurate than simple estimates of REE in mechanically ventilated patients. It may be particularly useful in the evaluation of patients who do not respond adequately to estimated nutritional needs.

CASE STUDIES

CASE 9-1

HISTORY

M.M. is a 39-year-old woman who has recently experienced episodes of "choking and coughing." She was referred by an industrial health specialist who suspected reactive airway involvement. M.M. relates that cigarette smoke and strong odors seem to bring on the episodes. She has never smoked and has no history of lung disease. She had some childhood allergies that disappeared at puberty. There is no history of lung disease in her immediate family. M.M. is not currently taking any medications.

PULMONARY FUNCTION TESTS

Personal Data

Sex: Female
Age: 39 yr
Height: 66 in
Weight: 130 lb

Spirometry

	Before Drug	**Predicted**	**%**
FVC (L)	3.71	3.8	98
FEV_1 (L)	2.96	2.97	99
$FEV_1\%$ (%)	80	78	—
$FEF_{25\%-75\%}$ (L/sec)	2.99	3.34	90
MVV (L/min)	106.4	109.7	97
Raw (cm H_2O/L/sec)	2.37	0.6-2.4	—
SGaw (L/sec/cm H_2O/L)	0.14	0.14-0.56	—

Methacholine Challenge*

Methacholine (mg/ml)	FEV_1	%Control	SGaw	%Control
Baseline	2.96	—	0.14	—
Control	2.92	100	0.14	—
0.0625	2.93	100	0.13	93
0.25	2.90	99	0.11	79
1.0	2.75	94	0.11	79
4.0	2.41	83	0.09	64
16.0	1.99	68	0.08	57

*5-breath dosimeter method.

TECHNOLOGIST'S COMMENTS

All spirometry and body box efforts were acceptable and reproducible.

QUESTIONS

1. What is the interpretation of:

   ■ Spirometry?
   ■ Airway resistance and conductance?

2. What is the interpretation of the methacholine challenge?
3. What is the cause of the patient's symptoms?
4. What treatment might be recommended based on these findings?

DISCUSSION

Interpretation (Prechallenge Pulmonary Function)

Spirometry before and during the inhalation challenge was performed acceptably, as were maneuvers in the body plethysmograph. Spirometry results are within normal limits. Raw and SGaw are close to the limits of normal, consistent with some airflow obstruction.

Interpretation (Methacholine Challenge)

The methacholine challenge test is positive with a PC_{20} of approximately 5.2 mg/ml. The test was terminated because the patient's FEV_1 decreased below 80% of the control value with the final dose of methacholine. SGaw decreased in a similar fashion, with a 36% decrease (64% of control) at the 4 mg/ml dose and a 43% decrease (57% of control) at the maximal inhaled dose. Wheezing was present on auscultation for the last two methacholine doses, and the patient experienced symptoms similar to her chief complaint when the test became positive.

Impression: Normal lung function with a positive methacholine challenge, consistent with hyperreactive airway disease.

Cause of Symptoms

This patient is an ideal candidate for a bronchial challenge test. Her baseline pulmonary function studies are normal. Her complaint of episodic coughing and choking suggests some form of hyper-reactive airway abnormality. Many patients who develop an asthmatic response to inhaled irritants complain of cough as the primary symptom; wheezing may or may not be present.

If obvious airway obstruction were present on the baseline spirometry, the challenge test would have been contraindicated. A simple before- and after-bronchodilator trial may have been sufficient to demonstrate reversible obstruction. Methacholine challenge testing may be used in patients with known obstruction to quantify the degree of airway hyperreactivity. In this case, the objective of the test was to determine whether the patient had hyperreactivity.

FEV_1 is commonly used as the index of obstruction for inhalation challenge tests because it is simple to perform and highly reproducible. Raw and SGaw are sometimes used to define the extent of airway reactivity. SGaw is sensitive and reproducible and is often used to quantify changes occurring during challenge testing. A decrease of 35% to 45% in SGaw is usually considered indicative of a positive response. As in this patient, SGaw may actually decrease more rapidly than FEV_1. In some instances, PEF may decrease as the challenge is performed, particularly if the large airways are involved.

Results of a methacholine challenge test should be interpreted cautiously. The patient should be free of symptoms at the time of the test. β-Adrenergic, anticholinergic, or methylxanthine bronchodilators that may influence the results must be withheld before testing (Table 9-2). These conditions were met in this patient. Because both FEV_1 and SGaw fell markedly with a PC_{20} less than 8 mg/ml, the test can be interpreted as positive with some certainty. The cause of the patient's symptoms appears to be asthma triggered by inhaled irritants as described in her history.

Treatment

The patient was started on an inhaled corticosteroid (fluticasone). She was also given a portable peak-flow meter (see Chapter 10). The patient was instructed in its use, and her PEF while using it correlated well with that measured during spirometry. She was told to use the device every morning and evening or when symptoms appeared. Any significant change in PEF was treated using a β-adrenergic bronchodilator via a metered-dose inhaler. Subsequent reports indicated that her peak flow fell in excess of the level demonstrated on the challenge, but symptoms were promptly relieved with use of the inhaler.

CASE 9-2

HISTORY

R.I. is a 38-year-old woman whose presenting complaint is shortness of breath while jogging or playing tennis. She has been physically active for several years but recently had a "chest cold" that took 4 weeks to resolve. She smoked for approximately 2 years while in high school. She works as a teacher and has no unusual environmental exposures. Family history includes an older sister who has chronic bronchitis. She is not currently taking any medications. Her HMO referred her for evaluation of possible exercise-induced bronchospasm.

PULMONARY FUNCTION TESTS

Personal Data

Sex: Female
Age: 38 yr
Height: 62 in
Weight: 119 lb

Eucapnic Voluntary Hyperventilation (see also Figure 9-6)

	Baseline	5 min	10 min	15 min	Postbronchodilator
FEV_1 (Pred: 2.64 L)	1.97	1.25			1.92
% Predicted	75	47			73
% Change	0	−37			−3
FVC (Pred: 3.37 L)	2.71	2.07			2.8
% Predicted	81	61			83
% Change	0	−24			3
PEF (Pred: 6.03 L/sec)	5.48	2.77			3.65
% Predicted	91	46			61
% Change	0	−49			−33

TECHNOLOGIST'S COMMENTS

All spirometry maneuvers were performed acceptably before and after hyperventilation. The patient hyperventilated at 60 L/min for 6 minutes. There were audible wheezes immediately after hyperventilation.

QUESTIONS

1. What is the interpretation of:

    ■ Baseline spirometry?
    ■ Response to EVH?
    ■ Response to bronchodilator?

2. What is the cause of the patient's symptoms?
3. What other tests might be indicated?
4. What treatment might be recommended based on these findings?

DISCUSSION

Interpretation

All spirometric maneuvers were performed acceptably. Baseline spirometry results are borderline, with a mildly decreased FEV_1. After EVH, there were significant decreases in FEV_1, FVC, and peak flow at 5 minutes. After an inhaled bronchodilator, FEV_1 returned to prechallenge levels and FVC increased. Peak-flow recovery was somewhat slower.

Impression: Borderline normal spirometry results with a positive EVH test consistent with hyperreactive airways.

Cause of Symptoms

This patient is typical of an adult who begins experiencing breathlessness with increased physical activity and seeks medical attention. Her complaints suggest exercise-induced bronchospasm. The development of this problem may or may not be related to her recent chest infection.

EVH is an appropriate way to challenge the airways in cases such as this. The patient breathed a mixture of 5% CO_2, 21% O_2, and balance N_2 for 6 minutes. The target level of ventilation was set at 30 times her FEV_1, or approximately 60 L/min. Spirometry was repeated 5 minutes after hyperventilation. In this case, the patient experienced a significant decrease in FEV_1, FVC, and PEF (Figure 9-6). Because of the marked decrease in FEV_1, additional postchallenge measurements (at 10 and 15 minutes) were omitted. Two inhalations of albuterol via metered-dose inhaler reversed the obstruction, although PEF recovered only partially.

Other Tests

EVH challenges the airways by inducing heat and water loss with increased ventilation. This is the same physical stimulus that may be responsible for exercise-induced bronchospasm. The patient in this case could have been tested using exercise as the challenge agent. However, EVH is simpler and takes less time. In addition, EVH may be more sensitive in detecting exercise-induced asthma than exercise testing itself. Exercise tests are often performed with patients working at 80% to 90% of their maximal HR for 6 to 8 minutes. In many patients, particularly if they are sedentary, the workload that produces this elevation in HR may not induce a high enough level of ventilation to

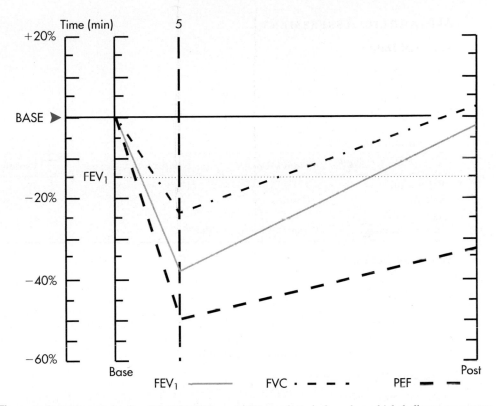

Figure 9-6 *EVH graph for Case 9-2.* FVC, FEV$_1$, and PEF are plotted after a bronchial challenge maneuver. In this patient, there was a marked decrease in all three variables at 5 minutes (a positive test). The graph also plots the reversal of the induced bronchospasm by inhaled bronchodilator.

provoke bronchospasm. EVH, using a target of 30 times the FEV$_1$, produces a level of ventilation that is approximately 75% of MVV.

Treatment

The patient was given a β-adrenergic bronchodilator to be used as pretreatment before exercise. She reported significant improvement in her symptoms. A trial regimen of cromolyn sodium also reduced the occurrence of symptoms associated with athletic activities.

CASE 9-3

HISTORY

J.P. is a 53-year-old woman who suffered multiple abdominal injuries in a motor vehicle accident. After surgical repair of a perforated bowel, acute renal failure developed, followed by respiratory failure. She was placed on mechanically supported ventilation and became increasingly dependent on the ventilator. After 13 days, a metabolic study was requested to assess the adequacy of parenteral nutrition.

Metabolic Assessment

Personal Data

Sex: Female
Age: 53 yr
Height: 62 in
Weight: 110 lb

Nutritional Information

	Total Calories	Nonprotein Calories	Protein (g)
Parenteral	1717	1393	75
Enteral	(None)	—	—
24-hour UN	9 g	—	—
Basal metabolic rate 1176 kcal/24 hours (estimated)			

Ventilator Settings

FIO_2 0.35
V_T 750 ml
Rate   10
Mode   SIMV*
Status   Awake, resting
*Synchronized intermittent mandatory ventilation.

Metabolic Measurements

$\dot{V}CO_2$ (ml/min)   205
$\dot{V}O_2$ (ml/min)   200
RER (RQ)   1.03
$\dot{V}_E$ (L/min)   10.2
REE   1442 kcal/day
RQ_{NP}*   1.07
*Nonprotein RQ; see text.

Energy Substrate Use

Carbohydrate   1480 kcal/day
Fat   289 kcal/day
Protein   243 kcal/day

Blood Gases

pH   7.37
$PaCO_2$ 51
PaO_2 71
HCO_3^- 29

Questions

1. What is the interpretation of:

   ■ REE?
   ■ Substrate utilization?

2. Why does the patient have an RER (RQ) greater than 1?

3. Are the data representative of the patient's caloric requirements?

4. What changes in therapy (ventilator settings, nutritional support) are indicated?

DISCUSSION

Interpretation

Exhaled gases for this study were collected over 26 minutes and appear to represent a steady state. A UN sample was collected for 24 hours before the test. The patient was receiving 1717 kcal/day of parenteral nutrition. REE as determined by metabolic assessment indicates a requirement of 1442 kcal/24 hours. Substrate utilization showed carbohydrate oxidation (104%). The negative value for fat utilization is consistent with lipogenesis. Replacement of glucose with lipids and reduction of total calories to approximately 1450 kcal/day is recommended. The patient should be reassessed within 24 hours.

Cause of Elevated RER (RQ)

This study involves factors commonly encountered in the nutritional support of critically ill patients. These elements include the patient's clinical status, estimated and actual caloric requirements, and the role of nutritional status in ventilatory support.

The patient was critically ill and required ventilatory support. Parenteral nutrition was being supplied approximately 45% above the estimated resting caloric requirements. Estimation of caloric requirements is often performed by calculating the basal rate using the Harris-Benedict equations (see Metabolic Measurements: Indirect Calorimetry section). BMR is then adjusted using factors that consider the clinical status of the patient (i.e., disease state, trauma).

The metabolic study indicated that the patient required fewer calories per day than were currently being given. In addition, carbohydrates were supplying the entire caloric need. The negative value calculated for fat utilization indicates that some of the carbohydrates were probably being stored as fat (i.e., lipogenesis). When carbohydrates are oxidized, CO_2 is produced. The RER of 1.03 supports an excess CO_2 production in relation to metabolic demands.

The metabolic assessment was performed with the patient on a ventilator. The patient's $\dot{V}_E$ during the assessment was 10.2 L, slightly higher than the ventilator settings. Difficulty weaning this patient from mechanically supported ventilation may have been caused by the CO_2 load induced by parenteral nutrition in excess of metabolic demand. The arterial blood gas analysis supports increased CO_2 production. $Paco_2$ is increased in spite of mechanical support of ventilation. The patient was unable to ventilate enough to return her $Paco_2$ to near 40 mm Hg. Excess CO_2 apparently contributed to the difficulty weaning the patient from mechanical ventilation.

Valid Data (Steady State)

The interpretation notes that the data were representative of a steady state. Steady-state measurements are essential to estimate caloric requirements for an entire 24-hour period. Each metabolic assessment should include adequate data so that steady-state conditions can be verified. The length of the study should be appropriate to establish that a steady state existed. Analysis of the variability of $\dot{V}o_2$ and $\dot{V}co_2$ may be helpful. O_2 consumption and CO_2 production ideally should vary during measurements of less than 10% and 6%, respectively. RER values outside the normal range of 0.70 to 1.00 should be carefully evaluated to ensure that measurement errors did not occur. Difficulty measuring $\dot{V}o_2$ in patients receiving supplemental O_2 is well documented. Calorimetry using open-circuit methods is usually limited to measurements when FIo_2 is 0.60 or less.

Changes in Therapy

J.P. was switched to a 50/50 mixture of lipid and carbohydrate. The total caloric intake was also reduced to 1450 kcal/day. Her ventilation decreased, and ventilatory support was gradually reduced. An additional metabolic study indicated agreement between the prescribed nutritional support and her metabolic demands. RER on the subsequent study was 0.79 with an REE of 1395 kcal/day. This RER value compares favorably with 0.82, which is a target value for metabolism of appropriate amounts of carbohydrate, fat, and protein. She was successfully weaned from the ventilator 4 days after the initial assessment.

▍ SELF-ASSESSMENT QUESTIONS

Entry-level

1. *A patient is referred for an evaluation of exercise-induced asthma (EIA). Which of the following protocols would be most appropriate?*

   a. Cycle ergometer ramp test at 50 W/min
   b. Treadmill exercise for 4 to 6 minutes at 85% of predicted maximal HR
   c. Treadmill exercise with increasing speed/slope to exhaustion
   d. EVH for 1 minute at 30% of MVV

2. *A patient with suspected asthma performs a methacholine challenge according to the 5-breath dosimeter protocol. The following data are recorded:*

	FEV_1
(Baseline)	4.1 L
(Diluent)	4.0 L
0.0625 mg/ml	3.5 L
0.250 mg/ml	3.0 L
1.0 mg/ml	2.7 L
4.0 mg/ml	2.2 L

   Which of the following best describes these findings?

   a. The test was negative.
   b. The test was positive after the first dose of methacholine.
   c. The test was positive after the 4.0 mg/ml dose.
   d. The test should have been stopped after the second dose of methacholine.

3. *A patient has an EVH test to evaluate bronchial hyperreactivity. FEV_1 is 2.5 L, and FVC is 3.1 L, with a PEF of 7.0 L/sec. For the hyperventilation challenge, the patient should breathe at approximately:*

   a. 75 L/min for 6 minutes
   b. 93 L/min for 4 minutes
   c. 210 L/min for 2 minutes
   d. 75 L/min for 30 seconds

4. *Following inhalation of methacholine, a patient has airway resistance (Raw) and specific conductance (SGaw) measured. Which of the following changes is consistent with increased airway reactivity?*

   a. An increase in Raw of 10%
   b. A decrease in Raw of 35% to 45%
   c. An increase in SGaw of 15%
   d. A decrease in SGaw of 35% to 45%

5. *Before performing a bronchial challenge study, patients should withhold short-acting bronchodilators, such as albuterol, for:*

   a. 4 hours
   b. 8 hours
   c. 24 hours
   d. 48 hours

Advanced

6. *A patient referred for exercise-induced asthma performs a treadmill exercise test at 86% of his predicted maximal HR for 6.5 minutes. The following data are recorded:*

	Base-line	5 min Post	10 min Post	15 min Post
FEV_1 (L)	4.20	3.99	4.07	4.10
FVC (L)	5.10	5.05	4.99	5.12
PEF (L/sec)	10.5	11.2	9.7	10.7

Which of the following is the most appropriate interpretation of these findings?

a. There is a positive response based on the change in FEV_1.
b. There is a positive response based on the change in FVC.
c. The test is negative for exercise-induced bronchospasm.
d. The patient was malingering based on the PEF.

7. *A patient with a history of pulmonary fibrosis is being evaluated for disability. His FEV_1 is 0.95 L (40% of predicted), and his DL_{CO} is 12.2 ml CO/min/mm Hg (50% of predicted). Which of the following tests is most appropriate to perform next?*

a. Lung volumes by plethysmography
b. Room air arterial blood gases
c. Treadmill exercise test with pulse oximetry
d. Maximal inspiratory/expiratory pressures

8. *A 154-lb patient has a metabolic study performed while on a mechanical ventilator with an FIO_2 of 0.40. These data are obtained, averaged over a 20-minute interval:*

	$\dot{V}CO_2$ (ml)	$\dot{V}O_2$ (ml)	RQ	REE kcal/ 24 hr
Average	222	403	0.55	2630
SD	9	52	0.06	525

The results suggest that:

a. The patient is being overfed
b. The patient is malnourished
c. The CO_2 analyzer is malfunctioning
d. The O_2 analyzer is malfunctioning

9. *For metabolic studies, steady-state data should be collected for at least:*

a. 24 hours
b. 8 hours
c. 1 hour
d. 10 to 15 minutes

10. *Which of the following are required for disability testing:*

   I. Flow spirometers should be calibrated at three different flows
  II. FVC maneuvers must be recorded at 10 mm/sec
 III. Two acceptable FEV_1 maneuvers must be within 5% or 0.1 L, whichever is greater
 IV. Postbronchodilator tests should be performed if FEV_1 is less than 70% of predicted

a. I and III
b. II and IV
c. I, II, and III
d. I, III, and IV

SELECTED BIBLIOGRAPHY

Bronchial Challenge

Argyros GJ, Roach JM, Hurwitz KM, et al: Eucapnic voluntary hyperventilation as a bronchoprovocation technique, *Chest* 109:1520-1524, 1996.

Assoufi BK, Dally MB, Newman-Taylor AJ, et al: Cold-air test: a simplified standard method for airway reactivity, *Clin Respir Physiol* 22:349-357, 1986.

Cockcroft DW, Killian DN, Mellon JJA, et al: Bronchial reactivity to inhaled histamine: a method and clinical survey, *Clin Allergy* 7:235-243, 1977.

Eliasson AH, Phillips YY, Rajagopal KR, et al: Sensitivity and specificity of bronchial provocation testing: an evaluation of four techniques in exercise induced bronchospasm, *Chest* 102:347, 1992.

Haas F, Axen K, Schicchi JS: Use of maximum expiratory flow-volume curve parameters in the assessment of exercise induced bronchospasm, *Chest* 103:64-68, 1993.

Irvin CG: Bronchial challenge testing, *Respir Clin North Am* 1:265-285, 1995.

Pepys G, Hutchcroft BJ: Bronchial provocation tests in etiologic diagnosis and analysis of asthma, *Am Rev Respir Dis* 112:829, 1975.

Perpina M, Pellicer C, deDiego A, et al: Diagnostic value of the bronchial provocation test with methacholine in asthma: Bayesian analysis approach, *Chest* 104:149-154, 1993.

Randolph C: Exercise-induced asthma: update on pathophysiology, clinical diagnosis, and treatment, *Curr Probl Pediatr* 27:53-77, 1997.

Preoperative Pulmonary Function Testing

Epstein SK, Faling LJ, Daly BD, et al: Predicting complications after pulmonary resection: preoperative exercise testing vs a multifactorial cardiopulmonary risk index, *Chest* 104:694-700, 1993.

Ferguson MK: Preoperative assessment of pulmonary risk, *Chest* 115(suppl 5):58S-63S, 1999.

Ferguson MK, Durkin AE: Preoperative prediction of the risk of pulmonary complications after esophagectomy for cancer, *J Thorac Cardiovasc Surg* 123:661-669, 2002.

Fisher BW, Majumdar SR, McAlister FA: Predicting pulmonary complications after nonthoracic surgery: a systematic review of blinded studies, *Am J Med* 112:219-225, 2002.

Fuso L, Cisternino L, Di Napoli A, et al: Role of spirometric and arterial gas data in predicting pulmonary complications after abdominal surgery, *Respir Med* 94:1171-1176, 2000.

Kearney DJ, Lee TH, Reilly JJ, et al: Assessment of operative risk in patients undergoing lung resection: importance of predicted pulmonary function, *Chest* 105:753-759, 1994.

Respiratory Impairment for Disability

Gaensler EM, Wright GW: Evaluation of respiratory impairment, *Arch Environ Health* 12:146, 1966.

Harber P, Schnur R, Emery J, et al: Statistical "biases" in respiratory disability determinations, *Am Rev Respir Dis* 128:413, 1983.

Morgan WKC: Pulmonary disability and impairment: can't work? won't work? Basics of RD, *Am Thoracic Soc* 10:5, 1982.

U.S. Department of Health and Human Services: *Guide to pulmonary function studies under the Social Security disability programs: disability evaluation under Social Security*, SSA Publication No 64-055, 1999.

Metabolic Measurements (Indirect Calorimetry)

Askanazi J, Nordenstrom J, Rosenbaum SH, et al: Nutrition for the patient with respiratory failure: glucose vs fat, *Anesthesiology* 54:373, 1981.

Battezzati A, Vigano R: Indirect calorimetry and nutritional problems in clinical practice, *Acta Diabetol* 38:1-5, 2001.

Branson RD: The measurement of energy expenditure: instrumentation, practical considerations and clinical application, *Respir Care* 35:640-659, 1990.

Consolazio CF, Johnson RE, Pecora LJ: *Physiological measurements of metabolic functions in man*, New York, 1963, McGraw-Hill.

Harris JA, Benedict FG: *Biometric studies of basal metabolism in man*, Carnegie Institute of Washington, Publication No 279, 1919.

Makita K, Nunn JF, Royston B: Evaluation of metabolic measuring instruments for use in critically ill patients, *Crit Care Med* 18:638-644, 1990.

Mascarenhas MR, Zemel B, Stallings VA: Nutritional assessment in pediatrics, *Nutrition* 14:105-115, 1998.

Weir JB: New methods for calculating metabolic rate with special reference to protein metabolism, *J Physiol* 109: 1-9, 1949.

Weissman C, Kemper MA, Askanazi J, et al: Resting metabolic rate of the critically ill patient: measured versus predicted, *Anesthesiology* 64:673-679, 1986.

Guidelines and Standards

American Association for Respiratory Care: Clinical practice guideline: metabolic measurement using indirect calorimetry during mechanical ventilation, *Respir Care* 39:1170-1175, 1994.

American Association for Respiratory Care: Clinical practice guideline: methacholine challenge testing 2001 revision & update, *Respir Care* 46:523-530, 2001.

American Thoracic Society: Guidelines for methacholine and exercise challenge testing—1999, *Am J Respir Crit Care Med* 161:309-329, 2000.

Chai H, Farr RS, Froelich LA, et al: Standardization of bronchial inhalation challenge procedures, *J Allergy Clin Immunol* 56:323, 1975.

Sterk PJ, Fabbri LM, Quanjer PH, et al: Airway responsiveness: standardized challenge testing with pharmacological, physical and sensitizing stimuli in adults: Statement of the European Respiratory Society, *Eur Respir J* 6(suppl 16):53-83, 1993.

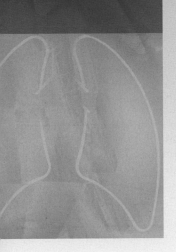

C H A P T E R   10

PULMONARY FUNCTION TESTING EQUIPMENT

OBJECTIVES

After studying this chapter and reviewing its tables and figures, you should be able to do the following:

Entry-level

1. Describe at least one type of volume displacement spirometer
2. List at least two principles used by flow-sensing spirometers to measure volume
3. Select a directional breathing valve for a specific testing situation
4. State how different types of gas analyzers are used in the pulmonary function laboratory

Advanced

1. Explain the causes of common blood gas electrode problems
2. Contrast and compare measurement of oxygen saturation by multiwavelength and pulse oximeters
3. Describe the basic components of the body plethysmograph
4. List the advantages of a relational database for storing pulmonary function records

This chapter describes pulmonary function equipment used for common testing applications. Included are volume-displacement and flow-sensing spirometers, peak flow meters, breathing valves, pulmonary gas analyzers, blood gas electrodes and oximeters, body plethysmographs, and computerized pulmonary function systems.

Hutchinson introduced the precursor of the modern spirometer around 1844. This spirometer was a water-sealed volume-displacement device. Some aspects of the original device are still evident in today's spirometers. Flow-sensing spirometers have become much more common with the advent of sophisticated electronics and software that can integrate flow signals to measure volume. Microprocessor-based spirometers are now small enough to be handheld.

Analysis of respiratory gases by volumetric methods was pioneered by Haldane in the early part of the twentieth century. Modern gas analyzers use indirect means (e.g., electrodes or sensors) to measure partial pressures of gases. Most instruments in the pulmonary function laboratory today combine physical transducers, analog-to-digital converters, and computer software to process and record physiologic data. Some devices, such as the pulse oximeter, are based almost entirely on electronic components. Computers eliminate many tedious calculations, allowing the technologist to concentrate on obtaining high-quality data.

Volume Displacement Spirometers

WATER-SEAL SPIROMETERS

For many years, the water-seal spirometer was the basic tool used to measure lung volumes and flows. The spirometer consists of a large bell (7 to 10 L) suspended in a container of water with the open end of the bell below the surface of the water (Figure 10-1). A breathing circuit into the interior of the bell allows for accurate measurement of gas volumes. The patient breathes into the spirometer, moving the bell up during expiration and down with inspiration. Each spirometer bell has a "bell factor" relating the vertical distance moved to a

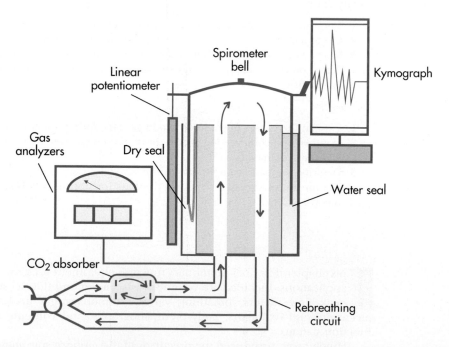

Figure 10-1 *Cutaway view of water-seal and dry-seal spirometers.* The spirometer bell "floats" in a well. A water seal (*right*) and a dry rolling seal (*left*) are shown. (*See text.*) Also shown is a rebreathing breathing circuit with CO_2 absorber and gas analyzers, as might be used for closed-circuit FRC determination. Although not widely used, a kymograph was often attached so that excursions of the bell traced a volume-time spirogram on moving graph paper. The convention of plotting expiratory volume in an upward direction can be traced to this type of spirometer/kymograph setup. A linear potentiometer provides analog outputs for volume and flow.

specific volume (milliliters or liters). Movement of the bell can be recorded using a pen to make a tracing on a rotating drum called a *kymograph*. Volumes can be measured from the kymograph tracing by using paper that incorporates the bell factor for the spirometer. Volumes measured in this way reflect the gas in the spirometer that is at ambient temperature, pressure, and saturation (ATPS). These volumes, such as vital capacity (VC), must be corrected to BTPS.

The spirometer bell can also activate a potentiometer. A potentiometer is a device that produces an analog DC voltage signal depending on its position, much like a dimmer switch connected to a light. The analog output (in volts) is proportional to the position of the bell. For example, 10 volts may equal 10 L in the spirometer. This analog signal can be used to drive a mechanical recorder such as a strip-chart recorder. More commonly, however, the analog signal is digitized using an analog-to-digital (A/D) converter. The digitized signal from the spirometer can then be stored and processed by a computer. Some potentiometers also produce analog signals representing the speed of movement of a volume-displacement spirometer. This signal is proportional to flow. All volume-displacement spirometers use some type of potentiometer or position encoder to produce signals that can be digitized and stored by a computer.

For simple spirometry, a single large-bore tube can be used for both inspiration and expiration. For rebreathing studies, the breathing circuit incorporates a CO_2 absorber (soda lime). Inspiratory and expiratory circuits are separated with one-way valves to reduce dead space. Water-seal spirometers are typically used for spirometry. They may also be used to measure ventilation, including $\dot{V}_E$, V_T, and respiratory rate. With an appropriate potentiometer and recorder or computer, water-seal spirometers can be used to obtain flow-volume (F-V) curves. By including the rebreathing apparatus described, lung volumes by helium dilution can be obtained. In combination with an appropriate reservoir for the test gas, water-sealed spirometers can be used to perform diffusing capacity tests, both single-breath and rebreathing. The water-seal spirometer can be used as a reservoir for special gas mixtures such as those used for DL_{CO} tests.

The Stead-Wells water-seal or dry-seal spirometer is still used. The Stead-Wells spirometer uses a lightweight plastic bell (Figure 10-2). The water-sealed bell "floats" in the water well, rising and falling with breathing excursions. In the dry-seal version, a rubberized seal connects the bell to the internal wall of the spirometer well. The rubber seal then "rolls" over itself, much the same as the dry rolling-seal spirometer (see next section). The spirometer bell can carry a recording pen mounted against a variable-speed (32, 160, and 1920 mm/min) kymograph, although this technique is seldom used. Expiration is traced upward on the volume-time graph (see Figure 2-2, Chapter 2). The Stead-Wells bell is usually attached to a linear potentiometer. The linear potentiometer provides analog signals proportional to volume and flow. These signals are passed to a computer through an A/D converter. The Stead-Wells design is capable of meeting the minimum requirements for flow and volume accuracy recommended by the American Thoracic Society (see Chapter 11).

Although most laboratories use computer-derived measurements, the capability to perform tests manually may be useful for quality assurance or for calibration. The "waterless" version of this type of spirometer allows the device to be transported more easily. In addition, periodic draining is eliminated and cleaning of the spirometer is simplified.

Problems with water-seal (and dry-seal) spirometers are usually caused by leaks in the bell or in the breathing circuit. Gravity causes the spirometer to lose volume in the presence of leaks. Leaks in the spirometer, tubing, or valves can be detected by raising the bell and plugging the patient connection. Any change in volume can be detected easily by recording the spirometer volume over several minutes. Small weights can be added to the top of the bell to enhance detection of small leaks. During patient testing, improper positioning of the

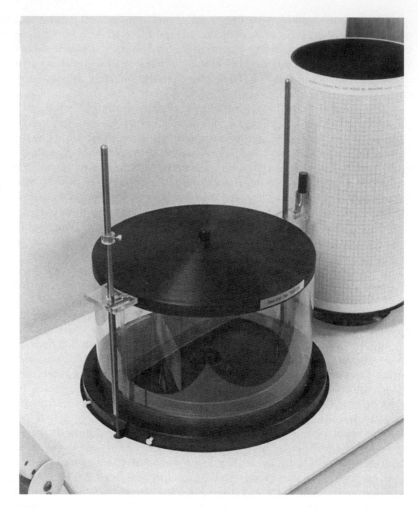

Figure 10–2 *Stead-Wells dry-seal spirometer.* The conventional Stead-Wells spirometer used a lightweight plastic bell that floated in water. This version uses a silicon seal similar to that found in the dry rolling-seal spirometer. The spirometer bell carries a pen that traces directly on a rotating kymograph. With appropriate circuitry and gas analyzers, He dilution FRC determinations and DL_{CO} measurements are easily performed. (*Courtesy Warren E. Collins, Inc., Braintree, Mass.*)

spirometer can cause inaccurate measurements. If positioned too high, the bell can rise out of the water or reach the top of its travel range. This causes the volume-time tracing to appear abruptly flattened. The pattern observed may be mistaken for a normal end-of-expiration. If a Stead-Wells spirometer is positioned too low, it may empty completely. This may result in water being drawn into the breathing circuit, gas analyzer, or other system components. Inadequate water in the device may also lead to erroneous readings that are sometimes difficult to detect. The size of the water-seal spirometer and its weight when filled with water make it somewhat difficult to transport. The waterless version of the spirometer eliminates the last consideration.

The use of volume-displacement spirometers accounts for some of the conventions employed in spirometry today. Plotting expiratory volume in the upward direction mimics the graph made by the pen of a Stead-Wells-type spirometer on a rotating kymograph. Plotting MVV as an accumulated volume over time originated from the chain-driven pulley of a water-sealed bell.

Maintenance of water-seal spirometers includes routine draining of the water well. Both wet and dry versions of the Stead-Wells spirometer must be checked for cracks or leaks in the bell. Chemical absorbers for water vapor must be routinely checked. Water absorbers can be rapidly exhausted because the gas in the spirometer is almost completely saturated with water vapor.

Infection control of water-seal spirometers typically involves replacing breathing hoses and mouthpieces after each patient. Although the patient's expired gas comes into direct contact with the water in the spirometer, cross-contamination is not common. Some systems allow use of low-resistance bacteria filters to protect from contamination the parts of the breathing circuit that are not changed after patient use. Such filters should be used with caution for flow-dependent maneuvers. Water condensation in the filter element may significantly alter its resistance. The volume of these filters may need to be considered when calculating system volume or system dead space.

Because of the problems and maintenance required for water-seal spirometers, few of these devices are used in clinical practice.

DRY ROLLING-SEAL SPIROMETERS

Another type of volume-displacement spirometer is the dry rolling-seal spirometer. A typical unit consists of a lightweight piston mounted horizontally in a cylinder. A rod that rests on frictionless bearings supports the piston (Figure 10-3). The piston is coupled to the cylinder wall by a flexible plastic seal. The seal rolls on itself rather than sliding as the piston moves. A similar type of rolling-seal may also be used with a vertically mounted, lightweight piston that rises and falls with breathing. The maximum volume of the cylinder with the piston fully displaced is usually 10 to 12 L. The piston has a large diameter so that excursions of just a few inches are all that is necessary to record large volume changes. The piston is normally constructed of lightweight aluminum to reduce inertia. Mechanical resistance is kept to a minimum by the bearings supporting the piston rod and by the rolling seal itself.

Although they can be used with a paper recorder, most dry rolling-seal spirometers use linear or rotary potentiometers. The potentiometer responds to piston movement to produce DC voltage outputs for volume and flow. For example, a 10-V potentiometer attached to a 10-L spirometer may produce an output of 1 V/L. On a separate channel, a flow of 1 L/sec may produce an output of 1 V. Flow in this case is proportional to the speed of the moving piston. These analog outputs for volume and flow are digitized so that a computer can store the data.

The piston of the standard dry rolling-seal spirometer (Figure 10-4) travels horizontally, eliminating the need for counterbalancing. The vertically mounted version (Figure 10-2) depends on a lightweight piston and the rolling seal to reduce resistance to breathing. Temperature corrections (from ATPS to BTPS) are made by applying a correction factor to the digital value stored in the computer. A one-way breathing circuit and CO_2 scrubber may be added so that dry rolling-seal spirometers can be used for rebreathing tests in much the same way as water-seal spirometers.

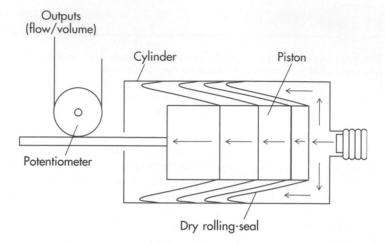

Figure 10-3 *Cutaway view of a dry rolling-seal spirometer.* An exaggerated view of the rolling seal, which actually fits closely between the piston and cylinder wall. The piston has a large surface area, so horizontal movement is minimized. This allows recording of normal breaths and maximal respiratory excursions with little resistance. The piston is supported by a rod that activates a rotary potentiometer. Rotation of the potentiometer generates analog signals for flow and volume. (*From Form 370, Datex, Ohmeda, Inc., Madison, Wis.*)

To perform studies such as the open-circuit nitrogen washout test, a "dumping" mechanism is attached to the spirometer. The dumping device empties the spirometer after each breath or after a predetermined volume has been reached. Addition of an automated valve and alveolar sampling device allows the dry rolling-seal spirometer to be used for single-breath diffusion studies. Dry rolling-seal spirometers are typically capable of meeting the minimum standards recommended by the ATS (see Chapter 11).

Common problems encountered with dry rolling-seal spirometers are sticking of the rolling-seal and increased mechanical resistance in the piston-cylinder assembly. These difficulties can usually be avoided by adequate maintenance of the spirometer. Infection control of the dry rolling-seal involves disassembling the piston-cylinder. The interior of the cylinder and the face of the piston are usually wiped with a mild antibacterial solution. The rolling-seal itself is also wiped with disinfectant. Alcohol or similar drying agents may cause deterioration of the seal and should not be used. The seal may be lubricated with cornstarch to prevent sticking, but care must be taken to avoid excessive powder being left in the spirometer. The seal should be routinely checked for leaks or tears. After reassembly, the piston should be positioned at the maximum volume position. When the rolling-seal is extended completely, the material of the seal is less likely to develop creases that can result in uneven movement of the piston. With the previously described reservations, bacteria filters may be used to avoid contamination of the spirometer.

BELLOWS-TYPE SPIROMETERS

A third type of volume-displacement spirometer is the bellows or wedge bellows. Both devices consist of a collapsible bellows that folds or unfolds in response to breathing excursions. The conventional bellows design is a flexible accordion-type container. One end is stationary and the other end is displaced in proportion to the volume inspired or expired. The wedge bellows operates similarly except that it expands and contracts like a fan

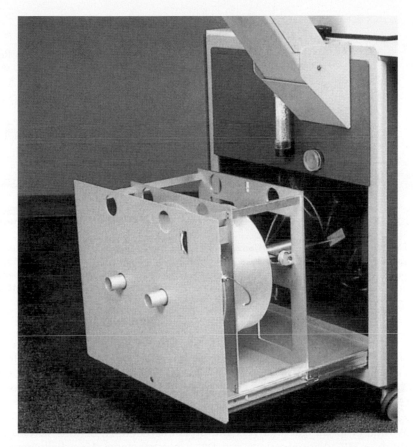

Figure 10-4 *Dry rolling-seal spirometer.* A typical dry-seal spirometer consisting of a large aluminum piston mounted in a cylinder, with two ports to accommodate simple spirometry, as well as rebreathing maneuvers with a CO_2 absorber (Figure 10-3).

(Figure 10-5). One side of the bellows remains stationary; the other side moves with a pivotal motion around an axis through the fixed side. Displacement of the bellows by a volume of gas is translated either to movement of a pen on chart paper or to a potentiometer. For mechanical recording, chart paper moves at a fixed speed under the pen while a spirogram is traced. For computerized testing, displacement of the bellows is transformed into a DC voltage by a linear or rotary potentiometer. The analog signal is routed to an A/D converter and then to a computer.

The conventional and wedge bellows may be mounted either horizontally or vertically. The horizontal bellows is mounted so that the primary direction of travel is on a horizontal plane. This design minimizes the effects of gravity on bellows movement. The horizontal bellows (either conventional or wedge) with a large surface area offers little mechanical resistance. This type is normally used in conjunction with a potentiometer to produce analog volume and flow signals. Several types of small (approximately 7 L to 8 L), vertically mounted bellows are available and may be used for portable spirometry and bedside testing. Most of these types offer simple mechanical recording and/or digital data reduction by means of a small, dedicated microprocessor.

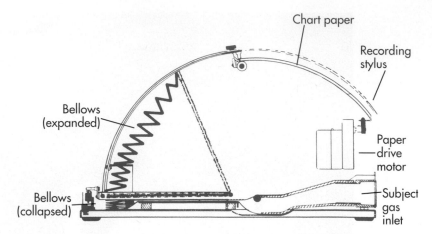

Figure 10-5 *Cross-sectional diagram of a wedge-bellows–type spirometer.* Fanlike movements of the wedge bellows cause the recording stylus to move across graph paper. Some manufacturers suspend the bellows so that the primary movement is in a horizontal rather than vertical plane. Large wedge-bellows offer little resistance and are comparable to dry-seal or water-seal spirometers in accuracy and linearity. (*Modified from Vitalograph Medical Instrumentation, Product Brochure, Lenexa, Kan.*)

Both bellows-type spirometers (Figure 10-6) can be used to measure vital capacity and its subdivisions, as well as FVC, FEV_1, expiratory flows, and MVV. Some bellows-type spirometers, especially those that are mounted vertically, are designed to measure expiratory flows only. These types expand upward when gas is injected, then empty spontaneously under their own weight. Horizontally mounted bellows can usually be set in a mid-range to record both inspiratory and expiratory maneuvers. This allows measurements such as F-V loops to be made. With appropriate gas analyzers and breathing circuitry, bellows systems may be used for gas dilution FRC determinations and DL_{CO} measurements. Most bellows-type spirometers meet ATS recommendations for flow and volume accuracy.

One problem that may occur with bellows-type spirometers is inaccuracy resulting from sticking of the bellows. The folds of the bellows may adhere because of dirt, moisture, or aging of the bellows material. Some bellows-type spirometers require the bellows to be partially distended when not in use. This technique allows moisture from exhaled gas to evaporate and prevents deterioration of the bellows. Leaks may also develop in the bellows material or at the point where the bellows is mounted. Leaks can usually be detected by filling the bellows with air, plugging the breathing port, and attaching a weight or spring to pressurize the contained gas.

Infection control of bellows-type spirometers depends on the method of construction. In some instruments, the bellows can be entirely removed; in others, the interior of the bellows must be wiped clean. Many bellows are made from rubberized or plastic-based material that can be cleaned with a mild detergent and dried thoroughly before reassembly. Bacteria filters may be used to avoid contamination of the bellows, with the reservations described previously.

The volume-displacement spirometer was once the main device used for pulmonary function testing. Many such devices are still in use, and some manufacturers continue to produce sophisticated spirometers based on the volume-displacement principle. However, use of flow-sensing spirometers has become increasingly common, both in the pulmonary function laboratory and in small portable devices for bedside or clinic use.

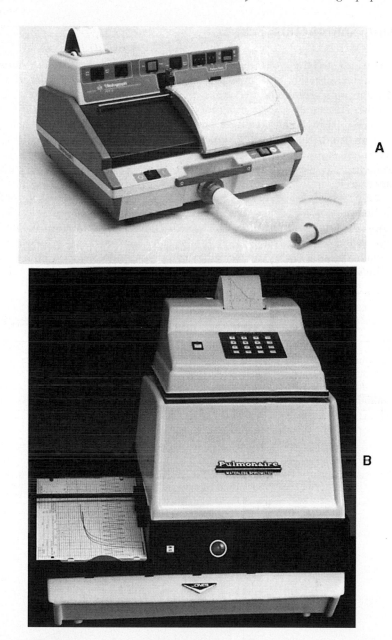

Figure 10-6 *Two types of bellows spirometers.* **A,** Wedge-bellows spirometer with direct writing recorder, digital displays, and built-in printer for automated data reduction. **B,** Conventional bellows-type spirometer, with the bellows mounted horizontally and driving a pen across moving graph papers. A potentiometer allows analog output to a dedicated microprocessor with built-in printer for automatic data reduction. (*A courtesy Vitalograph Medical Instrumentation, Lenexa, KS; B courtesy Jones Medical Instrument Co., Oakbrook, IL.*)

Flow-Sensing Spirometers

In contrast to the volume-displacement spirometer is the flow-sensing spirometer, or pneumotachometer. The term *pneumotachometer* describes a device that measures gas flow. Flow-sensing spirometers use various physical principles to produce a signal proportional to gas flow. This signal is then integrated to measure volume in addition to flow. Integration is a process in which flow (volume per unit of time) is divided into a large number of small intervals (time). The volume from each interval is summed (Figure 10-7). Integration can be performed easily by an electronic circuit or by computer software. Accurate volume measurement by flow integration requires an accurate flow signal, accurate timing, and sensitive detection of low flow.

One type of device that responds to bulk flow of gas is the turbine or impeller. Integration may be unnecessary because the turbine directly measures gas volumes. Some turbine spirometers produce volume pulses in which each "pulse" equals a fixed volume. These spirometers count pulses very accurately. Most flow-sensing spirometers use tubes through which laminar airflow is possible (see Appendix E). Four basic types of flow sensors are commonly used: turbines, pressure-differential flow sensors, heated-wire flow sensors, and Pitot tube flow sensors.

Most spirometers utilize a flow sensor. Flow-sensing spirometers have several advantages over volume-displacement devices. They are smaller, easier to maintain, easier to clean, and can even use disposable sensors. Their small size makes them ideal for portable systems, making simple spirometry a powerful diagnostic tool that can be used in settings outside of the traditional pulmonary function laboratory.

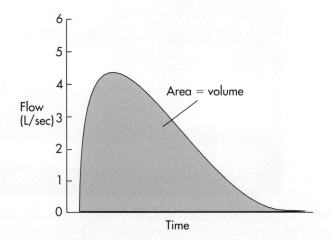

Figure 10-7 *Volume measurement by flow integration.* The flow signal from many types of flow-sensing spirometers is integrated to compute volume. Flow is measured against time. The area under the flow-time curve is subdivided into a large number of small sections. Each section represents a small interval of time. Volume is equal to the sum of the areas of all sections. By dividing the curve into a large number of sections, even irregular flow curves can be accurately integrated. Integration is usually performed by a dedicated electronic circuit or by software.

TURBINES

The simplest type of flow-sensing device is the turbine, or respirometer. This instrument consists of a vane connected to a series of precision gears. Gas flowing through the body of the instrument causes the vane to rotate, registering a volume (Figure 10-8). The respirometer can be used to measure vital capacity. It can also be used for ventilation tests such as V_T and $\dot{V}_E$. One such device is the Wright respirometer. This respirometer can measure volumes accurately at flows between 3 and 300 L/min. At flows greater than 300 L/min (5 L/sec), the vane is subject to distortion. Because of this limitation, it should not be used to measure FVC when the patient is capable of flows greater than 300 L/min. At low flows (less than 3 L/min), inertia of the vane-gear system may underestimate volume.

The special advantage of this type of respirometer is its compact size and usefulness at the bedside. Most respirometers can register a wide range of volumes using multiple scales. The standard Wright respirometer measures 0.1 to 1 L on one scale, and up to 100 L on another scale. Turbine devices are also widely used for bulk measurements in various dry gas meters.

An adaptation of the turbine flow device includes a photo cell and light source that is interrupted by the movement of the vane or impeller (Figure 10-9). Rotation of the vane interrupts a light beam between its source and the photo cell. This produces a pulse, with each pulse equivalent to a fixed gas volume. The pulse count is summed to obtain the volume of gas flowing through the device. The signal produced may not be linear across a wide range of flows because of inertia or distortion of the rotating vane.

The accuracy of turbine flow devices is usually limited by the factors described. For this reason, most turbine devices do not meet the ATS minimum recommendations for diagnostic

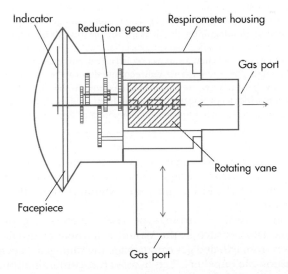

Figure 10-8 *Cutaway view of a turbine-type flow sensor.* The Wright respirometer is shown. A rotating vane mounted on jeweled bearings drives reduction gears connected to the main indicator arm. Two gas ports allow flow through the housing for measurement of volume. Although the vane turns in only one direction, inspired or expired volumes can be measured by attachment to the appropriate port. Not pictured is a small indicator arm, which marks volumes larger than 1 L on the face, so that accumulated volumes can be measured. The instrument also features controls for engaging or disengaging the vane and for resetting the indicators to zero. (*From the British Oxygen Co., Ltd. Operating Instructions, Wright Respirometer, Print No 630207, Issue 3:6, Aug 1971.*)

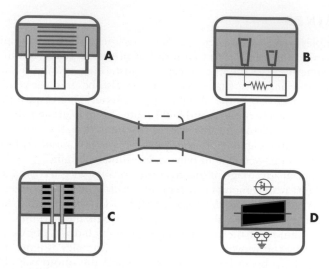

Figure 10-9 *Common flow-sensing devices (pneumotachometers).* Each flow sensor is mounted in a tube that promotes laminar flow (*center*). **A,** Pressure-differential pneumotachometer in which a resistive element causes a pressure drop proportional to the flow of gas through the tube. A sensitive pressure transducer monitors the pressure drop across the resistive element and converts the differential to an analog signal. The resistive element may be a mesh screen or capillary tube; it is usually heated to 37° C or higher to prevent condensation of water from expired gas. **B,** Heated-wire pneumotachometer contains heated elements of small mass that respond to gas flow by heat loss. An electrical current heats the elements. Gas flow past the elements causes cooling. In one element, current is increased to maintain a constant temperature; the other element acts as a reference (Figure 10-11). The current change is proportional to gas flow, and a continuous signal is supplied to an integrating circuit as for the pressure differential flow sensor. **C,** Pitot tube flow sensor uses a series of small tubes that are placed at right angles to the direction of gas flow. Sensitive pressure transducers detect changes in gas velocity. Pitot tubes are mounted in struts in the flow tube; separate devices face either way so that bidirectional flow can be measured (Figure 10-12). **D,** Electronic rotating-vane flow sensor. A vane or impeller is mounted in the flow tube. An LED is mounted on one side of the vane, and a photodetector on the other side. Each time the vane rotates, it interrupts the light from the LED reaching the detector. These pulses are counted and summed to calculate gas volume.

spirometers. These devices may be used for monitoring or screening. Because of their simplicity and small size, several such devices are marketed for home use. This type of spirometer allows FVC, FEV_1, and peak expiratory flow (PEF) to be monitored outside the usual clinical setting.

Infection control of turbine-type respirometers depends on their construction and intended use. Devices such as the Wright respirometer usually must be gas sterilized. Water condensation from exhaled gas can damage the vane-gear mechanisms. Some turbine spirometers use disposable impellers. This avoids cross-contamination, but accuracy is limited by the quality of the disposable sensor.

▮ PRESSURE DIFFERENTIAL FLOW SENSORS

The most common implementation of flow sensing consists of a tube containing a resistive element. The resistive element allows gas to flow through it but causes a pressure decrease (Figure 10-9, *A*). The pressure difference across the resistive element is measured by means of a sensitive pressure transducer. The transducer usually has pressure taps on either side of the element (Figure 10-10, *A*). The pressure differential across the resistive element is proportional to gas flow as long as flow is laminar. This flow signal is integrated to measure volume (Figure 10-7). Turbulent gas flow upstream or downstream of the resistive element may interfere with development of true laminar flow. Most pneumotachometers attempt to reduce turbulent flow by tapering the tubes in which the resistive elements are mounted.

Although there are many designs for resistive elements, two types are commonly used. The Fleisch-type pneumotachometer uses a bundle of capillary tubes (or similar material) as the resistive element. Laminar flow is ensured by size and arrangement of the capillary tubes. The cross-sectional area and length of the capillary tubes determines the actual resistance to flow through the Fleisch pneumotachometer. The dynamic range of the Fleisch device must be matched to the range of flows to be measured. Different sizes (i.e., resistances) of pneumotachometers may be used to accurately measure high or low flows.

The other common type of pressure differential flow sensor is the Silverman (or Lilly) type. The Silverman pneumotachometer uses one or more screens to act as a resistive

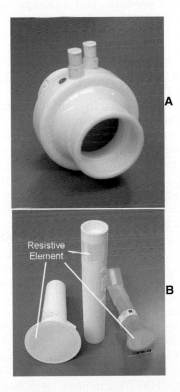

Figure 10-10 *Pressure differential flow sensors (pneumotachometers).* **A,** Small reusable pressure differential flow sensor is shown. This pneumotachometer consists of an unheated screen that acts as a resistive element. Two Luer-type fittings provide for connection to a pressure transducer so that the pressure drop across the resistive element can be measured. **B,** Three disposable pressure differential flow sensors are shown. Each device uses a porous paper or plastic screenlike material to act as a resistive element. A single pressure tap upstream of the resistive element allows pressure to be measured and compared to ambient pressure. Disposable flow sensors are calibrated at the time of manufacture. Some manufacturers print a calibration code or calibration bar code on the disposable sensor that can be used by the spirometer software to achieve accurate measurement of flow and volume.

element. A typical arrangement has three screens mounted parallel to one another. The middle screen acts as the resistive element with the pressure taps on either side, whereas the outer screens protect the middle screen and help ensure laminar flow. The Silverman pneumotachometer has a wider dynamic flow range than the Fleisch type. As a result, it is better suited for measuring widely varying flows.

Most Fleisch and Silverman pneumotachometers use a heating mechanism to warm the resistive element to 37° C or higher. Heating the resistive element prevents condensation of water vapor from exhaled gas on the element. Condensation or other debris lodging in the resistive element changes the resistance across it, thus changing its calibration. A change in the resistive element such as condensation or a hole causes a change in the pressure-flow relationship. Pneumotachometers need to be recalibrated after cleaning or similar maintenance.

Some flow-sensing spirometers use resistive elements such as porous paper, rendering the flow sensor disposable (Figure 10-10, B). These devices usually have a single pressure tap upstream of the resistive element. Pressure measured in front of the resistive element is referenced against ambient pressure. This technique requires that the flow sensor be carefully "zeroed" before making any flow measurements. The accuracy of these types of spirometers often depends on how carefully the disposable resistive elements are manufactured. If the resistance varies widely from sensor to sensor, each unit may need to be calibrated before use to ensure accuracy. Some manufacturers calibrate their disposable sensors and provide a calibration code with each sensor. This code is then used to identify a particular sensor by the software that makes the measurements. One method of identifying the correct calibration factor for individual flow sensors is to imprint the sensor with a bar code (Figure 10-10, B). The spirometer then includes a simple bar code reader to identify the appropriate calibration factors. Some portable spirometer systems that use precalibrated flow sensors do not provide for user calibration. However, verification of accuracy (using a 3-L syringe) is usually possible, even if the manufacturer has not provided for this in the software accompanying the spirometer.

Systems that use permanent pressure-differential flow sensors usually meet or exceed the ATS minimal recommendations for diagnostic spirometers. Spirometers that use disposable sensors can meet or exceed the minimal requirements, depending on the quality of the sensor and the application software responsible for signal processing. Gas composition affects the accuracy of flow measurements in pressure-differential pneumotachometers. Correction factors for gases other than air can be applied by software so that these types of flow sensors can be used for most types of pulmonary function tests.

Infection control of pressure-differential flow sensors depends on their placement in the spirometer. In open-circuit systems in which only exhaled gas is measured, only the mouthpiece needs to be changed between patients. If inspiratory and expiratory flows are measured, the flow sensor may need to be disinfected between patients. Disassembly and cleaning of flow sensors usually require that the spirometer be recalibrated. Disposable or single-use sensors avoid this problem. In-line filters may be used to isolate the pneumotachometer from potential contamination. The spirometer should meet all ATS requirements for range, accuracy, and flow resistance with the filter in place (see Chapter 11). If a filter is used, calibration with the filter in-line may be required. The effect of bacteria filters on spirometric measurements has not been well defined.

■ HEATED-WIRE FLOW SENSORS

A third type of flow-sensing spirometer is based on the cooling effect of gas flow. A heated element, usually a thin platinum wire, is situated in a laminar flow tube (Figure 10-9). Gas flow past the wire causes a temperature decrease so that more current must be supplied to

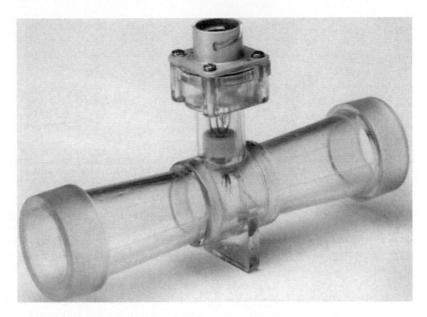

Figure 10-11 *Heated-wire flow sensor.* A flow tube contains very thin, paired stainless steel wires. The wires are maintained at two temperatures exceeding body temperature and are connected by a Wheatstone bridge. The tube streamlines gas flow into laminar flow. The temperature of the wires decreases in proportion to the mass of the gas and its flow. Two wires are used; one measures expiratory flow and the other serves as a reference. (*Courtesy VIASYS Healthcare Critical Care Division, Palm Springs, Calif.*)

maintain a preset temperature. The current needed to maintain the temperature is proportional to flow. The heated element usually has a small mass so that very slight changes in gas flow can be detected. The flow signal is integrated electronically or by software to obtain volume measurements. The heated wire is usually protected behind a screen to prevent impaction of debris on the element. Debris or moisture droplets on the element can change its thermal characteristics. Some systems use two wires (Figure 10-11). One measures gas flow, and the second serves as a reference. Most heated-wire flow sensors maintain a temperature higher than 37° C. Heating prevents condensation from expired air that might interfere with sensitivity of the element.

Most heated-wire flow sensors meet or exceed ATS recommendations for accuracy and precision. Gas composition may affect the accuracy of flow measurements. Correction factors for gases other than room air can be applied via software. This allows heated-wire devices to accurately measure gases for pulmonary function tests using helium, oxygen, and other gases. Heated-wire sensors can be used for routine pulmonary function tests, exercise testing, and metabolic studies. Infection control for heated-wire sensors is similar to that for pressure-differential devices. Disposable or single-use devices avoid cross-contamination even when the sensor is located proximal to the patient's airway.

PITOT TUBE FLOW SENSORS

A fourth type of flow sensor uses the Pitot tube principle. The pressure of gas flowing against a small tube is related to the gas's density and velocity. Flow can be measured by placing a series of small tubes in a flow sensor and connecting them to a sensitive pressure transducer

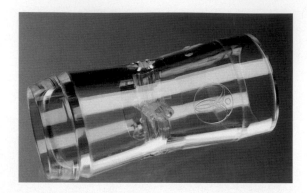

Figure 10–12 *Pitot tube flow sensor.* A series of small tubes is mounted on struts in the flow tube. The tubes are connected to very sensitive pressure transducers (*not shown*). Using a series of transducers allows a wide range of flows to be accurately measured. Pitot tubes are mounted with struts facing both directions so that inspiratory and expiratory flow can be detected. (*Courtesy Medical Graphics, Inc., St. Paul, Minn.*)

(Figure 10-9). The pressure signal must be linearized and integrated as described for other flow-sensing devices. In practice, two sets of Pitot tubes are mounted in the same sensor so that bidirectional flow can be measured (Figure 10-12). A wide range of flows can be accommodated by using two pressure transducers with different sensitivities. Because this type of flow-sensing device is affected by gas density, software correction for different gas compositions is necessary. This is accomplished by sampling the gas, analyzing O_2 and CO_2, and applying the necessary correction factors. Software corrections for test gases used for various pulmonary function tests (e.g., DL_{CO}) can be easily applied.

Pitot tube flow sensors meet or exceed ATS recommendations for accuracy and precision. Their practical applications include routine pulmonary function tests, metabolic measurements, and exercise testing. Infection control for this type of device includes single-use, or disposable flow meters.

Flow-sensing spirometers have some advantages over volume-displacement systems. When combined with appropriate gas analyzers and breathing circuits, flow-sensing spirometers can be used to perform lung volume determinations by the open-circuit or closed-circuit methods. Diffusing capacity can be measured with flow-sensing spirometers as well. Pressure-differential, heated wire, and Pitot tube pneumotachometers are used to measure flow and volume in body plethysmographs, exercise testing systems, and metabolic carts. Because flow sensors require electronic circuitry to integrate flow or sum volume pulses, flow-based spirometers are usually microprocessor controlled. Some flow-sensing spirometers provide their analog signal (flow, volume, or both) to a strip chart or X-Y recorder. However, most flow sensors use computer-generated graphics to produce volume-time or flow-volume tracings.

Most flow-based spirometers can be easily cleaned and disinfected. Some flow sensors can be immersed in a disinfectant without disassembly. As noted, many systems use inexpensive, disposable sensors that can be discarded after one use. The use of in-line bacteria filters to prevent contamination of flow-based spirometers may result in changes in the operating characteristics of the spirometer. Any resistance to airflow through the filter will be added to the resistance of the spirometer. For this reason, the spirometer may need to be calibrated with the filter in place. Although the resistance offered by most filters is low, it may change with use. This may occur if water vapor from expired gas condenses on the filter media. Use of barrier filters does not eliminate the need for routine decontamination of spirometers.

Most of the flow sensors described produce a signal that is not linear across a wide range of flows. Some systems use two separate flow sensors to accommodate both low and high flows. Better accuracy can be obtained for flow and volume by matching the flow range of the sensor to the physiologic signal. Most flow-based spirometers "linearize" the flow signal electronically or by means of software corrections. In many systems, a "look-up table" is stored in the computer. The flow signal is continuously checked against the table and corrected. By combining a calibration factor (see Chapter 11) with the look-up table corrections, very accurate flow and integrated volume measurements are possible. Flows and volumes are corrected before variables such as FEV_1 are measured.

Turbine, pressure-differential, heated-wire, and Pitot tube flow-sensing spirometers are affected by the composition of the gas being measured. Changes in gas density or viscosity require correction of the transducer signal to obtain accurate flows and volumes. In most systems, these corrections are performed by computer software using a stored table. A flow-sensing spirometer may be calibrated with air but then used to measure mixtures containing helium, neon, oxygen, or other test gases. Some gases cause a linear shift in flow proportional to their concentrations. Corrections are usually made by applying a simple multiplier to the signal.

The accuracy of flow-based spirometers depends on the electronics and/or software that processes the flow signal. Pulmonary function variables measured on a time base (e.g., FEV_1 or FEV_6) require precise timing as well as accurate flow measurement. The timing mechanism in flow-based spirometers is critical in the detection of the start or end of the test. Timing is usually triggered by a minimum flow or pressure change. Signal integration begins when flow reaches a threshold limit, usually 0.1 to 0.2 L/sec. Spirometers that initiate timing in response to volume pulses usually have a similar threshold that must be achieved to begin recording. Contamination of resistive elements, thermistors, or Pitot tubes by moisture or other debris can alter the flow-sensing characteristics of the transducer and interfere with the spirometer's ability to detect the start or end of test.

Problems related to electronic "drift" require flow sensors to be "zeroed" frequently. Many systems "zero" the flow signal immediately before a measurement. Zeroing corrects for much of the electronic drift that occurs. A true zero requires no flow through the flow sensor. Hence the flow sensor must be held still or occluded during the zero maneuvers. Most flow-based systems use a 3-L syringe for calibration. By calibrating with a known volume signal, the accuracy of the flow sensor and the integrator can be checked with one input. Calibration and quality-control techniques for volume-displacement and flow-sensing spirometers are included in Chapter 11.

▉ PORTABLE SPIROMETERS

Many flow-sensing spirometers interface directly with small personal computers (Figure 10-13). Some spirometers use an interface that plugs directly into a personal computer (PC). With the appropriate software installed on the PC, spirometry can be performed. Other spirometers contain the electronic hardware in the flow sensor head. This implementation allows the flow sensor to be connected to a serial or USB (universal serial bus) port, which is standard on most computers. The pressure transducer and electronics for flow-based spirometry can also be mounted on a removable card (i.e., a PCMCIA card). These cards (Figure 10-14) allow spirometry to be performed with handheld computers, laptop computers, or personal digital assistants (PDAs). Other flow-based spirometers use dedicated microprocessors incorporated in a small package (Figure 10-15, *A*). This allows the unit to be handheld and portable.

Many portable spirometers utilize disposable flow sensors. Disposable sensors can provide accurate measurements if they are manufactured according to rigid specifications. Disposable

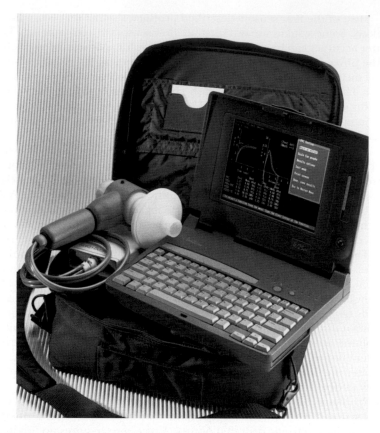

Figure 10-13 *Flow-sensing spirometer interfaced to a laptop computer.* A pressure-differential pneumotachometer with its interface electronics connects to the serial port of a laptop PC. The laptop computer runs software that provides calculations, data storage, and printing of results. (*Courtesy Pulmonary Data Service Instrumentation, Louisville, Colo.*)

flow sensors may be precalibrated at the time of manufacture. Some manufacturers include calibration codes (or bar codes) on the sensor to be used in conjunction with the spirometer software. Ideally, each spirometer should provide a means for calibration using a 3-L syringe. As a minimum, the software in portable spirometers should allow verification of volumes, even if precalibrated flow sensors are used.

Interfacing a flow sensor to a PC or laptop computer makes spirometry available in a variety of clinical settings. Handheld or PC-based systems provide a relatively inexpensive

Most portable spirometers include software features to help the user obtain high-quality data. These features include prompts to direct the patient's efforts, along with messages regarding the quality of data obtained. These quality indicators are usually based on ATS recommendations for spirometry. Many spirometers also include a grading system to assess the overall acceptability and reproducibility of the patient's efforts.

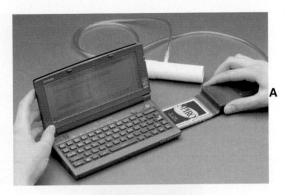

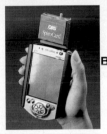

Figure 10-14 *Portable spirometers using plug-in cards.* **A,** Using a disposable flow sensor and a small pressure transducer mounted on a plug-in card, spirometry can be performed with a handheld computer. **B,** A similar plug-in card can be used with a personal digital assistant (PDA). (*Courtesy QRS Diagnostics, Plymouth, Minn.*)

way to perform spirometry, before and after bronchodilator studies, and even bronchial challenges. Precalibrated disposable flow sensors can provide accurate measurements of important spirometric variables. Increasingly sophisticated software allows spirometric data to be stored, manipulated, and displayed graphically.

The National Lung Health Education Program (NLHEP) has provided recommendations for office spirometers to be used in primary care settings. The goal of these spirometers is to allow early detection of COPD. Office spirometers are simple and small (Figure 10-15, *B*), designed to measure primarily FEV_1 and FEV_6. In order to provide accurate measurements, office spirometers should display automated messages describing the acceptability and reproducibility of efforts. Automated interpretation of simple spirometry can be performed if test quality is acceptable and appropriate reference values are used. Display or printouts of spirograms are optional. In general, office spirometers should meet the accuracy recommendations of the ATS (see Chapter 11).

Peak Flow Meters

PEF can be measured easily with most spirometers, either volume-displacement or flow-sensing types. Many devices are available that measure PEF exclusively. PEF has become a recognized means of monitoring patients who have asthma (see Chapter 2). By incorporating a simple measurement into an inexpensive package, portable peak flow meters allow monitoring of airway status in a variety of settings.

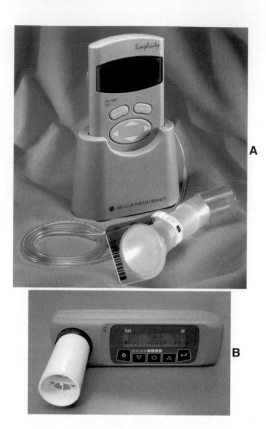

Figure 10-15 *Handheld "office" spirometers.* **A,** Small handheld spirometer designed for screening spirometry according to NLHEP recommendations. The disposable flow sensor has a bar-coded calibration factor that is read by a bar-code scanner built into the spirometer. **B,** Another small, handheld spirometer designed for office screening by measuring FEV_1 and FEV_6. (*A courtesy Nellcor Puritan Bennett, Inc., Pleasanton, Calif; B courtesy SDI Diagnostics, South Easton, Me.*)

Most peak flow meters use similar designs. The patient expires forcefully through a resistor or flow tube that has a movable indicator attached (Figure 10-16). An orifice provides the resistance in most devices. The movable indicator is deflected in proportion to the velocity of air flowing through the device. PEF is then read directly from a calibrated scale. Because these devices are nonlinear, different flow ranges are usually available. High-range peak flow meters typically measure flows as high as 850 L/min. Low-range meters measure up to 400 L/min (Table 10-1). Low-range peak flow meters are useful for small children or for patients who have marked obstruction.

The absolute accuracy of portable peak flow meters is less important than precision. These devices are intended to provide serial measurements of peak flow as a guide to treatment. Normal patients who are carefully instructed should be able to reproduce their peak flow measurements within 10%. However, asthmatics may not be able to reproduce PEF. PEF meters must be easy to use and easy to read. Scale divisions of 5 L/min for low-range devices and 10 L/min for high-range devices allow small changes in PEF to be detected. The scale should be calibrated to read flow in BTPS units. Corrections for altitude should be included because PEF meters tend to underestimate flow as altitude increases (i.e., approximately 7% per 100 mm Hg change in barometric pressure).

Although the simple design of portable peak flow meters allows them to be used repeatedly, moisture or other debris can cause sticking of the movable indicator. This can be problematic because it may suggest that the patient's asthma has worsened. Some instruments can be cleaned, but may need to be replaced periodically. Because portable peak flow meters may have a limited life span, reproducibility between same-model instruments should be 5% (ATS recommendations suggest 10% or 20 L/min). This allows the patient to continue monitoring with a new device. Clear instructions on how to use and maintain the peak flow meter should come with each device. Most peak flow meters comply with the National Asthma Education Program's "color zone" scheme for identifying clinically significant changes (see Chapter 2).

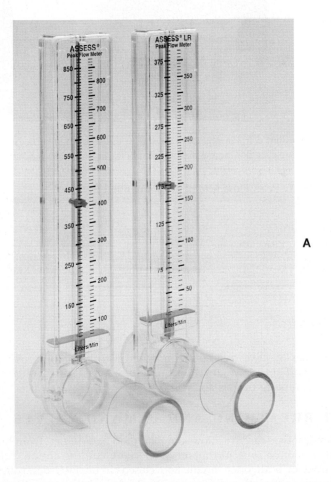

A

Figure 10-16 *Portable peak flow meters.* **A,** Portable peak flow meters for measuring PEF outside of the pulmonary function laboratory. The patient exhales forcefully through the mouthpiece at the bottom. Pressure generated by the flow of gas deflects the movable indicator up the scale. Two flow ranges are available, for normal and reduced peak flows. (*Courtesy Respironics, Inc., Murrysville, Pa.*)

Figure continued on next page

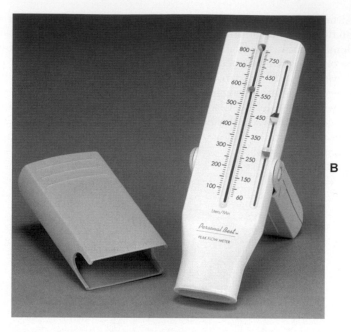

Figure 10-16—Cont'd B, Portable peak flow meter in which exhaled flow is directed against a movable indicator. Two separate flow ranges are provided in the same device. (*Courtesy Respironics, Inc., Murrysville, Pa.*)

TABLE 10-1 **Peak Flow Meter Recommended Ranges**

	Children	Adults
National Asthma Education Program	100-400 L/min ± 10%	100–700 L/min ± 10%
American Thoracic Society	60-400 L/min ± 10% or 20 L/min, whichever is greater	100–850 L/min ± 10% or 20 L/min, whichever is greater

Breathing Valves

Various types of valves are commonly used with both volume-displacement and flow-sensing spirometers. These valves direct inspired or expired gas through the spirometer or provide a means of sampling for gas analysis.

▉ FREE BREATHING AND DEMAND VALVES

The simplest type of valve allows the patient to be switched from breathing room air to breathing gas contained in a spirometer or special breathing circuit. Free breathing valves are routinely used in both open-circuit and closed-circuit FRC determinations. The free breathing valve is designed so that the patient can be "switched in" to the system either manually or by computer control at a specific point in the breathing cycle.

The typical free breathing valve consists of a body with two or more ports. A drum in the valve body rotates to connect different combinations of ports. Because these valves are used mainly for tidal breathing or slow vital capacity (SVC) maneuvers, resistance to flow is not critical. Most have ports with diameters of 1.5 to 3 cm. For studies involving gas analysis, such as FRC determination, the valve must be free of leaks.

Some systems use a "breathing manifold" that consists of multiple ports and valves. The ports allow inspired or expired gas to be directed to the spirometer or gas-sampling devices. The valves may be electrical or gas-powered solenoids, balloon valves that inflate with compressed air, or scissors-type valves that pinch flexible tubing to control flow. With computer control, different combinations of valves and ports are opened and closed. This type of manifold permits spirometry, gas-dilution lung volumes, and DL_{CO} tests to be performed with the same breathing circuit. A similar manifold is used in many body plethysmograph systems to permit measurement of V_{TG} and Raw along with DL_{CO}.

Infection control of free breathing valves and multiple-port manifolds involves disassembly, cleaning, and disinfection or sterilization. Because cleaning between patients may not be practical, in-line filters may be used to prevent contamination of these devices.

The most common problem encountered in breathing circuits that use valves is failure of the valves to operate correctly. Ballon-type valves often develop leaks. Demand valves sometimes stick or require excessive inspiratory pressure to open. Solenoid-type valves have O-rings that must be properly lubricated to prevent leaks. Directional valves (one-way and two-way) may have leaflets that stick or have been assembled incorrectly.

Demand valves are used in many circuits in which the patient inspires a test gas (e.g., DL_{CO}, N_2 washout). The primary considerations for demand valves are the pressure required to trigger gas flow and the adequacy of flow once the valve opens. Most demand valves consist of a valve body that contains a diaphragm. The diaphragm moves in response to the patient's inspiratory effort, opening the valve and allowing gas to flow. Maximal flow is controlled by the valve but may depend on the driving pressure (usually 20 to 50 psi). Demand valves are often adjustable, allowing the sensitivity to be set so that minimal pressure is needed to trigger gas flow. Problems typically encountered with demand valves include inadequate source pressure (turned off or not connected) and sticking or incorrectly adjusted diaphragms. Demand valves used in DL_{CO} circuits should be able to deliver 6 L/sec flow with less than 10 cm H_2O pressure.

DIRECTIONAL VALVES

Directional (one-way and two-way) valves are used in many types of breathing circuits. The simplest type consists of a flap or diaphragm that opens in only one direction. The valve is then mounted in a rigid tube that can be inserted in a breathing circuit. Because gas is only permitted to flow in one direction, these valves are called one-way valves.

A more common design is that used to separate inspired from expired gas, often called a two-way nonrebreathing valve. This type of directional valve consists of a T-shaped body with three ports and two separate diaphragms (Figure 10-17). The diaphragms allow gas to flow in only one direction. The patient connection is between the diaphragms, effectively separating inspired from expired gas. Two-way nonrebreathing valves are used in exercise testing, metabolic studies, or any procedure requiring collection, measurement, or analysis of exhaled gas. The valve body may contain a tap for connection of gas sample tubing. This tap is typically placed between the diaphragms so that both inspired and expired gas can be sampled.

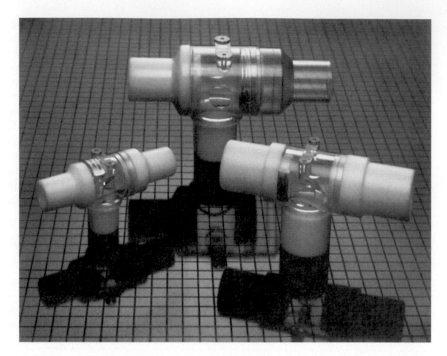

Figure 10–17 *Two-way nonrebreathing valves.* Three differently sized valves used for measurement of expired gas are shown. Each valve consists of a T-shaped body containing two diaphragms that separate inspired and expired gas. The smaller valves have less dead space but higher resistance to flow; the large valve has low flow resistance but more dead space. The small and medium valves are used for studies in which low flows are encountered, such as metabolic measurements. The large valve is appropriate for high flow rates such as those occurring during maximal exercise testing. (*Courtesy Hans Rudolph, Inc., Kansas City, Mo.*)

Two factors must be considered in the selection of appropriate directional valves: dead space volume and flow resistance. In one-way valves, only flow resistance is a concern. In two-way nonrebreathing valves, dead space is the volume contained between the two diaphragms along with the volume of any connectors (e.g., a mouthpiece). Most manufacturers supply information about the dead space of individual valves. Sometimes the dead space value is printed on the valve body. Unknown dead space can be determined by blocking two of the three ports and measuring the water volume required to fill the dead space portion of the valve.

Low dead space valves (less than 50 ml) may be required if the patient already has increased dead space, particularly if only tidal breathing is being assessed. Valves with large-bore ports and low-resistance diaphragms usually have larger dead space volumes. During exercise testing, large-bore nonrebreathing valves are used to minimize resistance at high flows. These valves usually have a large dead space volume. Selection of the appropriate-sized nonrebreathing valve should be based on the maximal flow anticipated during the test. For example, a maximal exercise test for a healthy adult patient may include flows greater than 100 L/min. A large-bore valve would be selected to accommodate the high flow. Valve dead space would be less of a concern because large tidal volumes are necessary to generate the increased flow. Mechanical (i.e., valve) dead space must be accurately determined for use in calculations involving gas analysis, such as physiologic dead space measurements.

Low resistance to flow is also a critical characteristic of one-way and two-way valves. Resistance to flow through most valves is nonlinear and depends on the cross-sectional area of valve leaflets or diaphragms (Figure 10-18). Resistance is usually not critical for tests in which flows of less than 1 L/sec occur. Small-bore (15 to 22 mm) directional valves can be selected based on an appropriate dead space volume. Most small-bore nonrebreathing valves have a resistance in the range of 1 to 2 cm H_2O/L/sec at flows of up to 1 L/sec (60 L/min). If the patient breathes through the valve for long intervals, even a small resistance may result in respiratory muscle fatigue and changes in the ventilatory pattern. Applications such as exercise testing often involve increased flows. Large-bore two-way valves are indicated when flows greater than 1 L/sec (60 L/min) can be expected to develop. Pressures lower than 3 cm H_2O can be maintained even at flows of 5 L/sec (300 L/min) with large-bore valves. Saliva may build up in valves during prolonged tests (e.g., exercise or eucapnic hyperventilation). Valves with "saliva traps" may be needed for these procedures. Valves used in a spirometry circuit must have very low resistance to meet the ATS recommendation of less than 1.5 cm H_2O/L/sec at flows of 12 L/sec. Valves used in a $D_{L_{CO}}$ circuit should produce a total resistance of less than 1.5 cm H_2O/L/sec at flows of 6 L/sec.

Any valve can cause increased resistance if not properly maintained. Rubber, plastic, or silicon leaflets and diaphragms can stick or become rigid with age. Valves should be disassembled and cleaned after each use according to the manufacturer's directions and allowed to dry thoroughly before reassembly. Care must be taken when reassembling valves to ensure

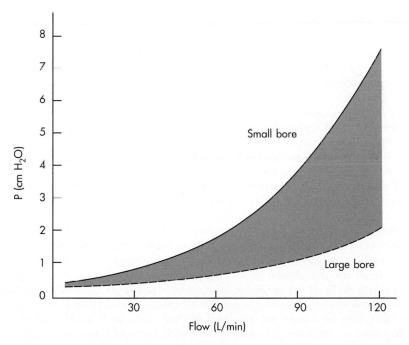

Figure 10-18 *Breathing valve resistance.* A graph plotting pressure developed across two different-sized valves in relation to gas flow through the valves. For small-bore valves (Figure 10-17), pressures of less than 1 cm H_2O are generated up to approximately 60 L/min (1 L/sec). Large-bore valves have less resistance (pressure per unit of flow) and are typically used for studies in which the patient develops high flow rates. Other factors affecting resistance include the design and material used for the diaphragms in the valve and whether the diaphragms move freely. Resistance increases nonlinearly in all types of valves; high resistance can occur even in large-bore valves at very high flows.

that all diaphragms are oriented properly. Valves should be visually inspected to make sure diaphragms open and close correctly before being used.

GAS-SAMPLING VALVES

Specialized valves may be used to sample gas during tests such as the single-breath DL_{CO}. Many gas-sampling valves use electrical or pneumatically powered solenoids to direct flow to a spirometer or sample bag. Other systems employ scissors valves to pinch compressible tubing. The primary concern with gas-sampling valves is smooth operation with appropriate direction of the gas to be sampled. Electrically activated solenoids may deteriorate with age, particularly if exposed to high-humidity conditions (e.g., expired air). Replacement of O-rings or similar types of seals may be necessary to ensure uncontaminated gas samples. Some sampling valves use balloons that inflate to block or direct the gas flow. These balloons require periodic replacement because a small leak can prevent the balloon from "seating." When this occurs, gas may not be directed to the appropriate device. Scissors-type valves offer an advantage in that the compressible tubing can be changed easily between patients.

Infection control for sampling valves usually requires disassembly and cleaning. Some complex valve manifolds may be difficult or impossible to disassemble. In such devices, an in-line filter may be needed to avoid cross-contamination.

Pulmonary Gas Analyzers

Various types of gas analyzers are used in pulmonary function testing. O_2 and CO_2 are analyzed during metabolic studies and exercise testing. Helium analysis is used for closed-circuit functional residual capacity (FRC) determinations and for several types of DL_{CO} tests. N_2 analysis is used in the open-circuit FRC method. CO measurements are integral to all of the diffusion capacity methods currently used. Analyses of neon, argon, methane, and acetylene are used in specialized tests for diffusion, lung volume measurements, and cardiac output determination.

How rapidly a gas analyzer can detect and display a change in gas concentration is termed *response time*. Response time is commonly measured in seconds or milliseconds (thousandths of a second). Manufacturers of gas analyzers list response time as the interval required for an analyzer to measure some fraction of a step change in gas concentration. For example, an O_2 analyzer might require 2 seconds to respond to an increase in O_2 concentration from 21% to 100%. The response time may be listed as the time required for 90% of the total change to be detected. Response time of an analyzer often depends on the size of the change in gas concentration. A related factor is transport time. *Transport time* is how long it takes to move the gas from the sample site to the analyzer itself. How rapidly a gas (e.g., O_2) can be analyzed depends on both the response time and the transport time of the instrument. In some tests, such as breath-by-breath gas analysis, response and transport times are critical and rapidly responding analyzers are required. Other tests, such as He dilution FRC measurement, require very accurate gas analysis but rapid response is not necessary.

OXYGEN ANALYZERS

Oxygen analysis can be performed by several different methods. Table 10-2 lists some types of O_2 analyzers available. Two types are used for rapid analysis of O_2 such as breath-by-breath exercise tests: the polarographic electrode and zirconium fuel cell. The other O_2 analyzers listed are used for specialized applications, including patient monitoring.

TABLE 10-2 Oxygen Analyzers

Type	Applications	Advantages/Disadvantages
Paramagnetic	Monitoring	Discrete sampling only
Polarographic electrode	Monitoring, exercise testing, metabolic studies	Discrete or continuous sampling; requires special electronic circuitry for fast response (200 msec)
Galvanic cell (fuel cell)	Monitoring	Continuous sampling; similar to polarographic but does not require polarizing voltage
Zirconium cell	Breath-by-breath exercise and metabolic studies	Heated (700° to 800° C) fuel cell; fast response useful for continuous sampling; thermal stabilization required
Gas chromatograph	Exercise testing, monitoring, metabolic measurements	Discrete sampling; response time ~30 seconds; very accurate; multiple gas analysis

Polarographic Electrodes

The polarographic electrode is similar to the blood gas O_2 electrode (see Blood Gas Electrodes, Oximeters, and Related Devices section). For gas analysis, a platinum cathode is used without a membrane covering the tip. A gas pump draws the sample past the polarized electrode at a constant flow. Oxygen is reduced in proportion to its partial pressure. The electrode is calibrated by exposing it to known fractional concentrations of O_2 at a known barometric pressure. A response time of approximately 200 msec can be attained by using special electronic circuitry. Rapid response allows continuous analysis for breath-by-breath measurements. Contamination of the electrode can degrade its response time and cause difficulty with calibration.

Zirconium Fuel Cells

An electrode is formed by coating a zirconium element with platinum. The zirconium, when heated to 700° to 800° C, acts as a solid electrolyte between the platinum coating on either side. When the two sides of the electrode are exposed to different partial pressures of O_2, gas traverses the electrode, creating a voltage proportional to the difference in concentrations. Sample gas is drawn past the element at a constant low flow. This allows rapid, continuous analysis without altering the temperature of the electrode. Electrode temperature must be held constant, so the electrode requires adequate insulation. A warm-up period of 10 to 30 minutes is typically required to reach thermal equilibrium at the elevated temperature. Response times of less than 200 msec are possible with the zirconium fuel cell, making it useful for breath-by-breath measurements.

A zirconium fuel cell, like the polarographic electrode, measures partial pressure of oxygen. Pressure changes in the sampling circuit can affect the concentration measurement. Such pressure changes can be caused by gas flow in a breathing circuit or by positive pressure in a mechanical ventilator circuit. The presence of water vapor in the sample affects both electrodes similarly. Oxygen concentration is measured accurately but is diluted in proportion to the water vapor pressure present in the sample. Zirconium fuel cells eventually degrade in

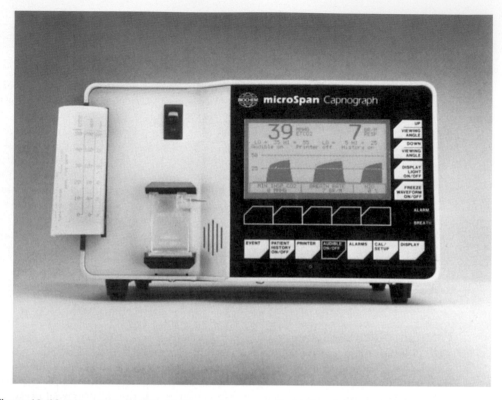

Figure 10–19 *Infrared CO$_2$ monitor.* A microprocessor-controlled infrared CO$_2$ analyzer as used for critical care monitoring. A liquid crystal display (LCD) allows presentation of end-tidal CO$_2$ values, breathing rate, and CO$_2$ waveforms. This capnograph includes a printer and alarms, along with a water trap to remove condensation from the sample line. (*Courtesy BCI, Inc., Waukesha, Wis.*)

relation to the volume of O$_2$ analyzed. The cell may be refreshed by passing a current through it, thus reversing the oxygen uptake process.

■ INFRARED ABSORPTION (CO$_2$, CO) ANALYZERS

Several types of respiratory gas analyzers are based on absorption of infrared radiation to measure gas concentrations. Infrared absorption is used in CO analyzers for DL$_{CO}$ tests. Infrared CO$_2$ analyzers are used for exercise testing, metabolic studies, and bedside monitoring (capnography) in critical care (Figure 10-19).

Certain gases (e.g., CO$_2$ and CO) absorb infrared radiation. A common type of infrared analyzer uses two beams of infrared radiation directed through parallel cells. One cell contains sample gas, whereas the other contains a reference gas. The two beams converge on a single infrared detector (Figure 10-20). A small motor rotates an interrupter or "chopper" between the infrared source and the cells. The chopper blades alternately interrupt the infrared radiation passing through the sample and reference cells. If the sample and reference gases have the same concentration, the radiation reaching the detector is constant. However, when a sample with a different gas concentration is introduced, the radiation reaching the detector varies in a rhythmic fashion. This causes a vibration in the detector that is translated into a pulsatile signal proportional to the difference between the two beams.

Infrared analyzers can measure small changes in gas concentrations such as the difference between inspired and expired CO in DL_{CO} tests. Infrared analyzers respond rapidly once the gas has been transported to the measuring chamber. Gas can be sampled either continuously or discretely with infrared analyzers. For continuous sampling, the gas flow must be constant. The analyzer must be calibrated using the same flow at which measurements are made. Pump settings and the sample line should not be altered after calibration. Condensation of water in the sample line can significantly alter the flow rate and affect the accuracy of the measurement. Water vapor in the sample will dilute the gas being analyzed. Water vapor can be removed if response time is not critical. For rapid response times, as required for breath-by-breath analysis, the effects of water vapor can be corrected mathematically by assuming that expired gas is fully saturated.

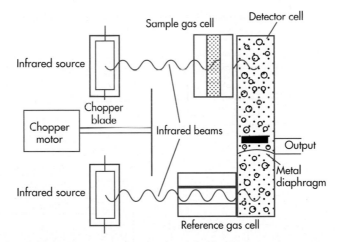

Figure 10–20 *Infrared absorption gas analyzer.* Components of an infrared analyzer used to measure CO_2 are depicted. Infrared sources emit beams that pass through parallel cells. One cell contains a reference gas; the other contains a gas sample to be analyzed. A rotating blade "chops" the infrared beams in a rhythmic fashion. When both reference and sample cells contain the same gas, the radiation reaching each half of the detector cell is the same. When a gas sample is introduced, it absorbs some infrared radiation. Different amounts of radiation reach the two halves of the detector cell, causing the diaphragm separating the compartments of the detector to oscillate. This oscillation is transformed into a signal proportional to the difference in gas concentrations. The infrared analyzer is ideal for determining small changes in concentration in gas samples. (*From Beckman Instruments, Inc., Medical gas analyzer LB-2: operating instructions, FM-149997-301, Schiller Park, Ill.*)

The most common problems occurring with infrared analyzers involve the chopper motor, sample cell, and infrared detector. Motors turning the chopper blades may wear out or work intermittently. Some analyzers use a nonmechanical means of alternating the infrared beams, thus eliminating the problem. The sample cell can easily become contaminated. Water condensation or other debris can contaminate the cell "window," interfering with transmission of the infrared beam. Infrared detector cells degrade over time and become less sensitive. Both contamination of the sample cell and detector aging can alter response time or make the analyzer impossible to calibrate.

■ EMISSION SPECTROSCOPY ANALYZERS

The single-breath and multiple-breath N_2-washout tests (open-circuit FRC determination) use N_2 analysis. The Giesler tube ionizer is an N_2 analyzer based on the principle of emission spectroscopy (Figure 10-21). This instrument consists of an enclosed ionization chamber that contains two electrodes and a photocell. A vacuum pump creates a constant low pressure in the ionization chamber by bleeding gas through a needle valve. The needle valve draws gas to be sampled from a breathing circuit. When current is supplied to the electrodes, the N_2 between them is ionized and emits light. After being filtered, this light is monitored by a photo detector. The intensity of the light is directly proportional to the concentration of N_2 in the sample. The current, distance between electrodes, and gas pressure must remain constant. The photo detector converts the light signal into a DC voltage. This analog signal is then amplified, linearized, and directed to an appropriate meter or analog-to-digital converter. The Giesler tube ionizer allows continuous and rapid analysis of N_2 with response times of less than 100 msec.

Analyzers using emission spectroscopy usually require a vacuum pump. Vacuum pressure must be maintained at a stable level to ensure accuracy and linearity. Leaks in the seals around

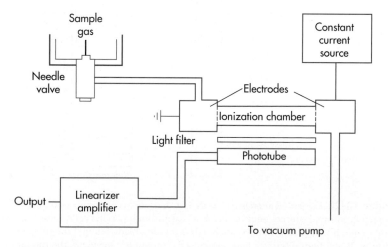

Figure 10–21 *Emission spectroscopy-type gas analyzer.* The optical emission analyzer (Giesler tube) is commonly used for N_2 analysis. A vacuum pump draws a small gas sample through a needle valve (usually in the breathing circuit). The gas sample passes through an ionization chamber, where the ionized gas emits light. All light except that from the desired gas is filtered out, and the remaining light is monitored by a phototube or similar detector. The detector transmits a signal proportional to the intensity of the light, allowing rapid gas analysis. (*From Hewlett-Packard, Application Note AN 729, San Diego, Calif.*)

the needle valve or in the pump itself may occur. Inability to zero or span the analyzer (i.e., adjust the gain) often indicates a leak or faulty vacuum source. The photo detector, ionizing electrodes, and light filter all degrade over time. Periodic linearity checks allow adjustment for small changes in these components.

■ THERMAL CONDUCTIVITY ANALYZERS

Measurement of FRC by the closed-circuit method requires He analysis. Some DL_{CO} systems also analyze helium as the tracer gas. Thermal conductivity analyzers measure gas concentrations in a sample by detecting the rate at which different gases conduct heat. Heated wires or beads (thermistors) are exposed to the gas sample. The concentration of a specific gas can be detected by measuring the change in electrical resistance of the thermistors. Two glass-coated thermistors serve as sensing elements connected by a Wheatstone bridge circuit (Figure 10-22). Thermistors change temperature and electrical resistance as a function of the molecular weight of the gases surrounding them. One thermistor serves as a reference. A difference in the concentration of gases between two thermistors can be detected because differences in heat conducted away alter the electrical resistance in the circuit. He analyzers use a reference cell containing no helium (He). Other gases can be analyzed by means of thermal conductivity if no interfering gases are present. Thermal conductivity analyzers are

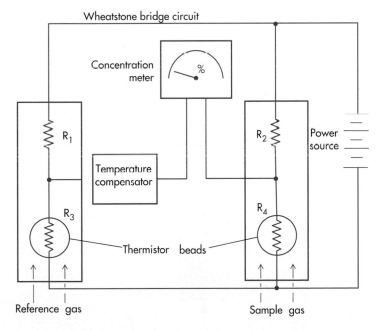

Figure 10-22 *Thermal conductivity analyzer.* A thermal conductivity gas analyzer, as used for He analysis or gas chromatography, is shown. Two thermistor beads (temperature-sensitive electrical resistors) are connected in a Wheatstone bridge circuit. When the thermistors are subjected to the same gas concentrations, their electrical resistances are equal and the meter registers zero (by calibration). When a gas is applied to the sample thermistor (R_4) and the reference thermistor submitted to a reference gas, an electrical potential occurs. This deflects the meter (i.e., a voltmeter) by an amount proportional to the difference in gas concentrations. (*From Bourns, Inc., Life systems operations instruction manual, Model LS114-5, Riverside, Calif.*)

used in conjunction with gas chromatography (see Gas Chromatography section). Water vapor and CO_2 are usually removed before He analysis. Thermal conductivity analyzers can be used for continuous or discrete measurements but have response times in the range of 10 to 20 seconds. Thermal conductivity analyzers cannot be used to detect rapid changes in gas concentration.

Thermal conductivity analyzers are very stable. Unless the thermistor in the sampling chamber is contaminated or physically damaged, the analyzer remains accurate for an extended period. Water vapor or CO_2 in the sample circuit (caused by malfunctioning absorbers) is a common cause of errors with this type of analyzer. Some He analyzers also use a water absorber in line with the reference thermistor. This allows dry room air to be used to zero the analyzer. Exhaustion of this absorber can result in calibration errors.

GAS CHROMATOGRAPHY

Gas chromatography combines a means of separating a sample into component gases and a detector for measuring concentrations of the components. The detector is usually a thermal conductivity analyzer as previously described. Most chromatographs use the principle of column separation to segregate the component gases of the sample (Figure 10-23). The

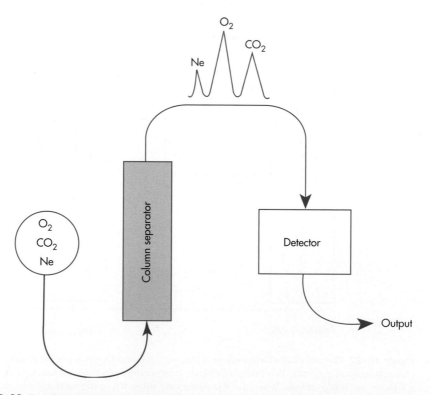

Figure 10–23 *Gas chromatograph.* Diagram of the components of a gas chromatograph for analyzing respiratory gases. The gas sample moves through a separator column via a carrier gas, usually He. Gases of different molecular sizes pass through the column at different rates and are monitored sequentially by a thermal conductivity detector. Gases can be analyzed very accurately by using appropriate separator columns.

chromatograph column contains a packing material that impedes movement of gas molecules, depending on their size. The material is usually a high-surface-area inorganic or polymer packing. Some columns also use materials that combine chemically with specific gases. A combination of columns allows a wide range of gases to be analyzed with a single detector. He is used as a carrier gas because of its high thermal conductivity. The sample gas, along with the He carrier gas, is injected into the column. Component gases exit the column at varying rates and are detected by a thermal conductivity analyzer. The concentrations of each gas can be determined by comparing the output of the thermal conductivity analyzer with a known calibration gas. Because He is used as the carrier gas, it cannot be used as an inert indicator for lung volume determinations or diffusing capacity measurements. Neon, which is relatively insoluble, may be substituted for He in these tests. Water vapor and CO_2 are usually removed from the sample to prevent contamination of the separator column.

Gas chromatographs are well suited to applications requiring analysis of multiple gases, such as DL_{CO} determinations. Chromatography is very accurate and is widely used for analysis of certified reference gases. Gas chromatograph response times are from 15 to 90 seconds, depending on the gas to be detected and the flow of carrier gas.

Gas chromatographs that are properly maintained are very accurate. Column material must be replaced when exhausted to maintain accuracy. Some chromatographs heat the column to enhance separation. Failure of the heating mechanism can lead to inaccurate analyses. Exhaustion of water or CO_2 absorbers can also cause the column to become contaminated.

■ GAS-CONDITIONING DEVICES

Interference from water vapor or CO_2 in expired gas is common to many types of gas analyzers. These two gases are usually removed by chemical "scrubbers."

CO_2 may be absorbed by passing the sample through granules containing either barium hydroxide $(Ba(OH)_2)$ or sodium hydroxide $(NaOH)$. Granules containing $NaOH$ have a light brown appearance that changes to white when saturated with CO_2. The $Ba(OH)_2$ (Baralyme) scrubber is usually supplied with an indicator (ethyl violet), which changes from white to purple when saturated with CO_2. Both $NaOH$ and $Ba(OH)_2$ are mildly corrosive and may generate heat if exposed to high concentrations of CO_2. Both generate water as a product of combination with CO_2. Therefore, they should be placed upstream of any water vapor absorber used in the same circuit.

Water vapor is absorbed by passing the humidified gas over granules of anhydrous calcium sulfate $(CaSO_4)$ (Drierite) or silica gel. These substances are termed *desiccants*. $CaSO_4$ usually contains an indicator that changes from blue to pink when saturated with water vapor. Some analyzers use silica gel to remove water vapor.

Conditioning of gas that contains water vapor may also be accomplished using special sample tubing (Nafion). This tubing is permeable to water vapor. Sample gas passing through the tubing equilibrates its water vapor pressure with that of the surrounding atmosphere. Water vapor is not removed; it remains constant at a known level. If wet gas (e.g., expired air) is passed through the tubing, the sample falls to ambient humidity. If dry gas (e.g., calibration gas) is passed through the tubing, the sample rises to ambient humidity. This allows corrections for water vapor pressure to be accurately applied, as long as the ambient humidity level is known.

Failure to adequately remove water vapor or CO_2 from a gas sample results in dilution of the remaining gases. Dilution lowers the fractional concentration of the gas being analyzed. Chemical scrubbers or permeable tubing should always be replaced according to the manufacturer's recommendations.

Blood Gas Electrodes, Oximeters, and Related Devices

Measurements of arterial or mixed venous blood gases include determination of P_{O_2}, P_{CO_2}, and pH. Calculation of arterial oxygen concentration (SaO_2), bicarbonate (HCO_3^-), total CO_2, base excess, and other variables depends on measurements derived from one or more of the three primary electrodes. Oxyhemoglobin saturation is measured using a multiwavelength oximeter; it may also be estimated using a pulse oximeter. Other methods of assessing blood gases rely on transcutaneous electrodes, intraarterial and extraarterial optodes, and reflective spectrophotometry.

▄ pH ELECTRODES

The glass pH electrode contains a solution of constant pH on one side of a glass membrane. The sample to be analyzed is brought into contact with the other side of the pH-sensitive glass (Figure 10-24). The difference in pH on either side of the glass causes a potential difference, or voltage. To measure this potential, two half-cells are used: one for the constant solution and one for the sample. The constant solution half-cell (i.e., the measuring electrode) is usually a silver–silver chloride wire. The external half-cell is usually a saturated calomel (i.e., approximately

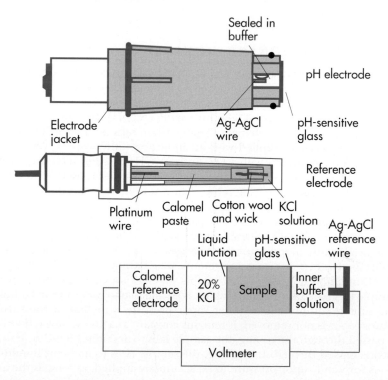

Figure 10–24 *pH and reference electrodes.* The pH electrode is a microelectrode, shown here with its plastic jacket. At the tip is a silver–silver chloride wire in a sealed-in buffer behind pH-sensitive quartz glass. The reference electrode contains a platinum wire in calomel paste that rests in a 20% KCl solution. The blood sample is introduced in such a way that it contacts the measuring electrode tip and the KCl. A voltmeter measures the potential difference across the sample, which is proportional to the pH.

20% KCl) electrode called the reference electrode. The reference electrode makes contact with the unknown solution by means of a permeable membrane or a liquid junction. These half-cells are connected to a voltmeter calibrated in pH units. The voltage difference between the two electrodes is proportional to the pH difference of the solutions. Because the pH of one solution is constant, the developed potential is a measure of the pH of the sample.

Protein contamination of the pH-sensitive glass is a common problem and increases with the number of specimens analyzed. Routine cleaning with a proteolytic agent (e.g., bleach) reduces buildup of protein on the electrode tip. KCl depletion or blockage of the reference junction can also cause pH electrode malfunction. Contamination of reagents used for pH electrode calibration may also result in measurement errors. Daily (or more frequent) use of suitable quality control (QC) materials can detect these and other problems (see Chapter 11).

■ P_{CO_2} ELECTRODES

The P_{CO_2} electrode (Severinghaus electrode) measures P_{CO_2} potentiometrically using an adaptation of the pH electrode (Figure 10-25). A combined pH-reference electrode is placed inside of a membrane-tipped plastic jacket. The jacket is filled with a bicarbonate electrolyte. The membrane is usually Teflon or a similar material permeable to CO_2 molecules. A spacer or wick made of nylon is sometimes placed between the pH-sensitive glass and the membrane. The spacer ensures that a thin layer of bicarbonate electrolyte is in contact with the electrode. When the blood sample is introduced at the tip of the electrode, CO_2 diffuses across the membrane. CO_2 is hydrated in the electrolyte according to the following equation:

$$CO_2 + H_2O \leftrightarrow H_2CO_3 \leftrightarrow H^+ + HCO_3^-$$

The higher the P_{CO_2}, the more the equation is driven to the right. The change in H^+ concentration is proportional to the change in P_{CO_2}. The electrode detects the change in P_{CO_2} as a change in pH of the electrolyte. The voltage developed is exponentially related to P_{CO_2}. A tenfold increase in P_{CO_2} is approximately equal to a decrease of 1 pH unit. Partial pressure of CO_2 can be determined by calibrating the pH change when the electrode is exposed to gases with known P_{CO_2} values.

PF Tips

Modern blood gas analyzers do an excellent job of detecting common electrode problems. Automated calibration allows tracking of electrode performance. The sensitivity of each electrode is monitored against a known range to detect sudden changes in performance. The drift between calibrations is also monitored to detect more subtle changes (trends) in electrode performance. If either sensitivity or drift exceeds specified limits, an alert is displayed.

The most common problem with the P_{CO_2} electrode is degradation or contamination of the permeable membrane. Protein or debris deposited on the membrane slows diffusion of CO_2. Equilibrium between the sample and electrode may not be achieved. Electrolyte depletion or exhaustion in the jacket around the electrode may also occur with extended use.

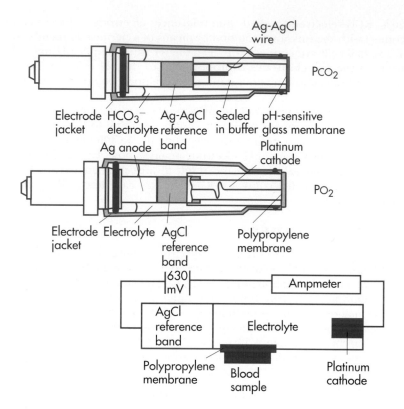

Figure 10-25 *Pco_2 and Po_2 electrodes.* The Pco_2 (Severinghaus) electrode is a modified pH electrode. The electrode has a sealed-in buffer; an Ag-AgCl reference band is the other half-cell. The entire electrode is encased in a Lucite jacket filled with a bicarbonate electrolyte. The jacket is capped with a Teflon membrane that is permeable to CO_2. A nylon mesh (*not shown*) covers the pH-sensitive glass, acting as a spacer to maintain contact with the electrolyte. CO_2 diffuses through the Teflon membrane, combines with the electrolyte, and alters the pH (*see text*). The change in pH is displayed as partial pressure of CO_2. The Po_2 (polarographic or Clark) electrode contains a platinum cathode and a silver anode. The electrode is polarized by applying a slightly negative voltage of approximately 630 mV. The tip is protected by a polypropylene membrane that allows O_2 molecules to diffuse but prevents contamination of the platinum wire. O_2 migrates to the cathode and is reduced, picking up free electrons that have come from the anode through a phosphate–potassium chloride electrolyte. Changes in the current flowing between the anode and cathode result from the amount of O_2 reduced in the electrolyte and are proportional to partial pressure of O_2.

Careful attention to shifts in electrode performance, during either calibration or control runs, can detect these common problems. Routine maintenance includes replacing the membrane and refilling the electrode with fresh electrolyte. Most manufacturers provide a kit that contains a disposable jacket with a membrane and fresh electrolyte. Guidelines for QC of blood gas electrodes are included in Chapter 11.

Po₂ ELECTRODES

The Po_2 electrode (Clark electrode) consists of a platinum cathode that is usually a thin wire encased in plastic or glass, together with a silver–silver chloride (Ag-AgCl) anode (Figure 10-25). Both anode and cathode are placed inside a plastic jacket that is tipped with a polypropylene or polyethylene membrane. This membrane is semipermeable and allows diffusion of oxygen molecules. The jacket is filled with phosphate–potassium chloride buffer. A polarizing voltage of approximately 630 mV is applied to the electrode. The cathode is slightly negative with respect to the anode. Because the electrode is polarized, it is often called a *polarographic* electrode. Oxygen is reduced (i.e., takes up electrons) at the cathode according to the following equation:

$$O_2 + 2H_2O + 4e^- \rightarrow 4OH^-$$

Electrons (*e* in the equation above) are supplied by the Ag-AgCl anode. Electrons flow from the anode to the cathode with a current proportional to the number of molecules of O_2 reduced. Each O_2 molecule can take up four electrons, and the greater the number of O_2 molecules present, the greater the current. The membrane causes a diffusion limitation to the number of molecules reaching the electrode. The greater the partial pressure on the sample side of the membrane, the higher the rate of diffusion. The measurement of the current developed within the electrode is therefore proportional to P_{O_2}.

As with the P_{CO_2} electrode, contamination or degradation of the membrane alters diffusion of O_2 and can result in erratic measurements. Most polarographic electrodes use a platinum wire of small diameter to reduce the actual consumption of O_2 at the tip of the electrode. The exposed surface of the platinum cathode gradually becomes plated with metal ions and must be periodically polished to maintain its sensitivity. The platinum wire can be polished by brushing or by abrading with a coarse substance such as pumice.

Because the membrane causes a diffusion limit to O_2 molecules reaching the cathode, the electrode performs differently when exposed to liquid versus gas samples. Many blood gas systems use gas to calibrate the P_{O_2} electrode. Noticeable differences may result when the electrode is then used to analyze the tension of O_2 dissolved in a liquid (e.g., blood). These differences are usually compensated for by correcting the P_{O_2} with an empirically determined gas-to-liquid factor.

▪ BLOOD GAS ANALYZERS

Laboratory Analyzers

Although the gas-measuring (P_{O_2} and P_{CO_2}) electrodes and the pH electrode system can each be used separately, all three are usually implemented together in a blood gas analyzer (Figure 10-26). The three electrodes are mounted in a single measuring chamber. This allows a small blood sample (200 µl or less) to be analyzed. Most blood gas analyzers are microprocessor-controlled. Sample aspiration, rinsing, and calibration can all be done automatically with program control. Standardization of these functions, especially calibration, reduces measurement error and improves precision. The microprocessor can calculate other blood gas values derived from pH, P_{CO_2}, and P_{O_2}, including HCO_3^-, total CO_2, and base excess (BE). In addition, computerized analyzers can monitor automated calibrations and electrode performance to alert the technologist of existing or impending problems. The computer can monitor the level of reagents and calibrating solutions/gases as well.

▪ POINT-OF-CARE ANALYZERS

To provide rapid results of critical analytes (i.e., blood gases and electrolytes), portable or bedside analyzers are available (Figure 10-27). These devices are designed for use in the emergency department or critical care unit. Most can be battery-operated, but some

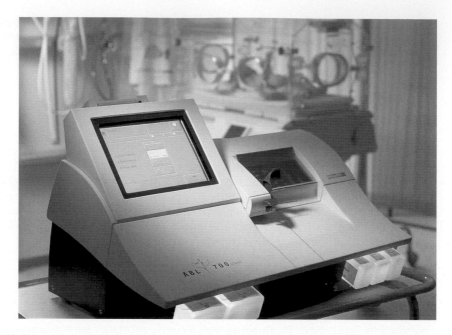

Figure 10–26 *Automated blood gas analyzer, including spectrophotometric oximeter.* This system provides automatic sample handling, flushing, and calibration. Results of sample analysis and calibrations are displayed using an integrated computer and display terminal. pH, Pco_2, and Po_2 are measured; HCO_3^-, total CO_2, standard bicarbonate, and other variables are calculated. This system also incorporates a spectrophotometric oximeter for analysis of Hb, O_2Hb, COHb, and MetHb. Base excess is calculated using HCO_3^- calculated from the blood gas analysis and Hb measured by the oximeter. Additional parameters can include bilirubin, electrolytes, glucose, and lactate. (*Courtesy Radiometer America, Westlake, Ohio.*)

point-of-care (POC) instruments require standard power. Blood gas measurement techniques differ slightly among models. Some POC blood gas analyzers use microelectrodes similar to those described previously, whereas others use electrochemical film methods. Reagents and calibration materials are contained in disposable packages. Some POC systems use cartridges that allow a fixed number of analyses. others use a single-patient sample chamber. Calibrations for POC systems that use multiple-specimen cartridges are usually performed in the traditional manner (see Chapter 11). Single-use devices often have the sample chamber precalibrated by the manufacturer. Some POC instruments use aqueous buffers in the single-patient chamber to perform calibration immediately before sample analysis.

The accuracy and precision of most POC blood gas analyzers appear comparable to that obtained with standard laboratory instruments. Routine analysis of multiple levels of QC material is required to assess precision. Analysis of unknown specimens and comparison with other instruments or laboratories (proficiency testing) is required to determine accuracy. Many POC instruments include ion-specific electrodes for analysis of potassium (K^+), sodium (Na^+), and calcium (Ca^{++}).

▉ TRANSCUTANEOUS Po_2 ELECTRODES

The transcutaneous O_2 electrode ($tcPo_2$) operates on a principle similar to that of the polarographic electrode. The $tcPo_2$ electrode consists of a ring-shaped silver anode heated by a coil to increase blood flow at the skin placement site. Inside the circular anode is a series of thin

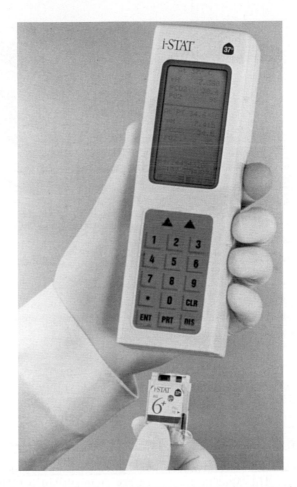

Figure 10-27 *POC blood gas analyzer.* This handheld POC blood gas analyzer uses microelectrodes. It is battery powered, so it can be used in a variety of clinical settings. (*Courtesy i-Stat Corp., East Windsor, NJ.*)

platinum cathodes (Figure 10-28). All elements are enclosed in a plastic case. The face of the sensor is covered by a Teflon membrane. Electrolyte (KCl) is placed between the membrane and the sensor. A second layer of electrolyte and a cellophane membrane are added to form a double membrane. The current between the silver anode and platinum cathodes is proportional to the Po_2 diffusing through the skin and membrane. A feedback controller keeps the temperature constant at the skin site. This also compensates for changes in capillary blood flow and stabilizes the measurement.

The gradient between $tcPo_2$ and Pao_2 is relatively constant in patients with normal cardiac output. In neonates there is a close correlation between transcutaneous and Pao_2. In hemodynamically stable adults, $tcPo_2$ is approximately 80% of Pao_2. Measurement of $tcPo_2$ can trend oxygenation when this gradient has been established. In patients with reduced cardiac output, the gradient between $tcPo_2$ and Pao_2 widens. Conditions that affect perfusion to the skin may also alter the gradient between arterial and $tcPo_2$.

Most transcutaneous monitors heat the skin site from 40° to 45° C. The increased temperature "arterializes" capillary blood flow. However, this necessitates moving the

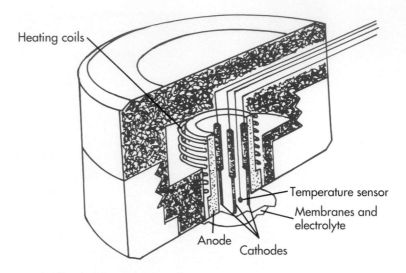

Figure 10–28 *Transcutaneous Po₂ electrode.* Cross-sectional diagram of the tcPO₂ electrode shows a circular anode around a series of cathodes and a temperature sensor. A heating coil causes local hyperemia so that skin PO₂ closely resembles PaO₂. A double membrane separates the electrode proper from the skin. Because the electrode warms the skin, it must be moved periodically.

electrode every 3 to 4 hours to prevent burns. Changing sensor sites is particularly important in neonates because of the reduced thickness of their epidermis. Periodic recalibration of the electrode is necessary even if the sensor site has not been changed. After placement of the electrode, an interval of 5 to 30 minutes may be required for equilibration to be reached.

■ SPECTROPHOTOMETRIC OXIMETERS

The spectrophotometric oximeter uses light absorption to analyze saturation of hemoglobin (Hb) with O_2. The concentration of carboxyhemoglobin (COHb) or other forms of Hb (e.g., methemoglobin, sulfhemoglobin) can also be determined. This type of spectrophotometer is sometimes called a *co-oximeter.*

The blood oximeter analyzes the absorption of light in a blood sample at multiple wavelengths. At certain wavelengths, two or more forms of Hb have similar absorbances (Figure 10-29). These common wavelengths are termed *isobestic points.* An isobestic point for oxyhemoglobin (O_2Hb), reduced Hb (RHb), and COHb is 548 nm. At this wavelength, the absorbance of a mixture of the three pigments is directly proportional to the total concentration of Hb. An isobestic point for O_2Hb and RHb is 568 nm. The absorbance of COHb at this point is considerably higher. A change in absorbance at 568 nm compared with 548 nm indicates a change in the concentration of COHb relative to the sum of the concentrations of the other two species. The isobestic point for RHb and COHb is 578 nm, with O_2Hb absorbance being considerably greater. The difference in absorbance at 578 nm indicates the concentration of O_2Hb relative to the other two pigments. The total Hb concentration, O_2Hb, COHb, and methemoglobin (MetHb) saturation can be determined by analyzing absorbances and solving simultaneous equations.

The spectrophotometric oximeter provides the true O_2Hb saturation (see Oxygen Saturation section, Chapter 6). This is particularly important if increased concentrations of COHb, MetHb, or other abnormal hemoglobins are present. Most automated blood gas

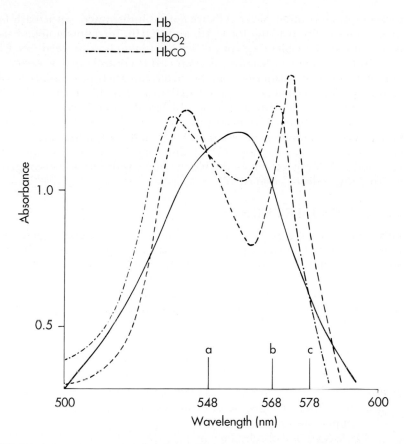

Figure 10-29 *Principle of spectrophotometric oximetry.* Absorbance measurements are made at three or more distinct wavelengths (548, 568, 578 nm) as light passes through a sample of hemolyzed blood. At 548 nm, all three forms of Hb (Hb, O_2Hb, and COHb) have identical absorbances. At 568 nm, only Hb and HbO_2 coincide, whereas at 578 nm, Hb and COHb coincide. The solution of simultaneous equations provides the relative proportions of each species, as well as total Hb (*see text*).

analyzers calculate O_2Hb saturation. Calculated saturation is based on the measured Po_2 and pH at 37° C. This calculation assumes that the Hb has a normal P_{50} (see Chapter 6). Calculated O_2Hb significantly overestimates true saturation in the presence of COHb or methemoglobin. The co-oximeter provides the most accurate estimate of the actual O_2 saturation. Combination blood gas analyzers and co-oximeters are available. These instruments combine conventional pH and blood gas electrodes with spectrophotometric measurements of Hb saturation, all performed with the same blood sample.

A co-oximeter may give erroneous Hb, O_2Hb, or COHb readings if forms of hemoglobin are present that the instrument does not recognize. For example, blood from a newborn (i.e., containing fetal Hb) will give erroneous values if analyzed by an oximeter set up for adult blood. Substances that cause light scattering in the specimen (e.g., lipids resulting from lipid therapy) may also cause false readings. To function properly, the blood oximeter must hemolyze the sample so that Hb molecules are suspended in solution rather than contained within the red cells. Hemolysis is accomplished by chemical or mechanical disruption of red cell membranes. Incomplete hemolysis results in light scattering within the sample rather than simple absorption. Sickle cells are not easily disrupted, particularly by chemical lysis, and may result in false readings for O_2Hb and COHb. Incomplete hemolysis may be difficult to detect unless whole-blood QC or proficiency testing is performed (see Chapter 11).

Most co-oximeters feature microprocessor control so that errors such as incomplete hemolysis or light scattering can be detected. Microprocessor-controlled oximeters also provide options so that fetal or animal Hb can be analyzed. In addition to measurements of O_2Hb, COHb, and MetHb saturations, the blood oximeter can calculate oxygen content and P_{50}. P_{50} can be estimated by measuring the actual saturation of a specimen (usually a venous sample with a saturation of less than 90%) and comparing this value with the calculated saturation based on Po_2 and pH of the same blood. This simplified method compares favorably with tonometering of the blood sample with various low-oxygen concentrations and constructing a dissociation curve.

◼ PULSE OXIMETERS

Pulse oximeters (Figure 10-30) are commonly used to assess oxygenation noninvasively. The pulse oximeter's immediate predecessor was a fiberoptic oximeter that passed multiple wavelengths of light through the earlobe and measured the absorption to derive oxygen saturation of Hb.

Pulse oximeters treat Hb as a filter that allows only red and near-infrared light to pass. Beer's law relates total absorption in a system of absorbers to the sum of their individual absorptions:

$$A_{total} = E_1C_1L_1 \quad E_2C_2L_2 \ldots E_nC_nL_n$$

where:
A_{total} = absorbance of a mixture of substances at a specific wavelength
E_n = extinction of substance n
C_n = concentration of substance n
L_n = length of light path through substance n

In principle, the pulse oximeter measures absorption of a mixture of just two substances, O_2Hb and RHb. The concentration of either one can be determined if their extinction is measured while the path length stays constant. The wavelengths of light used in pulse oximetry are near 660 nm in the red region of the spectrum and near 940 nm in the near infrared region. Extinction curves for O_2Hb and RHb show that reduced Hb has absorption 10 times higher than oxyhemoglobin at 660 nm, whereas O_2Hb has a higher absorbance (2 to 3 times) at 940 nm. Calculating all possible combinations of the two forms of Hb (i.e., varying the saturation from 0% to 100%) allows the ratio of absorbances at the two wavelengths to be determined. As a result, a calibration curve can be constructed. The capillary bed does not follow the optical principles exactly as described by Beer's law, so the calibration curve is derived empirically. The ratio of absorbances at the two distinct wavelengths is expressed as follows:

$$R = A_{660\,nm}/A_{940\,nm}$$

A series of R values (i.e., the calibration curve) is determined by relating the ratio to actual saturation measurements. Unlike the spectrophotometric oximeter, which measures absorption in a hemolyzed blood sample, the pulse oximeter measures light passing through living tissue. The transmitted light is not only absorbed but also refracted and scattered. This causes the absolute accuracy of the pulse oximeter to be less than the blood oximeter.

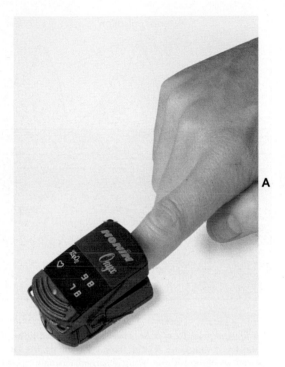

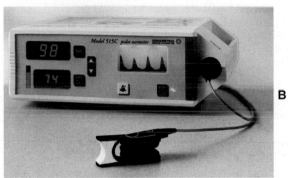

Figure 10-30 *Pulse oximeters.* Each oximeter provides a digital display of oxygen saturation and pulse rate. **A,** A small, portable pulse oximeter that fits over the patient's finger. Miniaturized components allow a device of this size to be easily transported. **B,** An LCD included with this oximeter allows the user to visualize pulse waveforms and monitor signal quality, both of which may be helpful in detecting conditions that interfere with accurate saturation determinations. Alarms for high and low saturations or pulse rates may be set. (*A courtesy Nonin Medical, Inc., Plymouth, Minn; B courtesy Novametrix Medical Systems, Inc., Wallingford, Conn.*)

The transmitted light at each wavelength consists of two components, the AC and DC components (Figure 10-31). The AC component varies with the pulsation of blood. The DC component represents light absorbed by tissue and venous blood. The DC component is larger than the AC and is relatively constant. The amplitude of both AC and DC levels depends on the intensity of the incident light. The AC component represents the arterial blood because the arterioles pulsate in the light path. By dividing the AC level by the DC level

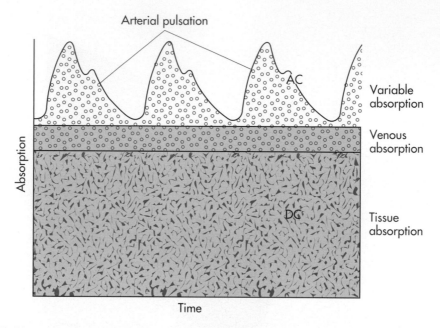

Figure 10–31 *Measurement principle of pulse oximetry.* Transmitted light (at wavelengths of 660 and 940 nm) consists of an AC and DC component. A large fixed component, the DC component, represents light passing through tissue and venous blood without being absorbed. A smaller portion is pulsatile in nature and changes absorption as blood pulses through the arterioles; this is represented as the AC component. The pulse oximeter divides the AC signal by the DC signal at each wavelength, effectively cancelling the DC component. The ratio of the AC signals at the two wavelengths is then a function of the relative absorptions of O_2Hb and RHb (*see text*). Modern pulse oximeters include sophisticated digital filters to better distinguish the AC and DC components of the signal.

at each of the two wavelengths, the AC component is effectively corrected. The AC component then becomes a function of the extinction of O_2Hb and RHb. The ratio just described then becomes:

$$R = \frac{(AC_1/DC_1)}{(AC_2/DC_2)}$$

where:
1 = red wavelength (660 nm)
2 = near-infrared wavelength (940 nm)

Correcting the pulsatile component (AC) in this manner allows the pulse oximeter to "ignore" absorbances caused by venous blood, tissue, and skin pigmentation.

The light source used in pulse oximetry is the light-emitting diode (LED). LEDs are capable of emitting a very bright light near the 660-nm and 940-nm wavelengths required for analysis of Hb saturation. Light intensity is controlled by a feedback circuit that regulates the driving current to the LED. The greater the DC component resulting from pigmentation or venous blood, the greater the current supplied to the LED. One problem with LEDs is that the exact wavelength of light emitted varies with individual diodes. Each LED has its own center wavelength that may differ from 660 or 940 nm by as much as 15 nm. To overcome this variation, each oximeter must have a series of calibration curves programmed into it so that it can accommodate a range of LEDs. The extinction curves for RHb and O₂Hb are steep and quite different at 660 nm, so 10 or more calibration curves are typically required for the red-light range. Slight variations in center wavelength are less critical in the 940-nm region because the extinction characteristics of O_2Hb and RHb are the same from 800 nm to 1000 nm.

A photo diode detects transmitted light in the pulse oximeter. A single photo diode senses both red and near-infrared light. The microprocessor that controls the oximeter cycles the LEDs on and off separately 400 to 500 times per second. The oximeter also turns both LEDs off during each cycle. This allows the photo diode to detect ambient light caused by scattering and to offset the LED signals.

Pulse oximeter accuracy tends to decrease at low saturations. Low saturations occur as the concentration of RHb increases. RHb has a much higher absorbance at 660 nm than does O_2Hb. Therefore, slight variations in the center wavelength of the red LED (as described) exaggerate the error in measured saturation. This is one reason that pulse oximeters exhibit decreasing accuracy at lower saturations.

Pulse oximeters measure the saturation of available hemoglobin at two wavelengths. The presence of COHb causes absorption at wavelengths similar to O_2Hb, and the pulse oximeter tends to read higher than the true saturation. MetHb causes increased absorption at both red and infrared wavelengths. This causes the ratio of the absorptions to be close to unity, and the pulse oximeter tends to read 85%.

Because the AC, or pulsatile component, is usually much smaller than the DC component, detecting it can sometimes cause problems. Low perfusion or poor vascularity can cause the oximeter to be unable to measure the pulsatile component. Most oximeters display a warning message if the photo detector senses inadequate light levels. Motion artifact can also cause inaccuracy with pulse oximeters. Movement, especially shivering, often occurs in the same frequency range as the signal to be detected (i.e., arterial pulsations). If the motion is consistent and lasts long enough, it introduces a signal of approximately the same amplitude into both red and infrared channels. The pulse oximeter senses motion artifact as part of the DC component. This adds a large value to both the numerator and denominator of the ratio (R). The motion signal forces R toward a value of 1, which is equal to a saturation of 85% on the typical oximeter calibration curve. Some oximeters use multiple digital filters to discriminate motion artifact and produce a more reliable signal.

Most pulse oximeters use the AC signal from one channel (660 nm or 940 nm) to calculate pulse rate. An algorithm implemented by the microprocessor locates peaks in the waveform of the AC signal and counts them (Figure 10-31). Some oximeters use this signal to display graphic representations of pulse waveforms. Pulse detection may be enhanced by the addition of a single electrocardiograph (ECG) lead. The additional input may allow the microprocessor to distinguish motion artifact or noise from the true signal.

REFLECTIVE SPECTROPHOTOMETERS

Reflective spectrophotometry is based on the variable reflection of light by O₂Hb and RHb at different wavelengths. Just as the light absorbed by O₂Hb and RHb is a function of wavelength, so is the intensity of reflected or back-scattered light. Carefully spaced optical fibers can be used as transmitting and receiving paths for light. Reflective spectrophotometry can be used to monitor arterial saturation in a manner similar to that of pulse oximetry. It can also be incorporated into a pulmonary artery catheter to measure mixed venous oxygen saturation ($S\bar{v}O_2$).

A reflective sensor can be placed at a site where a thin layer of tissue covers bone, such as the forehead. The oximeter then measures O_2Hb in a manner similar to that used for pulse oximetry, but using reflected rather than absorbed light. Pulse oximeters are available that can utilize either the regular sensor (i.e., pulse) or a reflective sensor.

A specially designed pulmonary artery (Swan-Ganz) catheter contains fiberoptic bundles (Figure 10-32). This catheter has regular pressure-sensing ports, a balloon tip for flotation through the right side of the heart, and a thermistor for thermodilution cardiac output determinations. Three LEDs, similar to those used in pulse oximeters, illuminate blood flowing past the tip of the catheter via one of the optical fibers. A photodetector senses the reflected light and converts its intensity into a signal. A microprocessor calculates two independent ratios of reflected light intensities from the three wavelengths. Combining two reflected light intensity ratios reduces the instrument's sensitivity to pulsatile blood flow or changing hematocrit. This design also minimizes changes caused by light scattering from red cell surfaces and the walls of the blood vessel. $S\bar{v}O_2$ is calculated from the light ratios using programmed calibration curves, similar to those used for a pulse oximeter. As in a pulse oximeter, saturation measured is the saturation of functional Hb (see Chapter 6). $S\bar{v}O_2$ determination by this method will be higher than that measured by a co-oximeter, especially if large amounts of COHb or MetHb are present. $S\bar{v}O_2$ is then displayed and may be printed using a trend recorder (Figure 10-33).

The reflective spectrophotometer must be routinely calibrated to ensure that observed changes in $S\bar{v}O_2$ are the result of physiologic phenomena rather than instrument drift. The catheter is usually standardized by calibrating it against an absolute color reference before insertion. After the catheter is in place, calibration is accomplished by adjusting the output to match saturation measured by a co-oximeter. This type of calibration is accurate at the time

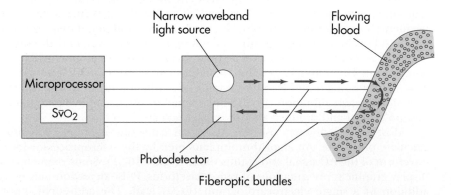

Figure 10-32 *Principle of reflective spectrophotometry.* A diagrammatic representation of the components of the optical pulmonary artery catheter. This type of catheter (Swan-Ganz) is used for continuous monitoring of $S\bar{v}O_2$. LEDs provide a narrow waveband light source. Light is transmitted along one fiberoptic filament to blood flowing past the tip of the catheter. Light reflected from the blood is transmitted back to a photodiode by the second fiberoptic bundle. The light intensity signals are then evaluated by a microprocessor to calculate light intensity ratios. These ratios (usually two ratios are determined from three wavelengths) determine the $S\bar{v}O_2$. The principle of reflective absorption can also be used for pulse oximetry.

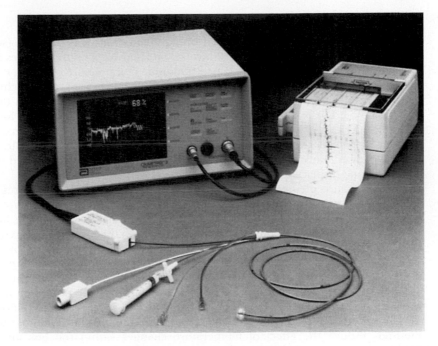

Figure 10-33 *Reflective spectrophotometer and pulmonary artery catheter.* A microprocessor-controlled reflective spectrophotometer. The pulmonary artery catheter contains fiberoptic bundles for continuous measurement of $S\bar{v}O_2$, as well as the usual pressure-measuring ports and thermistors for thermodilution cardiac output. The instrument displays mixed venous saturation digitally and as a trend graph that can be printed. High and low saturation alarms are included along with a "light intensity" alarm to detect artifact caused by catheter motion or problems with the fiberoptics. (*Courtesy Abbott Critical Care Systems, Mountain View, Calif.*)

it is performed, but may change if there are shifts in pH or hematocrit. Because reflective spectrophotometers measure reflected light in whole blood that is flowing rather than transmitted light in a hemolyzed blood sample, their absolute accuracy is less than that of a co-oximeter.

Body Plethysmographs

Whole-body plethysmographs are used in many pulmonary function laboratories. Two types of body plethysmographs are commonly used: the constant-volume, variable-pressure plethysmograph and the flow or variable-volume plethysmograph. These are sometimes called the pressure and flow plethysmographs, respectively. Whole-body plethysmographs are also called body boxes. Both designs are used to measure thoracic gas volume (V_{TG}) (see Chapter 3) and airway resistance (Raw) and its derivatives (see Chapters 2 and 3). Both types of box use a pneumotachometer to measure flow and a mouth pressure transducer with a shutter to measure alveolar pressure. They differ in the method used to measure volume change in the box, and hence in the lungs.

PRESSURE PLETHYSMOGRAPHS

The pressure plethysmograph is based on an adaptation of Boyle's law (see Appendix E). Volume changes in a sealed box are inversely related to pressure changes if temperature is constant. A sensitive pressure transducer monitors box pressure changes. Pressure change is related to volume change by calibration (see Chapter 11 for calibration techniques). Pressure changes result from compression and decompression of gas within both the patient's chest and the box. If box temperature remains constant, each unit of pressure change equals a specific volume change. For example, a volume change of 15 ml may result in a pressure change of 1 cm H_2O. After the box has been calibrated empty, the calibration factor changes slightly when a patient enters the plethysmograph. This change is easily corrected using an estimate of the volume displaced by the patient.

The pressure plethysmograph must be essentially leak-free. Most pressure boxes use a solenoid to vent the box and maintain thermal equilibrium. In some implementations, the vent remains open until the pressure measurement begins, so that the box is continually being vented. Making V_{TG} and Raw measurements with the patient panting reduces unwanted pressure changes caused by thermal drift, leaks, or background noise. Some pressure plethysmograph systems use a "slow" leak to facilitate thermal equilibrium. This type of leak may be created by connecting a long length of small-bore tubing to the box. The leak allows gas to escape as the interior of the box warms, but does not interfere with high frequency changes such as those that occur with panting. Similarly, connecting the atmospheric side of the box pressure transducer to a container within the box dampens the effects of thermal drift. Both methods reduce the effect of temperature changes within the box and maintain good frequency response. Pressure plethysmographs are best suited to maneuvers that measure small volume changes (i.e., 100 ml or less). Measurements of VC or FVC can usually be made only with the door open or the box adequately vented to the atmosphere.

FLOW PLETHYSMOGRAPHS

The flow plethysmograph uses a flow transducer in the box wall to measure volume changes in the box. Gas in the box is compressed or decompressed, causing flow through the opening in the box wall. Flow through the wall is integrated, corrections are applied, and volume change is recorded as the sum of the volume passing through the wall and the volume compressed. In one implementation, the patient breathes through a pneumotachometer connected to the room (transmural breathing). The transmural pneumotachometer allows larger gas volumes (i.e., the VC or flow-volume curves) to be measured while the patient is enclosed in the plethysmograph. The transmural flow is redirected to the plethysmograph for Raw measurements so that the ratio of flow to box volume can be plotted. For V_{TG} measurements, the flow transducer in the plethysmograph wall is blocked so that the device works like a pressure box. The flow-type plethysmograph requires computerization so that the pressure, volume, and flow signals can be measured in phase. Although thermal changes must be accounted for, the flow plethysmograph does not need to be rigorously airtight. The flow box's primary advantage is the ability to measure flows at absolute lung volumes (i.e., corrected for gas compression).

In both types of plethysmograph, a pneumotachometer is needed to measure airflow at the mouth (Figure 10-34). Flow measurement is required to compute Raw. The integrated flow signal (i.e., volume) is also used to determine end-expiration for shutter closure in V_{TG} measurements. The pneumotachometer must be linear across the range of flows encountered in spontaneous breathing and panting (–2 to +2 L/sec). Heated Fleisch or Silverman types of pressure-differential pneumotachometers are usually implemented in the plethysmograph. Pitot tube or heated-wire flow transducers can also be used.

A mouth pressure transducer is normally coupled to a shutter mechanism. The shutter can be an electrical solenoid, a scissors-type valve, or a balloon valve. The transducer records mouth pressures in the range of –20 to +20 cm H_2O when the airway is occluded. Some systems require the technologist to close the shutter by remote control at end-expiration. This may be accomplished by observing the tidal breathing maneuver on a display and actuating the shutter at end-expiration. Computerized systems automatically close the shutter at a preselected point in the breathing cycle. The technologist initiates a sequence in which the computer monitors flow and closes the shutter when expiratory flow becomes zero. Automated shutters allow the airway to be occluded for a fixed length of time or for a specified number of panting breaths.

Recording of plethysmographic maneuvers is usually performed by a computer. Breathing efforts are displayed in real time, allowing the technologist to elicit proper maneuvers from the patient. The real-time display assists in ensuring that panting maneuvers are performed correctly; some systems display prompts or flags so that the patient can be coached to pant at the correct frequency. The computer then stores the data and performs the necessary calculations to compute thoracic gas volume and airway resistance. Because the computer can track volume changes in the body box, V_{TG} and airway resistance are often measured from the same maneuver. The patient breathes normally to establish the end-expiratory level, then pants. When an appropriate pattern of panting is obtained (i.e., correct frequency and volume), the shutter closes and the thoracic gas volume is measured. The volume change between the established end-expiratory level and the point at which the shutter was closed is then used to "correct" the measured V_{TG} so that it equals the patient's FRC.

Computerized plethysmographs draw a "best-fit" line to determine the slope (i.e., tangent) of the open-shutter and closed-shutter panting maneuvers. The technologist can

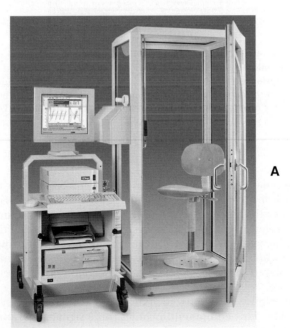

A

Figure 10–34 *Body plethysmograph.* **A,** Modern plethysmograph setup, with a highly transparent box, self-contained calibration equipment, and computerized data reduction and display. (*Courtesy SensorMedics Corp., Yorba Linda, Calif.*)   *Figure continued on next page.*

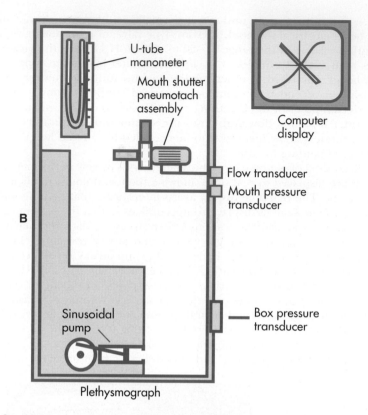

Figure 10–34—Cont'd B, Diagram of plethysmograph components. A pneumotachometer with an automatic shutter mechanism is mounted at a height that is comfortable for a patient sitting in the plethysmograph. Pressure transducers for flow, mouth pressure, and box pressure provide signals that are digitized and processed by a computer. A sinusoidal pump allows calibration of the box pressure signal; a small, known volume change can be repeatedly generated. A pressure manometer (U-tube) or similar device is used to calibrate the mouth pressure transducer. A 3-L syringe is used to calibrate the pneumotachometer.

also manipulate the tangent via the computer keyboard or mouse. This allows some degree of correction for efforts in which the patient panted incorrectly. Computerized plethysmographs offer the advantage of providing lung volume and airway resistance data immediately after completion of the maneuver. This aids in selecting appropriate maneuvers to report. The test can also be repeated as required when questionable values are obtained. Computerization also allows panting frequency to be calculated and displayed. Using computer-displayed panting frequency, the technologist can coach the patient to maintain a desired rate.

Most plethysmographs include the hardware to perform physical calibration (see Chapter 11). This equipment includes three signal-generating devices. A pressure manometer or U-tube may be mounted on the box for calibration of the mouth pressure transducer. A volume-displacement device such as a 30-ml to 50-ml syringe driven by an electric motor allows box pressure calibration. The motorized pump usually produces a sine-wave flow with frequency that can be varied. This allows checking of box calibration at various frequencies.

A flow generator and rotameter (i.e., a flow meter) may be included for pneumotachometer calibration. However, most computerized plethysmographs simply use a standard 3-L syringe to calibrate the pneumotachometer or flow sensor. Computerized plethysmograph systems provide automated calibration of transducers. The output of the transducer (i.e., its amplified signal) is measured, and the computer generates a software correction factor. This correction is then applied to every measurement made with the transducer. A few manufacturers also supply QC devices such as an isothermal lung analog (see Chapter 11). These devices provide QC to verify calibration of transducers and appropriateness of software correction factors.

Most patients can perform plethysmographic measurements acceptably, even if they experience claustrophobia. Modern body plethysmographs use Plexiglas or similar transparent material so that the subject does not feel confined. Plethysmographic measurements can be made quickly, reducing the length of time spent with the door closed. Plethysmography may not be possible for some patients who have orthopedic impairments, or for those who are receiving IV infusions by pump.

The ease with which a patient can enter the plethysmograph and perform the required maneuvers is an important feature. Some patients may experience claustrophobia when inside the plethysmograph. Older boxes used a plywood cabinet to provide the necessary rigidity so that pressure changes were not attenuated. Boxes made of durable plastics are largely transparent and less confining for the patient (Figure 10-34) while maintaining the necessary rigidity. Most plethysmographs contain 500 to 700 L of volume and can accommodate even large patients. Careful design allows the patient to easily enter the box. Some plethysmographs are large enough to accommodate patients in wheelchairs. Others use a clamshell design so that the patient may be seated and the box closed around him or her. Most plethysmographs provide an internal switch or mechanism that allows the patient to open the box from inside if they become uncomfortable.

Equally important is a communication system that allows both voice and visual contact with the patient. Panting against a closed shutter may be difficult for some individuals, and continuous coaching is often necessary to elicit valid maneuvers. An intercom system that provides continuous two-way communication is essential.

Computerized Pulmonary Function Systems

All modern pulmonary function equipment uses computers in one form or another. Most systems use either a dedicated microprocessor (Figure 10-35) or a PC (Figure 10-36). Computerized pulmonary function systems allow very sophisticated data handling and storage, graphic display of maneuvers, accurate calculations, and enhanced reporting capabilities. Some laboratories use minicomputers or mainframe computers interfaced to spirometers and gas analyzers, or networked with PC-based systems. Both dedicated microprocessor systems and PC-based systems use similar components.

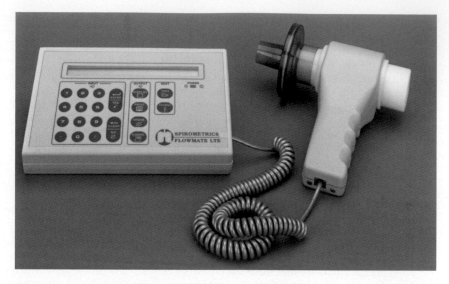

Figure 10–35 *Spirometer with dedicated microprocessor.* Many modern spirometers use a dedicated microprocessor. This system uses a pressure differential pneumotachometer interfaced with the microprocessor. The computer executes instructions stored in read-only memory (ROM). A simple keypad provides user access to various functions. Stored data may be downloaded to another computer or to a printer. The entire unit is small enough to be easily transported to the bedside. (*Courtesy Spirometrics, Gray, Me.*)

DATA ACQUISITION AND INSTRUMENT CONTROL

Computerized pulmonary function systems process analog signals from spirometers, pneu-motachometers, and gas analyzers. Equally important is the computer's capacity to control instrument functions, such as switching valves or recording signals. Computer control allows the technologist to manage complex test maneuvers. Data acquisition and instrument control are implemented with an interface (Figure 10-37) between the computer and pulmonary function equipment. Similar principles are applied in large laboratory systems and in small handheld spirometers.

An important component of the pulmonary equipment interface is the A/D converter. An A/D converter accepts an analog signal (such as pressure or flow) and transforms it into a digital value. The analog signal is usually a DC voltage in the range of either 0 to 10 V, or –5 to +5 V. A/D converters are classified by the number of bits (binary digits) into which they convert the signal. The higher the number of bits, the greater the resolution of the input signal in the resulting digital value. A 12-bit converter can transform a voltage into a number represented by 000000000000 to 111111111111 as a binary number. In the decimal notation, this corresponds to a range of 0 to 4096, or 2^{12}. For example, a 10-L spirometer may produce an analog signal ranging from 0 V to 10 V (i.e., 1 V = 1 L). If the spirometer is connected to a 12-bit converter, the signal can be divided into 4096 parts. This provides a resolution of approximately 0.0024 V or 2.4 ml over the 10-L volume range. The smallest volume change that can be detected by the computer is 2.4 ml for this spirometer system. For most volume and flow sampling applications, 12-bit converters are adequate. For greater resolution, a 16-bit A/D converter may be used. Sometimes 8-bit and 10-bit converters are used for

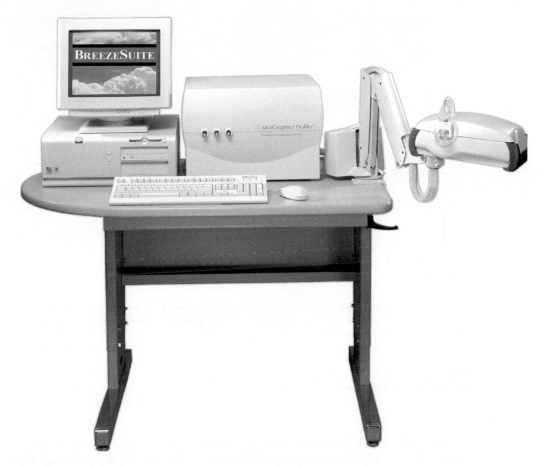

Figure 10-36 *Computerized pulmonary function system.* Modern laboratory systems utilize PCs interfaced to spirometers, gas analyzers, body plethysmographs, and associated breathing circuitry. This automated system includes a Pitot tube flow sensor, gas analyzers, and a computer-controlled breathing circuit. The PC allows rapid and accurate processing of data, including calculation of test variables, calibration, BTPS and STPD corrections, and graph display. Data can be stored locally on a high-capacity hard disk or on a networked server. The computer's capacity to store large volumes of data allows trending and recall of individuals or groups of patients. (*Courtesy Medical Graphics, Inc., St. Paul, Minn.*)

functions that do not require high resolution. Some modern systems use transducers (i.e., pressure or flow) that directly produce a digital output. These transducers do not require an A/D converter, simplifying the measurement.

The rate at which data are sampled also affects accuracy. Most A/D converter systems use 8 to 16 distinct channels. Each channel is capable of accepting a separate analog input. For tests such as an FVC maneuver, conversions may be performed on just one channel. High-speed converters can perform more than 20,000 conversions per second on a single channel. As more channels are included in the conversion, the rate for each channel is reduced.

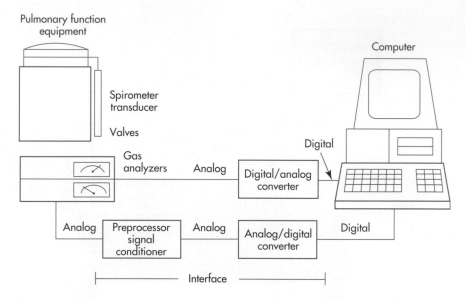

Figure 10-37 *Computer interface for pulmonary function equipment.* Components of a typical interface between a spirometer, gas analyzers, and a PC are shown. Analog signals from the pulmonary function equipment are preprocessed and then passed to an A/D converter. The A/D converter transforms a voltage (usually DC) into digital form. Digital data are then processed by the computer for calculations, display, and storage. Some systems use digital transducers that combine all of these functions and can communicate directly with the PC. For the computer to control various instrument functions, a D/A converter transforms digital data into appropriate analog signals to control system functions, such as opening valves in the breathing circuit.

Most computerized pulmonary function systems sample data 100 times/sec (i.e., 100 Hz) or greater. These high rates exceed the frequency bandwidth of breathing maneuvers by a factor of more than two. Accuracy is attained by matching analog output of a device (e.g., a spirometer) to an A/D converter with appropriate sampling rate and voltage resolution.

Another means of sampling volume or flow signals is measuring the time required for a known change in volume or flow. For example, the number of clock ticks that occur for a volume change of 100 ml can be counted and flow calculated. This technique requires a spirometer that uses a position encoder or that generates pulses for each volume increment. The accuracy of encoder-pulse systems depends on clock resolution and volume increment, especially when measuring high flows.

Most devices (e.g., pulse oximeters or capnographs) use a dedicated microprocessor and A/D board to process data. These instruments often include a communication port so that data can be sent to a PC or to a printer. Most computers have serial ports that can be used to interface various instruments. Serial data ports are often used when a small amount of data is transmitted or timing is not critical. For large volumes of data, USB or Ethernet-type communications are commonly employed. Parallel ports are typically used for interconnection with printers.

Another function of the interface is to allow the computer to "control" the test equipment (e.g., spirometer, valves). A D/A converter provides this ability. The D/A converter acts as a relay switch between the computer and an instrument. A digital signal from the computer can be used to control functions such as recording volumes and flows, or opening valves to deliver O_2 or other test gases.

PULMONARY FUNCTION DATA STORAGE AND PROGRAMS

Computerized pulmonary function systems, even small portable spirometers, generate large volumes of patient data. Managing these large amounts of data is relatively easy via computer networks.

Most PC-based systems are capable of *multitasking*, or simultaneously running multiple programs. Multitasking permits the user to perform one task in the foreground while the computer performs other tasks in the background. For example, a multitasking testing system allows spirometry to be performed on one patient while the report from another patient is being printed. Multitasking also allows several programs to operate simultaneously. This allows the user to transfer data between programs easily.

Almost all PC-based systems support networking to some extent. Networked computers allow multiple users to share data, as well as peripheral devices such as printers. The network typically consists of a primary computer or server. Other microcomputers are then linked by one of several types of networks. Data can be transferred between any two computers linked by the system. The server usually maintains programs and data that all of the networked users need.

The combination of multitasking and multiuser capabilities offers numerous possibilities to enhance laboratory data management. Some multitasking systems permit the user to perform diagnostic testing in real time while the computer prints reports or transmits data to another system in the background. A network allows pulmonary function testing to be performed at one terminal while blood gas data are entered at a second terminal, physicians review test results at a third station, and clerical staff print final reports at a fourth station.

The format in which test data are stored is determined by (1) complexity of the data, (2) number of tests done per month or year, and (3) how data will be accessed. Three methods for data management are used with computerized pulmonary function systems:

Temporary Storage or No Data Storage

Some portable spirometers provide only temporary storage of patient data. In these systems, a microprocessor performs calculations and then displays or prints the results, but patient data are not stored. Some microprocessor-based spirometers store tests in RAM (random access memory) for viewing and printing. These instruments permit tests from multiple patients to be stored; data can be recalled whenever the system is operating. Data can usually be transferred to a host computer or to a printer. Some monitoring devices (e.g., pulse oximeters) also provide limited data storage with interfaces for host computers or printers.

Permanent Individual Patient Data Files

Patient data records are stored by creating individual files, usually on the PC's hard disk. The volume of data stored in files of this type is limited only by the computer's operating system and the physical capacity of the storage device. A commonly used format stores patient information and test results in one file, with graphic data (e.g., flow-volume curves) in a separate file. Graphic data often require more disk space than tabular data, depending on the format in which they are stored. Modern systems support large hard drives, so a large volume of test data can be stored on a desktop or laptop PC. Because so much data can be stored on a single physical device, an appropriate backup mechanism is required.

Database Storage

Many pulmonary function systems use a relational database format. Tests from different patients are stored as individual records in a file. Files (sometimes called *tables*) are then "linked" to form a database. One file may contain all spirometry records, a second file all lung volume records, a third file DL_{CO} measurements, and so on. Complete tests are linked across files by an index using patient number or test date. A database structure allows sorting, selecting, searching, and editing of patient data. Some applications of a database system for pulmonary function data include the following:

- Serial comparisons of multiple tests on a single patient may be extracted to plot a trend.
- Data from longitudinal studies on groups of patients may be extracted for statistical analysis or export to an external program.
- Queries may be performed to extract data that match selected criteria.
- An unlimited number of report formats may be generated.
- Reference equations may be stored in a database format. This structure allows input of user-defined equations for predicting normal values.

Relational database systems support a special command language called Structured Query Language (SQL). SQL databases provide a standardized means for the user to enter and retrieve data, generate reports, and perform functions such as importing or exporting records. SQL databases can be easily restructured, so that additional information can be added to existing databases.

Pulmonary function software often includes interpretation programs. Interpretation programs use algorithms for identifying obstructive, restrictive, combined, or normal patterns of pulmonary function. The algorithms can evaluate spirometry, lung volumes, and DL_{CO}, comparing measured and reference values. Although algorithms use logic similar to that of a clinician, they are usually not able to consider the patient's clinical history or other laboratory findings. Some programs are very sophisticated and can diagnose obstruction or restriction reasonably well. An incorrect computer interpretation may occur if test data are invalid because of poor patient effort or technical problems. However, computerized spirometers routinely include software that assesses the acceptability and reproducibility of efforts. If the computerized interpretation considers data quality, an accurate interpretation is possible. Even if computerized interpretation is not implemented, computer-generated statements regarding test quality can be very useful for traditional interpretation. Computer interpretation in no way substitutes for evaluation by a qualified clinician. It may be helpful when an immediate report of abnormalities is necessary, such as for screening purposes. Computer interpretation can also be used in an educational setting If a computer interpretation is included in the final report, it should be clearly labeled as such.

Blood gas interpretation by computer uses algorithms to evaluate acid-base and oxygenation status. Computerized blood gas interpretation may be useful when rapid interpretation to exclude abnormal findings is required. Because a computer can routinely evaluate all measured and calculated blood gas variables, it may suggest abnormalities that a casual interpreter may overlook. Computer-assisted blood gas interpretations should be considered preliminary until verified by a qualified interpreter.

A related area in which computer-assisted interpretation may be useful is QC of blood gas analyzers. Evaluation of controls requires statistical calculations involving large volumes of data (see Chapter 11). Most QC programs compute means and standard deviations (see Appendix G) for multiple levels of pH, Pco_2, Po_2, and Hb. Controls may be run daily or more often on multiple instruments. Computerized management of data and statistics can simplify record keeping in a busy laboratory. An added advantage is that a computer can interpret QC data in real time. This allows the technologist to quickly determine the status of individual blood gas electrodes (see Chapter 11).

Summary

This chapter examines various devices commonly found in the pulmonary function laboratory, as well as in other clinical settings. These include spirometers that use either volume-displacement or flow-sensing principles. Spirometers are used in many different pulmonary function tests. Small computerized spirometers are available for testing in many areas outside of the traditional pulmonary function laboratory. Peak flow meters are also common. Small portable peak flow devices have been developed and are widely used in clinical and home settings. Body plethysmographs are also more widely used than in the past; their design and methodology have benefited from advances in electronics and computerization.

Different types of pulmonary gas analyzers are also described. Their principles of operation are discussed along with how they are used for pulmonary function testing. Breathing valves and related devices are also discussed, with particular attention to selection and maintenance. Blood gas electrodes, oximeters, and related monitors are described. Advantages and disadvantages of various methods of blood gas monitoring are also considered.

Computers, especially PC-based systems and dedicated microprocessors, have become a primary component of almost every type of pulmonary function system. Monitoring devices such as pulse oximeters rely almost completely on computerization. This chapter presents information on the components of computer systems, data acquisition and storage, and specific interfaces to pulmonary function equipment.

■ SELF-ASSESSMENT QUESTIONS

Entry-level

1. *Which of the following statements describe a Stead-Wells type of spirometer?*

    I. It can be used to measure He dilution lung volumes.
    II. It uses the wedge bellows design.
    III. Water-sealed and waterless versions are available.
    IV. Leaks do not affect spirometric measurements.

    a. I and III
    b. II and IV
    c. I, II, and III
    d. II, III, and IV

2. *A 3-L syringe is used to calibrate a dry rolling-seal spirometer, and the following results are obtained:*

    Calibration 1:   3.30 L
    Calibration 2:   3.32 L
    Calibration 3:   3.34 L

    Which of the following best explains these findings?

    a. The calibration syringe has a leak.
    b. The spirometer has a leak.
    c. Automatic BTPS correction is turned on.
    d. The calibration injections were performed too rapidly.

3. *Which of the following devices integrate flow to measure volume?*

    I. Turbine respirometer
    II. Wedge bellows spirometer
    III. Pressure differential pneumotachometer
    IV. Heated-wire sensor

    a. I and II
    b. III and IV
    c. I, III, and IV
    d. I, II, and III

4. *Fleisch and Silverman pneumotachometers both use a:*

    a. Hot-wire sensor
    b. Rotating vane with photodetector
    c. Pitot tube
    d. Resistive element

5. *Which of the following valves should be used for a maximal exercise test on a patient with an MVV of 90 L/min?*

   a. Large-bore one-way directional valve
   b. Small-bore two-way nonrebreathing valve
   c. Large bore two-way nonrebreathing valve
   d. Free breathing valve with low-resistance bacteria filter

6. *Which of the following gas analyzers is commonly used to measure carbon dioxide concentration during exercise testing?*

   a. Emission spectroscopy-type analyzer
   b. Polarographic electrode
   c. Fuel cell analyzer
   d. Infrared analyzer

7. *Which of the following are components of a gas chromatograph?*

   I. Column separator
   II. Chopper motor
   III. Thermal conductivity detector
   IV. Carrier gas

   a. I and IV
   b. II and III
   c. II, III, and IV
   d. I, III, and IV

8. *A gas analyzer circuit uses a dessicant column to remove water vapor from exhaled gases; if the dessicant column contains blue granules, the most appropriate action would be to:*

   a. Proceed with testing
   b. Replace the dessicant because it is exhausted
   c. Replace the granules with barium hydroxide
   d. Replace the granules with fresh sodium hydroxide

Advanced

9. *Which of the following problems commonly affect Po_2 electrode performance in a blood gas analyzer?*

   a. Depletion of the bicarbonate buffer
   b. Metal ions plating the platinum cathode
   c. Reference electrode malfunction
   d. Contamination of the KCl buffer

10. *A blood gas analyzer reports "excessive drift" for the Pco_2 electrode following automatic calibration. One hour earlier, the same analyzer had an acceptable calibration and controls were within established limits. Ten specimens were analyzed during the hour between the two calibrations. The most appropriate first step would be to:*

    a. Replace the electrode
    b. Clean with a proteolytic agent (bleach) and recalibrate
    c. Replace the reference electrode
    d. Refill the electrode with phosphate-potassium buffer

11. *A patient in the emergency department has his O_2 saturation measured by pulse oximetry, and an Spo_2 of 85% is recorded. Blood gases are drawn immediately, and the Sao_2 (by co-oximetry) is reported as 98%. A possible explanation of these findings is that the patient:*

    a. Had an elevated level of COHb
    b. Was shivering
    c. Was hyperventilating
    d. Had severe anemia

12. *Which of the following are measured by a spectrophotometric oximeter (co-oximeter)?*

    I. O_2Hb
    II. COHb
    III. MetHb
    IV. Pao_2

    a. I and IV
    b. II and III
    c. I, II, and IV
    d. I, II, and III

13. *The box pressure transducer in a variable pressure plethysmograph is calibrated using a(n):*

    a. U-tube manometer
    b. 50-ml sinusoidal pump
    c. 3-L syringe
    d. Isothermal lung analog

14. *When selecting a body plethysmograph, which of the following are important factors?*

    I. "Hands-off" intercom system
    II. Internal volume less than 299 L

III. Patient access to plethysmograph

IV. Internal door control

a. I and II

b. III and IV

c. II and III

d. I, III, and IV

15. *A pulmonary function lab is planning to participate in a research protocol that will track*

multiple tests on a large number of patients over 2 years. Which of the following methods would be the most practical?

a. Spirometers with a large amount of RAM

b. Printed data files

c. Individual patient files stored on disk

d. SQL database

SELECTED BIBLIOGRAPHY

Spirometers

American Thoracic Society: Standardization of spirometry—1994 update, *Am J Respir Crit Care* 152:1107-1136, 1995.

Banks DE, Wang ML, McCabe L, et al: Improvement in lung function measurements using a flow spirometer that emphasizes computer assessment of test quality, *J Occup Environ Med* 38:270-283, 1996.

Ferguson GT, Enright PL, Buist AS, et al: Office spirometry for lung health assessment in adults: a consensus statement from the National Lung Health Education Program, *Chest* 117:1146-1161, 2000.

Gardner RM, Hankinson JL, West BJ: Evaluating commercially available spirometers, *Am Rev Respir Dis* 121:73-78, 1980.

Hankinson JL: Pulmonary function testing in the screening of workers: guidelines for instrumentation, performance, and interpretation, *J Occup Med* 28:1081-1092, 1986.

Hankinson JL: Instrumentation for spirometry. In Eisen JE, ed: *Occupational medicine: state of the art reviews*, Philadelphia, 1993, Hanley and Belfus.

Johns DP, Ingram C, Booth H, et al: Effect of a microaerosol barrier filter on the measurement of lung function, *Chest* 107:1045-1048, 1995.

Porszaz J, Barstow TJ, Wasserman K: Evaluation of a symmetrically disposed Pitot-tube flowmeter for measuring gas flow during exercise, *J Appl Physiol* 77:2651-2665, 1994.

Pulmonary Function Standards for Cotton Dust, 29 Code of Federal Regulations; 1910.1043 Cotton Dust, Appendix D, Occupational Safety and Health Administration, 1980.

Ruppel GL: Spirometry, *Respir Care Clin North Am* 3:155-181, 1997.

Sullivan WJ, Peters GM, Enright PL: Pneumotachographs: theory and clinical applications, *Respir Care* 29:736, 1984.

Townsend MC: ACOEM position statement: spirometry in the occupational setting. American College of Occupational and Environmental Medicine, *J Occup Environ Med* 42:228-245, 2000.

Peak Flow Meters

Folgering H, vander Brink W, van Heeswijk O, et al: Eleven peak flow meters: a clinical evaluation, *Eur Respir J* 11:188-193, 1998.

Irvin CG, Martin RJ, Chinchilli VM, et al: Quality control of peak flow meters for multicenter clinical trials. The Asthma Clinical Research Network (ACRN), *Am J Respir Crit Care Med* 156:396-402, 1997.

Jackson AC: Accuracy, reproducibility, and variability of portable peak-flow meters, *Chest* 107:648-651, 1995.

Jensen RL, Crapo RO, Berlin SL: Effect of altitude on hand-held peak flowmeters, *Chest* 109:475-479, 1996.

Koyama H, Nishimura K, Ikeda A, et al: Comparison of four types of portable peak flow meters (Mini-Wright, Assess, Pulmo-graph and Wright Pocket meters), *Respir Med* 92:505-511, 1998.

Gas Analyzers

Erdmann K, Jantzen JP, Etz C, et al: Evaluation of two oxygen analyzers by computerized data acquisition and processing, *J Clin Monit* 2:105-113, 1986.

Macfarlane DJ: Automated metabolic gas analysis systems: a review, *Sports Med* 31:841-861, 2001.

Norton AC: Accuracy in pulmonary measurements, *Respir Care* 24:131, 1979.

Rebuck AS, Chapman KR: Measurement and monitoring of exhaled carbon dioxide. In Nochomovitz ML, Cherniack NS, eds: *Non-invasive respiratory monitoring*, New York, 1986, Churchill Livingstone.

Blood Gas Electrodes, Oximeters, and Related Devices

Barker SJ, Shah NK: The effects of motion on the performance of pulse oximeters in volunteers (revised publication), *Anesthesiology* 86:101-108, 1997.

Barker SJ, Tremper KK: Pulse oximetry: applications and limitations. In Tremper KK, Barker SJ, eds: *International anesthesiology clinics,* Boston, 1987, Little, Brown.

Cariou A, Monchi M, Dhainaut JF: Continuous cardiac output and mixed venous oxygen saturation monitoring, *J Crit Care* 13:198-213, 1998.

Franklin ML: Transcutaneous measurement of partial pressure of oxygen and carbon dioxide, *Respir Care Clin North Am* 1:119-131, 1995.

Gehring H, Hornberger C, Matz H, et al: The effects of motion artifact and low perfusion on the performance of a new generation of pulse oximeters in volunteers undergoing hypoxia, *Respir Care* 47:48-60, 2002.

Kozlowski-Templin R: Blood gas analyzers, *Respir Care Clin North Am* 1:35-46, 1995.

Peruzzi WT, Shapiro BA, eds: Blood gas measurements, *Respir Care Clin North Am* 1:1-157, 1995.

Pologue JA: Pulse oximetry: technical aspects of machine design. In Tremper KK, Barker SJ, eds: *International anesthesiology clinics,* Boston, 1987, Little, Brown.

Severinghaus JW: The invention and development of blood gas analysis apparatus, *Anesthesiology* 97:253-256, 2002.

Severinghaus JW, Bradley AF: Electrodes for blood PO_2 and PCO_2 determination, *J Appl Physiol* 13:515, 1958.

Tremper KK, Waxman KS: Transcutaneous monitoring of respiratory gases. In Nochomovitz ML, Cherniack NS, eds: *Noninvasive respiratory monitoring,* New York, 1986, Churchill Livingstone.

Villanueva R, Bell C, Kain ZN, et al: Effect of peripheral perfusion on accuracy of pulse oximetry in children, *J Clin Anesth* 11:317-322, 1999.

Plethysmographs

American Association for Respiratory Care: Clinical practice guideline: body plethysmography, *Respir Care* 39:1184-1190, 1994.

Bargeton D, Barres G: Time characteristics and frequency response of body plethysmographs. International Symposium on Body Plethysmography, Nijmegen, *Prog Respir Res* 4:2, 1969.

DuBois AB, Bothello SY, Bedell GN, et al: A rapid plethysmographic method for measuring thoracic gas volume: a comparison with nitrogen-washout method for measuring functional residual capacity in normal subjects, *J Clin Invest* 35:322, 1956.

DuBois AB, Bothello SY, Comroe JH: A new method for measuring airway resistance in man using a body plethysmograph: values in normal subjects and in patients with respiratory disease, *J Clin Invest* 35:327, 1956.

Quanjer PH, Tammeling GJ, Cotes JE, et al: Lung volumes and forced ventilatory flows: report of the Working Party for Standardization of Lung Function Tests, European Community for Steel and Coal, *Eur Respir J* 16(suppl):5-40, 1993.

Computers

American Thoracic Society, Committee on Proficiency Standards for Clinical Pulmonary Laboratories: Computer guidelines for pulmonary laboratories, *Am Rev Respir Dis* 134:628, 1986.

Ellis JH, Perera SP, Levin DC: A computer program for the interpretation of pulmonary function studies, *Chest* 68:209, 1975.

Scanlan C, Ruppel GL: Computer applications in respiratory care. In Scanlan C, ed: *Egan's fundamentals of respiratory care,* St Louis, 1995, Mosby.

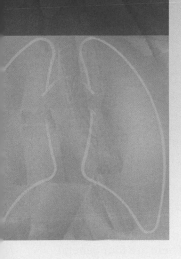

CHAPTER 11

QUALITY ASSURANCE IN THE PULMONARY FUNCTION LABORATORY

OBJECTIVES

After studying this chapter and reviewing its tables and figures, you should be able to do the following:

Entry-level

1. Describe acceptable calibration of a spirometer using a 3-L syringe
2. Determine whether a blood gas analyzer is "in control" using a control chart
3. Describe universal precautions to be applied during blood gas specimen collection and analysis
4. Suggest appropriate technologist comments to include with a pulmonary function report

Advanced

1. List at least three of the minimal requirements of an acceptable spirometer for diagnostic testing
2. Use results obtained from biologic control subjects to troubleshoot pulmonary function equipment
3. Describe how to check the linearity of a gas analyzer
4. Identify potential sources of cross-contamination in pulmonary function equipment

This final chapter discusses issues related to quality assurance. General concepts include equipment standards for spirometers and blood gas analyzers. Proper instrument maintenance and calibration are bases for obtaining acceptable and reproducible data. The chapter also deals with quality control (QC) for equipment used for pulmonary function testing and blood gas analysis. Problems commonly encountered with various types of equipment are listed to guide in troubleshooting.

Special attention is given to methods by which the pulmonary function technologist can assess data quality. Documentation of pulmonary function data

417

quality (i.e., acceptability and reproducibility) is discussed. Those who perform pulmonary function tests must make decisions during testing that often determine the quality of data obtained.

Safety and infection control are discussed as they relate to patients and to those performing pulmonary function tests. As in previous chapters, self-assessment questions are included.

Elements of Laboratory Quality Control

Quality control is one aspect of quality assurance. QC is essential in the operation of a pulmonary function laboratory to obtain valid and reproducible data. There are four general elements to consider in regard to a quality assurance program.

METHODOLOGY

The type of equipment used (e.g., volume- versus flow-based spirometer) often determines which procedures are required for calibration and QC. For example, both flow- and volume-based spirometers require calibration using a 3-L syringe, but only volumetric spirometers need to be checked for leaks. The number and complexity of the tests performed may also dictate which equipment and methods are used. Methods and equipment that have been validated in the scientific literature should be used whenever possible. QC is usually easier to perform when standardized techniques are used.

EQUIPMENT MAINTENANCE

The type and complexity of instrumentation for a specific test determine the long-term and short-term maintenance that will be required. Preventive maintenance is scheduled in anticipation of equipment malfunction to reduce the possibility of equipment failure. Corrective maintenance or repair is unscheduled service that is required to correct equipment failure. This failure is often signaled by QC procedures or extreme test results. Familiarity with the operating characteristics of spirometers, gas analyzers, plethysmographs, and computers requires manufacturer support and thorough documentation. A procedure manual (Table 11-1) and accurate records are essential to a comprehensive maintenance program. Documentation of procedures and repairs is required by most accrediting organizations.

CONTROL METHODS

A *control* is any known test signal for an instrument that can be used to determine its accuracy and precision. Controls or control materials must be available for spirometers, gas analyzers, blood gas analyzers, and other instruments. Because many laboratories use computerized pulmonary function or blood gas analyzers, controls are required to ensure that both software and hardware are functioning within acceptable limits. Control methods may vary from use of 3-L syringes for spirometers to tonometered blood for blood gas analyzers. *Biologic controls* are test subjects for whom specific variables have been determined.

TESTING TECHNIQUE

A primary means of ensuring data quality is to rigidly control the procedures by which data are obtained. For pulmonary function testing, this refers to the technologist's ability to conduct the procedure and to elicit subject cooperation in the test maneuvers. Technologist

TABLE 11–1 Pulmonary Function Procedure Manual

Items to be included in a typical procedure manual for a pulmonary function laboratory. For each procedure performed, the following should be present:

1. *Description* of the test and its purpose
2. *Indications* for ordering the test and contraindications, if any
3. Description of the *general method(s)* and any specific equipment required
4. *Calibration* of equipment required before testing (manufacturer's documentation may be referenced)
5. *Patient preparation* for the test, if any (e.g., withholding medication)
6. Step-by-step procedure for both computerized and manual *measurement/calculation* of results
7. *Quality control* guidelines with acceptable limits of performance and corrective actions to be taken
8. *Safety precautions* related to the procedure (e.g., infection control, hazards) and alert values that require physician notification
9. *References* for all equations used for calculating results and for predicted normals, including a bibliography
10. Documentation of *computer protocols* of calculations and data storage; guidelines for computer downtime
11. Dated *signatures* of medical and technical directors

and subject performance, as well as proper equipment function, must be evaluated on a test-by-test basis. This may be accomplished by using appropriate criteria to judge the acceptability of results.

Each pulmonary function laboratory should have a written quality assurance program that includes the following:

- Methods used for specific tests
- Limitations of each procedure (if any)
- Indications or schedules for maintenance
- QC materials or signals to be used
- Action to be taken if controls exceed specified limits
- Specific guidelines as to how tests are to be performed

The quality assurance program should be included as part of the laboratory procedure manual (Table 11-1).

Two concepts that are central to quality assurance are accuracy and precision. *Accuracy* may be defined as the extent to which measurement of a known quantity results in a value approximating that quantity. For most laboratory tests, repeated measurements of a control are made and a *mean,* or average, is calculated. If the *mean value* approximates the *known value* of the control, the instrument is considered accurate.

Precision may be defined as the extent to which repeated measurements of the same quantity can be reproduced. If a control is measured repeatedly and the results are similar, the instrument may be considered precise.

Accuracy and precision may not always be present together in the same instrument. For example, a spirometer that consistently measures a 3-L test volume as 2.5 L is precise, but not very accurate. A spirometer that evaluates a 3-L test volume as 2.5, 3.0, and 3.5 L on repeated maneuvers produces an accurate mean of 3.0 L, but the individual measurements are not precise. Determining both the accuracy and precision of instruments such as spirometers is important because many pulmonary function variables are effort-dependent. The largest observed value, rather than the mean, is often reported as the *best test* (see Chapter 2). Reporting the largest result observed is based on the rationale that the subject cannot overshoot on a test that is effort-dependent.

For instruments such as blood gas analyzers, accuracy is determined by measuring an unknown control and comparing the results with other analyzers or laboratories. This is commonly referred to as *proficiency testing*. Precision is determined by checking the day-to-day variability of controls and expressing the variability in terms of the standard deviation (see Appendix G).

Calibration and Quality Control of Pulmonary Function Equipment

Calibration is the process in which the signal from an instrument is adjusted to produce a known output. This may be accomplished by one of several methods:

1. Adjustment of the analog output signal from the primary transducer (i.e., spirometer bell, flow sensor, gas analyzer)
2. Adjustment of the sensitivity of the recording device
3. Software correction or compensation

Calibration involves adjustment of the instrument (or its signal). It should not be confused with verification or QC. QC assesses function of the instrument after it has been calibrated. Most pulmonary function systems use software calibration.

▆ SPIROMETERS

Spirometers that produce a voltage signal by means of a potentiometer (see Chapter 10) normally allow some form of "gain" adjustment so that the analog output can be matched to a known input of either volume or flow. For example, a 10-L volume-displacement spirometer may be equipped with a 10-V potentiometer. The potentiometer amplifier would be adjusted so that 0 V equals 0 L (zero), and 10 V equals 10 L (gain). The calibration could be verified by setting the spirometer at a specific volume and noting the analog signal (i.e., 5 L should equal 5 V).

A second technique is adjustment of the sensitivity of the recording device. This method is used for older spirometers equipped with kymographs, X-Y plotters, or strip chart recorders. In these devices, a known volume is injected into the spirometer and deflection of the recording device is adjusted to match the volume. For example, a strip chart recorder is turned on and has its pen adjusted to read 0 L when the spirometer is empty. A 3-L volume is then injected. The gain of the recorder is adjusted so that the tracing deflects to the 3-L mark on the graph paper. This method is appropriate when the recorded tracing is to be manually measured. This method is seldom used because most modern spirometers use computerized output (display or printer). The ability to evaluate a spirometer's accuracy using a mechanical recorder may be useful for checking a computerized system.

Most spirometer systems are computerized (see Chapter 10). In computerized systems, the signal produced by the spirometer is often corrected by applying a software calibration factor. A known volume or flow is injected into the spirometer using a large-volume (usually 3-L) syringe. A correction (i.e., calibration) factor is calculated based on the measured versus expected values:

$$\text{Correction factor} = \frac{\text{Expected volume}}{\text{Measured volume}}$$

The correction factor derived by this method is then stored, usually in memory and on the computer's hard disk. The correction is applied to all subsequent volume measurements. For example, if a syringe with a volume of 3.00 L were injected into a spirometer and a volume of 2.97 L recorded, the correction factor would be as follows:

$$1.010 = \frac{3.00\ L}{2.97\ L}$$

The correction factor 1.010 would then be used to adjust subsequent measured volumes. This method assumes that the spirometer's output is linear and that the same factor would be correct for any volume, large or small. Most automated spirometers allow the correction factor to be verified by reinjecting a known volume, usually 3 L. After calibration, the spirometer should display an accuracy of 3% or 50 ml, whichever is larger. Three percent of a standard 3-L syringe means that the spirometer should read 3.00 ± 0.09 L (range, 2.91 to 3.09 L).

Care should be taken that the gas in the syringe, which is at ambient temperature (ATPS) is not "temperature corrected" by the software. Many computerized spirometers provide software functions specifically for calibration and verification. This allows the use of a 3-L syringe without applying corrections that are necessary when patients are tested. Inappropriate temperature correction produces an erroneously high measured value and a low correction factor. Ambient temperature should be available from an accurate thermometer, both for calibration and for testing. If the ambient temperature changes significantly, the temperature used by the software should be updated, or recalibration may be needed. The calibration syringe should be maintained at the same environmental conditions as the spirometer.

(PF *Tips*)

Most spirometers provide a means of verifying the volume calibration. This step typically uses the 3-L calibration syringe. After calibration, additional injections and withdrawals of a known volume (usually 3 L, but other volumes may be used) can be used to verify that the spirometer produces a known output. The verification step should include a range of flows to demonstrate volume accuracy that is independent of flow.

Other factors that may influence establishment of the software correction value include the accuracy of the large-volume syringe and the speed with which injections are performed. An inaccurate syringe or leaks in the connection to the spirometer may produce erroneous software corrections. Accuracy of calibration syringes should be verified annually. Syringes can be checked for leaks simply by occluding the port and trying to empty the syringe. Some laboratories use two syringes: one to calibrate and another to verify volume accuracy.

Some spirometers, particularly those that are flow-based, may require that the calibration volume be injected within certain flow limits. Volume calibration at different flows can be accomplished by injecting 3 L at flows between 2 and 12 L/sec. Varying the flow at which 3 L is injected permits the software to generate correction factors to accommodate a range of flows. Similarly, volume-displacement spirometers may be calibrated (or verified) using a range of flows. Ideally, volume accuracy (i.e., 3% or 50 ml) should be maintained across the flow range of the spirometer. Flow-based spirometers that measure both inspiratory and expiratory volumes require the syringe volume to be injected and withdrawn. This allows separate correction factors for inspired and expired gas to be generated. Many flow-sensing spirometers also require a "zero" before measuring exhaled volume. This means that the flow sensor must be held motionless (so there is no flow through it) while the software adjusts the output of the sensor to equal zero. If an in-line bacteria filter will be used for testing, calibration should be performed with the device in place.

QC of spirometers is closely related to calibration, and the two are sometimes confused. An important distinction is that calibration (i.e., adjustment) may or may not be needed, but QC must be applied on a routine basis. Calibration, whether it includes the output of the spirometer, recorder sensitivity, or generation of a software correction factor, involves *adjusting* of the device to perform within certain limits. QC is a *test* performed to determine the accuracy and/or precision of the device using a known standard or signal. Various control methods (i.e., signal generators) are available for spirometers.

Simple Large-Volume Syringe

A syringe of at least 3-L volume (Figure 11-1) should be used to generate a control signal for checking spirometers. A 3-L syringe can be used to verify volume-displacement spirometers and associated deflection of mechanical recorders. A large-volume syringe may also be used to check the volume accuracy of flow-based spirometers. The 3-L syringe should be accurate to within 15 ml. Syringes with other volumes should be accurate to within 0.5%. Computerized systems often have the user inject (or withdraw) a 3-L volume to calibrate the spirometer, and then immediately perform additional injections to verify the calibration. Some portable flow-based spirometers do not provide for calibration, but do allow checking or verification of a stored calibration.

QC for spirometer volume measurements should be performed at least once each day that the device is to be used. For field studies, accuracy should be checked every 4 hours that the device is used. Frequent checks are recommended for industrial applications or

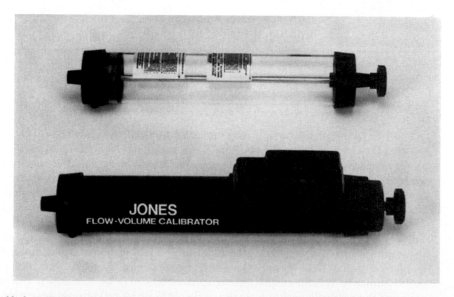

Figure 11-1 *Calibration syringes.* Standard 3-L syringe is used for volume calibration of volume-based and flow-based spirometers (*top*). The same syringe may be used for FRC and DL_{CO} quality control. A 3-L syringe is recommended for both calibration and quality control. Computerized FVC simulator uses a microprocessor to measure FEV_1 and other flows during injection of a 3-L volume (*bottom*). The volumes and flows delivered can be compared with those reported by the spirometer. (*Courtesy Jones Medical Instrument Co., Oakbrook, Ill.*)

epidemiologic research, especially if the spirometer is moved or used for a large number of tests.

Spirometer linearity should be verified at least quarterly. Volume-displacement spirometers should be checked in 1-L increments across their volume range. A 3-L syringe injection performed when the spirometer is nearly empty or nearly full should yield comparable results. The linearity of flow-sensing spirometers should be tested over a range of flows. Different flows can be generated by varying the speed at which the syringe is emptied. Applying different flows and measuring the resulting volumes may indicate if the spirometer (and its software) is accurate at low and high flows. For example, three different injection times, 0.5 to 1.0 seconds, 1.0 to 1.5 seconds, and 5.0 to 6.0 seconds, may be used with a 3-L syringe to simulate a wide range of flows.

Computerized syringes (Figure 11-1) are available for assessing the accuracy of commonly measured parameters such as forced expiratory volume (FEV_1) and $FEF_{27\%-75\%}$. These syringes use a built-in microprocessor to time the volume injection and calculate the flows. The microprocessor displays volume and flows for comparison with those produced by the spirometer. A computerized syringe provides a 3-L volume for calibration or volume checks, and tests accuracy for commonly reported flows.

QC for spirometers should be performed as if a patient were being tested. The 3-L syringe should be connected to the patient port, with the circuitry used for the actual test. Spirometer temperature correction may need to be set to 37° C (i.e., no correction applied). Most computerized spirometers provide a specific routine for volume checks or calibration that disables temperature corrections. In some systems, temperature correction cannot be disabled. In these spirometers, injection of 3 L at ATPS results in a reading greater than 3 L because the system attempts to "correct" the volume to body temperature (BTPS). For water-seal spirometers, the syringe should be filled and emptied several times to allow equilibration with the humidified air in the device. Some flow-sensing spirometers require a length of tubing between the flow sensor and syringe to reduce artifact caused by turbulent flow in the syringe. If an in-line bacteria filter is used, volume verification should be performed with it in place.

The accuracy of any spirometer can be calculated as follows:

$$\% \text{ Error} = \frac{\text{Expected volume} - \text{Measured volume}}{\text{Expected volume}} \times 100$$

where:
Expected volume = known syringe volume (usually 3 L)
Measured volume = volume recorded for the test

The maximum acceptable error for diagnostic spirometers, according to American Thoracic Society (ATS) recommendations, is ±3% or ±0.05 L, whichever is larger (Table 11-2). For monitoring spirometers, maximum allowable error is ±5% or ±0.1 L, whichever is greater (Table 11-3). If the percentage of error exceeds the allowable limits, careful examination of the spirometer, recording device, software, most recent calibration, and testing technique should be performed (Quality Assurance 11-1).

Biologic Controls

Biologic controls are test subjects who are available for repeated tests. These controls can be laboratory personnel or other individuals who can be tested repeatedly. Using biologic controls does not eliminate other control devices such as large-volume syringes. Although a 3-L syringe can verify volume and flow accuracy of a spirometer, biologic controls can evaluate an entire system, including spirometers, gas analyzers, plethysmographs, and software.

TABLE 11-2 Minimal Recommendations for Spirometers (Diagnostic)

A 3-L calibration syringe is recommended for testing VC and FVC. Twenty-four standardized waveforms are available for validating FVC, FEV_1, and $FEF_{25\%-75\%}$. Twenty-six standard flow waveforms are available for validating PEF. Other flows require manufacturer's proof of performance. A sine-wave pump is recommended for MVV validation.

Test	Range/Accuracy (BTPS)	Flow Range (L/sec)	Time (sec)	Resistance/ Back Pressure
VC	0.5-8 L ± 3% of reading or ±0.05 L, whichever is greater	0-14	30	N/A
FVC	0.5-8 L ± 3% of reading or ±0.05 L, whichever is greater	0-14	15	<1.5 cm H_2O/L/sec
FEV_1	0.5-8 L ± 3% of reading or ±0.05 L, whichever is greater	0-14	1	<1.5 cm H_2O/L/sec
Time zero	Time point for calculating all FEV_T values, using back-extrapolation	N/A	N/A	N/A
PEF	Accuracy: ±10% of reading or ±0.4 L/sec, whichever is greater Precision: ±5% of reading or ±0.2 L/sec, whichever is greater	0-14	N/A	<1.5 cm H_2O/L/sec
$FEF_{25\%-75\%}$	7.0 L/sec ± 5% of reading or ±0.2 L/sec, whichever is greater	−14 + 14	15	<1.5 cm H_2O/L/sec
$\dot{V}$	±14 L/sec ± 5% of reading or ±0.2 L/sec, whichever is greater	0-14	15	<1.5 cm H_2O/L/sec
MVV	250 L/min at V_T of 2 L ± 10% of reading or ± 15 L/min, whichever is greater	−14 + 14 ± 3%	12-15	<(±)10 cm H_2O at V_T of 2 L at 2.0 Hz

Adapted from Standardization of spirometry—1994 update, *Am J Respir Crit Care Med* 152:1107-1136, 1995.
VC, vital capacity; *FVC,* forced vital capacity; *PEF,* peak expiratory flow; *MVV,* maximal voluntary ventilation.

A disadvantage of using biologic controls is that pulmonary function varies from day to day. However, by establishing means and measures of variability from repeated tests, real problems with most pulmonary function equipment can be identified (Quality Assurance 11-2).

Control subjects should have normal lung function (i.e., no asthma or other respiratory symptoms) and span a range of values. For example, a 64-inch-tall female and a 72-inch-tall male will provide a wide range of values for most pulmonary function parameters. Pulmonary function studies on controls should be performed on a regular basis (weekly or monthly). All tests should use the same protocols applied to the patient population. Control measurements

TABLE 11-3   Minimal Recommendations for Monitoring Spirometers and Peak Flow
Meters

Requirement	FVC, FEV$_1$ (BTPS)*	PEF (BTPS)
Range	High: 0.50-8 L	High: 100 L/min to ≥700 L/min but "850 L/min
	Low: 0.50-6 L	Low: 60 L/min to ≥275 L/min but "400 L/min
Accuracy	±5% of reading or ±0.1 L, whichever is greater	±10% of reading or ±20 L/min, whichever is greater
Precision	±3% of reading or ±0.05 L, whichever is greater	Intradevice: "5% of reading or "10 L/min, whichever is greater Interdevice: "10% of reading or "10 L/min, whichever is greater
Linearity	Within 3% over range	Within 5% over range
Resolution	High: 0.05 L Low: 0.025 L	High: 10 L/min Low: 5 L/min
Resistance	<2.5 cm H$_2$O/L/sec, from 0-14 L/sec	<2.5 cm H$_2$O/L/sec, from 0-14 L/sec

Adapted from Standardization of spirometry—1994 update, *Am J Respir Crit Care Med* 152:1107-1136, 1995.
*High and low refer to spirometers or peak flow meters with either a high or low range.

QUALITY ASSURANCE 11-1   Common Spirometer Problems

Some problems detected by routine quality control of spirometers include the following:

- Creaks or leaks (in volume-displacement spirometers)
- Low water level (in water-seal spirometers)
- Sticking or worn bellows
- Inaccurate or erratic potentiometers
- Obstructed or dirty flow tubes (flow sensors)
- Mechanical resistance (in volume-displacement spirometers)
- Leaks in tubes and connectors
- Faulty recorder timing
- Inappropriate signal correction (BTPS)
- Improper software calibration (corrections)
- Defective software or computer interface

should meet all criteria for acceptability and reproducibility. Tests should be performed at the same time of day to minimize diurnal variation. If the laboratory has multiple pulmonary function systems, controls may be tested on each instrument on the same day to provide a check of interinstrument bias.

To provide useful statistics, at least 10 sets of measurements should be recorded. However, means and standard deviations (SDs) from controls with fewer sets may be used. Pulmonary function variables that are not derived from other measurements should be recorded. These include FVC, FEV$_1$, FRC, and DL$_{CO}$. Calculated values such as TLC or D$_L$/V$_A$ can be used as controls; however, if subsequent tests show significant differences, it may be unclear which component test is at fault. A calculator or a computer spreadsheet may be used to perform the simple statistics required (Table 11-4). Most spreadsheets have built-in functions to

Quality Assurance 11-2   How to Use Biologic Controls

1 *Performance of a single instrument.* Test biologic controls on a regular basis. Compare variables (e.g., FEV_1) to the established mean. Control values should fall within a range of ± 2 SDs of the mean (at least 95% of the time). If the value is outside of this range, the cause of the change should be identified. Was the last calibration performed correctly? Have any modifications been made to the spirometer hardware? Have any software upgrades or modifications been made? If the source of the problem is found and corrected, the control should be retested to confirm that the instrument performs as expected.

2 *Establish precision of the system.* Include data in the control database that falls within the 2-SD limit. Data outside of 2 SDs may be included if it is clearly caused by variability and not an equipment problem. This may be verified by repeating the test. If the second test produces another result more than 2 SDs from the mean, there is likely an equipment or procedural error. By calculating SDs from repeated measures, the precision of a particular instrument or system can be established.

3 *Use CV to reduce variability.* The CV for most pulmonary function variables should be approximately 5% or less. Some measures, such as $FEF_{25\%-75\%}$ are variable even in healthy individuals and may show CV values closer to 10%. If the CV is greater than 10%, calibration and testing procedures should be reviewed to see if sources of error can be eliminated.

4 *Compare instruments or laboratories.* Biologic controls can be used to perform interinstrument or interlaboratory evaluation. Similar devices should produce similar control results. However, if different instruments (i.e., a flow-based and a volume-based spirometer) are compared, slightly different values for the same control may be obtained. This difference is termed *bias*. The true value (e.g., FVC) may be considered the average of the means for the two instruments or labs. Alternatively, one instrument may be considered the "gold standard"; the other instrument can be described as having a negative or positive bias, depending on whether its measurement is less than or greater than the gold standard.

5 *Compare methods.* Biologic controls may also be used to compare different methodologies within the same laboratory. For example, FRC might be measured using a gas dilution technique and by plethysmograph. The means, SDs, and CVs of each method can then be compared.

6 *Troubleshooting.* Biologic controls can be used to troubleshoot a problem instrument. For example, if a system produces low DL_{CO} values on several otherwise normal patients, a problem might exist. Test a biologic control; if the control value is within expected limits, the low DL_{CO} values may be valid.

calculate mean ($\bar{X}$) and SD, and to allow data to be graphed. The coefficient of variation (CV) is calculated by dividing one SD by the mean. Separate statistics should be calculated for each control and for separate instruments. Data more than 1 or 2 years old should be replaced with more recent measurements to account for changes in pulmonary function that occur over time.

Other Calibration/Quality Control Tools
Sine-Wave Rotary Pump
This device produces a biphasic volume signal. A biphasic or sine-wave signal may be useful for checking volume and flow accuracy for both inspiration and expiration. A rotary-drive syringe may be useful for checking the frequency response of a spirometer, or to evaluate a spirometer's ability to adequately record tests such as the MVV. Sine-wave pumps are also commonly used in the calibration of body plethysmographs (see Figure 10-34).

TABLE 11-4 Example Spreadsheet for a Biologic Control*

Control subject: J.S.

Date	FVC	FEV$_1$	FRC	DL$_{CO}$
1/15/97	4.51	3.93	3.51	25.1
2/15/97	4.61	3.99	3.55	26.2
3/14/97	4.49	3.95	3.65	27.2
3/19/97	4.40	3.90	3.50	25.5
4/21/97	4.57	3.89	3.60	26.0
5/1/97	4.50	3.94	3.66	27.2
5/15/97	4.55	3.95	3.65	27.0
Mean	4.52	3.94	3.59	26.3
SD	0.06	0.03	0.06	0.78
CV	1.38%	0.79%	1.77%	2.97%

*Most spreadsheet programs have built-in functions to calculate means and standard deviations; additional calculations, such as coefficient of variation, can be entered by the user. Additional data can be entered by inserting more lines. Quality control charts may be constructed using mean and standard deviation data for each variable.

Computer-Driven Syringes

These devices incorporate large-volume syringes with a computer-controlled motor drive. Computerized syringes are usually used only by equipment manufacturers or for research applications. The ATS has developed a series of standard waveforms that may be used to drive a computer-controlled syringe. These waveforms are used to validate spirometers.

Explosive Decompression Devices

Explosive decompression simulates the exponential flow pattern of a forced expiratory maneuver. Such devices use compressed gas, such as CO_2, released through an orifice. The gas from the device is injected into a spirometer to generate a simulated forced exhalation. The primary advantage of these devices is that they allow flow and volume signals to be reproduced. When the control signal can be reproduced, both accuracy and precision can be assessed. Using a gas other than air may not work properly with certain types of flow-sensing spirometers.

In addition to checking the volume and flow accuracy of spirometers, several other important aspects of QC require routine evaluation.

Leak Checks

For volume-displacement spirometers, a check for leaks should be performed daily before assessing volume accuracy. Fill the device with air to approximately half of its volume range and apply a constant pressure by means of a weight or spring. No change in the volume tracing should be noted while the pressure is applied. The spirometer should return to its original volume baseline when the pressure is removed.

Flow Resistance

The "back pressure" from a spirometer should be less than 1.5 cm H_2O up to a flow of 14 L/sec. Resistance to flow is measured by placing an accurate manometer or pressure transducer at the patient connection and applying a known flow. This is easily accomplished with flow-sensing devices but somewhat difficult with volume-displacement devices. Measurement of flow resistance is normally performed only when there is some reason to suspect that the spirometer is causing undue resistance. The total resistance requirement must be met with all tubing, valves, and filters in place.

Frequency Response

Frequency response refers to the spirometer's ability to produce accurate volume and flow measurements across a wide range of frequencies. Frequency response is most critical for peak expiratory flow (PEF) and maximal voluntary ventilation (MVV) maneuvers. Frequency response is usually evaluated by means of a sine-wave pump or computer-driven syringe. It should be measured as part of the manufacturer's validation and rechecked if the spirometer is suspect.

Flow

Flow-sensing spirometers directly measure flow and indirectly calculate volume by integration or counting volume pulses. It may be necessary to assess the flow accuracy of such devices. Inaccurate measurement of flow usually results in inaccurate volume determinations. A rotameter (a large calibrated flow-metering device) may be used in conjunction with an adjustable compressed gas source to supply a gas at a known flow to the device. A weighted volume-displacement spirometer, such as a water-seal type, can also be used to generate a known flow. Most commercial flow-sensing spirometers use a volume signal (i.e., a 3-L syringe) to perform software calibration as previously described. It may be useful to check the flow signal from the spirometer at different known flows if the volume accuracy is observed to vary with flow.

Recorder/Displays

Printed records or computer-generated displays of spirometry signals are required for diagnostic functions, validation, or when waveforms are to be measured manually. Table 11-5 lists recommended scale factors for recorders and displays. Hard-copy recordings of volume-time or flow-volume tracings should be available for diagnostic spirometry. Flow-volume curves should be plotted with expired flow in the positive direction on the vertical axis and expired volume from left to right on the horizontal axis. A flow-to-volume scale ratio of 2:1 should be maintained (i.e., 2 L/sec flow for each 1 L of volume). Accurate recorder speed and volume sensitivity are particularly important if FEV_1 or other flows are calculated manually. Recorder accuracy should be checked at least quarterly. Paper speed of strip chart recorders can be easily checked with a stopwatch. Kymographs and similar mechanical recording devices may require repair or replacement of drive motors if paper speed is determined to be inaccurate. Most modern pulmonary function systems are computerized, and printed tracings are generated by ink-jet, dot matrix, or laser printers. The output of these devices should adhere to the recommended scale factors but often do not. In effect, computer-generated tracings cannot be used to check spirometer functions such as timing, etc.

TABLE 11-5 Minimum Recommended Scale Factors for Recorders and Displays

	Resolution	Scale factor
Volume	0.025 L	10 mm/L
Flow	0.100 L/sec	5 mm/L/sec
Time	0.20 sec	2 cm/sec

Adapted from Standardization of spirometry—1994 update, *Am J Respir Crit Care Med* 152:1107-1136, 1995.

GAS ANALYZERS

Accurate analysis of inspired and expired gases is required to measure lung volumes, DL_{CO}, and gas exchange during exercise or metabolic testing. The validity of these tests depends on accuracy of both the spirometer and gas analyzers used. Various types of gas analyzers are commonly used in pulmonary function testing (see Chapter 10). Calibration refers to the process of adjusting analyzer output to match the input of a known gas concentration. QC refers to a method for routinely checking the accuracy and precision of the gas analyzer. Calibration techniques for gas analyzers include the following:

Physiologic Range

Many gas analyzers are not linear or exhibit poor accuracy over a wide range of gas concentrations. Analyzers should be calibrated to match the physiologic range over which measurements will be made. For example, an O_2 analyzer may be used to measure fractional concentrations from 0.00 to 1.00, representing a wide physiologic range. If the O_2 analyzer is to be used for exercise tests in subjects breathing room air, an appropriate calibration range should be from 0.12 to 0.21. This narrow interval represents the physiologic range of expired O_2 likely to be encountered during an exercise test in a patient breathing air. Reducing the physiologic range of an analyzer generally allows greater accuracy and precision. Some types of analyzers provide range adjustments for this purpose. Calibration gases should represent the extremes of the physiologic range. In the example of the O_2 analyzer described, room air and a gas containing 12% oxygen would be appropriate.

Sampling Conditions

Gas analyzers must be calibrated under the same conditions that will be encountered during the test. Analyzers that are sensitive to partial pressure (see Chapter 10) may be affected by the sample flow rate. For certain tests, gas is sampled continuously from the breathing circuit using a pump (e.g., breath-by-breath gas analysis during exercise). Sample flow through the pump must be adjusted *before* calibration, then left unchanged during sampling. If gas flow stops before analysis is actually performed (e.g., some types of DL_{CO} systems), sample flow is usually not critical. A gas analyzer in this type of system must be calibrated under conditions of zero flow. Measurement errors may occur if an analyzer is calibrated and then configuration of the sampling circuit is changed. This may happen if tubing, valves, or stopcocks are added or changed. Any gas-conditioning devices, such as those used for CO_2, H_2O, or dust, should be in place during calibration as well. If a CO_2 or H_2O absorber is changed, calibration should be repeated.

Two-Point Calibration

The most common technique for analyzer calibration involves introducing two known gases. One gas is typically used to "zero" or adjust the low end of the range, whereas the second gas is used to "span" or adjust the high end of the range. Adjusting the "span" is actually setting the gain of the analyzer, so that a known input produces a known output. For some pulmonary function tests, the gas to be analyzed is not normally present in expired air (e.g., helium, CO, or neon). For such tests, room air may be used to zero the analyzer. Calibration gas (cal gas) representing the other end of the physiologic range may be used to span the analyzer. He dilution FRC and DL_{CO}sb are examples of such tests. He and CO analyzers are zeroed by drawing room air into the measuring chambers. He and CO are assumed to be absent from the atmosphere. Then calibration gas containing a known concentration of the gas to be analyzed is introduced. The analyzer gain is adjusted to match the known concentration. The calibration gas approximates the concentration to be analyzed during the test. The analyzer may then be rezeroed, and the entire process repeated to verify the calibration. A similar technique may be used with two gases of known concentration if the expirate normally contains varying concentrations of the gas. For example, room air and 12% oxygen may be used to perform a two-point calibration of an O_2 analyzer for exercise testing. Depending on the stability of the analyzer, calibration may need to be repeated before each test or measurement. Gas analyzers should be calibrated before each patient for gas dilution lung volumes, DL_{CO}, exercise tests, and metabolic studies. Gas analyzers used for monitoring (e.g., capnographs) should be calibrated on a schedule appropriate for the extent of use. Calibration should be performed according to the manufacturer's recommendations. The accuracy of the calibration gas should reflect the necessary accuracy of the measurements involved. For exercise or metabolic studies, calibration gases should be accurate to at least two decimal places (i.e., hundredth of a percent). Calibration gases may require verification by an independent method.

Multiple-Point (Linearity) Calibration

An assumption made by a two-point calibration is that analyzer output is linear between the points used. To verify linearity or to determine the pattern of nonlinearity, three or more calibration points must be determined (Figure 11-2). A multiple-point calibration is performed in a manner similar to the two-point calibration except that concentrations of known gases across the range to be analyzed are checked and plotted. If multiple points are determined, regression analysis may be used to determine the slope (or type of curve) relating the measured gas concentrations to the expected gas concentrations. A spreadsheet or graphing calculator can be used to analyze the data points. If the analyzer is linear, the points plotted fall in a straight line. A minimum of three points (i.e., gases) is required to demonstrate linearity. If the analyzer is nonlinear, a calibration curve must be constructed to correct the results. In most instances, an equation describing a nonlinear curve can be generated. This equation can then be used either manually or by software to correct analyzer readings. Most nonlinear analyzers incorporate electronics that linearize their output. Linearity of analyzers used for DL_{CO}, lung volumes, exercise, and metabolic studies should be assessed at least quarterly.

PF Tips

The 3-L calibration syringe can often be used as a lung model to evaluate the accuracy of gas analyzers used for lung volumes or DL_{CO} tests. For example, a DL_{CO} test can be simulated by setting the calibration syringe to a volume of 1 L, and then connecting it to the patient port of the pulmonary function system. The syringe is then withdrawn to "inspire" 2 L of test gas. After a 10-second breath hold, the syringe is emptied. This simulates a lung with a total volume (TLC) of 3 L and an inspired volume (VC) of 2 L. The DL_{CO} using this technique should be close to zero because no diffusion occurred in the syringe.

QC of gas analyzers can be performed by submitting known concentrations of gases to the analyzer, by testing a lung analog, or by using biologic controls. Several gases with concentrations spanning the range of the analyzer can be maintained. This can be a costly means of QC for pulmonary function laboratories. A simpler technique is to prepare serial dilutions of a known gas using a large-volume syringe. The syringe may be the type used for volume calibration. For example, 100 ml of He and 900 ml of air may be mixed in a syringe to produce

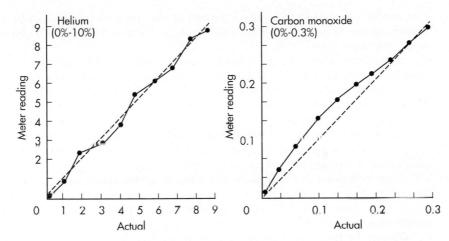

Figure 11-2 *Calibration and linearity check of gas analyzers.* Two plots of varying gas concentrations (for He and CO) are shown. Each graph plots the meter reading of the analyzers against the actual concentration of the gas. Different dilutions of each gas are prepared and then analyzed. The He analyzer shows good linearity in the comparison of measured versus expected concentrations. The CO analyzer shows a nonlinear pattern, typical of an infrared analyzer. If enough points are determined, a calibration curve can be generated to correct meter readings. Computerized systems often use an equation or a table of points representing a calibration curve. This allows an analyzer to be calibrated using only two points. Three or more points (gas concentrations) are required to demonstrate linearity.

a 10% He mixture, then injected into the analyzer. Subsequently, 100 ml of He may be diluted in 1000 ml, then 1100 ml, and so on, with the expected concentrations calculated as follows:

$$\text{Expected \% test gas} = \frac{\text{Volume of test gas}}{\text{Total volume of gas}} \times 100$$

where:

$$\text{Total volume of gas} = \text{test gas} + \text{added air} + \text{syringe dead space}$$

As each dilution is analyzed, the meter reading is recorded and plotted against the expected percentage (Figure 11-2). This method is simple and available in most laboratories. Care must be taken when preparing samples so that air does not leak into the syringe, further diluting the test gas. The volume of air in the syringe connectors (i.e., dead space) must be included when calculating the dilution of the test gas. Some calibrated syringes include their dead space volume.

A second method of verifying analyzer performance involves simulating either lung volume or DL_{CO} tests. This may be accomplished using a lung analog. A lung analog is simply an airtight container of known volume. The lung volume simulator is attached at the patient connection with the system set up for a lung volume or DL_{CO} test. A large-volume syringe is used to "ventilate" the lung analog, mimicking the patient's breathing. The resulting lung volume (e.g., FRC) is compared with the known volume of the analog system. A calibration syringe may also be used as the lung analog. Many calibration syringes feature a locking collar that can be adjusted so that only a portion of the syringe's volume can be emptied. With a known volume of air in the syringe, the test is performed by filling and emptying the syringe to the starting volume.

Simulation of the $DL_{CO}sb$ maneuver using a lung analog can check analyzer linearity. Both the tracer gas (He, Ne, CH_4) and CO are diluted equally in the lung analog, and their relative concentrations should be identical. This causes the calculated $DL_{CO}sb$ to be near zero. If the two analyzers are not linear in relation to one another, the ratio of tracer gas to CO will not equal 1. Calculated $DL_{CO}sb$ will be either above or below zero. This method tests not only the gas analyzers, but also the volume transducer, breathing circuit, and software. Temperature or gas corrections should be disabled. A linearity check at different dilutions can be performed by varying the volume of the lung analog.

Some computerized systems do not allow lung simulators to be used. The software may be designed to make all necessary corrections for human subjects, giving erroneous results when a simulator is used. However, if the software reports gas analyzer values, the accuracy and linearity of various dilutions can be checked.

Testing biologic controls (Quality Assurance 11-2) is a third means of evaluating gas analyzers. This method may not detect small changes in analyzer performance because of day-to-day variability of lung volumes, DL_{CO}, or resting energy expenditure. Despite variability as high as 10% for DL_{CO} or exercise parameters in healthy patients, gas analyzer malfunctions can be detected. Biologic controls may be the simplest means of checking automated exercise/metabolic systems that depend on accurate gas analysis. Abnormal results from biologic controls can suggest which component of the gas analyzer may be faulty (Quality Assurance 11-3).

BODY PLETHYSMOGRAPHS

The calibration techniques described here apply primarily to variable-pressure, constant-volume plethysmographs. Flow-based plethysmographs may require slightly different calibration procedures for the box transducer. Mouth pressure and pneumotachometer calibrations are similar for both types of plethysmographs.

QUALITY ASSURANCE 11-3   Common Gas Analyzer Problems

Some problems detected by routine calibration or quality control of gas analyzers include the following:

- Leaks in sample lines or connectors
- Blockage of sample lines
- Exhausted water vapor or CO_2 absorbers
- Contamination of photocells or electrodes
- Improper mechanical zeroing (taut band display)
- Inadequate warm-up time
- Deterioration or contamination of column packing material (gas chromatographs)
- Poor vacuum pump performance (emission spectroscopy analyzers)
- Chopper motor malfunction (infrared analyzers)
- Electrolyte or fuel cell exhaustion (O_2 analyzers)
- Aging of detector cells (infrared analyzers)
- Poor optical balance (infrared analyzers)

Mouth Pressure Transducer

Calibration is done by connecting the pressure transducer to a water manometer or some other device that can generate an accurate pressure. The manometer is a U-shaped tube with a calibration scale that allows very accurate pressures to be generated (see Chapter 10, Figure 10-34). Some plethysmographs use a weighted piston to produce a calibration pressure signal. The range of the mouth pressure transducer should be ±20 to ±50 cm H_2O. Air is injected into one port of the U-tube manometer. For example, a small volume of air may be introduced to cause a deflection of 5 cm. In effect, this creates a difference of 10 cm between the two columns of the manometer. The gain of the mouth pressure amplifier is then adjusted so that its signal display deflects by an amount equivalent to 10 cm H_2O per centimeter. The display device is most commonly a computer screen. The deflection then becomes the calibration factor for the mouth pressure transducer. In the previous example, a pressure change of 10 cm H_2O results in a 1-cm deflection on the display. In computerized systems, the analog output of the transducers is measured and a software correction factor is determined. The correction (or calibration) factor is calculated in a manner similar to that used for spirometer output (see Spirometers section). The correction factor is then applied by the software as the signals are acquired.

Box Pressure Transducer

Calibration of the box pressure transducer is accomplished by closing the plethysmograph's door and applying a volume signal comparable to what occurs during patient testing. In a 500- to 600-L plethysmograph, a volume signal of 25 to 50 ml is typical. The box pressure transducer (for a 500-L pressure box) should have a range of ±2 cm H_2O. An adjustable sine-wave pump connected to a small syringe is ideal for box calibration (see Chapter 10, Figure 10-34). The volume is pumped in and out of the box. With the pump operating, the gain of the box pressure transducer is adjusted so that volume change in the box causes a specific deflection on the display. For example, the pressure signal generated by a 30-ml volume might be adjusted to cause a 2-cm deflection on the display. The box pressure calibration factor would then become 15 ml/cm. For computerized systems (most plethysmographs), a calibration factor is derived rather than an actual adjustment of the displayed signal. In other words, no actual adjustment of the output of the box pressure transducer is necessary; the software correction is simply applied to all signals generated during measurements. The calibration procedure may be repeated by adjusting the pump speed from 0.5 to 5.0 cycles/sec (Hz). Varying the frequency allows the frequency response of the box and transducer to be checked. The volume deflection or calibration factor should not change at different frequencies. Flow-based plethysmographs may be calibrated similarly. The output of the box flow transducer is adjusted rather than that of a pressure transducer. The plethysmograph is normally calibrated empty. A volume correction for the patient is then applied in the calculation of results (see Appendix F).

Flow Transducer

The pneumotachometer (flow sensor) may be calibrated by applying either a known flow or a known volume. A precise flow may be generated using a rotameter or similar calibrated flow meter. Most systems, however, calibrate the pneumotachometer using a 3-L syringe. The flow is integrated, and the gain of the flow signal is then adjusted until the output of the integrator matches the 3-L volume. As for the box and mouth pressure transducers, a software calibration factor may be computed rather than physically adjusting the output of the flow sensor. Pressure-differential, heated-wire, or Pitot tube flow sensors may be used (see Chapter 10). Once the flow sensor is calibrated, both volumes and flows (as needed for measurement of Raw) can be measured.

QC of body plethysmographs may be accomplished using one or more of the following: an isothermal lung analog, known resistors, biologic controls, or comparison with gas dilution or radiologic lung volumes.

An isothermal volume analog can be constructed from a 4- or 5-L glass bottle filled with metal wool, usually copper or steel. The metal wool acts as a heat sink (Figure 11-3). The mouth of the bottle is fitted with two connectors. One connector attaches to the mouth shutter (or the patient connection). The other is attached to a rubber bulb with a volume of 50 to 100 ml (i.e., the bulb from a blood pressure cuff). The actual volume of the lung analog can be determined by subtracting the volume of the metal wool from the volume of the bottle. The volume occupied by metal wool is calculated from its weight times its density. Alternately, the gas volume of the bottle may be measured by filling it with water from a volumetric source. The volume of the connectors and rubber bulb should be added to the total volume.

The accuracy check is performed with an assistant seated in the sealed plethysmograph. The isothermal volume device is connected to the mouthpiece. The mouth shutter is then closed. While the assistant holds his or her breath, the bulb is squeezed at a rate of 1 to 2 times per second. A P_{MOUTH}/P_{BOX} tangent is recorded just as would be done testing a patient.

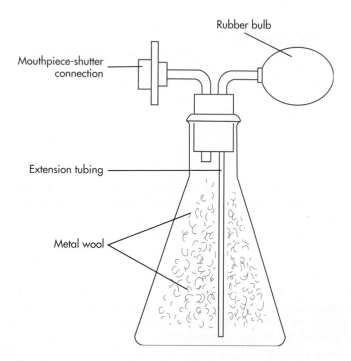

Figure 11-3 *Isothermal lung analog.* A schematic of an isothermal lung analog for quality control of the body plethysmograph. A 3- to 4-L jar or flask is fitted with a stopper with two openings. One opening connects to the mouthpiece shutter apparatus; the other is connected to a rubber hand bulb with an extension tube to the bottom of the jar. Copper or steel wool is used to fill the container. The metal wool acts as a heat sink so that pressure changes in the bottle cause only minimal changes in gas temperature. A patient sits in the plethysmograph, holds his or her breath, and squeezes the bulb. This simulates a VTG maneuver. The P_{MOUTH}/P_{BOX} angle may be recorded, and the volume of the jar calculated. The measured volume should be within 5% of the actual volume. The true volume is determined by filling the container with water and subtracting the volume of the metal wool. The volume of metal wool may be calculated by multiplying its density and its weight. The volumes of the connectors and rubber bulb should be considered as well.

Thoracic gas volume (V_{TG}) is calculated as usual, except that PH_2O is not subtracted (see Appendix F). The V_{TG} calculated should equal the volume of the isothermal lung analog (as measured previously) within ±5%. Correction should be made for the assistant's volume (based on body weight) plus the known volume of the isothermal lung analog. The procedure may be repeated at frequencies of 0.5 to 5.0 cycles/sec to check the frequency response of the box. If the box's frequency response is "flat," tangents should not change when the bulb is squeezed at different rates. The lung analog must contain a sufficient volume of metal wool to act as a heat sink (i.e., isothermal). The metal wool "absorbs" changes in temperature that would result from the compression and decompression of gas in the bottle. If there is not enough metal wool, small temperature changes may affect the volume determination.

The accuracy of the box for measuring airway resistance (Raw) can be assessed using known resistances. A resistor can be made using a plug with a small-diameter orifice. Alternately, a resistor can be constructed from capillary tubes arranged lengthwise in a flow tube. In either case, the pressure drop across the resistor is measured at a known flow rate. Some manufacturers supply resistors with known resistances. The resistor is then inserted in front of the pneumotachometer/mouth shutter assembly. A patient whose Raw has been previously measured then has Raw measured with the resistor in place. The increase in measured Raw should approximate that of the resistor.

Another means of checking plethysmograph function is to measure V_{TG} and/or Raw from a biologic control (Quality Assurance 11-2). A series of 10 box measurements provides an appropriate mean value for comparison with subsequent results. Day-to-day variability in trained subjects is usually less than 10%. This method allows checking of the box, the transducers, the recording devices, and the software. A discrepancy between the established mean and an individual QC trial may not indicate which component is causing the problem. For example, a control whose V_{TG} has been established as 3 L is measured again and the V_{TG} is calculated to be 2 L. The biologic control establishes that there is a problem, but the cause of the discrepancy requires further investigation. In this example, either incorrect calibration of box or mouth pressure transducers, or a leaky door seal, may be the cause (Quality Assurance 11-4).

A third method of checking plethysmograph accuracy is to compare the V_{TG} with FRC determined by gas dilution. Correlations greater than 0.90 have been demonstrated between gas dilution and plethysmograph lung volumes in healthy individuals. Differences greater than 10% (in healthy individuals) for volumes measured by plethysmograph and gas dilution are not specific but may indicate equipment malfunction. This method, as well as use of

QUALITY ASSURANCE 11-4   Common Plethysmograph Problems

Some problems detected by routine quality control of body plethysmographs include the following:

- Leaks in door seals or connectors (pressure boxes)
- Improperly calibrated pressure transducers
- Obstructed or perforated pneumotachometers
- Excessive thermal drift
- Poor frequency response
- Excessive vibration (poorly mounted transducers)
- Inappropriate software calibration factors
- Procedural errors (e.g., testing before thermal equilibrium reached)

biologic controls, is based on measurements of healthy individuals with normal day-to-day variability. It is important that control individuals perform the breathing maneuvers correctly (see Chapter 3).

Calibration and Quality Control of Blood Gas Analyzers

Modern blood gas analyzers rely on a microprocessor or computer to control functions such as calibration. The user selects a "calibration schedule" appropriate for the complexity and number of tests performed. For example, in a laboratory that performs many blood gas analyses, automated calibration may be performed every 30 minutes. Government agencies and some voluntary credentialing organizations have specific schedules for the frequency and type of calibrations that may be required.

Calibrating blood gas electrodes involves exposing the gas electrodes (i.e., Po_2, Pco_2) to one or two gases with known partial pressures of O_2 and CO_2. If only one gas is used, the calibration is termed a "one-point calibration"; if two gases are used, it is called a "two-point calibration." Similarly, one or two known buffers may be used to calibrate the pH electrode. Calibration gases spanning the physiologic ranges of the Po_2, and Pco_2 electrodes are used just as for gas analyzers. Typical combinations include one calibration gas with a fractional O_2 concentration of 0.20 (20%) and a fractional CO_2 concentration of 0.05 (5%). A second calibration gas may have a CO_2 concentration of 0.10 (10%) with an O_2 concentration close to zero. If blood with a very high Po_2 is to be analyzed (e.g., a shunt study), the analyzer may be calibrated with a gas that has a high fractional concentration of O_2. However, this may require an analyzer that allows manual calibration.

Calibration gases may be bubbled through water at 37° C to saturate them with water vapor before entering the measuring chamber. The partial pressures of O_2 and CO_2 in the calibration gases depend on local barometric pressure. For each gas, the partial pressure is calculated as follows:

$$P_{GAS} = F_{GAS} \times (P_B - 47)$$

where:
P_{GAS} = partial pressure of calibration gas, mm Hg
F_{GAS} = fractional concentration of the same gas
P_B = local barometric pressure, mm Hg
47   = partial pressure of water vapor (PH_2O) at 37° C, mm Hg

As for gas analyzers, a "low" gas is used to *zero* or *balance* each electrode. A "high" gas is used to *adjust the gain* (also called the slope) of the electrode's amplifier. "Electronic" zeroing may be done without exposing the electrode to a gas with a partial pressure of zero. Some blood gas analyzers use this method to zero the Po_2 electrode.

Calibration may consist of either a one-point or two-point calibration. One-point calibration exposes the gas electrodes to a single partial pressure of calibration gas and brings one buffer into contact with the pH electrode. Two-point calibration doubles the number of calibration gases and buffers. Most automated blood gas analyzers use a combination of one-point and two-point calibrations. Computerized systems allow the user to select how frequently and what type of calibration is performed on the gas and pH electrodes. The Po_2 electrode is usually calibrated over a range of 0 to 150 mm Hg. The Pco_2 electrode is usually calibrated for the range of 40 to 80 mm Hg. The pH electrode is usually calibrated using buffers with pH values of 6.840 (low) and 7.384 (high).

Most blood gas analyzers use precision gases to calibrate the gas electrodes, even though gas tensions are measured in liquid (i.e., blood). Some difference may exist when partial pressure of gas is analyzed in gaseous versus liquid medium, especially for O_2. The reduction of O_2 at the tip of the polarographic electrode occurs more rapidly in a gaseous medium than in a liquid. If the electrode is calibrated with a gas, its response when measuring a liquid will be to read slightly lower. This difference is termed the gas-liquid factor. Gas-liquid corrections may be clinically important when measuring high partial pressures of O_2, particularly above 400 mm Hg. Some computerized analyzers create solutions for calibration of the gas and pH electrodes. Calibration gases are bubbled through buffers in a process called "tonometering." The microprocessor calculates partial pressures of calibration gases based on an internal barometer. When the Pco_2 of the tonometered solution is calculated, pH of the solution can be determined. The built-in tonometer allows calibration materials for all three electrodes to be produced. Computerized blood gas analyzers often include a software correction for the difference in electrode response to gas and liquid. This allows the analyzer to be used to measure both liquid and gas specimens.

Computerized calibration brings calibration gases or buffers into contact with the electrodes. Electrode responses to the calibration gas or buffer are then stored. The microprocessor compares the measured responses to expected calibration values. The computer then "corrects" the zero and gain (for a two point calibration) so that measured and expected values match. Most computerized blood gas analyzers compare the current calibration results with the previous calibration. The difference between calibrations is termed *drift* and indicates an electrode's stability.

Automatic calibrations can be programmed to occur at predetermined intervals. Adjustments are performed automatically, based on the response of the electrodes. Because of this, all conditions for an acceptable calibration must be met before the procedure actually begins. Automated blood gas analyzers check most conditions that may affect accurate results, such as temperature of the measuring chamber. During automatic calibration, inadequate buffer or the wrong calibration gas may cause the microprocessor to correct inappropriately for an properly functioning electrode. A similar problem arises if protein contaminates the electrode tip, altering its sensitivity. The microprocessor adjusts the electrode's output in an attempt to bring it into range. This process works well for minor changes in electrode sensitivity. However, electrodes cannot be properly calibrated if they are contaminated with protein, if membranes are damaged, or if the electrolyte is depleted. The user must maintain reagents, calibration gases, and electrodes so that automatic calibration can occur successfully. Systematic errors can sometimes be masked by automatic calibration. Contamination of the calibration gases or buffers is a common example. If the microprocessor adjusts electrodes to match a contaminated calibration standard, the calibrations appear normal but analysis of control samples will show differences. Detection of these errors usually requires appropriate QC and proficiency testing (described later in this section). Automated blood gas analyzers reduce variability by controlling calibration as well as sample analysis but require careful attention to function appropriately.

Two methods of QC for blood gas analysis are used: tonometry and commercially prepared controls. Interpretation of blood gas QC is the same for either method.

TONOMETRY

A tonometer allows precision gas mixtures to be equilibrated with either whole blood or a buffer solution. One type of tonometer creates a thin film of blood or buffer by spinning it in a chamber flooded with precision gas. A second type bubbles gas through the blood or buffer;

the bubbles create a large surface for gas exchange. In both types, the tonometer is maintained at 37° C and the gas is humidified. The equilibration time is determined by gas flow and volume of control material. A portion of the blood or buffer is then injected into the blood gas analyzer. The expected gas tensions are calculated from fractional concentrations of the precision gas, as described for calibration. If whole blood is used as the control material, only Po_2 and Pco_2 can be checked because pH cannot be easily calculated. Blood is ideal for QC of the gas electrodes because its viscosity and gas-exchange properties are the same as those of patient samples. No other control material provides the oxygen-carrying capacity of whole blood. For the most precise control of the Po_2 electrode, tonometry is the method of choice. However, pH cannot be accurately calculated for whole blood because its buffering capacity is usually unknown. Tonometry of a bicarbonate-based buffer using a known fractional concentration of CO_2 allows both gas and pH electrodes to be quality controlled. The gas exchange characteristics of this type of buffer make it less useful than whole blood for QC of Po_2 and Pco_2.

Tonometry can be performed inexpensively using pooled waste blood and small amounts of precision gas. Using pooled blood requires special care. All blood specimens must be handled using universal precautions (see Infection Control and Safety section). QC of the pH electrode requires additional tonometry of a buffer. Three levels of control materials spanning the measuring range of the electrode are recommended. Three precision gas mixtures are therefore required.

Accuracy of tonometry is highly dependent on a standardized technique. Sampling syringes should be lubricated and then flushed with the precision gas. Careful attention to the preparation and sampling from the tonometer is required to obtain reproducible results. The values obtained using tonometry may depend on individual technique. Problems that occur with tonometry include contamination of the precision gas resulting from leaky connections, improper temperature control of the chamber, or inadequate gas flow to achieve equilibrium. Because of the complexity required for multilevel controls for all three electrodes, tonometry is not widely used.

■ COMMERCIALLY PREPARED CONTROLS

There are three types of commercially prepared controls: blood-based, aqueous, and fluorocarbon-based. The blood-based matrix consists of a solution containing buffered human red blood cells. The aqueous material is usually a bicarbonate buffer. The fluorocarbon-based control material is a perfluorinated compound that has enhanced oxygen-dissolving characteristics. Multiple levels (i.e., acidosis, alkalosis, normal) of these materials provide control over the range of blood gases seen clinically.

All three types of controls are packaged in sealed glass ampules of 2 to 3 ml volume. They require minimum preparation for use. Blood-based material must be refrigerated, then warmed to 37° C and agitated before use. Aqueous- and fluorocarbon-based controls can be stored under refrigeration for long periods or at room temperature for day-to-day use. Most aqueous- and fluorocarbon-based controls have shelf lives of 1 year. Each requires agitation for 10 to 15 seconds before use to ensure equilibration with the gas sealed in the ampule. Commercially prepared controls may cost more than samples prepared using tonometry. They are convenient to use, however, and may be less susceptible to handling errors than tonometered materials.

One problem with aqueous controls (and to a lesser extent with fluorocarbon solutions) is poor precision of Po_2. The oxygen-carrying capacity of these materials is much lower than that of whole blood. Consequently, the Po_2 in the control material changes rapidly on exposure to air. Controls with low PO_2 values (50 to 60 mm Hg) become quickly "contaminated" after opening. Aqueous or fluorocarbon controls may produce a wide range of "expected"

Most laboratories use commercially prepared controls. These controls should be prepared according to the manufacturer's instructions. This usually involves shaking the contents to mix the liquid and gaseous contents of the ampule. Once opened, the contents should be immediately injected into the analyzer. Delay in injecting blood gas controls results in Po_2 values drifting toward 150 mm Hg and Pco_2 values drifting toward zero. The temperature at which the ampule is stored may be needed to correct for small differences in the Po_2 of the control.

Po_2 values, limiting their usefulness in detecting an out-of-control electrode. Some of these difficulties may be overcome by careful statistical evaluation of Po_2 control data as described in this section.

A sound statistical method of interpreting "control runs" is necessary to detect blood gas analyzer malfunctions (Quality Assurance 11-5). The most commonly used method for detecting out-of-control situations is calculating the control mean ±2 SDs. A series of runs of the same control material is performed. Twenty to 30 runs provide an adequate base for calculation of the mean and SD (see Appendix F for a sample calculation). One SD on either side of the mean in a normal distribution includes approximately 67% of the data points. Two SDs include 95% of the data points in a normal distribution. Three SDs include 99% of the data points in a normal series. A QC value that falls within ±2 SDs of the mean can be considered in control. If the control value falls between 2 and 3 SDs from the mean, there is only a 5% chance that the run is in control. The normal variability that occurs when multiple measurements are performed is called *random error*. One of 20 control runs (i.e., 5%) can be expected to produce a result in the 2 to 3 SD range and still be acceptable. For example, if a control

QUALITY ASSURANCE 11-5   Common Blood Gas Analyzer Problems

Some problems detected by routine quality control or proficiency testing of blood gas analyzers include the following:

- *Electrode malfunction.* Protein deposited on membranes or electrodes is common and can usually be remedied by cleaning. Leaks in membranes and electrolyte depletion cause electrode drift or shifts in performance.

- *Temperature control.* Failure to maintain 37° C water or air bath, or thermometer inaccuracy causes QC results to be out of control.

- *Improper calibration.* Problems during calibration are almost always related to inadequate or contaminated buffer or calibration gas. QC data that are consistently high or low may indicate a problem with reagents.

- *Mechanical problems.* Leaks in pump tubing or poorly functioning pumps allow calibrating solutions, controls, and patient samples to be contaminated. Air bubbles introduced during analysis cause gas tensions to be in error. Inadequate rinsing may also occur with pump problems or improperly functioning valves. This usually results in blood clotting in the transport tubing or measuring chamber.

- *Improper sampling technique.* Failure to anaerobically collect arterial specimens or properly store samples in ice water, excessive heparin, or bubbles in the specimen all may result in questionable results. Another common problem related to sampling is inadvertently obtaining a venous specimen. Adequately functioning electrodes, as demonstrated by good QC, can distinguish poor sampling from actual clinical abnormalities.

run shows a value that is more than 2 SDs above the mean, the control is usually repeated. If the second run shows a value within 2 SDs of the mean, the first value was probably a random error.

Complex sets of rules have been developed to distinguish true out-of-control situations from random errors. A widely used set of rules is that proposed by Westgard (see References). The rules are selected to provide the greatest probability for detecting real errors and rejecting false errors. This approach to QC is termed the *multiple-rule method*. The multiple-rule method usually requires that two or more control levels be evaluated on the same measurement device (electrode). An example of the multiple-rule method may be applied as follows:

1. When one control observation exceeds the mean ±2 SDs, a "warning" condition exists.
2. When one control observation exceeds the mean ±3 SDs, an out-of-control condition exists.
   When two consecutive control observations exceed the mean +2 SDs or the mean −2 SDs, an out-of-control condition exists.
3. When the range of differences between consecutive control runs exceeds 4 SDs, an out-of-control condition exists.
4. When four consecutive control observations exceed the mean +1 SD or the mean −1 SD, an out-of-control condition exists.
5. When 10 consecutive control observations fall on the same side of the mean (±), an out-of-control condition exists.

These are just some of the rules that may be applied; not all rules have to be used at all times. Rules 1 and 2 detect marked changes in electrode performance, sometimes called a *shift*, by examining how far from the mean a single control value falls. Rule 3 looks for a shift by comparing two consecutive control runs. Rule 4 looks for shifts in electrode performance by noting excessive variability between consecutive runs. Rules 5 and 6 look for "trends" in electrode response by evaluating an unexpected pattern (i.e., multiple values on the same side of the mean) in the recent history of control runs. Similar rules may be applied by linking multiple levels (i.e., high, low, normal) of control material. For example, if three levels of controls all show values greater than 2 SDs above their respective means, it is likely that the electrode is out of control.

One problem with a strict statistical approach is that if *outliers* (i.e., values more than 2 SDs from the mean) are sometimes excluded, the SD becomes smaller with repeated calculation. Eventually, valid control data may be rejected. This situation can be managed by including data in the calculations that are clinically acceptable, although they may be more than 2 SDs above or below the mean.

When using the multiple-rule method, it is necessary not only to evaluate the mean and SD of the current control run, but to keep a control history as well. This is often accomplished by means of a control chart (Figure 11-4). A graph for each control is created with the mean ±2 SDs on the y-axis and control run number (or time) on the x-axis. Individual controls are then plotted as they are run to track electrode performance.

To provide adequate QC for a blood gas analyzer, three levels of control materials are normally used. Three levels of control for each of the three electrodes (i.e., pH, P_{CO_2}, and P_{O_2}) require that 9 means and 9 SDs must be calculated for each instrument. Controls may also be used for blood oximeters, and this adds more control histories to be managed. When controls are run several times daily, tracking multiple runs can become complex. To simplify this task, computerized QC programs are often used. Such programs are sometimes included in the software for automated blood gas analyzers. Many laboratory computer systems also support statistical databases for control data. The chief advantages of computerized QC are

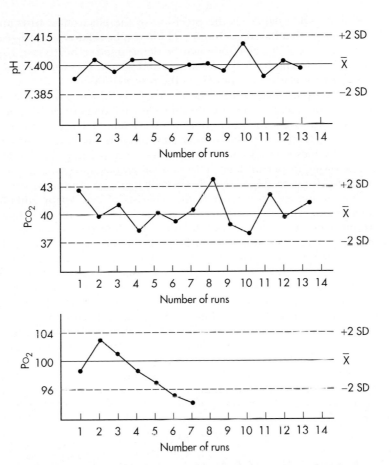

Figure 11-4 *Blood gas quality control charts.* Three examples of Shewhart/Levey-Jennings charts for pH, PCO_2 and PO_2. The mean for a specific control material is plotted as a solid line, and the +2 SD lines are dashed. The left y-axis on each graph is labeled with the actual mean and 2 SD values. Consecutive control runs are plotted on the horizontal x-axis. On the pH control chart (*top*) all values vary about the mean in a regular fashion; the electrode appears in control for the 13 measurements plotted. The PCO_2 chart (*middle*) shows somewhat more variability. Control run 8 shows a value outside of the ±2-SD range. This is probably a random error because it is the only control value outside the ±2-SD limits. Subsequent controls show normal variability about the mean, also suggesting that run 8 was a random error. The PO_2 chart (*bottom*) shows a trend of decreasing control values. Runs 6 and 7 both produce values of more than 2 SDs below the mean. This pattern suggests that the electrode is malfunctioning and needs to be serviced. By applying multiple rules (*see text*) to the interpretation of consecutive control runs, with or without charts, most out-of-control situations can be detected.

simplified data storage and maintenance of necessary statistics. Multiple rules can be applied easily to each new control run to detect problems. Computerized records and control charts can be printed. These types of QC records are required by many accrediting agencies. (See Appendix D for a list of regulatory agencies.)

QC of blood gas analyzers should be performed on a schedule appropriate for the number of specimens analyzed. In most laboratories, controls must be performed daily or more often. In busy laboratories, multiple levels of controls may be required on each shift. QC is also usually required after electrode maintenance is performed.

Routine QC establishes the precision of the electrodes. Instrument precision must be determined so that blood gas interpretation can be related to a range of values. For example, the variability of a Po_2 electrode may be determined to be ± 6 mm Hg (i.e., 2 SDs) around a mean of 50 mm Hg. Each Po_2 result (around 50 mm Hg) can then be interpreted with some certainty that it is within 6 mm Hg of the reported value.

Several other techniques related to QC of blood gas analyzers are commonly used. Interlaboratory comparison of control results can compare the performance of similar instruments for measuring the same lot of controls. Manufacturers of control materials and some voluntary credentialing bodies provide such interlaboratory databases. Each laboratory submits its control values for a specific period, usually once per month. The laboratory then receives a report showing its performance related to all participating laboratories. This type of comparison is useful for detecting systematic errors that may go unnoticed when running daily controls.

Interlaboratory proficiency testing consists of comparing unknown control specimens from a single source in multiple laboratories. This allows an individual laboratory to compare its results with other laboratories. Results using different methodologies (i.e., analyzers) may also be compared. Results of proficiency testing are usually reported as means and SDs for each instrument participating in the program. Proficiency testing does not measure precision, as does daily QC. However, it provides a measure of the absolute accuracy of the individual laboratory. A laboratory may have acceptable precision as determined by daily QC but be inaccurate when compared with other laboratories. Proficiency testing often detects systematic errors that occur because of improper calibration, contaminated reagents, or procedural problems. Multiple levels of unknowns are usually provided to check the range of values seen in clinical practice. Proficiency testing programs are available from professional organizations such as the College of American Pathologists, as well as from commercial vendors. Satisfactory performance on interlaboratory proficiency testing has been mandated by the U.S. Department of Health and Human Services under the Clinical Laboratory Improvement Amendment of 1988 (see Appendix D).

Criteria for Acceptability of Pulmonary Function Studies

Quality assurance in the pulmonary function laboratory requires not only appropriate calibration and QC, but also careful attention to the testing technique. Testing technique may be compared with "sampling" technique in other laboratory sciences. In pulmonary function testing, sampling refers to procedures used to obtain patient data. These include eliciting maximal effort and cooperation from the patient, as well as the correct performance of the equipment. Applying objective criteria to determine the validity of data is one means of providing high-quality results.

■ USING CRITERIA FOR ACCEPTABILITY

Criteria for assessing the validity of each test have been described in Chapters 2 through 8. Standards for pulmonary function testing have been published by the ATS, European Respiratory Society, British Thoracic Society, and American Association for Respiratory Care. Criteria for acceptability have three primary uses:

1. To provide a basis for decision making during testing. Standards or guidelines can be used to decide whether equipment is functioning properly, whether the patient is giving maximal effort, or whether testing should be continued or repeated. Standardized

criteria also help to characterize the types of problems known to occur during specific tests (e.g., poor effort, etc.).

2. To evaluate validity of pulmonary function data from an individual patient. Criteria may be applied either by the technologist performing the test, by computer software, or by the clinician responsible for interpretation. This may consist of assigning a grade or a code to individual efforts or tests.

3. To score or evaluate the performance of the technologist. Many pulmonary function tests, especially spirometry, depend on the interaction between technologist and patient. Criteria for acceptability can be used to gauge the performance of individual technologists and to provide objective feedback.

Implementation of a quality assurance program in the pulmonary function laboratory should use acceptability criteria during testing, both to evaluate individual tests and to rate technologists. For each of these, certain procedures will be similar:

Examine Printed Tracings or Displayed Graphics Whenever Available

Compare the observed tracing with the characteristics of an acceptable curve or pattern. Computer graphic displays make this particularly easy. Graphics may be superimposed or displayed side-by-side to assess patient effort and cooperation. Similarly, expected values can be displayed graphically along with each individual effort. The user should be able to modify the graphic display (e.g., change graphing scale) to allow for extremes such as very low flows or volumes. During testing, graphs of multiple efforts should be available. Storage of graphic data (all acceptable maneuvers) may be useful for assessing data quality after testing has been completed.

Look at Numerical Data

Are the highest values of multiple efforts within the accepted range of reproducibility? The decision to perform additional maneuvers is usually based on reproducibility. Many manufacturers provide software that applies standard guidelines for reproducibility. Data from multiple efforts should be maintained during testing to allow selection of appropriate results for the final report. Storage of all data may be necessary for subsequent review or editing.

Evaluate Key Indicators

Most pulmonary function tests have one or two features that determine whether the test was performed acceptably. For spirometry, the start of test and duration of effort are key indicators. For gas dilution lung volumes, absence of leaks and test duration are key indicators. For $DL_{CO}sb$, inspired volumes and breath-hold times are important. Key indicators vary with the methodology used for specific tests. In each instance, the important indicator should be assessed in relation to an accepted standard. During testing, these indicators help to determine whether additional patient instruction or tests are needed. Key indicators are also useful in assessing what factors might influence the interpretation of the test (e.g., the patient was unable to blow out for 6 seconds).

Check for Consistent Results

The results of various tests should be consistent with the clinical history and presentation of the patient. Spirometry, lung volumes, DL_{CO}, and blood gas values should all suggest a similar interpretation for a specific diagnosis. Discrepancies among tests may indicate a technical problem rather than a clinical condition.

■ TECHNOLOGIST'S COMMENTS

Scoring or grading the quality of a patient's test is an important component of quality assurance for pulmonary function testing. The technologist administering the test can accomplish this by adding notes. Some automated spirometers use software that grades test performance or that includes codes denoting problems with the test. Evaluation of spirometry, lung volumes, DL_{CO}, and any other tests performed should be included.

The technologist's comments or notes can usually be added to the test results. The commentary should be based on standardized criteria. If a particular test meets all criteria, that fact should be stated. Failure to meet any of the laboratory's criteria should be documented as well. The reason the patient was unable to perform the test acceptably should be explained whenever possible. Failure to meet criteria for acceptability does not necessarily invalidate a test. For some patients, their best performance may fail one or more of the criteria. Table 11-6 lists examples of statements that may be used to document test quality.

TABLE 11-6 Technologist's Comments*

Test	Comments
Spirometry	Meets all ATS recommendations.
	Poor start of test or patient effort.
	Expiration did not last 6 seconds, or there was no obvious plateau.
	Back-extrapolated volume was >5% of FVC.
	Patient was unable to continue to exhale because of _____.
	Two best FVC maneuvers were not within 200 ml.
	Two best FEV_1 maneuvers were not within 200 ml.
	MVV does not correlate with FEV_1.
Lung volumes (gas dilution)	Lung volumes by _____ (method) _____ were performed acceptably.
	Lung volumes reported were the average of ____(n)____ FRC determinations.
	Slow VC was (greater/less) than FVC (____ %).
	Lung volumes by gas dilution were unacceptable because of a leak.
	Equilibration not reached within 7 minutes—He dilution.
	Alveolar N_2 >1.5% after 7 minutes—N_2 washout.
Plethysmography	All plethysmographic measurements were performed acceptably.
	V_{TG} tangents were variable.
	Raw tangents were variable.
	Patient was unable to pant at the correct frequency.
DL_{CO}sb	Meets all ATS recommendations.
	DL_{CO} reported is average of ____(n)____ maneuvers.
	DL_{CO} corrected for an Hb of _____.
	Inspired volume <90% of best vital capacity (_____ %).
	Breath-hold time not within 9 to 11 seconds (_____ seconds).
	DL_{CO} values not within 3 ml CO/min/mm Hg or 10%.
	DL_{CO} not corrected for Hb or COHb.

*Values in parentheses may be filled in with appropriate values from the patient's data.

The technologist's comments should be added to the final report. Many automated systems provide for "free text" comments to be included with tabular data. Some software supports "canned text" functions that allow predetermined statements (Table 11-6) to be entered with a single keystroke. The technologist's name or initials should be included.

Some computerized spirometer systems automatically score FVC maneuvers. The score may be indicated by a letter or numeric code that is attached to each maneuver. For example, an FVC maneuver that meets all criteria (e.g., start-of-test) might be scored with an "A." Other systems allow the technologist to select a user-defined code to attach to individual maneuvers. Both techniques can be used to provide feedback that enhances quality assurance.

TECHNOLOGIST'S FEEDBACK

A well-trained and highly motivated technologist is a key component for obtaining valid data, particularly in tests that require patient instruction and encouragement. A quality assurance program based on established criteria for acceptability and reproducibility can be used to provide feedback on test performance to individual technologists.

Routine review of tests performed by each technologist is recommended. If criteria for acceptability have been recorded (as described in this section), these can be evaluated against raw data to determine the accuracy of results. This information forms the basis for reinforcing superior performance or correcting identified problems. Feedback should include the type and extent of unacceptable or nonreproducible tests. Feedback should also include what corrective action can be taken to improve performance.

Infection Control and Safety

Pulmonary function tests, including blood gas analysis, often involve patients with blood-borne or respiratory pathogens. Reasonable precautions applied to testing techniques and equipment handling can prevent cross-contamination among patients. Similar techniques can prevent infection of the technologist performing the tests.

POLICIES AND PROCEDURES

Each laboratory should have written guidelines defining safety and infection control practices. The guidelines should be part of a policy and procedure manual (Table 11-1). Procedures should include, but not be limited to, handwashing techniques, use of protective equipment such as laboratory coats and gloves, and guidelines for equipment cleaning. The handling of contaminated materials (e.g., waste blood) should be clearly described. Policies and procedures should include education of technologists regarding proper handling of biologic hazards. Department policies and procedures should be consistent with those mandated by individual hospitals or institutions. Most accrediting agencies require written plans for safety, waste management, and chemical hygiene. In the United States, the Occupational Safety and Health Administration (OSHA) has published strict guidelines regarding handling of blood and other medical waste (see Appendix D).

PULMONARY FUNCTION TESTS

Pulmonary function testing does not present a significant risk of infection for patients or technologists. However, some potential hazards are involved. Most respiratory pathogens are spread by either direct contact with contaminated equipment or by an airborne route.

Airborne organisms may be contained in droplet nuclei, on epithelial cells that have been shed, or in dust particles. The following guidelines can help reduce the possibility of cross-contamination or infection:

1. Disposable mouthpieces and nose clips should be used for spirometry. Reusable mouthpieces should be disinfected or sterilized after each use. Proper handwashing should be done immediately after direct contact with mouthpieces or valves. Gloves should be worn when handling potentially contaminated equipment. Hands should always be washed between patients.
2. Tubing or valves through which subjects rebreathe should be changed after each test. Any equipment that shows visual condensation from expired gas should be disinfected before reuse. This is particularly important for maneuvers such as the FVC, where there is a potential for mucus, saliva, or droplet nuclei to contaminate the device. Breathing circuit components should be stored in sealed plastic bags after disinfection.
3. Spirometers should be cleaned according to the manufacturer's recommendations. The frequency of cleaning should be appropriate for the number of tests performed. For open-circuit systems, only that part of the circuit through which air is rebreathed needs to be decontaminated between patients. Some flow-based systems offer pneumotachometers that can be changed between patients. These may be advantageous if patients with known respiratory infections must be tested. Pneumotachometers not located proximal to the patient are less likely to be contaminated by mucus, saliva, or droplet nuclei. Disposable flow sensors should not be reused. Volume-displacement spirometers should be flushed using their full volume at least five times between patients. Flushing with room air helps clear droplet nuclei or similar airborne particulates. Water-sealed spirometers should be drained at least weekly, allowed to dry completely, and refilled only with distilled water. Bellows and rolling-seal spirometers may be more difficult to disassemble but should be disinfected on a routine basis. After disassembly and disinfection, the spirometer may require recalibration.
4. Bacteria filters may be used in some circuits to prevent equipment contamination. Systems used for spirometry, lung volumes, and diffusing capacity tests often use breathing manifolds that are susceptible to contamination. Bacteria filters may be used to prevent contamination of these devices. Filters may impose increased resistance, thus affecting measurement of maximal flows. Some types of filters show increased resistance after continued use in expired gas. Spirometers with bacteria filters should be calibrated with the filter in line; the spirometer should meet the minimal recommendations in Table 11-2 with the filter in place. If filters are used for procedures such as lung volume determinations, their volumes must be included in the calculations. Filters may be useful in protecting equipment from contamination when patients with known respiratory pathogens must be tested.
5. Small-volume nebulizers, such as those used for bronchodilator administration or bronchial challenge, offer the greatest potential for cross-contamination. These devices, if reused, should be sterilized to destroy vegetative microorganisms, fungal spores, tubercle bacilli, and some viruses. Disposable single-use nebulizers are preferable but may not be practical for routines such as inhalation challenges. Metered-dose devices may be used for bronchodilator studies by using disposable mouthpieces or "spacers" to prevent colonization of the device.
6. Gloves or other barrier devices minimize the risk of infection for the technologist who must handle mouthpieces, tubing, or valves. The risk of transmission from subjects with hepatitis B, human immunodeficiency virus (HIV), or acquired immunodeficiency syndrome (AIDS) through respiratory secretions is slight. Special precautions should be

taken whenever there is evidence of blood on mouthpieces or tubing. There is a risk of acquiring infections such as tuberculosis or pneumonia caused by *Pneumocystis carinii* from infected patients. A mask should be worn by the technologist when testing subjects who have active tuberculosis or other diseases that can be transmitted by coughing. Masks may be required for "reverse isolation" when testing immunocompromised patients.

7. Patients with respiratory diseases such as tuberculosis may warrant specially ventilated rooms, particularly if many individuals need testing. Risk of cross-contamination or infection can be greatly reduced by filtering and increasing the exchange rate of air in the testing room. Equipment can be reserved for testing only infected patients. Patients with known pathogens can also be tested in their own room or at the end of the day (to facilitate equipment decontamination).

8. Surveillance should include routine cultures of reusable components, such as mouthpieces, tubing, and valves, after disinfection.

BLOOD GASES

The Centers for Disease Control and Prevention (CDC) has established universal precautions that apply to personnel handling blood or other body fluids containing blood. Universal precautions apply to blood, semen, vaginal secretions, cerebrospinal fluid, synovial fluid, pleural fluid, pericardial fluid, and amniotic fluid. Some of these fluids are commonly encountered in the blood gas laboratory. These fluids present a significant risk to the health care worker. Hepatitis B, HIV, and other blood-borne pathogens must be assumed to be present in these fluids.

PF *Tips*

The two most important practices for infection control in the pulmonary function laboratory are *proper use of gloves* and *handwashing*. Gloves should be worn any time blood is handled or drawn, including handling of blood-tinged mouthpieces. Handwashing is essential to prevent cross-contamination. Hands should be washed between patient contacts; any time mouthpieces, tubing, or nebulizers are handled; and when gloves are removed.

Body fluids to which the universal precautions do not apply include feces, nasal secretions, sputum, sweat, tears, urine, and vomitus, unless they contain visible blood. Some of these fluids may be encountered in the pulmonary function laboratory. These fluids present an extremely low or nonexistent risk for HIV or hepatitis B. However, they are potential sources for nosocomial infections from other non–blood-borne pathogens. Universal precautions do not apply to saliva, but infection control practices such as use of gloves and handwashing further minimize the risk involved in contact with mucous membranes of the mouth.

These universal precautions should be applied in the pulmonary function and/or blood gas laboratory:

1. Treat *all* blood and body fluid specimens as potentially contaminated.
2. Exercise care to prevent injuries from needles, scalpels, or other sharp instruments. Do not resheath used needles by hand. If a needle must be resheathed, use a one-handed technique or a device that holds the sheath. Do not remove used, unprotected needles from disposable syringes by hand. Do not bend, break, or otherwise manipulate used

needles by hand. Use a rubber block or cork to obstruct used needles after arterial punctures. Use needle safety devices (now used in almost all blood gas kits) as described by the manufacturer. Place used syringes and needles, scalpel blades, and other sharp items in puncture-resistant containers. Locate the containers as close as possible to the area of use.

3. Use protective barriers to prevent exposure to blood, body fluids containing visible blood, and other fluids to which universal precautions apply. Examples of protective barriers include gloves, gowns, laboratory coats, masks, and protective eyewear. Gloves should be worn when drawing blood samples, whether from a needle puncture or an indwelling catheter. Gloves cannot prevent penetrating injuries caused by needles or sharp objects. Gloves are also indicated if the technologist has cuts, scratches, or other breaks in the skin. Protective barriers should be used in situations where contamination with blood may occur. These situations include obtaining blood samples from an uncooperative patient, performing finger-heel sticks on infants, and receiving training in blood drawing. Examination gloves should be worn for procedures involving contact with mucous membranes. Masks, gowns, and protective goggles may be indicated for procedures that present a possibility of blood splashing. Blood splashing may occur during arterial line placement or when drawing samples from arterial catheters.

4. Wear gloves while performing blood gas analysis. Laboratory coats or aprons that are resistant to liquids should also be worn. Protective eyewear may be necessary if there is risk of blood splashing during specimen handling. Maintenance of blood gas analyzers, such as repair of electrodes and emptying of waste containers, should be performed wearing similar protective gear. Laboratory coats or aprons should be left in the specimen handling area. Blood waste products (e.g., blood gas syringes) should be discarded in clearly marked biohazard containers.

5. Immediately and thoroughly wash hands and other skin surfaces that are contaminated with blood or other fluids to which the universal precautions apply. Hands should be washed after removing gloves. Blood spills should be cleaned up using a solution of 1 part 5% sodium hypochlorite (bleach) in 9 parts of water. Bleach should also be used to rinse sinks used for blood disposal.

Summary

This chapter focuses on various elements of quality assurance as applied to pulmonary function testing. Calibration of spirometers, gas analyzers, and body plethysmographs is discussed. Special emphasis is placed on techniques to ensure that pulmonary function equipment meets established standards of accuracy. QC methods are reviewed, including the use of large-volume syringes and biologic controls.

Calibration and QC of blood gas analyzers are discussed, as well as advantages and disadvantages of automated calibration. Basic statistical concepts commonly used in laboratory situations are covered, including the application of multiple control rules.

Testing technique is a key element in ensuring the validity of pulmonary function data. Some guidelines for applying acceptability criteria (as listed throughout the text) are given. These include decision making during testing, assessing test quality for interpretive purposes, and providing feedback on technologist performance.

Infection control and safety issues are also presented. Cleaning of spirometers and related equipment, along with techniques to avoid cross-contamination, are listed. Universal precautions applicable to blood gas analysis and pulmonary function testing are reviewed. Case studies and self-assessment questions are also included.

CASE STUDIES

CASE 11-1

This case concerns the use of blood gas QC to detect analytical errors.

HISTORY

F.F. is a 30-year-old man referred for pulmonary function testing and arterial blood gas analysis as part of a 5-year physical examination required by his fire district. He has no extraordinary symptoms or history suggestive of pulmonary disease. He has never smoked. He performed all portions of the spirometry, lung volumes, and DL_{CO} maneuvers acceptably. All results were within normal limits for his age and height. Arterial blood gases were drawn for analysis.

Blood gases	(FIO_2 0.21)
pH	7.41
$PaCO_2$ (mm Hg)	39
PaO_2 (mm Hg)	54
SaO_2 (%)	96.0
COHb (%)	1.2
HCO_3^- (mEq/L)	24.1

Because of the low PaO_2 in an otherwise normal patient and because SaO_2 measured independently by co-oximetry showed normal saturation, the PO_2 electrode of the automated blood gas analyzer was questioned.

A review of the two most recent automatic calibrations revealed the following:

	Calibration	Expected	Drift
9 AM			
pH	7.387	7.384	0.003
PCO_2 (mm Hg)	39.1	38.6	0.5
PO_2 (mm Hg)	132	140.1	−8.1
10 AM			
pH	7.383	7.384	−0.001
PCO_2 (mm Hg)	38.4	38.6	−0.2
PO_2 (mm Hg)	151.2	140.1	11.1

For each automatic calibration, the instrument analyzes a calibration gas or buffer and compares the measured value with an expected value. Drift is the amount of adjustment applied to a particular electrode to bring it within calibration limits. The excessive drift exhibited by the PO_2 electrode prompted a review of the most recent QC runs performed on the analyzer.

Blood Gas Quality Control (Five Most Recent Runs)

Control	Mean (mm Hg)	SD	Runs 1	2	3	4	5
Level A	45	±2.1	46	47	49	42	50
Level B	100	±2.0	101	99	97	96	105
Level C	150	±3.1	147	151	151	149	143

*Control runs performed every 8 hours.

QUESTIONS

1. Why is the patient's Po_2 so low?
2. What is the interpretation of the 9 AM and 10 AM automated calibrations for the blood gas analyzer?
3. What do the routine QC runs show?
4. What corrective action, if any, is necessary?

DISCUSSION

Cause of the Low Po_2

The findings in this case regarding O_2-electrode function are not unusual. An abnormally low Pao_2 in an otherwise healthy person with normal lung function suggested that an analytical error might have occurred. If the patient had presented with evidence of lung disease or abnormalities in his pulmonary function test, the inaccuracy of the Pao_2 might have gone unnoticed or led to inappropriate therapy.

Automatic Blood Gas Analyzer Calibrations

Excessive drift of the oxygen electrode should have prompted the immediate attention of the technologist performing the blood gas analyses. A common problem with automated analyzers is their apparent simplicity. Because calibrations are performed automatically, corrections that the analyzer makes may be overlooked. Automated analyzers adjust the zero and gain of each electrode to correct for small changes that occur in electrode performance. These small changes may be caused by a buildup of protein at the tip, electrolyte depletion, or slight temperature alterations. If there is a large change in electrode performance, the instrument attempts to correct the electrode's output just as it would for small changes that occur normally. Some automated analyzers flag a large drift in electrode performance as an error, whereas others simply report the drift. In this case, the reported drifts signaled that the Po_2 electrode was fluctuating markedly. One calibration reading was high, and the next one read lower than the expected value.

Quality Controls

The change in electrode performance should have been detected by the routine QC run before the excessive drift was observed during automatic calibration. Blood gas QC used in this laboratory consisted of multiple levels of control materials. Means and SDs had been determined for each level.

Examination of control runs 1 through 4 reveal acceptable electrode performance. All values are within ±2 SDs of the mean. Run 5 (the most recent run) shows values that are all 2 SDs or more away from the mean. These control results may be expected to occur 5% of the time simply because of the random error associated with sampling. If run 5 is compared with the previous 4 runs and multiple rules are applied (see Calibration and Quality Control of Blood Gas Analyzers section), the electrode is clearly out of control. When multiple levels of controls are evaluated, more than one control value outside of the 2-SD limit suggests an out-of-control situation. For both levels A and B, there is a change of 4 SDs from run 4 to run 5. Changes of this magnitude are not consistent with random error and are detected only when a control history is kept. Similarly, there are inconsistencies within run 5 across the three levels of controls. Levels A and B both show control values that are more than 2 SDs *above* their respective means, whereas level C shows a value that is more than 2 SDs *below* its mean. This pattern suggests fluctuating electrode performance, as displayed during the automatic calibrations that followed.

Corrective Action

The Po_2 electrode was removed from the instrument. A new membrane was installed after the tip was polished with an abrasive to expose the platinum cathode. The electrode was refilled with fresh electrolyte. The instrument was recalibrated, and multiple levels of controls were repeated. All Po_2 values fell within 2 SDs of the established mean. The patient's blood, which had been kept in an ice-water bath, was reanalyzed, and a Pao_2 value of 89 mm Hg was obtained.

CASE 11-2

This case addresses the use of biologic controls in the pulmonary function laboratory.

HISTORY

Pulmonary function studies are performed on three consecutive patients, each of whom has a chief complaint of shortness of breath. The following data are obtained:

	Patient 1	Patient 2	Patient 3
FVC	4.04 (101%)	5.22 (97%)	3.90 (83%)
FEV_1	3.51 (99%)	4.10 (103%)	3.12 (82%)
$FEV_1\%$	87%	79%	80%
TLC	5.11 (98%)	6.96 (100%)	5.01 (81%)
DL_{CO}	14.3 (69%)	18.2 (65%)	10.2 (50%)

The pulmonary function technologist notices that each patient has apparently normal spirometry and lung volumes, but their DL_{CO} values are reduced.

QUESTIONS

1. Is the reduction in DL_{CO} representative of the actual lung function of each patient, or has a technical problem occurred?
2. What can be done to evaluate the accuracy of the DL_{CO} system?
3. What (if anything) needs to be done to correct the problem?

DISCUSSION

Has a Technical Problem Occurred?

This type of situation arises frequently in the pulmonary function laboratory when patients with possible pulmonary disease are being evaluated. The technologist is this case noticed a pattern in which three patients all had apparently normal results from spirometry and lung volume measurements but displayed reduced DL_{CO} values. Careful attention to inconsistencies in different categories of tests can often point to technical problems with spirometers, gas analyzers, or software. In this case, it is difficult to determine whether the low DL_{CO} values are due to physiologic abnormality or a technical problem with the DL_{CO} system.

Evaluating the DL_{CO} System

The first step in assessing a possible technical problem would be to look for problems with the measurement system. In this case, pretest calibrations and all other system functions were acceptable. This laboratory used a monthly program of testing laboratory personnel as biologic controls.

Each of three technologists performed spirometry, lung volumes, and DL_{CO} measurements on one another to establish representative means and standard deviations. The technologist in this case tested one of her co-workers before performing any further tests on patients. A DL_{CO} value of 26.8 ml CO/min/mm Hg (mean of two acceptable maneuvers) was obtained from the biologic control. The biologic control's DL_{CO} had been established as 27.1 ± 1.5 ml CO/min/mm Hg from a series of 10 previous measurements. This simple comparison suggests that the DL_{CO} values obtained from the three patients in question were most likely accurate.

What Needs to Be Done?

The use of a biologic control in this case demonstrated that the DL_{CO} system was functioning properly. This suggests that the low DL_{CO} values obtained from three apparently normal patients represent real physiologic abnormalities. Further testing of patients 1 and 2 revealed that both had significant anemia, and that patient 2 also had an elevated COHb from smoking. Patient 3 had been taking an antiarrhythmic medication for several months, which may have caused the reduction in DL_{CO}.

■ SELF-ASSESSMENT QUESTIONS

Entry-level

1. *Three injections using a 3-L syringe are required to calibrate a flow-sensing spirometer. The calibration produces the following results:*

   First injection: 2.99 L
   Second injection: 2.96 L
   Third injection: 2.94 L

   Which of the following best describes these results?

   a. Spirometer performance is acceptable.
   b. Spirometer shows excessive drift.
   c. Volume is being corrected to BTPS.
   d. Volumes were injected too rapidly.

2. *QC is performed on a blood gas analyzer. The Po_2 electrode shows the following results when plotted on a QC chart (Levy-Jennings):*

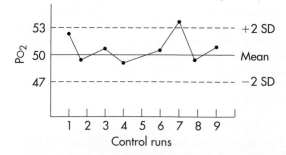

   Which of the following best describes the result of control run 8?

   a. Normal electrode performance
   b. A random error
   c. A trend
   d. An out-of-control situation

3. *A 3-L syringe is used to calibrate a dry rolling-seal spirometer; the spirometer reads a volume of 2.97 L. The software correction factor for this system would be:*

   a. Outside of acceptable limits
   b. 1.01
   c. 0.99
   d. +0.03

4. *Which of the following precautions should the pulmonary function technologist observe when drawing an arterial blood sample?*

   a. Determine if protective barriers are needed by checking the patient's history
   b. Carefully resheath used needles using the original protective covering
   c. Wear gloves while drawing and analyzing the blood
   d. Dispose of used needles in red plastic bags marked "biohazard"

5. *A patient performs eight FVC maneuvers, and these results are recorded from the three best efforts:*

	Trial 5	Trial 6	Trial 8
FVC (L)	5.0	5.1	4.7
FEV$_1$ (L)	1.9	1.6	1.8
PEF (L/sec)	3.7	4.4	3.9

Which of the following are appropriate to report in the technologist's comments?

a. "Spirometry meets all ATS criteria."
b. "FVC is not reproducible."
c. "FEV$_1$ is not reproducible."
d. "Peak flow is not reproducible."

Advanced

6. *According to ATS recommendations, diagnostic spirometers should have a range and accuracy of:*

a. 0 to 14 L with less than 1.5 cm H$_2$O/L/sec resistance
b. 0.5 to 8 L ±3% of reading or ±0.05 L, whichever is greater
c. 0.5 to 6 L ±5% of reading or ±0.1 L, whichever is greater
d. 0 to 5 L ±3% of reading or ±0.05 L, whichever is greater

7. *A biologic control subject performs multiple FVC maneuvers to check the accuracy of a portable spirometer. The control's established FVC is 4.90 L with an SD of 0.15 L. The following values are obtained from the control:*

Effort 1: 4.55 L
Effort 2: 4.45 L
Effort 3: 4.49 L

Based on these findings, the pulmonary function technologist should conclude that:

a. The portable spirometer values were corrected to BTPS.
b. Spirometer accuracy is questionable.
c. The control's efforts were submaximal.
d. Spirometer performance is within acceptable statistical limits.

8. *A pulmonary function technologist wants to check the linearity of an He analyzer used for closed-circuit FRC determinations. Which of the following should be used?*

a. A gas mixture containing 10% He, and room air
b. Gas mixtures of 10% He and 5% He
c. Gas mixtures of 5% He and 15% He
d. A gas mixture of 10% He, and a 3-L syringe

9. *Which of the following are true regarding infection control of pulmonary function equipment?*

I. Reusable mouthpieces should be disinfected between patients.
II. Bacteria filters should be removed before calibration.
III. Volume-displacement spirometers do not require cleaning.
IV. Tubing or valves through which the patient rebreathes should be changed between patients.
   a. I and II
   b. III and IV
   c. I and IV
   d. I, II, and IV

10. *QC of a body plethysmograph is performed using two biologic controls with the following results:*

	Expected V$_{TG}$	Quality Control V$_{TG}$
Biologic control 1	4.81	4.75
Biologic control 2	3.60	3.70

Based on these findings, the pulmonary function technologist should conclude that:

a. There is a leak in the door seal.
b. The box pressure transducer is malfunctioning.
c. Mouth pressure calibration was performed incorrectly.
d. The box is functioning acceptably.

SELECTED BIBLIOGRAPHY

General References

American Thoracic Society: *Pulmonary function laboratory management and procedure manual,* New York, 2002, American Thoracic Society.

Ruppel GL: Spirometry, *Respir Care Clin North Am* 3: 155-181, 1997.

Wanger J: Quality assurance, *Respir Care Clin North Am* 3:273-289, 1997.

Calibration and Quality Control

Hankinson JL: Pulmonary function testing in the screening of workers: guidelines for instrumentation, performance, and interpretation, *J Occup Med* 28:1081, 1986.

Kozlowski-Templin R: Blood gas analyzers, *Respir Care Clin North Am* 1:35-46, 1995.

Leary ET, Graham G, Kenny MA: Commercially available blood-gas quality controls compared with tonometered blood, *Clin Chem* 26:1309, 1980.

Leith DE, Mead J: *Principles of body plethysmography,* Bethesda, Md, 1974, National Heart, Lung, and Blood Institute, Division of Lung Diseases.

Linn WS, Solomon JC, Gong H Jr, et al: Standardization of multiple spirometers at widely separated times and places, *Am J Respir Crit Care Med* 153:1309-1313, 1996.

Olafsdottir E, Westgard JO, Ehrmeyer SS, et al: Matrix effects and the performance and selection of quality-control procedures to monitor Po_2 measurements, *Clin Chem* 42:392-396, 1996.

Westgard JO, Groth T, Aronsson T, et al: Performance characteristics of rules for internal quality control: probabilities for false rejection and error detection, *Clin Chem* 23:1857, 1977.

Westgard JO, Stein B, Westgard SA, et al: QC Validator 2.0: a computer program for automatic selection of statistical QC procedures for applications in healthcare laboratories, *Comput Methods Programs Biomed* 53:175-186, 1997.

Criteria for Acceptability of Pulmonary Function Studies

Enright PL, Johnson LJ, Connett JE, et al: Spirometry in the Lung Health Study: methods and quality control, *Am Rev Respir Dis* 143:1215-1223, 1991.

Ferris BG, ed: Epidemiology standardization project: recommended standardized procedures for pulmonary function testing, *Am Rev Respir Dis* 118(suppl 2):55, 1978.

Gardner RM, Clausen JL, Crapo RO, et al: Quality assurance in pulmonary function laboratories, *Am Rev Respir Dis* 134:626-627, 1986.

Gardner RM, Clausen JL, Epler GR, et al: Pulmonary function laboratory personnel qualifications, *Am Rev Respir Dis* 134:623-624, 1986.

Malmstrom K, Peszek I, Al Botto, et al: Quality assurance of asthma clinical trials, *Control Clin Trials* 23:143-156, 2002.

Infection Control

Centers for Disease Control and Prevention: Guidelines for preventing the transmission of *Mycobacterium tuberculosis* in health care facilities, *MMWR Morb Mortal Wkly Rep* 43:1-132, 1994.

Centers for Disease Control and Prevention: Recommendations for preventing transmission of human immunodeficiency virus and hepatitis B virus to patients during exposure-prone invasive procedures, *MMWR Recomm Rep* 40:1-9, 1991.

Centers for Disease Control and Prevention: Recommendations for prevention of HIV transmission in healthcare settings, *MMWR Morb Mortal Wkly Rep* 36:3S, 1987.

Garner JS, Favero MS: CDC guidelines for the prevention and control of nosocomial infections: guideline for handwashing and hospital environmental control, *Am J Infect Control* 14:110, 1986.

Johns DP, Ingram C, Booth H, et al: Effect of a microaerosol barrier filter on the measurement of lung function, *Chest* 107:1045-1048, 1995.

NIOSH: *Preventing needlestick injuries in health care settings,* DHHS (NIOSH) Publication No 2000-108, 1999.

Rutala DR, Rutala WA, Weber DR, et al: Infection risks associated with spirometry, *Infect Control Hospital Epidemiol* 12:89-92, 1991.

Tablan OC, Williams WW, Martone WJ: Infection control in pulmonary function laboratories, *Infect Control* 6:442, 1985.

Standards and Guidelines

American Association for Respiratory Care: Clinical practice guideline: blood gas analysis and hemoximetry: 2001 revision and update, *Respir Care* 46:498-505, 2001.

American Association for Respiratory Care: Clinical practice guideline: body plethysmography: 2001 revision and update, *Respir Care* 46:506-513, 2001.

American Association for Respiratory Care: Clinical practice guideline: sampling for arterial blood gas analysis, *Respir Care* 37:913-917, 1992.

American Association for Respiratory Care: Clinical practice guideline: spirometry, 1996 update, *Respir Care* 41:629-636, 1996.

American Association for Respiratory Care: Clinical practice guideline: static lung volumes 2001 revision and update, *Respir Care* 46:531-539, 2001.

American Association for Respiratory Care: Single-breath carbon monoxide diffusing capacity, 1999 update, *Respir Care* 44:539-546, 1999.

American Thoracic Society: Single-breath carbon monoxide diffusing capacity (transfer factor): recommendations for a standard technique—1995 update, *Am J Respir Crit Care Med* 152:2185-2198, 1995.

American Thoracic Society: Standardization of spirometry—1994 update, *Am J Respir Crit Care Med* 152:1107-1136, 1995.

British Thoracic Society and Association of Respiratory Technicians and Physiologists: Topical review: guidelines for the measurement of respiratory function, *Respir Med* 88:165-194, 1994.

National Committee for Clinical Laboratory Standards (NCCLS): *Protection of laboratory workers from infectious disease transmitted by blood, body fluids, and tissue,* ed 2, Publication M29-T2, 1992.

Quanjer PH, Tammeling GJ, Cotes JE, et al: Lung volumes and forced ventilatory flows: report of the working party, standardization of lung function tests; European Community for Steel and Coal—official statement of the European Respiratory Society, *Eur Respir* J6(suppl 16):9-40, 1993.

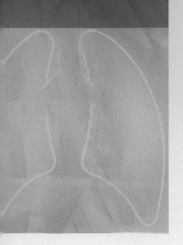

APPENDIX A

ANSWERS TO SELF-ASSESSMENT QUESTIONS

Chapter 1

■ ENTRY-LEVEL

1. d
2. b
3. c
4. b
5. c
6. d
7. c
8. c

■ ADVANCED

9. d
10. c
11. a
12. c
13. b
14. c

Chapter 2

■ ENTRY-LEVEL

1. c
2. b
3. b
4. c
5. c
6. b
7. d

■ ADVANCED

8. c
9. c
10. b
11. b
12. b
13. c
14. d

Chapter 3

■ ENTRY-LEVEL

1. b
2. a
3. c
4. c
5. a
6. d

■ ADVANCED

7. c
8. d
9. b
10. b
11. c
12. a

Chapter 4

ENTRY-LEVEL

1. c
2. a
3. c
4. d
5. b

ADVANCED

6. d
7. c
8. d
9. a
10. a

Chapter 5

ENTRY-LEVEL

1. c
2. b
3. c
4. c
5. b

ADVANCED

6. c
7. d
8. d
9. a
10. b

Chapter 6

ENTRY-LEVEL

1. b
2. a
3. c
4. c

ADVANCED

5. a
6. a
7. d
8. d
9. c
10. b

Chapter 7

ENTRY-LEVEL

1. c
2. b
3. c
4. b
5. b
6. d

ADVANCED

7. d
8. c
9. c
10. d
11. c
12. a

Chapter 8

ENTRY-LEVEL AND ADVANCED

1. c
2. d
3. a
4. c
5. d
6. d
7. c
8. a
9. d
10. d

Chapter 9

ENTRY-LEVEL

1. b
2. d
3. a
4. d
5. b

ADVANCED

6. c
7. b
8. d
9. d
10. d

Chapter 10

ENTRY-LEVEL

1. a
2. c
3. b
4. d
5. c
6. d
7. d
8. a

ADVANCED

9. b
10. b
11. b
12. d
13. b
14. d
15. d

Chapter 11

ENTRY-LEVEL

1. a
2. a
3. b
4. c
5. a

ADVANCED

6. b
7. b
8. d
9. c
10. d

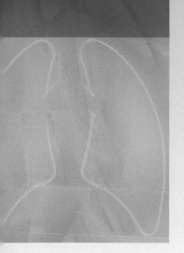

APPENDIX B

REFERENCE VALUES

Typical Values for Pulmonary Function Tests

Values are for a healthy young male, 1.7 m² body surface area.

Test	Value
Lung Volumes (BTPS)	
IC	3.60 L
ERV	1.20 L
VC	4.80 L
RV	1.20 L
FRC	2.40 L
V_{TG}	2.40 L
TLC	6.00 L
$(RV/TLC) \times 100$	20%
Ventilation (BTPS)	
V_T	0.50 L
Frequency	12 breaths/min
$\dot{V}_E$	6.00 L/min
V_D	0.15 L
$\dot{V}_A$	4.20 L/min
V_D/V_T	0.30
Pulmonary Mechanics	
FVC	4.80 L
FEV_1	4.00 L
$FEV_{1\%}$	83%
$FEF_{25\%-75\%}$	4.7 L/sec
$\dot{V}_{max50\%}$	5.0 L/sec
PEF	10.0 L/sec
MVV	160 L/min
C_L	0.2 L/cm H_2O
C_{LT}	0.1 L/cm H_2O

Test	Value
Raw	1.5 cm H_2O/L/sec
SGaw	0.25 L/sec/cm H_2O
MIP	130 cm H_2O
MEP	250 cm H_2O
Gas Distribution	
$\Delta N_{2_{750-1250}}$	<1.5% N_2
7-minute N_2	<2.5% N_2
Diffusion	
$DL_{CO}sb$	25 ml CO/min/mm Hg
DL/V_A	4.2 ml CO/min/mm Hg/L
Blood Gases and Related Tests	
pH	7.40
Pa_{CO_2}	40 mm Hg
HCO_3^-	24.0 mEq/L
Pa_{O_2}	95 mm Hg
Sa_{O_2}	97%
COHb	<1.5%
MetHb	<1.5%
$\dot{Q}_s/\dot{Q}_T$	<7%

Selecting and Using Reference Values

Reference values for pulmonary function tests are derived by statistical analysis of a group of normal individuals. These individuals are classified as *normal* (i.e., healthy) because they have no history of lung disease in themselves or their families. Minimal exposure to risk factors, such as smoking or environmental pollution, is usually considered in selecting these individuals.

All pulmonary function measurements vary in healthy individuals. Some tests vary much more than others. Arterial pH and Pa_{CO_2} have a very narrow range in healthy individuals. However, $FEF_{25\%-75\%}$ may vary by as much as ±2 L/sec. This variability becomes important when measured values are compared with reference values. Most measurements *regress;* that is, they vary in a predictable way in relation to one or more physical factors. The physical characteristics that most influence pulmonary function are as follows:

- Age
- Sex
- Height (standing/sitting)
- Race or ethnic origin
- Weight or body surface area

The altitude at which individuals reside may also influence their lung function. By analyzing each pulmonary function variable in regard to the individual's physical characteristics, regression equations can be generated to predict the expected value. Most regression analyses presume that lung function changes are linearly related to physical characteristics such as age and height. This may not be true in individuals who are very old or young, or very tall or short.

Race or ethnic origin influences stature and body proportions. Lung function, particularly lung volumes and diffusing capacity (DL_{CO}), differs significantly among races. Some computerized pulmonary function systems apply a "correction factor" to reference values for Whites to adjust expected values for a different race. Although differences in lung function among races are well documented, no single correction factor is applicable to all measurements. Some laboratories reduce reference values for volumes (e.g., FVC, TLC) by factors of 10% to 15% for African Americans. Separate regression equations derived from healthy individuals of each race tested are preferred. Race-specific reference values should be used if they are representative of the population the laboratory tests.

Several methods for applying reference values are used:

- Tables
- Nomograms
- Graphs
- Regression equations

When a computer is unavailable, tables, nomograms, or graphs may be used. Figures B-1 and B-2 are examples of nomograms used to obtain a reference value. A ruler is placed so that it intersects the height and age scales for the individual. The expected values can then be read from points where the ruler crosses the other scales. Figures B-3, B-4, and B-5 are graphs that may be used to obtain reference values for children. In these figures, lung function is graphed against height. The use of computers (or calculators) allows regression equations to be available in software. In most automated systems, the user selects sets of prediction equations best suited to the population being tested. Some software allows the user to enter or modify prediction equations. This provides a means of using new reference equations as they become available.

Establishing a lower limit of normal is done in one of several ways. Some clinicians use a fixed percentage of the reference value to determine the degree of abnormality. The measured value is divided by the reference value and multiplied by 100. Plus or minus 20% is often used as the limit of normal. This method is simple. It approximates lower limits of normal for adults of average age and height for FVC and FEV_1. Eighty percent of predicted is close to the fifth percentile in these individuals. Using a fixed percentage results in shorter, older individuals being classified as abnormal. Taller, younger individuals may be erroneously classified as normal, even though they have disease. Using a fixed percentage of reference produces erroneous lower limits for $FEF_{25\%-75\%}$ and for instantaneous flows ($\dot{V}_{max}$). The lower limit of normal for these flow measurements may be as low as 50% of the predicted value, depending on the reference set used. Fixed percentages may be acceptable in children if the variability is proportional to the predicted "mean" value.

A more precise approach bases the lower limit on the reference value and its variability. If lung function varies in normal fashion (a Gaussian or bell-shaped distribution curve), the mean ±1.96 standard deviations (SDs) defines the 95% confidence limits. Statistically, 95% of the healthy population falls within approximately 2 SDs of the mean. If an individual's measured value is outside of the range defined by his or her mean ±1.96 SDs, there is only a 5% chance that the test is normal. For some pulmonary function variables, only the lower limit of normal (i.e., below the mean) is significant. For example, it is not usually clinically significant if FVC is greater than predicted, only if it is lower. For such variables, 1.65 SDs may be used to define the lower limit of normal. Variables that can be abnormally high or low (e.g., RV, TLC, $Paco_2$) must use the 1.96 SD method.

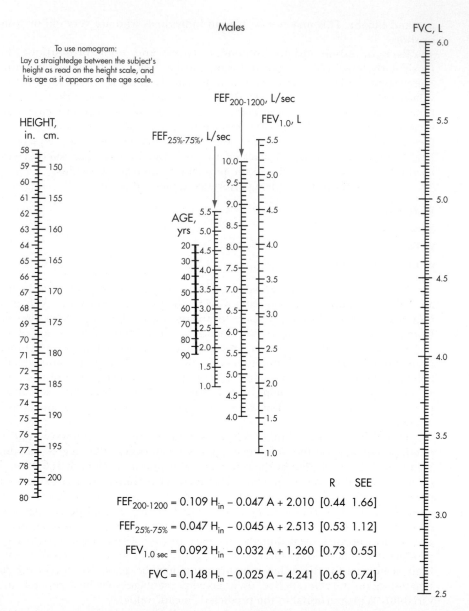

Figure B-1 Prediction nomograms (BTPS), spirometric values in normal males. *(From Morris JF, Koski WA, Johnson LD:* Am Rev Respir Dis *103[1]:57, 1971.)*

FEF$_{200-1200}$ = 0.109 H$_{in}$ − 0.047 A + 2.010 [0.44 1.66]

FEF$_{25\%-75\%}$ = 0.047 H$_{in}$ − 0.045 A + 2.513 [0.53 1.12]

FEV$_{1.0 sec}$ = 0.092 H$_{in}$ − 0.032 A + 1.260 [0.73 0.55]

FVC = 0.148 H$_{in}$ − 0.025 A − 4.241 [0.65 0.74]

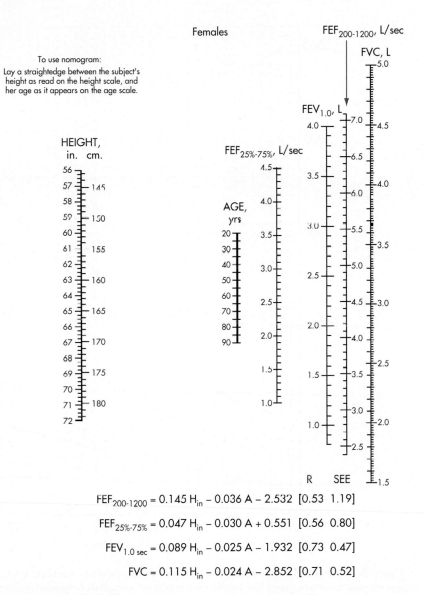

To use nomogram:
Lay a straightedge between the subject's
height as read on the height scale, and
her age as it appears on the age scale.

$FEF_{200\text{-}1200} = 0.145\ H_{in} - 0.036\ A - 2.532\ [0.53\ 1.19]$

$FEF_{25\%\text{-}75\%} = 0.047\ H_{in} - 0.030\ A + 0.551\ [0.56\ 0.80]$

$FEV_{1.0\ sec} = 0.089\ H_{in} - 0.025\ A - 1.932\ [0.73\ 0.47]$

$FVC = 0.115\ H_{in} - 0.024\ A - 2.852\ [0.71\ 0.52]$

Figure B-2 Prediction nomograms (BTPS), spirometric values in normal females. *(From Morris JF, Koski WA, Johnson LD:* Am Rev Respir Dis *103[1]:57, 1971.)*

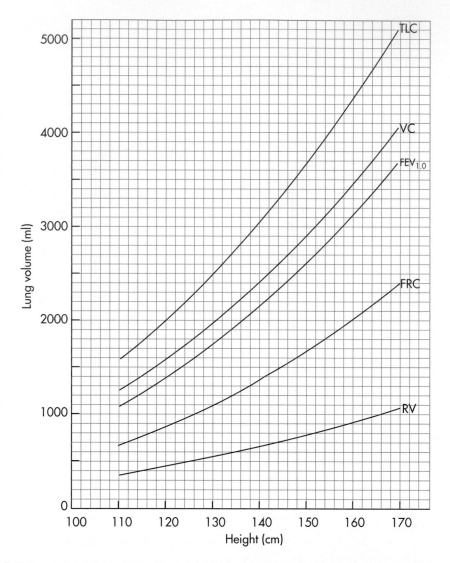

Figure B-3 Summary curves for lung volumes and FEV$_1$ in milliliters, for boys, as a function of height in centimeters. Summary curves are derived from regression equations from several different studies. *(From Polgar G, Promadhat V: Pulmonary function testing in children, Philadelphia, 1971, WB Saunders.)*

Abnormality may also be expressed as the difference between the individual's reference and measured values in terms of confidence intervals (CIs). The difference between the reference and measured values is divided by 1 CI (either 1.96 or 1.65 SDs). The result is expressed as a ratio:

$$\frac{Reference - Measured}{CI}$$

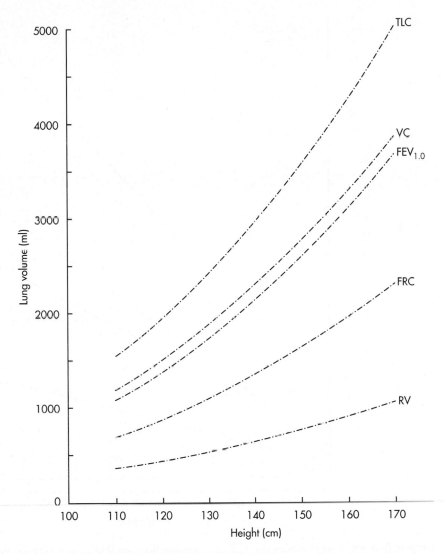

Figure B-4 Summary curves for lung volumes and FEV_1 in milliliters, for girls, as a function of height in centimeters. Summary curves are derived from regression equations from several different studies. *(From Polgar G, Promadhat V: Pulmonary function testing in children, Philadelphia, 1971, WB Saunders.)*

Using this method, a normal value is always less than or equal to 1.00, whereas abnormal values are greater. The extent of abnormality (obstruction or restriction) can also be described using the CI ratio. For example, $FEV_{1\%}$ may be evaluated as follows:

$FEV_{1\%}$	(CI)
Normal	<1 CI
Mild obstruction	>1 <2 CI
Moderate obstruction	>2 <4 CI
Severe obstruction	>4 CI

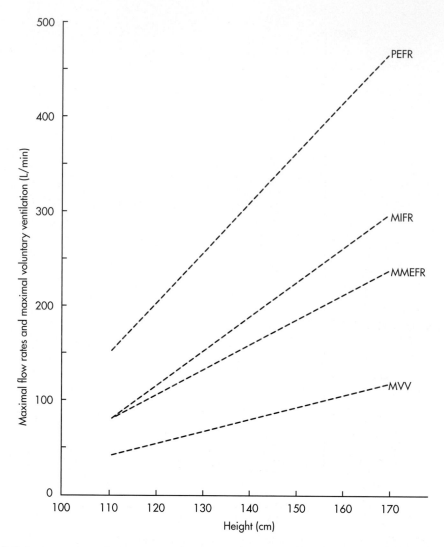

Figure B-5 Summary curves for maximal midexpiratory flow rate (FEF$_{25\%-75\%}$), peak expiratory flow (PEF), maximal voluntary ventilation (MVV), and maximal inspiratory flow rate (MIFT) in liters per minute, as a function of height for boys and girls. Summary curves are derived from regression equations from several different studies. *(From Polgar G, Promadhat V:* Pulmonary function testing in children, *Philadelphia, 1971, WB Saunders.)*

Each pulmonary function variable can be assessed using this method as long as its CI has been determined. Tests that are quite variable (e.g., FEF$_{25\%-75\%}$) have large CIs. In some instances, the CI may be larger than the expected value. As a result, the lower limit of normal may be zero or even a negative value. Although statistically valid, CI may not be applicable in every situation.

A third method for determining lower limits of normal uses the fifth percentile. The fifth percentile is the percent of the reference value above which 95% of the healthy population falls. The fifth percentile method requires a large sample population. However, it does not require the pulmonary function variable to be normally distributed in the population. Lower limits of normal using the fifth percentile are usually defined for specific age groupings. Both the CI and fifth percentile methods yield similar results for lower limits of normal, for variables that are normally distributed in the population.

Individual laboratories should try to choose reference studies from a population similar to that to be tested. The following factors may be considerations in selecting reference values:

1. *Type of equipment used for the reference study:* Does equipment comply with the most recent recommendations of the American Thoracic Society? (See Chapter 11.)
2. *Methodologies:* Were procedures used in the reference study similar to those to be used, particularly for spirometry, lung volumes, and DL_{CO}?
3. *Sample population:* What were the age ranges of the individuals? Did the study generate different regressions for different ethnic origins? Did the study include smokers or other "at-risk" individuals as normal individuals?
4. *Statistical data:* Are lower limits of normal defined? Are adequate data available (SD, CI) so that lower limits of normal can be calculated?
5. *Conditions of the study:* Was the study performed at a different altitude or under different environmental conditions?
6. *Published reference equations:* Do reference values generated using the study's regressions differ markedly from other published references?

Each laboratory should perform measurements on 20 to 40 individuals who represent a healthy cross-section of the population that the laboratory usually tests. Measured values from these individuals should be compared with expected values using various reference equations. Equations that produce the smallest average differences should be selected. Evaluation of a small number of individuals may not show much difference between equations for FVC and FEV_1. However, there may be noticeable discrepancies for DL_{CO} or maximal flows. Equations for spirometry, lung volumes, and DL_{CO} should be taken from a single reference, if possible. If healthy individuals fall outside the limits of normal, the laboratory should examine its test methods, how the individuals were selected, and the prediction equations.

There are no universally accepted reference values. Several excellent studies are available that address most of the considerations listed previously. The reference equations included here are widely used and compare favorably with other published studies. Other acceptable studies are included in the Selected Bibliography. Laboratories are encouraged to evaluate these and other equations in selecting references.

Prediction Regressions for Pulmonary Function Tests

Values are BTPS unless otherwise noted.

Tables B-1 to B-3 show coefficients for calculating predicted values and lower limits of normal using the equation format at the bottom of each table.

Tables B-4 and B-5 show regression equations for calculating various pulmonary function parameters; height is in inches and age is in years unless otherwise noted.

TABLE B-1 NHANES III[1] Prediction and Lower Limit of Normal Equations for Spirometric Parameters for Males* (Height in centimeters and age in years.)

Males	Intercept	Age	Age^2	Ht$_{PRD}$ (cm)^2	Ht$_{LLN}$ (cm)^2	R^2
Caucasian <20 Years of Age						
FEV$_1$	−0.7453	−0.04106	0.004477	0.00014098	0.00011607	0.8510
FEV$_6$	−0.3119	−0.18612	0.009717	0.00018188	0.00015323	0.8692
FVC	−0.2584	−0.20415	0.010133	0.00018642	0.00015695	0.8668
PEF	−0.5962	−0.12357	0.013135	0.00024962	0.00017635	0.7808
FEF$_{25\%\text{-}75\%}$	−1.0863	0.13939		0.00010345	0.00005294	0.5601
Caucasian 20 Years of Age						
FEV$_1$	0.5536	−0.01303	−0.000172	0.00014098	0.00011607	0.8510
FEV$_6$	0.1102	−0.00842	−0.000223	0.00018188	0.00015323	0.8692
FVC	−0.1933	0.00064	−0.000269	0.00018642	0.00015695	0.8668
PEF	1.0523	0.08272	−0.001301	0.00024962	0.00017635	0.7808
FEF$_{25\%\text{-}75\%}$	2.7006	−0.04995		0.00010345	0.00005294	0.5601
African American <20 Years of Age						
FEV$_1$	−0.7048	−0.05711	0.004316	0.00013194	0.00010561	0.8080
FEV$_6$	−0.5525	−0.14107	0.007241	0.00016429	0.00013499	0.8297
FVC	−0.4971	−0.15497	0.007701	0.00016643	0.00013670	0.8303
PEF	−0.2684	−0.28016	0.018202	0.00027333	0.00018938	0.7299
FEF$_{25\%\text{-}75\%}$	−1.1627	0.12314		0.00010461	0.00004819	0.4724
African American 20 Years of Age						
FEV$_1$	0.3411	−0.02309		0.00013194	0.00010561	0.8080
FEV$_6$	−0.0547	−0.02114		0.00016429	0.00013499	0.8297
FVC	−0.1517	−0.01821		0.00016643	0.00013670	0.8303
PEF	2.2257	−0.04082		0.00027333	0.00018938	0.7299
FEF$_{25\%\text{-}75\%}$	2.1477	−0.04238		0.00010461	0.00004819	0.4724
Mexican American <20 Years of Age						
FEV$_1$	−0.8218	−0.04248	0.004291	0.00015104	0.00012670	0.8536
FEV$_6$	−0.6646	−0.11270	0.007306	0.00017840	0.00015029	0.8657
FVC	−0.7571	−0.09520	0.006619	0.00017823	0.00014947	0.8641
PEF	−0.9537	−0.19602	0.014497	0.00030243	0.00021833	0.7530
FEF$_{25\%\text{-}75\%}$	−1.3592	0.10529		0.00014473	0.00009020	0.5482
Mexican American 20 Years of Age						
FEV$_1$	0.6306	−0.02928		0.00015104	0.00012670	0.8536
FEV$_6$	0.5757	−0.02860		0.00017840	0.00015029	0.8657
FVC	0.2376	−0.00891	−0.000182	0.00017823	0.00014947	0.8641
PEF	0.0870	0.06580	−0.001195	0.00030243	0.00021833	0.7530
FEF$_{25\%\text{-}75\%}$	1.7503	−0.05018		0.00014473	0.00009020	0.5482

*Ht$_{PRD}$ coefficient is used for prediction equation, and Ht$_{LLN}$ is used (replaces Ht$_{PRD}$) for the lower limit of normal equation.

Lung function parameter = $b_0 + b_1 \times$ age $+ b_2 \times$ age$^2 + b_3 \times$ height^2.

TABLE B-2 NHANES III[1] Prediction and Lower Limit of Normal Equations for Spirometric Parameters for Females* (Height in centimeters and age in years.)

Females	Intercept	Age	Age²	Ht_PRD (cm)²	Ht_LLN (cm)²	R²
Caucasian <18 Years of Age						
FEV_1	−0.8710	0.06537		0.00011496	0.00009283	0.7494
FEV_6	−1.1925	0.06544		0.00014395	0.00011827	0.7457
FVC	−1.2082	0.05916		0.00014815	0.00012198	0.7344
PEF	−3.0181	0.00044	0.016846	0.00018623	0.00012148	0.5559
$FEF_{25\%-75\%}$	−2.5284	0.52490	−0.015309	0.00006982	0.00002302	0.5005
Caucasian 18 Years of Age						
FEV_1	0.4333	−0.00361	−0.000194	0.00011496	0.00009283	0.7494
FEV_6	−0.1373	0.01317	−0.000352	0.00014395	0.00011827	0.7457
FVC	−0.3560	0.01870	−0.000382	0.00014815	0.00012198	0.7344
PEF	0.9267	0.06929	−0.001031	0.00018623	0.00012148	0.5559
$FEF_{25\%-75\%}$	2.3670	−0.01904	−0.000200	0.00006982	0.00002302	0.5005
African American <18 Years of Age						
FEV_1	−0.9630	0.05799		0.00010846	0.00008546	0.6687
FEV_6	−0.6370	−0.04243	0.003508	0.00013497	0.00010848	0.6615
FVC	0.6166	−0.04687	0.003602	0.00013606	0.00010916	0.6536
PEF	−1.2398	0.16375		0.00019746	0.00012160	0.4736
$FEF_{25\%-75\%}$	−2.5379	0.43755	−0.012154	0.00008572	0.00003380	0.3787
African American 18 Years of Age						
FEV_1	0.3433	−0.01283	−0.000097	0.00010846	0.00008546	0.6687
FEV_6	−0.1981	0.00047	−0.000230	0.00013497	0.00010848	0.6615
FVC	−0.3039	0.00536	−0.000265	0.00013606	0.00010916	0.6536
PEF	1.3597	0.03458	−0.000847	0.00019746	0.00012160	0.4736
$FEF_{25\%-75\%}$	2.0828	−0.03793		0.00008572	0.00003380	0.3787
Mexican American <18 Years of Age						
FEV_1	−0.9641	0.06490		0.00012154	0.00009890	0.7268
FEV_6	−1.2410	0.07625		0.00014106	0.00011480	0.7208
FVC	−1.2507	0.07501		0.00014246	0.00011570	0.7103
PEF	−3.2549	0.47495	−0.013193	0.00022203	0.00014611	0.4669
$FEF_{25\%-75\%}$	−2.1825	0.42451	−0.012415	0.00009610	0.00004594	0.4305
Mexican American 18 Years of Age						
FEV_1	0.4529	−0.01178	−0.000113	0.00012154	0.00009890	0.7268
FEV_6	0.2033	0.00020	−0.000232	0.00014106	0.00011480	0.7208
FVC	0.1210	0.00307	−0.000237	0.00014246	0.00011570	0.7103
PEF	0.2401	0.06174	−0.001023	0.00022203	0.00014611	0.4669
$FEF_{25\%-75\%}$	1.7456	−0.01195	−0.000291	0.00009610	0.00004594	4.4305

*Ht_PRD coefficient is used for prediction equation, and Ht_LLN is used (replaces Ht_PRD) for the lower limit of normal equation.

Lung function parameter = $b_0 + b_1 \times age + b_2 \times age^2 + b_3 \times height^2$.

TABLE B–3 NHANES III[1] Prediction and Lower Limit of Normal Equations for $FEV_1/FEV_6\%$ and $FEV_1/FVC\%$ for Male and Females* (Age in years.)

	Intercept$_{PRD}$	Age	Intercept$_{LLN}$	R^2
Males				
Caucasian				
$FEV_1/FEV_6\%$	87.340	−0.1382	78.372	0.2151
$FEV_1/FVC\%$	88.066	−0.2066	78.388	0.3448
African American				
$FEV_1/FEV_6\%$	88.841	−0.1305	78.979	0.0937
$FEV_1/FVC\%$	89.239	−0.1828	78.822	0.1538
Mexican American				
$FEV_1/FEV_6\%$	89.388	−0.1534	80.810	0.1711
$FEV_1/FVC\%$	90.024	−0.2186	80.925	0.2713
Females				
Caucasian				
$FEV_1/FEV_6\%$	90.107	−0.1563	81.307	0.3048
$FEV_1/FVC\%$	90.809	−0.2125	81.015	0.3955
African American				
$FEV_1/FEV_6\%$	91.229	−0.1558	81.396	0.1693
$FEV_1/FVC\%$	91.655	−0.2039	80.978	0.2284
Mexican American				
$FEV_1/FEV_6\%$	91.664	−0.1670	83.034	0.2449
$FEV_1/FVC\%$	93.360	−0.2248	83.044	0.3352

*Intercept$_{PRD}$ coefficient is used for prediction equation and intercept$_{LLN}$ is used (replaces intercept$_{PRD}$) for the lower limit of normal equation.
Lung function parameter = $b_0 + b_1 \times$ age.

TABLE B–4 Lung Volume Regression Equations (Height in inches and age in years, unless otherwise noted.)

Test		Regression Equation	SD	Source
VC (L)				
	Males	(Same as for FVC)		1
	Females	(Same as for FVC)		1
FRC (L)				
	Males	0.130H − 5.16	—	2
	Females	0.119H − 4.85	—	2
RV (L)				
	Males	0.069H + 0.017A − 3.45	—	3
	Females	0.081H + 0.009A − 3.90	—	3
Derived Lung Volumes				
		TLC (L) = VC + RV or		
		TLC (L) = FRC + IC		

TABLE B-5 Other Pulmonary Function Regression Equations (Height in inches and age in years, unless otherwise noted.)

Test		Regression Equation	SD	Source
$\dot{V}_{max75}$ (L/sec)				
	Males	$0.090H - 0.020A + 2.726$	—	4
	Females	$0.069H - 0.019A + 2.147$	—	4
$\dot{V}_{max50}$ (L/sec)				
	Males	$0.065H - 0.030A + 2.403$	—	4
	Females	$0.062H - 0.035A + 1.426$	—	4
$\dot{V}_{max25}$ (L/sec)				
	Males	$0.036H - 0.041A + 1.984$	—	4
	Females	$0.023H - 0.035A + 2.216$	—	4
MVV (L/min)				
	Males	$3.03H - 0.816A - 37.9$	—	4
	Females	$2.14H - 0.685A - 4.87$	—	4
CV/VC (%)				
	Males	$0.357A + 0.562$	4.15	5
	Females	$0.293A + 2.812$	4.90	5
CC/TLC (%)				
	Males	$0.496A + 14.878$	4.09	5
	Females	$0.536A + 14.420$	4.43	5
$D_{L_{CO}}sb$ (ml CO/min/mm Hg STPD)				
	Males	$0.250H - 0.177A + 19.93$	—	6
	Females	$0.284H - 0.177A + 7.72$	—	6
Maximal Expiratory Pressure (cm H_2O)				
	Males	$268 - 1.03A$	—	7
	Females	$170 - 0.53A$	—	7
Maximal Inspiratory Pressure (cm H_2O)				
	Males	$143 - 0.55A$	—	7
	Females	$104 - 0.51A$	—	7
$\dot{V}O_{2max}$ (L/min STPD)				
	Males	$4.2 - 0.032A$	0.4	8
	Females	$2.6 - 0.014A$	0.4	8
HR_{max} (beats/min)				
	Males and females	$210 - 0.65A$	10-15	8
Pa_{O_2} (mm Hg)				
	Males and females	$-0.279A + 0.113PB + 14.632$	—	9

TABLE B-6 Reference Values for Spirometry in Children (All values BTPS unless otherwise noted. Height in centimeters and age in years unless otherwise noted.)

Test	Regression Equation	SD	Source
Children, males 8-20 years of age, females 8-18 years of age			
FEV₁ (L)			
Males	See **Table B-1**		1
Females	See **Table B-2**		1
FEV₆ (L)			
Males	See **Table B-1**		
Females	See **Table B-2**		
FVC (L)			
Males	See **Table B-1**		1
Females	See **Table B-2**		1
PEF (L/sec)			
Males	See **Table B-1**		1
Females	See **Table B-2**		1
FEF₂₅%₋₇₅% (L)			
Males	See **Table B-1**		1
Females	See **Table B-2**		1
FEV₁/FVC			
Males	See **Table B-3**		1
Females	See **Table B-3**		1
MVV (L/min) children 42-78 inches, 5-17 years of age			
Males and females	$3.81 H_{in} - 134$	—	2

TABLE B-7 Lung Volumes,* RV/TLC%[†] and DL_{CO}* in Children. (All values BTPS unless otherwise noted. Height in centimeter and age in years unless otherwise noted.)

	a	b	SD[‡]	Source
Male Subjects, 5-18 Years of Age				
VC (ml)		Same as FVC		
FRC_{BOX} (ml)	−2.4915	+2.6523	0.0381	3
RV_{BOX} (ml)	−1.2720	+1.9427	0.838	3
TLC_{BOX} (ml)	−2.0018	+2.5698	0.0276	3
Female Subjects, 5-18 Years of Age				
VC (ml)		Same as FVC		
FRC_{BOX} (ml)	−2.4314	+2.6149	0.0538	3
RV_{BOX} (ml)	−2.0493	+2.3062	0.0819	3
TLC_{BOX} (ml)	−2.0377	+2.5755	0.0361	3
Males and Females				
RV/TLC_{BOX} (%)	34.6549	−0.0673	3.91	3
$DL_{CO}sb$ (ml CO/min/mm Hg STPD)	−3.2292	+2.0876	0.09	3

*Log(lung function parameter) = a+b(log height [cm]).

[†]Lung function parameter = a+b(height [cm]).

[‡]Upper/lower limit = antilog(a+[b±SD][log height (cm)]).

SELECTED BIBLIOGRAPHY

Prediction Regressions

1. Hankinson JL, Odencrantz JR, Fedan KB: Spirometric reference values from a sample of the general U.S. population. *Am J Respir Crit Care Med* 159:179-187, 1999.
2. Bates DV, Macklem PT, Christie RV: *Respiratory function in disease,* ed 2, Philadelphia, 1971, WB Saunders.
3. Goldman HI, Becklake MR: Respiratory function tests: normal values at median altitudes and the prediction of normal results, *Am Rev Tuberculosis* 79:457, 1959.
4. Cherniack RM, Raber MD: Normal standards for ventilatory function using an automated wedge spirometer, *Am Rev Respir Dis* 106:38, 1972.
5. Buist SA, Ross BB: Predicted values for closing volumes using a modified single-breath nitrogen test, *Am Rev Respir Dis* 111:405, 1975.
6. Gaensler EA, Wright GW: Evaluation of respiratory impairment, *Arch Environ Health* 12:146, 1966.
7. Black LF, Hyatt RE: Maximal respiratory pressures: normal values and relationships to age and sex, *Am Rev Respir Dis* 99:696, 1969.
8. Jones NL, Campbell EJM, Edwards RHT, et al: *Clinical exercise testing,* ed 2, Philadelphia, 1983, WB Saunders.
9. Morris AH, Kanner RE, Crapo RO, et al: *Clinical pulmonary function testing,* ed 2, Salt Lake City, 1984, Intermountain Thoracic Society.

Additional Recommended Sources for Pulmonary Function Predicted Values

General

American Thoracic Society: Lung function testing: selection of reference values and interpretive strategies, *Am Rev Respir Dis* 144:1202, 1991.

Spirometry

Crapo RO, Morris AH, Gardner RM: Reference spirometric values using techniques and equipment that meet ATS recommendations, *Am Rev Respir Dis* 123:659, 1981.

Knudson RJ, Slatin RC, Lebowitz MD: The maximal expiratory flow-volume curve: normal standards, variability, and effects of age, *Am Rev Respir Dis* 113:587, 1976.

Morris JF, Koski A, Johnson LC: Spirometric standards for healthy nonsmoking adults, *Am Rev Respir Dis* 103:57, 1971.

Quanjer PH, ed: Report of working party—European community for coal and steel: standardized lung function testing, *Bull Eur Physiopathol Respir* 19(suppl 5):7, 1983.

Schoenberg JB, Beck GJ, Bouhuys A: Growth and decay of pulmonary function in healthy blacks and whites, *Respir Physiol* 33:367, 1978.

Lung Volumes

Crapo RO, Morris AH, Clayton PD, et al: Lung volumes in healthy nonsmoking adults, *Bull Eur Physiopathol Respir* 18:419, 1982.

Grimby G, Soderholm B: Spirometric studies in normal subjects. III. Static lung volumes and maximum voluntary ventilation in adults with a note on physical fitness, *Acta Med Scand* 173:199, 1963.

Diffusing Capacity

Bates DV, Macklem PT, Christie RV. *Respiratory function in disease,* ed 2, Philadelphia, 1971, WB Saunders.

Crapo RO, Morris AH: Standardized single-breath normal values for carbon monoxide diffusing capacity, *Am Rev Respir Dis* 123:185, 1981.

Knudson RJ, Kaltenborn WT, Knudson DE, et al: The single-breath carbon monoxide diffusing capacity: reference equations derived from a healthy nonsmoking population and effects of hematocrit, *Am Rev Respir Dis* 135:805-811, 1987.

Miller A, Thornton JC, Warshaw R, et al: Single breath diffusing capacity in a representative sample of the population of Michigan, a large industrial state, *Am Rev Respir Dis* 127:270-277, 1983.

Paoletti P, Viegi G, Pistelli G, et al. Reference equations for the single breath diffusing capacity: a cross-sectional analysis and effect of body size and age, *Am Rev Respir Dis* 132:806-813, 1985.

Sources for Normal Values—Children

1. Hankinson JL, Odencrantz JR, Fedan KB: Spirometric reference values from a sample of the general U.S. population, *Am J Respir Crit Care Med* 159:179-187, 1999.
2. Dickman ML, Schmidt CD, Gardner RM: Spirometric standards for normal children and adolescents (ages 5 years through 18 years), *Am Rev Respir Dis* 104:680-689, 1971.
3. Zapletal A, Samanek M, Paul T: Lung function in children and adolescents: methods, reference values. In: *Progress in respiration research,* vol 22, Basel, 1987, Karger.

Additional Recommended Sources for Pulmonary Function Predicted Values

Hsu KHK, Bartholomew PH, Thompson V, et al: Ventilatory functions of normal children and young adults—Mexican-American, white, and black. I. Spirometry, *J Pediatr* 95:14, 1979.

Polgar G, Promadhat V: *Pulmonary function testing in children: techniques and standards,* Philadelphia, 1971, WB Saunders.

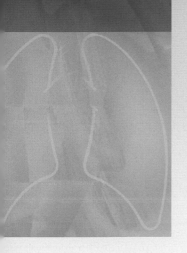

APPENDIX C

CONVERSION AND CORRECTION FACTORS

Converting Gas Volumes from ATPS to BTPS

$$\text{Volume (BTPS)} = \text{Volume (ATPS)} \times \frac{P_B - PH_2O}{P_B - 47} \times \frac{310}{273 + T}$$

where:

P_B = barometric pressure, mm Hg
PH_2O = vapor pressure of water at spirometer temperature
T = temperature in °C
47 = vapor pressure of water at 37° C
310 = absolute body temperature

Most factors in this equation can be combined into a single conversion factor. Local barometric pressure changes cause slight differences. The most significant differences occur with temperature changes.

Conversion Factor	Gas Temperature (°C)	PH₂O (mm Hg)
1.112	18	15.6
1.107	19	16.5
1.102	20	17.5
1.096	21	18.7
1.091	22	19.8
1.085	23	21.1
1.080	24	22.4
1.075	25	23.8
1.068	26	23.8
1.063	27	26.7
1.057	28	28.3
1.051	29	30.0
1.045	30	31.8
1.039	31	31.8
1.032	32	35.7
1.026	33	35.7
1.020	34	35.7
1.014	35	42.2
1.007	36	44.6
1.000	37	47.0

Converting Gas Volumes from ATPS to STPD

$$\text{Volume (STPD)} = \text{Volume (ATPS)} \times \frac{P_B - PH_2O}{760} \times \frac{273}{273 + T}$$

where:

P_B = barometric pressure, mm Hg
PH_2O = vapor pressure of water at spirometer temperature
T   = temperature in °C
760   = standard barometric pressure at sea level
273   = absolute temperature equal to 0° C

Calculating Water Vapor Pressure

$$PH_2O = 47.07 \times 10^{\left[\frac{6.36(T-37)}{232+T}\right]}$$

where:

PH_2O = vapor pressure of water at spirometer temperature
T   = temperature in °C, 0° to 40°

Calculating Barometric Pressure at Altitude

$$P_B = 760 \times [1 - (6.873 \times 10^{-6} \times \text{Altitude})]^{5.256}$$

where:

P_B = barometric pressure, mm Hg
Altitude = altitude, feet above sea level

Converting Temperature

$$°C = (°F - 32) / 1.8$$
$$°F = (1.8 \times °C) + 32$$
$$°K = °C + 273$$

SI (Système International) Units

The following table shows conversion factors for units of measurement commonly used in pulmonary function testing. Except for temperature, to convert a value from conventional to SI units, *multiply* conventional units by the conversion factor. To convert a value from SI to conventional units, *divide* by the factor.

Measurement	Conventional Unit	SI Unit	Conversion Factor
Temperature	°C	K	°C+273.15
Length	inch (in)	meter (m)	0.0254
	foot (ft)	m	0.3048
Area	in^2	cm^2	6.452
	ft^2	m^2	0.0929
Volume	ft^3	L	28.32
Pressure	cm H_2O	kilopascal (kPa)	0.09806
	mm Hg (torr)	kPa	0.1333
	pounds/in^2 (psi)	kPa	6.895
Work	kilogram meter (kg m)	joule (J)	9.807
Power	kg m/min	(J)	0.1634
Energy	kilocalorie (kcal)	(J)	4185
Compliance	L/cm H_2O	L/kPa	10.2
Resistance	cm H_2O/L/sec	kPa/L/sec	0.09806

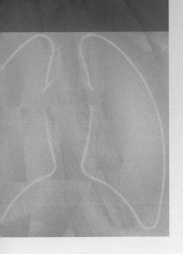

APPENDIX D

REGULATIONS AND REGULATORY AGENCIES

Several agencies regulate operations in pulmonary function and/or blood gas laboratories. These regulations concern laboratory procedures, infection control, safety, and reimbursement.

Occupational Safety and Health Administration

The Occupational Safety and Health Administration (OSHA) is a U.S. government agency that develops and implements policies to address hazards in the workplace. OSHA regulations apply to two main areas in pulmonary function and blood gas laboratories:

1. *Hazard communication* relates to all chemicals or substances used in the laboratory. Laboratories are required to maintain lists of hazardous substances. In addition, Material Safety Data Sheets (MSDSs) must be kept. Employees must be trained regarding, and kept informed of, hazardous chemicals in their workplace.
2. Training regarding *blood-borne pathogens* is mandated. Employees who may be exposed to blood or blood products must receive training regarding the transmission of blood-borne pathogens. Methods of preventing exposure, identification of tasks that cause risk of exposure, and actions to be taken must be documented. Plans for removal of blood and blood products are necessary, as are explanations of personal protective equipment, such as gloves and gowns.

Regulations mandated by OSHA are published in the *Federal Register* and are continually updated.

National Institute for Occupational Safety and Health

The National Institute for Occupational Safety and Health (NIOSH) is a U.S. government agency that enforces standards set by OSHA. NIOSH regulations concerning pulmonary function measurements are related to the "Cotton Dust Standard." Federal regulations (29 CFR: 1910.1043) describe how spirometry is to be performed in the examination of individuals exposed to cotton dust. The appendix to this statute lists standards for spirometers and recorders used, measurement techniques, interpretation of spirometry, and qualifications for personnel performing spirometry. Guidelines for minimal spirometry training are included. These NIOSH regulations regarding spirometry are often applied in areas of occupational exposure other than cotton dust, making them *de facto* standards.

Updates to NIOSH regulations are published in the *Federal Register.*

Health and Human Services

Health and Human Services (HHS) is a U.S. government department. Programs affecting pulmonary function and blood gas laboratories are administered by the Centers for Medicare and Medicaid Services (CMS). CMS was formerly the Health Care Financing Administration (HFCA).

■ CLINICAL LABORATORY IMPROVEMENT AMENDMENTS OF 1988

Clinical Laboratory Improvement Amendments of 1988 (CLIA 88) consist of regulations that ensure safe, accurate quality laboratory testing. Regulations 42 CFR, Part 493, HSQ-176 consist of standards regarding laboratory practices. These regulations include blood gas laboratories and may have ramifications for pulmonary function testing as well. Under CLIA 88 regulations:

1. Laboratories must register and apply for certification. Level of certification depends on the complexity of tests performed. Three categories of testing, based on complexity of the testing method, have been established:
   Waived tests: Waived tests include simple nonautomated tests such as pH measurement by dipstick method.
   Tests of moderate complexity: Tests of moderate complexity include automated tests or manual procedures with limited steps. Automated blood gas analyses that do not require operator intervention during the analytic process are included in the moderate complexity group.
   Tests of high complexity: Tests of high complexity include semiautomated or manual procedures that require multiple steps, preparation of complex reagents, and operator intervention in the analytic process.
2. Personnel requirements are linked to the complexity model for testing. For moderately complex tests, standards for laboratory directors, technical consultants, clinical consultants, and testing personnel are defined. For high-complexity tests, standards for technical and general supervisors are added to the list. The regulations list specific functions and qualifications for each position. Qualified individuals can fill more than one position in either moderate- or high-complexity testing.

3. Proficiency testing is required to externally evaluate each laboratory's performance. Each laboratory performing moderate- or high-complexity tests must participate in proficiency testing. Proficiency tests must be performed for each regulated analyte for which the laboratory reports results. Proficiency testing samples must include five samples for each analyte or test. The laboratory must participate in the program at least three times per year. A separate grading formula is established for each analyte. For most analytes or tests, a score of 80% (an acceptable measurement on four of five samples) is required. Laboratories that are unsuccessful (score less than 80%) on two of three tests will be subject to sanctions for the involved test.

4. Each laboratory must establish a quality control program. Regulations require that for tests of moderate complexity (e.g., blood gases) manufacturer's instructions be followed, a procedure manual be available, and calibrations be performed. Quality control runs with at least two levels must be performed daily. Instruments and test systems will be evaluated by the Food and Drug Administration (FDA) to determine the applicable levels of quality control required.

In addition to the laboratory regulations defined by CLIA 88, HHS sets standards for reimbursement under the DRG (Diagnosis Related Groups) system for Medicare inpatients and under the APC (Ambulatory Payment Classification) system for outpatients. Reimbursement requires that charges for procedures performed be correctly classified using Current Procedural Terminology (CPT) codes. HHS also lists requirements for disability according to the Social Security Administration (SSA). These regulations specify levels of pulmonary function impairment that qualify candidates for disability reimbursement (see Chapter 9).

Updates to CLIA 88 regulations are published in the *Federal Register*. Regulations related to reimbursement under CMS or SSA are published by the respective agencies.

Joint Commission on Accreditation of Healthcare Organizations

The Joint Commission on Accreditation of Healthcare Organizations (JCAHO) is a voluntary accrediting agency that develops standards of quality for health care organizations. JCAHO has published standards for all areas of the health care environment. Standards that affect pulmonary function laboratories are listed primarily under Respiratory Care Services. JCAHO standards require the following:

1. Pulmonary function and blood gas analysis capability should be appropriate for the level of respiratory care services provided and should be readily available to meet the needs of patients. Blood gases should be available 24 hours per day.

2. The scope of diagnostic services must be defined in writing and must be related to other hospital departments by an organizational plan.

3. Services provided from outside of the hospital must meet all necessary requirements.

4. Medical direction should be provided by a physician qualified by special training or interest in respiratory problems and should be readily available for consultation.

5. Trained personnel should be available to meet the needs of the patients served. Hazardous procedures (e.g., arterial puncture) must be authorized in writing according to medical staff policy.

6. There must be written policies and procedures for pulmonary function testing and for obtaining and analyzing blood samples. Policies and procedures should address equipment maintenance, safety, infection control, and administration of medications.

7. There must be sufficient facilities (equipment, space) for performing pulmonary function studies and blood gas analysis. Requirements regarding performance of pulmonary function or blood gas studies must be met regardless of which hospital department performs them. Equipment must be calibrated and maintained according to the manufacturer's specifications.

Standards developed by JCAHO are published annually in its document entitled *Accreditation Manual for Hospitals.*

Certifying and Standards Organizations

The following organizations offer certification or publish standards related to pulmonary function testing and/or blood gas analysis:

Organization and Web Address	Certification/Standards
American College of Sports Medicine (ACSM) www.acsm.org	Provides training courses and certification for exercise technologists; publishes guidelines for exercise testing and training
American Thoracic Society (ATS) www.thoracic.org	Publishes standards for spirometry, single-breath DL_{CO}, pulmonary function personnel qualifications, use of computers in pulmonary function testing, guidelines for quality assurance, and interpretive strategies; standards published in the *American Journal of Respiratory and Critical Care Medicine*
Centers for Disease Control and Prevention (CDC) www.cdc.gov	Promulgates standards related to infection control and disease prevention; regulations published in *Morbidity and Mortality Weekly Report*
College of American Pathologists (CAP) www.cap.org	Accredits clinical and research laboratories, including blood gas laboratories; provides quality control programs and proficiency testing survey materials
National Board for Respiratory Care (NBRC) www.nbrc.org	Provides national certification for respiratory care practitioners, including pulmonary function technologists; offers credentials of Certified Pulmonary Function Technologist (CPFT) for entry-level and Registered Pulmonary Technologist (RPFT) for advanced-level practitioners
National Committee for Clinical Laboratory Standards (NCCLS) www.nccls.org	Publishes standards for all areas of laboratory medicine, including blood gas laboratories

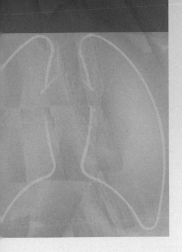

APPENDIX E

SOME USEFUL EQUATIONS

Alveolar Air Equation

It is often necessary to determine the partial pressure of O_2 in alveolar gas. One practical application of the alveolar air equation is determination of PaO_2 for calculation of the present shunt. The alveolar air equation is as follows:

$$PaO_2 = (FIO_2 \times (P_B - 47)) - PaCO_2 \left(FIO_2 + \frac{1 - FIO_2}{R} \right)$$

where:

FIO_2 = fractional concentration of inspired O_2
P_B = barometric pressure
47 = partial pressure of water vapor at $37°$ C
$PaCO_2$ = arterial CO_2 tension, presumed equal to alveolar CO_2 tension
R = respiratory exchange ratio ($\dot{V}CO_2 / \dot{V}O_2$)

If the fraction of inspired O_2 is 1.0, the factor in the parentheses on the right equals 1 and can be deleted. R varies, especially during exercise; it is often assumed to be 0.80.

Poiseuille's Law

Poiseuille's law relates variables that affect gas flow through a tube. The law has many applications in pulmonary physiology. It describes laminar gas flow through the conducting airways. It is also used in pneumotachography to relate flow and pressure changes within a tube. The law is stated as follows:

$$\Delta P \frac{\dot{V} 8 \eta l}{\pi r^4}$$

where:

ΔP = change in pressure from one end of the tube to the other
$\dot{V}$ = flow through the tube

η = coefficient of viscosity of the gas
l   = length of the tube
r   = radius of the tube

The equation can be rearranged as follows:

$$\Delta P \dot{V} = 8\eta l \pi r^4$$

The ratio of pressure differences at the end of the tube (ΔP) to flow through the tube ($\dot{V}$) defines *resistance*. Resistance varies directly with the length (l) of the conducting tube. It varies inversely with the fourth power of the radius (r^4). A twofold increase in length of the tube doubles resistance. A reduction of the radius by half increases the pressure difference 16 times. In the airways, narrowing caused by secretions or other lesions can significantly increase airway resistance. Poiseuille's law applies to any round tube in which laminar flow is possible. Pressure differential pneumotachography is based directly on this law (see Pressure-Differential Flow Sensors, Chapter 10). The length and radius of a pressure differential flow sensor remain constant. The viscosity of respiratory gases varies only slightly. The variables in Poiseuille's equation, except for ΔP and $\dot{V}$, can be reduced to a single constant. Flow can then be defined as follows:

$$\dot{V} = \frac{\Delta P}{K_R}$$

where:
K_R = resistance constant determined by length and radius of the flow tube

Using this equation, $\dot{V}$ can be measured by determining the pressure differential. This is easily accomplished by means of pressure transducers.

Thoracic Gas Volume Equation

Measurement of V_{TG} with the body plethysmograph is based on Boyle's law:

$$P_1 V_1 = P_2 V_2$$

or by expanding:

$$P_1 V_1 = (P_1 + \Delta P)(V_1 + \Delta V)$$

where:
P_1 = initial dry pressure in the lungs (713 mm Hg or 970 cm H_2O)
V_1 = V_{TG} or volume of gas in the thorax
ΔV = change in lung volume
ΔP = change in lung pressure

Then by rearranging:

$$P_1 \Delta P + V_1 \Delta P + \Delta V \Delta P = 0$$

Solving for V_1:

$$V_1 = -\frac{\Delta V}{\Delta P}(P_1 + \Delta P)$$

Because ΔP is small compared with P_1, $P_1 + \Delta P \approx P_1$; therefore:

$$V_1 = -\frac{P_1(\Delta V)}{\Delta P}$$

In terms of the plethysmographic method (and disregarding the sign):

$$V_{TG} = 970\frac{\Delta V}{\Delta P}$$

A sloping line is recorded on a computer screen or an oscilloscope. The slope represents the change in mouth pressure per unit change in box volume ($\Delta P/\Delta V$), or λV_{TG}, as the patient pants against an occluded airway. The equation then becomes:

$$V_{TG} = \frac{970}{\lambda V_{TG}}$$

This is the working form of the equation. Box pressure and mouth pressure calibration factors are also required to complete the calculation (see Appendix F). Measurement of the slope of the tracing allows rapid calculation of V_{TG}.

Fick's Law of Diffusion (Modified)

In reference to gas exchange across a membrane, Fick's law states that:

$$\dot{V}_{GAS} = \frac{A}{T} \times D \times (P_1 - P_2)$$

where:
A   = area of the membrane
T   = thickness of the membrane
$P_1 - P_2$ = pressure gradient across the membrane
D   = diffusion constant for a specific gas

D is related to the molecular weight and solubility of the gas to which it refers by:

$$D \propto \frac{\dot{V}_{GAS}}{\sqrt{\text{Molecular weight}}}$$

Because A and T remain relatively constant in the lungs:

$$D_L \propto \frac{\dot{V}_{GAS}}{P_A - P_C}$$

where:
D_L = diffusion constant for the lung
P_A = alveolar gas pressure
P_C = capillary gas pressure

When D_L is measured with carbon monoxide (CO), the capillary partial pressure is assumed zero thus:

$$D_L = \frac{\dot{V}_{CO}}{P_A CO}$$

All CO methods of measuring D_L use this basic equation. The single-breath and steady-state methods differ in that the former measures $\dot{V}_{CO}$ during breath holding, whereas the latter measures it during normal breathing. The steady-state methods vary by the way in which they measure $P_A CO$.

Fick Principle (Cardiac Output Determination)

The Fick principle relates $\dot{V}_{O_2}$ to arterial-mixed venous $\dot{V}_{O_2}$ content difference ($C[a - \bar{v}]_{O_2}$) to determine cardiac output ($\dot{Q}_T$):

$$\dot{Q}_T = \frac{\dot{V}_{O_2}}{CaO_2 - C\bar{v}O_2}$$

This equation forms the basis for determining various fractions of the cardiac output, namely, the shunt fraction ($\dot{Q}_S$) and the fraction participating in ideal gas exchange ($\dot{Q}_C$). The relationship between $\dot{Q}_S$ and the total cardiac output $\dot{Q}_T$ can be expressed as a ratio using the concept of O_2 content differences:

$$\frac{\dot{Q}_S}{\dot{Q}_T} = \frac{CcO_2 - CaO_2}{CcO_2 - C\bar{v}O_2}$$

where:
$CcO_2 - CaO_2$ = content difference between pulmonary end capillary blood, CcO_2, and arterial blood, CaO_2, which increases when blood passes through the pulmonary system without coming into contact with alveolar gas (a shunt)
$CcO_2 - C\bar{v}O_2$ = content difference between blood returning to the lungs by way of the pulmonary artery and the pulmonary end-capillary blood; the total change reflects the arterialization of mixed venous blood

If all pulmonary capillary blood equilibrates with alveolar gas, CcO_2 and CaO_2 become identical, no matter what the value of the denominator, so the ratio becomes zero and the shunt must be zero. If some blood does not equilibrate, the numerator becomes larger in relation to the denominator and an increased $\dot{Q}_S/\dot{Q}_T$ results.

Pulmonary end-capillary O_2 content (CcO_2) is impossible to sample and represents a mathematical entity rather than an actual phenomenon. A modified form of the equation is used clinically (as described in Chapter 6):

$$\frac{\dot{Q}_S}{\dot{Q}_T} = \frac{(P_AO_2 - PaO_2)(0.0031)}{(C[a-\bar{v}]O_2) + (P_AO_2 - PaO_2)(0.0031)}$$

where:

$P_AO_2 - PaO_2$ = difference in O_2 tension between alveoli and arterial blood
0.0031 = solubility factor to convert O_2 tension to volume percent

The equation is applied after the patient has breathed 100% O_2 long enough to completely saturate Hb (PaO_2 >150 mm Hg). The only difference between pulmonary end-capillary blood (assumed to be in equilibrium with PaO_2) and arterial blood exists in the difference in O_2 content in the dissolved form. This difference is related to the normal $a - \bar{v}$ content difference ($C[a-\bar{v}]O_2$) plus the actual dissolved content difference, denoted by the same term in both numerator and denominator. A ratio between the content difference of shunted blood and the total difference is derived using dissolved O_2 differences. PaO_2 is determined by the alveolar air equation outlined previously in this appendix.

Calculated Bicarbonate (HCO_3^-)

The bicarbonate concentration in plasma can be calculated using the Henderson-Hasselbalch equation if pH and PCO_2 are known:

$$pH = pK + \log\frac{HCO_3^-}{H_2CO_3}$$

The working form of the equation becomes as follows:

$$(HCO_3^-) = 0.0306 \times PCO_2 \times 10^{([pH-6.161]/[0.9524])}$$

where:
HCO_3^- = bicarbonate concentration, mEq/L
0.0306 = solubility coefficient for CO_2
6.161 = pK of carbonic acid
0.9524 = an empirically determined constant

Total CO_2 concentration can then be determined by summing HCO_3^- and dissolved CO_2:

$$TCO_2 = 0.0306 \times PCO_2 + (HCO_3^-)$$

Calculated Oxygen Saturation

Although it is preferable to measure oxygen saturation (see Chapter 6), saturation of Hb with O_2 can be calculated if pH and P_{O_2} are known. Assuming that Hb is normal (P_{50} of 26.6), saturation may be calculated as follows:

$$HbO_2 = \frac{Z^{2.60}}{(26.6)^{2.60} + Z^{2.60}} \times 100$$

where:

$$Z = P_{O_2} \times 10^{(-0.48[7.40 - pH])}$$

where:
P_{O_2} = partial pressure of O_2 in the sample
pH   = negative log of the hydrogen ion concentration in the sample
−0.48 = the Bohr factor (normal blood)

Because Hb is assumed normal, calculated saturation may be in error if the O_2 binding capacity of Hb is altered (see Chapter 6).

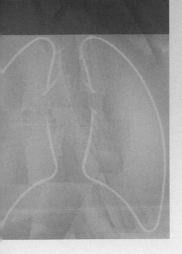

APPENDIX F

SAMPLE CALCULATIONS

Sample Calculations

■ OPEN-CIRCUIT FRC DETERMINATION (N_2 WASHOUT) (SEE CHAPTER 3)

FRC:	Unknown
$F_E N_{2final}$:	0.06
$F_A N_{2alveolar\ 1}$:	0.76
$F_A N_{2alveolar\ 2}$:	0.01
Volume expired (V_E):	27.5 L
Test time (T):	7 min
N_{2tiss}:	0.04 L/min (correction factor)
Spirometer temperature:	24° C

1. $\text{FRC} = \dfrac{[F_E N_{2final} \times (V_E + V_D)] - (T \times N_{2tiss})}{F_A N_{2alveolar1} - F_A N_{2alveolar2}}$

    $= \dfrac{[0.06 \times (27.5 + 1.0\,L)] - (7.0\,min \times 0.04\,L/min)}{0.76 - 0.01}$

    $= \dfrac{(0.06 \times 28.5) - (0.28\,L)}{0.75}$

    $= \dfrac{1.71\,L - 0.28\,L}{0.75}$

    $= \dfrac{1.43}{0.75}$

2. FRC = 1.91 L (ATPS)

   This value is ATPS and must be corrected to BTPS. The spirometer temperature was 24° C. Using the appropriate correction factor from p. 479:

3. FRC (BTPS) = 1.91 × 1.08
4. FRC (BTPS) = 2.06

CLOSED-CIRCUIT FRC DETERMINATION (HELIUM DILUTION) (SEE CHAPTER 3)

FRC:	Unknown
He added:	0.5 L
%He$_{initial}$:	9.5% (0.095 as a fraction)
%He$_{final}$:	5.5% (0.055 as a fraction)
He absorption correction:	0.1 L
Spirometer temperature:	24° C

1. $FRC = \left[\dfrac{(\%He_{initial} - \%He_{final})}{\%He_{final}} \times \text{System volume} \right] - \text{He correction}$

2. $\text{System volume} = \dfrac{He_{added}}{\%He_{initial}}$

    $= \dfrac{0.5\,L}{0.095}$

    $= 5.26\,L$

$FRC = \left[\dfrac{(0.095 - 0.055)}{0.055} \times 5.26\,L \right] - 0.1\,L$

$= (0.73 \times 5.25\,L) \times 0.1\,L$

$= 3.84\,L - 0.1\,L$

4. FRC = 3.74 L (ATPS)

Correcting to BTPS with appropriate correction factor from p. 479:

5. FRC (BTPS) = 3.74 × 1.08
6. FRC (BTPS) = 4.04 L

SINGLE-BREATH DL$_{co}$ (SEE CHAPTER 5)

Volume inspired (V$_I$):	4.0 L
F$_I$CO:	0.003
F$_A$CO$_{T2}$:	0.00125
F$_I$He:	0.10
F$_E$He:	0.075
P$_B$:	760 mm Hg
Breath-hold time (T$_2$ − T$_1$):	10.0 sec
Spirometer temperature:	25° C
Hb:	10.0 g/dl
CoHb:	5.5%

1. $DL_{CO}sb = \dfrac{V_A \times 60}{(P_B - 47)(T_2 - T_1)} \times Ln\left(\dfrac{F_A CO_{T1}}{F_A CO_{T2}} \right)$

2. $V_A = \dfrac{V_I}{F_E He / F_I He}$

    $= \dfrac{4.0\,L}{0.075/0.10}$

    $= 5.33\,L\,(5333\,ml)$

3. $F_ACO_{T1} = F_ICO \times F_EHe/F_IHe$

$$= 0.003 \times \frac{0.075}{0.10}$$

$$= 0.0025$$

4. $DL_{CO}sb = \dfrac{5333\ ml \times 60\ sec}{(713\ mm\ Hg) \times (10.0\ sec)} \times Ln\left(\dfrac{0.0025}{0.00125}\right)$

$$= \frac{319,980}{7130} \times Ln\,(1.8)$$

$$= 44.9\ ml/min/mm\ Hg \times 0.5878$$

5. $DL_{CO}sb = 26.38\ ml\ CO/min/mm\ Hg\ (ATPS)$

This value is ATPS and is normally converted to STPD (0° C), 760 mm Hg, dry. The correction factor is calculated as follows:

6. $STPD\ correction\ factor = \dfrac{273}{273 + T°\,C} \times \dfrac{P_B - PH_2OT°\,C}{760}$

where:

$T°\,C$ = spirometer temperature
$PH_2O\ T°\,C$ = partial pressure of water vapor at the spirometer
    temperature, in this case 24 mm Hg at 25° C

7. $STPD\ correction\ factor = \dfrac{273}{273 + 25} \times \dfrac{760 - 24}{760}$

$$= 0.916 \times 0.968 = 0.887$$

$$= 0.887$$

8. $DL_{CO}sb = (26.38\ ml\ CO/min/mm\ Hg) \times (0.887)$

$$= 23.4\ ml\ CO/min/mm\ Hg\ (STPD)$$

This value should also be corrected for the Hb, in this case 10 g/dl:

9. $Hb\ correction = \dfrac{10.22 + Hb}{1.7 \times Hb}$

$$= \frac{10.22 + 10.0}{1.7 \times 10.0}$$

$$= 1.19$$

10. $DL_{CO}sb\ (corrected) = 1.19 \times 23.4$

$$= 27.9\ ml\ CO/min/mm\ Hg\ (STPD)$$

If the COHb level is known, the $DL_{CO}sb$ can be corrected for the back pressure of CO:

11. $COHb\ adjusted\ DL_{CO} = Measured\ DL_{CO} \times \left(1.00 + \dfrac{\%COHb}{100}\right)$

$$= 27.9 \times \left(1.00 + \frac{5.5}{100}\right)$$

12. $COHb\ adjusted\ DL_{CO} = 29.4\ ml\ CO/min/mm\ Hg\ (STPD)$

■ THORACIC GAS VOLUME (V_{TG}) (SEE CHAPTER 3)

Data for V_{TG} and Raw are from the same patient.

V_{TG}:	Unknown
V_{TG} tangents:	0.71 (angle 35.4)
	0.73 (angle 36.1)
	0.73 (angle 36.1)
P_B:	755 mm Hg
Patient weight:	71 kg
P_{MOUTH} calibration:	10 cm H_2O/cm
P_{BOX} calibration:	30 ml/cm
Dead space correction:	100 ml
Plethysmograph volume:	530 L

1. Average V_{TG} tangent (TAN) $= \dfrac{(0.71 + 0.73 + 0.73)}{3}$

$$= 0.72$$

The barometric pressure correction is calculated as follows:

2. $P_{Bcorr} = (P_B - 47) \times 1.36$

$\quad\quad = (755 \text{ mm Hg} - 47 \text{ mm Hg}) \times 1.36$

$\quad\quad = 963 \text{ cm } H_2O$

The patient volume correction (K) is calculated as follows:

3. $K = \dfrac{[\text{Pleth volume} - (\text{Patient weight}/1.07)]}{\text{Pleth volume}}$

$\quad = \dfrac{[530 \text{ L} - (71 \text{ kg}/1.07)]}{530 \text{ L}}$

$\quad = 0.874$

4. $V_{TG} = \left(\dfrac{P_{Bcorr}}{TAN} \times \dfrac{P_{BOXcal}}{P_{MOUTHcal}} \times K \right) - \text{Dead space}$

$\quad\quad = \left(\dfrac{963 \text{ cm } H_2O}{0.72} \times \dfrac{30 \text{ ml/cm}}{10 \text{ cm } H_2O/\text{cm}} \times 0.874 \right) - 100 \text{ ml}$

After canceling like terms in the numerator and denominator (cm, cm H_2O):

5. $\quad = (1338 \times 3 \text{ ml} \times 0.874) - 100 \text{ ml}$

$\quad V_{TG} = 3408 \text{ ml} (3.41 \text{ L})$

■ AIRWAY RESISTANCE (Raw) AND CONDUCTANCE (SGaw) (SEE CHAPTER 2)

Raw:	Unknown
P_{MOUTH}/P_{BOX} TAN:	0.61 (angle = 31)
$\dot{V}/P_{BOX}$ TAN:	3.0 (angle = 72)
P_{MOUTH} calibration:	10 cm H_2O/cm
P_{BOX} calibration:	30 ml/cm
$\dot{V}$ calibration:	1.0 L/sec/cm
R_{sys}:	0.25 cm H_2O/L/sec

1. $\text{Raw} = \left(\dfrac{P_{MOUTH}/P_{BOX}\,TAN}{\dot{V}/P_{BOX}\,TAN} \times \dfrac{P_{MOUTHCal}}{\dot{V}_{cal}} \right) - R_{sys}$

$= \left(\dfrac{0.61}{3.0} \times \dfrac{10\,\text{cm H}_2\text{O/cm}}{1.0\,\text{L/sec/cm}} \right) - 0.25$

$= (0.203 \times 10) - 0.25$

2. $\text{Raw} = 1.78 \text{ cm H}_2\text{O/L/sec}$

Several repetitions of the panting maneuver are usually performed. Unlike the V_{TG} maneuver, however, tangents are not averaged. Because flow and volume tangents influence each other, Raw is calculated and then averaged. To calculate SGaw (specific airway conductance), the volume at which each Raw maneuver was performed is calculated as for V_{TG}, using the P_{MOUTH}/P_{BOX} tangent from the specific maneuver. In this example:

1. $\text{SGaw} = (1/\text{Raw})/V_{TG}$

2. $V_{TG} = \left(\dfrac{963\,\text{cm H}_2\text{O}}{0.61} \times \dfrac{30\,\text{ml/cm}}{10\,\text{cm H}_2\text{O/cm}} \times 0.874 \right) - 100$

$= (1579 \times 3\,\text{ml} \times 0.874) - 100$

$= 4040 \text{ ml } (4.04 \text{ L})$

Calculating the SGaw:

3. $\text{SGaw} = \dfrac{1/1.78\,\text{cm H}_2\text{O/L/sec}}{4.04\,\text{L}}$

4. $= 0.14 \text{ cm H}_2\text{O/L/sec/L}$

The average of three to five maneuvers is usually reported, after the SGaw for individual efforts has been calculated.

EXERCISE STUDY (SEE CHAPTER 7)

Volume exhaled (V):   20.0 L (ATPS)
Collection time (sec):   60 sec
Temperature (T):   24° C
F_EO_2:   0.17
F_ECO_2:   0.03
f_b: 25/min
HR: 100/min
PaO_2:   95 mm Hg
$PaCO_2$:   35 mm Hg
P_B: 750 mg Hg
Mechanical V_D: 18 ml (0.018 L)
Patient's weight: 55 kg

The first step is to calculate conversion factors to correct ventilation and gas exchange measurements to BTPS and STPD, respectively. This STPD factor is for conversion from BTPS:

1. $\text{BTPS factor} = \dfrac{P_B - P_{H_2O}}{P_B - 47} \times \dfrac{273 + 37}{273 + T}$

$= \dfrac{721}{703} \times \dfrac{310}{297}$

$= 1.07$

2. $\text{STPD factor} = \dfrac{P_B - 47}{760} \times \dfrac{273}{273 + 37}$

$\qquad\qquad\quad = \dfrac{703}{760} \times 0.881$

$\qquad\qquad\quad = 0.815$

Next, parameters of ventilation are calculated as follows:

3. $\dot{V}_E \text{ (BTPS)} = \dfrac{V_{exhaled} \times 60}{\text{Collection time in seconds}} \times \text{BTPS factor}$

$\qquad\qquad\quad = \dfrac{20.0\,\text{L} \times 60}{60} \times 1.07$

$\qquad\qquad\quad = 21.4\,\text{L (BTPS)}$

4. $V_T \text{ (BTPS)} = \dfrac{\dot{V}_E \text{ (BTPS)}}{f_b}$

$\qquad\qquad\quad = \dfrac{21.4}{25}$

$\qquad\qquad\quad = 0.856\,\text{L (BTPS)}$

5. $V_D \text{ (BTPS)} = V_T \text{ (BTPS)} \times \left[1 - \dfrac{F_E CO_2 \times (P_B - 47)}{Paco_2} \right] - V_{Dmech}$

$\qquad\qquad\quad = 0.856 \times \left[1 - \dfrac{0.03 \times 703}{35} \right] - 0.018$

$\qquad\qquad\quad = (0.856 \times 0.397) - 0.018$

$\qquad\qquad\quad = 0.340 - 0.018$

$\qquad\qquad\quad = 0.322\,\text{L}$

6. $\dot{V}_A \text{ (BTPS)} = \dot{V}_E \text{ (BTPS)} - [f_b \times V_D \text{ (BTPS)}]$

$\qquad\qquad\quad = 21.4 - [25 \times 0.322]$

$\qquad\qquad\quad = 21.4 - 8.05$

$\qquad\qquad\quad = 13.4\,\text{L}$

7. $V_D / V_T = \dfrac{0.322}{0.856}$

$\qquad\qquad\quad = 0.38$

Next, gas exchange parameters are calculated as follows:

8. $\dot{V}_E \text{(STPD)} = \dot{V}_E \text{(BTPS)} \times \text{STPD factor}$

$\qquad\qquad\quad = 21.4 \times 0.815$

$\qquad\qquad\quad = 17.4\,\text{L}$

9. $\dot{V}_{O_2} \text{ (STPD)} = \left[\left(\dfrac{1 - F_E O_2 - F_E CO_2}{1 - F_I O_2} \times F_I O_2 \right) - F_E O_2 \right] \times \dot{V}_E \text{ (STPD)}$

$\qquad\qquad\quad = \left[\left(\dfrac{1 - 0.17 - 0.03}{1 - 0.2093} \times 0.2093 \right) - 0.17 \right] \times 17.4$

$\qquad\qquad\quad = \left[\left(\dfrac{0.80}{0.79} \times 0.2093 \right) - 0.17 \right] \times 17.4$

$\qquad\qquad\quad = [(1.01 \times 0.2093) - 0.17] \times 17.4$

$\qquad\qquad\quad = [0.212 - 0.17] \times 17.4$

$\qquad\qquad\quad = 0.042 \times 17.4$

$\quad \dot{V}_{O_2} \text{ (STPD)} = 0.731\,\text{L}$

co-oximeter A spectr
analyzing the various
carboxyhemoglobine
CO$_2$ absorber A devi
from a breathing cir
CO$_2$ narcosis Sleepir
high levels of carbon
CO$_2$ production Mea
carbon dioxide excre
usually measured du
COHb Carboxyhemo
by carbon monoxide
compliance The dist
change per unit of p
conscious sedation A
can be easily reverse
agent, and in which
responsiveness to en
control A system or
and measuring actua
results
COPD Chronic obst
cor pulmonale Right
lung disease
corticosteroids Any
couplet Two premat
in a row
cromolyn sodium A
presumably by stabil
preventing release o
CV In statistics, coef
deviation divided by
measurement
cyanosis Bluish colo
associated with hypo
of reduced hemoglo
cycle ergometer A st
specifically for exerc
to be estimated
cystic fibrosis A her
glands characterized
enzymes and respira
damping Attenuatio
accurately represent
dead space The volu
but not perfused by
deconditioned Refe
usually including el
pressure and muscu
defibrillator A devic
fibrillation is presen
demand valve A dev
volume, flow, or pre
denervated Having
disabled or cut

10. $\dot{V}_{CO_2}\,(STPD) = (F_E CO_2 - 0.0003) \times \dot{V}_E\,(STPD)$
$= (0.03 - 0.0003) \times 17.4$
$= 0.297 \times 17.4$
$= 0.517\,L$

11. $R = \dfrac{\dot{V}_{CO_2}\,(STPD)}{\dot{V}_{O_2}\,(STPD)}$
$= \dfrac{0.517}{0.731}$
$= 0.71$

12. $\dot{V}_E/\dot{V}_{O_2} = \dfrac{\dot{V}_E\,(BTPS)}{\dot{V}_{O_2}\,(STPD)}$
$= \dfrac{21.4}{0.731}$
$= 29.3\,L/L\,\dot{V}_{O_2}$

13. $\dot{V}_{O_2}/HR = \dfrac{\dot{V}_{O_2}\,(STPD)}{HR} \times 1000$
$= \dfrac{0.731\,L/min}{100\,beats/min} \times 1000$
$= 7.31\,ml\,O_2/beat$

The calculation of energy expenditure at any particular workload is described by the term *METS*, for multiples of the resting $\dot{V}_{O_2}$. The MET level for any workload is calculated by one of two methods. In each method:

14. $METS = \dfrac{\dot{V}_{O_2}\,(STPD)\,exercise}{\dot{V}_{O_2}\,(STPD)\,rest}$

but the means of estimating $\dot{V}_{O_2}\,(STPD)$ at rest differs. $\dot{V}_{O_2}\,(STPD)$ at rest can be measured, or it may be estimated as 0.0035 L/min/kg (3.5 ml/kg). Using the second method in this example:

$$METS = \dfrac{0.731\,L/min}{0.0035\,L/min/kg \times 55\,kg}$$
$$= 3.80$$

If patient's measured $\dot{V}_{O_2}$ at rest had been 0.225 L/min (STPD), then:

$$METS = \dfrac{0.731\,L/min}{0.225\,L/min}$$
$$= 3.25$$

asbestosis Fibrotic l
of asbestos fibers
asthma Obstructive
reversible airway na
inflammation, and
atelectasis A state o
AT Anaerobic thres
which energy needs
by aerobic pathways
ATPS Ambient tem
(water vapor)
ATS American Tho
β-Adrenergic Stimul
system β-receptors
β-Blocker A drug th
in the sympathetic
back pressure Press
a tube or vessel
balance To bring in
instrument, to adju
berylliosis Fibrotic l
inhalation of dust fi
bias In statistics, the
measurement cause
also error
bicarbonate A buffe
other body solution
bidirectional In two
positive and negativ
biologic control Use
standard for measu
instrument or proce
black lung Legal ter
disease in a coal mii
bleomycin A potent
the management of
BMR Basal metabol
oxygen consumptio
bolus A large mass
one large dose
Borg scale One of s
perceived exertion
brachial Refers to th
puncture
breath-by-breath Re
variables on each br
breathing kinetics T
respiratory rate and
exercise
bronchiectasis A pu
characterized by de
bronchiolitis obliter
which small airways
destroyed; also calle
syndrome (BOS)

emboli Multiple blood clots that travel from their site of origin to lodge in another blood vessel
emphysema Obstructive airway disease characterized by destruction of alveolar walls and collapse of small airways; may be accompanied by air trapping and hyperinflation of the lungs
end-tidal Refers to gas collected at the end of a quiet breath, usually assumed to represent alveolar gas
endotracheal tube An artificial airway used to manage a patient's airway, often used in an emergency
enteral Passing through the stomach and intestines
eucapnic Maintaining a normal level of carbon dioxide in the lungs and blood
explosive decompression A process or device that uses rapid expansion of gas to generate a known flow
extrathoracic Outside of the thorax or chest cavity
exudate A fluid accumulation caused by infection or inflammation
false negative The result of a test or examination in which a diagnosis is incorrectly overlooked
false positive The result of a test or examination in which the diagnosis is incorrectly supported
febrile Having a fever
fibrillation Rapid, tremulous contractions of muscles; often used to describe a serious cardiac arrhythmia
fibrosis Scarring of tissue caused by chemical or biologic agents, repeated infection, or inflammation, as in pulmonary fibrosis
fibrotic Refers to the presence of scar tissue or fibrous changes related to inflammation and healing
Fick method A means of determining cardiac output by measuring oxygen consumption and arteriovenous oxygen content difference
FIo$_2$ Fractional concentration of inspired oxygen
flow limitation The characteristic of gas movement in the airways when increases in driving pressure do not result in further increases in flow
flow-volume loop A plot of maximal inspiratory and expiratory flows versus FVC and FIVC on a single graph or display
fractional Used to describe the concentration of one or more gases in a mixture, expressed as a decimal fraction
frequency response The ability of an instrument to detect a changing signal, dependent on the signal's frequency
full scale Refers to the entire range over which an instrument is capable of measuring
gain The amplification of a signal from an instrument
glottis Elongated space between the vocal cords; also the structure surrounding this space
glycolysis The energy-yielding conversion of glucose to lactic acid
goiter Enlargement of the thyroid gland

gradient Difference in a quantity between two fixed points of reference
Guillain-Barré A progressive disease of the peripheral nerves
half-life The time required for half of a substance to deteriorate
Hb Hemoglobin concentration, usually expressed in ml/dl
hematocrit Ratio of volume of packed red blood cells to volume of whole blood
hemoglobin An iron-containing conjugated protein respiratory pigment occurring in the red blood cells of vertebrates
hemolysis The process or condition in which red blood cells are broken open
hemoptysis Coughing up of blood
hemorrhage Copious discharge of blood from blood vessels
heparin A substance that inhibits blood clotting, also used to preserve blood specimens
hilar Related to the hilum, or roots, of the lungs
histamine Chemical compound ($C_5H_9N_3$) that causes dilatation and increased permeability of blood vessels that play a role in allergic reactions
honeycombing Resembling or having a honeycomb pattern; usually seen on chest x-ray examination
hypercapnia Higher than normal level of carbon dioxide; usually greater than 45 mm Hg in arterial blood
hyperinflation Overinflation of the lungs; usually denoted by an increased total lung capacity above the upper limit of normal (120%)
hyperpnea Rapid breathing
hyperreactive Excessively responsive to stimulation
hypertensive Having a blood pressure that is greater than normal
hyperventilation Ventilation in excess of CO_2 production resulting in respiratory alkalosis
hypocapnia A low level of carbon dioxide in arterial blood
hypotension Low blood pressure, usually less than 90/50
hypothermic Having a temperature below normal; usually below 37°C
hypoventilation Inadequate ventilation to remove CO_2 resulting in respiratory acidosis
hypoxemia Abnormally low level of oxygen in the blood
hypoxia Inadequate oxygen to meet tissue demands
idiopathic Describing a finding or syndrome that is self-originated or arising spontaneously from an unknown cause
in vivo Refers to measurements or observations made in the living organism

incremental Refers to exercise tests that increase the workload by fixed amounts over given intervals

infiltrate The abnormal fluid that fills tissues or spaces; to pass through tissues or spaces

infrared Radiation outside the visible spectrum at its red end

inspiratory limb The portion of a flow-volume loop that depicts flow during maximal inhalation

integration The operation of solving a differential equation; specifically to find the area under a curve

interstitial lung disease A group of lung disorders characterized by infiltrates, inflammation of the alveolar walls, loss of lung volume, and exertional dyspnea

intrathoracic Inside the thorax or chest cavity

ischemic Having decreased blood flow

isobestic Refers to a common wavelength at which two or more chemical compounds absorb light, as measured by a spectrophotometer

isocapnia A normal level of carbon dioxide, usually in the blood

isothermal lung analog A glass jar or container filled with copper or steel wool, used for quality control of a body plethysmograph

ketosis The presence or process of ketones in the body or blood

kilopascal Unit of pressure measurement in the International System; 1 mm Hg ~ 0.133 kilopascals

kinetics The activity of some object; in exercise testing, refers to gas exchange patterns (oxygen uptake, CO_2 production)

kpm Kilopond-meters; the work of moving a 1-kg mass 1 m vertically against the force of gravity

Kreb's cycle The main source of energy in the mammalian body and the end toward which carbohydrate, fat, and protein metabolism are directed; citric acid cycle

kymograph A recording device, usually a rotating drum, on which a graph of motion or pressure may be traced

kyphoscoliosis A combination of anterior-posterior and lateral curvature of the spine

kyphosis Abnormal curvature of the spine anteriorly

lactate See *lactic acid*

lactic acid An acid produced by anaerobic metabolism at high levels of work

laminar flow Streamline flow in a viscous fluid or gas near a solid boundary

large airway obstruction Any process or disease that limits flow in the upper airway, trachea, or mainstem bronchi

laryngoscope A device used to visualize the larynx and vocal cords, specifically for intubating the trachea

learning effect The phenomenon in which a subject performs better after multiple attempts at a test or procedure

LED Light-emitting diode

leukotriene antagonists A class of drugs used in the treatment of asthma; these drugs block the release of leukotrienes that potentiate inflammatory mediators

linear Refers to a system in which a given input produces a consistent output

linear regression A statistical procedure in which an equation is computed that represents a linear (one-to-one) relationship between two variables

linearity The ability to produce a proportional output for a given input across a fixed range

lipogenesis Formation of fat, usually from carbohydrate

lobectomy Surgical excision of the lobe of an organ such as the lung

logarithm The exponent that indicates the power to which a number is raised to produce a given number

luminescence An emission of light produced by physiologic or chemical processes

lung reduction A surgical procedure in which poorly perfused lung tissue is removed; also lung volume reduction surgery (LVRS)

lung transplantation Removal of one or both native lungs and replacement with lungs from a donor

lupus erythematosus Slowly progressive systemic disease characterized by degenerative changes of the collagenous tissues

manometer A device for measuring pressure using a tube marked with a scale and containing a fluid (mercury or water); level of the fluid varies with the pressure applied above it

maximal expiration The point at which no further air can be exhaled from the lungs

maximal inspiration The point at which the lungs are completely filled

MDI Metered-dose inhaler; a small canister containing a propellent gas to deliver bronchodilator or other respiratory medications

mediastinal Located in or near the mediastinum

medullary centers Those areas of the medulla oblongata that are responsible for controlling the rate and depth of breathing

metabolic acidosis An acid-base imbalance characterized by a pH less than 7.35 resulting from accumulation of acid (other than that produced by CO_2) or loss of base

metabolic alkalosis An acid-base imbalance characterized by a pH greater than 7.45 resulting from accumulation of base or loss of acid (other than that produced by CO_2)

metabolism The process of breaking down food substrates to produce energy

methacholine A potent chemical that increases parasympathetic muscle tone in the airways when inhaled; used to induce bronchoconstriction to test for hyperreactivity of the airways

MetHb Methemoglobin; the fraction of Hb in which the iron atoms have been oxidized to the Fe state

METS Metabolic equivalents based on a multiple of resting oxygen consumption; usually equal to an oxygen consumption of 3.5 ml/min/kg of body weight

microprocessor An integrated circuit capable of performing logical and mathematical calculations; the primary component of a computer

minute ventilation The total volume of gas moved in and out of the lungs each minute; also called the minute volume

mixed expired Refers to gas collected that includes dead space and alveolar gas; usually collected in a bag, balloon, or spirometer

mixing chamber A container with baffles for collecting expired gas for analysis

molar Units of measure for concentration of solute in a solvent based on the number of moles (gram molecular weight) of solute

morbidity The state or quality of being affected by disease

mouthpiece A device that connects a patient to the breathing circuit for pulmonary function tests

MRI Magnetic resonance imaging; a type of scan that evaluates structures subjected to strong magnetic fields

Müller's maneuver Production of negative intrathoracic pressure by closing the glottis and making a forced inspiratory effort

multifocal Refers to ectopic beats of the heart arising from different locations (foci)

multiwavelength Refers to an instrument or measurement made at two or more wavelengths, as in a spectrophotometer

myasthenia gravis A disease of the neuromuscular system characterized by progressive weakness, often episodic; neck, throat, and facial muscles may be primarily affected

myocardial Related to the heart muscle

myxedema A dry, waxy swelling of the skin or other tissues associated with hypothyroidism

natural logarithm A logarithm with e (2.71828) as its base

neoplasm Cancer, usually a tumor

neuromuscular Related to the nerves, muscles, or the junction of the two

NO nitric oxide; a normally occurring gas found in exhaled air and related to inflammatory processes within cells

nodal Refers to cardiac rhythms originating in the A-V node

normal distribution In statistics, the even distribution of data points on either side of the mean; a Gaussian distribution

normoxia An adequate level of oxygen, usually an F_{IO_2} of 0.21

nose clip A springlike device used to compress the nose and prevent nasal breathing during pulmonary function testing

O_2 consumption Measurement of the volume of oxygen used by the tissues per minute; usually measured during exercise or metabolic studies

O_2 pulse The volume of oxygen (ml) consumed or delivered per heartbeat

O_2Hb Oxyhemoglobin saturation; the fraction of Hb bound with oxygen

obesity-hypoventilation A syndrome characterized by chronic respiratory acidosis in a patient who is overweight

obstruction Any process that interferes with air flow into or out of the lungs

obstructive sleep apnea (OSA) A syndrome in which an individual experiences cessation of airflow caused by blockage of the upper airway during sleep

occlusion pressure The pressure generated during the first 100 msec of a breath against an occluded airway; also called P_{100} or $P_{0.1}$

occupational lung disease Pulmonary disease related to exposure in the workplace

optode An optical electrode

orthopnea Difficulty breathing related to body position; especially shortness of breath while lying supine

oscillometry Measurements of airflow mechanics made using pressure oscillations generated by sound waves of various frequencies

OSHA Occupational Safety and Health Administration

out-of-control The state or condition in which an instrument does not perform measurements accurately or precisely

oxidation-reduction A chemical process in which one element gives up electrons (oxidation) while another element receives them (reduction)

oximetry The measurement, either directly or indirectly, of the oxygen saturation of the blood

oxygen uptake $\dot{V}O_2$ or the volume of oxygen consumed per minute

pallor Lack of color, paleness

paradoxical Refers to a change or movement that is contrary to what is expected

parasympathetic Relating to that part of the autonomic nervous system that contains chiefly cholinergic fibers and increases the tone/contractility of smooth muscle

parenchyma The essential and distinctive tissue of an organ such as the lung

parenteral Nourishment occurring outside of the stomach and intestines

pathogen Any microorganism capable of producing disease

PC$_{20}$ Provocative concentration of a drug at which a specified variable (such as FEV$_1$) changes by exactly 20%

PD$_{20}$ Provocative dose of a drug at which a specified variable changes by 20% or more

peak flow meter A device that can register PEF

pectus excavatum An abnormal depression of the sternum

percent grade Refers to a treadmill or similar device; describes the slope of the walking surface

percutaneously Through the skin

pericarditis Inflammation of the pericardium

PET Positron emission tomography; a type of scan capable of imaging metabolically active organ structures

pH Negative logarithm of the hydrogen ion concentration used as a positive number

phase delay The time interval between when an event occurs and when it is registered by an instrument or analyzer; also, the delay between the response times of two separate instruments

phlegm Mucus that is coughed up

Pitot tube A tube that has a short, right-angled bend placed vertically in a moving body of air; the mouth of the bent part is directed upstream and uses a manometer to measure velocity of flow (Henri Pitot, 1771)

plethysmograph From the Greek *plethys* for pressure; any device for recording pressure. In pulmonary function testing, a booth in which the patient sits to measure pressure and volume changes in the lung

pleura The lining of the lungs and thoracic cavity

pleurisy Inflammation of the pleural surfaces

pneumoconiosis Lung disease related to inhalation of dust

Pneumocystis carinii A microorganism that causes pneumocystosis, a type of interstitial cell pneumonitis

pneumonectomy Surgical excision of a lung

pneumonitis Inflammation of airways and alveoli caused by irritants or infection

pneumotachometer Any device used to measure gas flow; in pulmonary function testing, a device used to measure flow and its integral volume

pneumothorax A partial or total collapse of the lung caused by entry of air into the pleural space

polarographic Refers to an electrode that is polarized by applying a voltage between an anode and cathode in order to make a measurement

potentiometer An instrument for measuring electromotive forces

precision The extent to which an instrument measures a known value repeatedly; reproducibility

precordial Refers to the position of ECG leads on the patient's chest over the heart

predicted value The expected or reference value for a lung function test; usually derived from studying a large population of healthy individuals

preload The pressure and/or volume of blood entering the atrium or ventricle

proficiency testing The process of comparing measurements of a known value from different sources to establish a level of accuracy

pulmonary embolism A blood clot arising in the venous system that breaks loose and then lodges in the pulmonary vascular system

pulmonary hypertension Elevated blood pressure in the pulmonary vascular system; usually a mean pulmonary artery pressure greater than 30 to 35 mm Hg

pulsatile Refers to a signal or phenomenon that rises and falls, as a pulse

pulse oximetry Estimation of arterial saturation by analysis of light absorption of blood pulsing through a capillary bed (finger or earlobe)

PVC Premature ventricular contraction

quality control The process of establishing the accuracy, precision, or other desired output of a procedure or measurement

RR interval The distance or time between successive R waves on the ECG; used to calculate heart rate

radiation therapy The use of radioactive substances to treat disease, often used in cancer therapy

ramp test An exercise test in which the workload is increased continuously rather than incrementally

random error Variability of a measurement outside of accepted limits that occurs in a nonreproducible fashion

rebreathing Refers to or describes a system that allows the patient to breathe continuously while measurements are made

REE Resting energy expenditure; the caloric needs of the body estimated from oxygen consumption and carbon dioxide production usually expressed in kcal/24 hours

reference equation An equation used to predict an expected value for a particular test parameter

refractory period An interval that is resistant to treatment or change

regression A statistical method for estimating one variable based on the progression of another variable

resection Surgical removal of part of an organ or structure

respiratory acidosis An acid-base imbalance characterized by a pH less than 7.35 because of an increased level of carbon dioxide in the blood

respiratory alkalosis An acid-base imbalance characterized by a pH greater than 7.45 because of excessive ventilation

respirometer A device for measuring breathing

restriction Any process that interferes with the bellows action of the lungs or chest, usually with a loss of lung volume

restrictive disease Any process or disease that interferes with the bellows action of the lungs, the chest wall, or both

reverse isolation Isolation procedures designed to protect the patient from infectious organisms carried by staff or visitors

RPE Relative perceived exertion, usually measured by a numeric scale (see *Borg scale*)

RQ Respiratory quotient; the ratio of carbon dioxide produced to oxygen consumed at the cell level

RQnp Nonprotein RQ; the respiratory quotient produced by metabolism of fats and carbohydrates

RTC Rapid thoracoabdominal compression; use of a squeeze jacket to cause forced expiration in infants

ST segment A portion of the electrical conduction pattern of the ECG; used to assess cardiac ischemia

sarcoidosis Chronic disease of unknown origin characterized by formation of nodules resembling true tubercles, especially in lymph nodes, lungs, bones, and skin

scleroderma A disease primarily of the skin, characterized by thickening and hardening of subcutaneous tissues

scoliosis Abnormal lateral curvature of the spine

sedation The act of calming, especially by the administration of a sedative

SD Standard deviation; in statistics, a mathematical statement of dispersion of a set of values from the mean

sensitivity In medicine, the ability of a test or examination to detect the presence of disease

shunt A bypass; in the lungs, an area in which blood flows through the lungs without coming into contact with alveolar gas

signal-to-noise ratio The relationship between a wanted signal and other unwanted signals (noise); in measurement theory, the ability to distinguish between wanted and unwanted signals or data

silicosis Fibrotic lung disease caused by inhalation of silica dust

sine-wave pump A pump that uses a circular motion, such as a flywheel, to produce output that varies above and below a set level in a regular fashion

slope To adjust the output or gain of an instrument

small airways In the lungs, airways less than 2 mm in diameter; these airways are supported by surrounding alveolar structures

SOB Abbreviation for "shortness of breath"

solenoid A cylinder containing a wire coil with a movable core; the core moves when an electrical current is applied

solubility coefficient A number that describes the volume of one substance that will dissolve in another substance under given conditions

span To adjust or confirm the measuring range of an instrument

specificity In medicine, the ability of a test or examination to exclude those who do not have a specific disease or disorder

spectrophotometer A device for analyzing chemical composition by measuring light intensity at various wavelengths

spirometer Any device used to measure lung volumes and flows

spreadsheet In computing, a program that allows entry of data and formulas to provide calculations

steady-state test In exercise testing, refers to tests conducted long enough for cardiopulmonary variables to reach a state of equilibrium

sternotomy A surgical procedure that involves opening the chest cavity through the sternum

STPD Standard temperature (0° C), pressure (760 mm Hg), dry

stridor High-pitched noise from the upper airway, usually on inspiration

suppurative To form or discharge mucus or pus

SV Stroke volume

Swan-Ganz catheter A balloon-tipped catheter that can be floated through the right atrium and ventricle into the pulmonary artery

systolic Refers to the blood pressure during ventricular contraction (systole)

tachyarrhythmia Any abnormal heart rhythm that includes an increased heart rate, usually greater than 100 beats per minute

tachycardia Rapid beating of the heart, usually applied to rates over 100 beats per minute

tangent A number that describes the slope of a line

tension pneumothorax A pneumothorax in which the pressure within the chest exceeds atmospheric pressure

theophylline A drug related to caffeine and theobromine that promotes bronchodilatation

thermistor A resistor that is sensitive to temperature changes; used for measurement of gas or blood flow

thermodilution Refers to a method of determining cardiac output by measuring temperature change of a solution injected into the right atrium and passing into the pulmonary artery

thoracotomy A surgical procedure in which the thorax is opened

thrombophlebitis Inflammation of a vein, developing before the formation of a thrombus

thrombi Formation of a blood clot

tidal volume The volume of gas moved in and out of the lung with each breath

tonometer An instrument used to measure or establish pressure of a gas in a liquid

tonometering The process of equilibrating a gas dissolved in a solution

tracer Refers to an element used to track or measure another element, as in a tracer gas

tracheal malacia Degeneration of elastic and connective tissue of the trachea; also trachcomalacia

transcutaneous Refers to a measurement made through the skin

transducer Any device that produces a signal (electrical voltage or current) in response to a physiologic phenomenon such as pressure or sound

transmural Across a wall or boundary

transudate A fluid accumulation caused by pressure imbalance

treadmill A device that incorporates a motor-driven belt on which walking, jogging, or running can be performed

trigger Something that sets another thing in motion; in asthma, the agent that causes the reaction to begin

tuberculosis A chronic granulomatous infection caused by an acid-fast bacillus, *Mycobacterium tuberculosis*, usually affecting the lungs and transmitted by droplet nuclei

universal precautions Standards for handling blood or specimens containing blood when there is possibility of infection

UUN Urinary urea nitrogen; the amount of nitrogen excreted in the urine over a 24-hour period

Valsalva maneuver High intrathoracic pressure caused by closing the glottis and constricting the abdominal and chest muscles

valvular insufficiency Inadequate function of one or more of the valves of the heart, allowing backward flow or leakage

vasoconstriction A reduction in the lumen of a blood vessel

VCD Vocal cord dysfunction

ventilatory reserve The difference between maximal exercise ventilation and the MVV, sometimes expressed as a ratio or percentage, or as an absolute volume

ventilatory threshold The workload at which ventilation and $\dot{V}co_2$ increase at a more rapid rate, indicative of anaerobic metabolism

ventricular Refers to cardiac rhythms originating in the ventricles

watt A measure of power; 1 watt equals 6.12 kilopond meters per minute

Wheatstone bridge A bridge for measuring electrical resistances, consisting of a conductor joining two branches of a circuit (Sir Charles Wheatstone, 1875)

wheezing High-pitched or musical breath sounds, usually on expiration; associated with airway narrowing

zirconium A tetravalent metallic element with a high melting point used in alloys and ceramics

Index

Note: Page numbers followed by f indicate figures; those followed by t indicate tables; those followed by b indicate boxed material.

Maximum voluntary ventilation (MVV) *(Continued)*
    interpretive strategies for, 69b
    measurement technique for, 67, 67b, 68f
    pediatric, 296
    reference values for, 461
        regression equations for, 473t
        summary curve with, 468f
    significance and pathophysiology of, 68–69, 69b
    summary curve reference values for, 468f
Mean, calculation of, 499–500
MEFV curve. *See* Maximal expiratory flow-volume curve.
MEP. *See* Maximal expiratory pressure (MEP).
MET (metabolic unit), 506
    calculation of, 216, 216b, 497
    exercise testing role of, 216, 216b
    oxygen consumption relation to, 216b, 236
Metabolic measurements, 338–346
    basal metabolic rate former role in, 8, 342
    calorimetry in, 338–340
        calculations for, 342–343
        closed-circuit, 340
        criteria for acceptability of, 344b
        indications for, 345t
        indirect, 338–340, 339f, 341f, 344b
        interpretive strategies for, 344b
        open-circuit, 339–340, 339f, 341f
        significance and pathophysiology of, 344–346
    measurement technique for, 339f, 340–342
    nutritional assessment in, 343
        case study for, 352–354
    REE (resting energy expenditure) in, 338, 341–342, 341f
Metered-dose inhaler (MDI), 505
    before and after bronchodilator studies using, 70, 70b
    technique for use of, 70b
Methacholine bronchial challenge test, 317–326
    5-breath method for, 321–322, 321t
    case study for, 347–349
    dosing schedules for, 318–321, 319t, 321t
    medications withheld prior to, 318, 319t
    2-minute tidal breathing method for, 322–324, 323f
    nebulizer and dosimeter for, 319–322, 320f
    provocative concentration calculation in, 323–324, 323f
    technical factors affecting, 324–326
Methemoglobin, 186f, 189
Minute ventilation
    acceptability criteria for, 129b
    description of, 128
    exercise effect on, 229–232, 230f, 231f, 232f
    measurement technique for, 128–129, 128b, 129b
    significance and pathophysiology of, 129–130, 129b
MIP. *See* Maximal inspiratory pressure (MIP).
MMFR (maximum midexpiratory flow rate), 43
    summary curve reference values for, 468f
Motion artifact, exercise causing, 219f, 220
Müller's maneuver, 506
MVV. *See* Maximum voluntary ventilation (MVV).
Myasthenia gravis, 20, 24

N

National Institute for Occupational Safety and Health, 482
Nebulizer, bronchial challenge testing with, 319–322, 320f
Negative inspiratory force (NIF), 296
Neoplasia, large airway obstructed by, 19–20
Neuromuscular disorders
    amyotrophic lateral sclerosis in, 24
    Guillain-Barré syndrome in, 24
    myasthenia gravis in, 20, 24
    ventilation restricted by, 24
NIF (negative inspiratory force), 296
NIOSH (National Institute for Occupational Safety and Health), 482
Nitric oxide exhalation, 308
Nitrogen, gas analyzer equipment for, 386–387, 386f
Nitrogen washout method
    lung volume measurement with, 97–100, 98f, 99b, 99f, 104f
    single-breath form of, 113–116, 114f, 115b, 116b
Nutrition
    case study in assessment of, 352–354
    metabolic calculations related to, 343

O

Obesity
    case study for, 117–119, 119f
    chest wall affected by, 23
    hypoventilation syndrome of, 23
Obstructive airway disease. *See* Chronic obstructive pulmonary disease (COPD).
Occlusion pressure (P100), 127, 134, 506
Open-circuit (nitrogen washout) method, 97–100, 98f, 99b, 99f, 104f
Organizations, regulatory, 481–484
Orthopnea, neuromuscular disorders with, 24
OSHA (Occupational Safety and Health Administration), 481
Oximeters
    arterial catheter used with, 401–403, 402f, 403f
    pulse, 398–401, 399f, 400f
    spectrophotometric, 396–398, 397f
        reflective, 401–403, 402f, 403f
Oxygen. *See also* Pulse oximetry.
    gas analyzer measurement of, 382–384, 383t
    transcutaneous electrode for, 394–396, 396f
    ventilation response test with, 134–139, 136f, 137b, 138b
    ventilatory equivalent for, 231f, 241, 242f
Oxygen consumption, 236–238
    calculation of, 227f, 237
    criteria for acceptability of, 236b
    exercise effect on, 221f, 230f, 236–238
    gas analyzer measurement and, 227f, 237
    interpretive strategies for, 240b
    minute ventilation related to, 232f
    oxygen pulse calculated from, 242–243
    pediatric, 289–290
    ventilatory reserve role of, 232f

Vital capacity (VC). *See also* Forced vital capacity (FVC).
  acceptability criteria for, 41, 41b
  description of, 40, 40f
  measurement technique for, 40f, 41, 41b
  predicted value formula for, 42b
  reference values for, 461, 466f
  significance and pathophysiology of, 41–43, 43b
Vocal cords
  airway obstructive disease affecting, 19
  pediatric, 281–284

W

Walking, 6-minute test using, 211t, 212–213, 212b, 213t
Wang-Dockery reference set, 306
Water vapor pressure, conversion factors related to, 477–478
Water-seal spirometer, 358–361, 358f

Watts, exercise testing role of, 216
Weight (body), patient measurement for, 28, 28b
Weir equation, 342
Wheatstone bridge, 509
Wheezing, asthma causing, 17
Work
  exercise testing definition of, 216
  units of, 479
Workload
  exercise testing role of, 213–217, 216b, 216t
  MET's in, 216, 216b
  quantitative expression of, 216, 216b
  varying of, 213–216, 214f, 215f, 215t, 216t

Z

Zirconium cells, 383–384